Management of Cardiac Arrhythmias

CONTEMPORARY CARDIOLOGY

CHRISTOPHER P. CANNON, MD
SERIES EDITOR

ANNEMARIE M. ARMANI, MD
EXECUTIVE EDITOR

For other titles published in this series, go to
http://www.springer.com/series/7677

MANAGEMENT OF CARDIAC ARRHYTHMIAS

Edited by

GAN-XIN YAN, MD, PhD

Main Line Health Heart Center
Wynnewood, PA, USA

PETER R. KOWEY, MD

Jefferson Medical College
Philadelphia, PA, USA

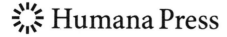 Humana Press

Editors
Gan-Xin Yan, MD, PhD
Main Line Health Heart Center
and
Lankenau Institute for Medical Research
Wynnewood, PA, USA
yanganxin@comcast.net

Peter R. Kowey, MD
Jefferson Medical College
Philadelphia, PA, USA
and
Main Line Health Heart Center
Wynnewood, PA, USA
koweypr@mlhheart.org

ISBN 978-1-60761-160-8   e-ISBN 978-1-60761-161-5
DOI 10.1007/978-1-60761-161-5
Springer New York Dordrecht Heidelberg London

Library of Congress Control Number: 2010934347

Printed on acid-free paper

Humana Press is part of Springer Science+Business Media (www.springer.com)

Preface

It is safe to say that few areas of medicine have moved faster than cardiac electrophysiology. In three short decades, our field has grown from its infancy to a highly sophisticated subspecialty of cardiology, complete with its own societies, scientific meetings, and board examination. Key to our successes has been a progressively more in-depth understanding of pathophysiology from our basic science laboratories. Burgeoning knowledge has been accompanied by a blitzkrieg of technology that has allowed us to treat what used to be lethal rhythm disturbances and to improve the quality of life of millions of people the world over. In 2010, we stand on the threshold of an even more impressive leap forward as we wrestle with defining how the genetic code predisposes to, or even causes, cardiac arrhythmias.

The price to pay for such rapid expansion of information is an ever-widening knowledge gap. It is obvious that practitioners who spend their time caring for patients find it difficult to keep up with the latest developments in our field. The number of articles and journals that come across our desks every month is mind numbing. And few have the sophistication to understand the myriad of discoveries that are unwrapped at each of our congresses. Clearly there is a need to have complex information presented in an efficient and user-friendly way.

We believe that condensed texts represent one of the best ways for colleagues to stay current. We also think that there are individuals in our field, as in any endeavor, who are particularly skilled in taking a complex mass of information, condensing and formulating it, and producing a state-of-the-art manuscript that makes clinical sense. Consequently, we agreed to recruit a stellar group of authors and edit the text you are about to read. Its organization is standard, proceeding from basic science to diagnostic and therapeutic techniques, before ending in a discussion of specific patient types and syndromes. We added an historical perspective that should be particularly gratifying to our younger readers. Since the time frame of development was short, the information is as current as possible and should bring the interested reader up to speed rather quickly. We have tried to feature issues that will be of continuing interest in our field over the next few years in order to provide a frame of reference for journal reading. Finally, we have kept the level of science high to appeal to physicians and health-care professionals, or those in training, who have a deep interest in cardiac arrhythmias.

There are several we would like to acknowledge and thank, including our colleagues who helped us with their knowledge and experience, our families who allowed us the time to write and edit, our staff who provided technical support, and the research foundations and granting agencies that keep us afloat. But most of all, we thank our patients who, by their courage and perseverance, inspire us to dig deeper so we can ultimately conquer the diseases that disrupt and end their lives.

Gan-Xin Yan, MD, PhD
Peter R. Kowey, MD

Acknowledgments

We wish to acknowledge Ms. Rose Well and Drs. Ying Wu and Xiaoqing Quan for their assistance in editing this book. We also wish to acknowledge American Heart Association, the W.W. Smith Charitable Trust, the Sharpe-Strumia Research Foundation, and the Albert M. Greenfield Foundation for their generous support of our research and education in cardiac electrophysiology.

Contents

Contributors

MICHAEL J. ACKERMAN, MD, PHD, *Departments of Medicine, Pediatrics, and Molecular Pharmacology & Experimental Therapeutics/Divisions of Cardiovascular Diseases and Pediatric Cardiology/Windland Smith Rice Sudden Death Genomics Laboratory, Mayo Clinic, Rochester, MN, USA*

KHALID ALMUTI, MD, *Division of Cardiology, Lankenau Hospital, Wynnewood, PA, USA*

CHARLES ANTZELEVITCH, PHD, *Masonic Medical Research Laboratory, Utica, NY, USA*

DAVID G. BENDITT, MD, *Cardiac Arrhythmia Center, Cardiovascular Division, Department of Medicine, University of Minnesota Medical School, Minneapolis, MN, USA*

BABAK BOZORGNIA, MD, *Naples Heart Rhythm Specialists, Naples, FL, USA*

ALFRED E. BUXTON, MD, *Department of Medicine, Rhode Island and Miriam Hospitals, The Warren Alpert Medical School of Brown University, Providence, RI, USA*

HUGH CALKINS, MD, *Department of Medicine and Cardiology, The Johns Hopkins Hospital, Baltimore, MD, USA*

DAVID J. CALLANS, MD, *Section of Cardiology, Department of Medicine, The Hospital of the University of Pennsylvania, Philadelphia PA, USA*

ILKNUR CAN, MD, *Cardiac Arrhythmia Center, Cardiovascular Division, Department of Medicine, University of Minnesota Medical School, Minneapolis, MN, USA*

DAWOOD DARBAR, MD, *Department of Medicine, Vanderbilt University School of Medicine, Nashville, TN, USA*

N.A. MARK ESTES III, MD, *New England Cardiac Arrhythmia Center, Division of Cardiology, Department of Medicine, Tufts Medical Center, Boston, MA, USA*

JOHN FIELD, MD, *Penn State Hershey Heart & Vascular Institute, Penn State Milton S. Hershey Medical Center, Hershey, PA, USA*

MICHAEL R. GOLD, MD, PHD, *Division of Cardiology, Medical University of South Carolina, Charleston, SC, USA*

KATHLEEN HICKEY, RN, DOCTOR OF NURSING, *Columbia University Medical Center, New York, NY, USA*

JONATHAN N. JOHNSON, MD, *Department of Pediatrics, Division of Pediatric Cardiology, Mayo Clinic, Rochester, MN, USA*

MARK E. JOSEPHSON, MD, *Division of Cardiology, The Beth Israel – Deaconess Hospital, Boston, MA, USA*

JOHN A. KALIN, MD, *New England Cardiac Arrhythmia Center, Division of Cardiology, Department of Medicine, Tufts Medical Center, Boston, MA, USA*

RONALD KANTER, MD, *Division of Cardiology, Department of Padiatrics and Medicine, Duke University, Durham, NC, USA*

ARTHUR C. KENDIG, MD, *Department of Medicine, University of Iowa Hospitals, Iowa City, IA, USA*

EDMUND C. KEUNG, MD, *Cardiology Section, San Francisco Veterans Affairs Medical Center, University of California, VA Medical Center, San Francisco, CA, USA*

DUSAN KOCOVIC, MD, *Division of Cardiology, Lankenau Hospital, Main Line Health Heart Center, Wynnewood, PA, USA*

PETER R. KOWEY, MD, *Main Line Health Heart Center, Wynnewood, PA, USA; Division of Cardiovascular Diseases, Jefferson Medical College, Philadelphia, PA, USA*

WEI WEI LI, MD, *Department of Medicine, University of Iowa Hospitals, Iowa City, IA, USA*

JIANFANG LIAN, MD, PHD, *Main Line Health Heart Center, Ning Bo Medical Center Li Hui Li Hospital, Medical School, Ning Bo University, Ning Bo, P.R. China*

MARK S. LINK, MD, *New England Cardiac Arrhythmia Center, Division of Cardiology, Department of Medicine, Tufts Medical Center, Boston, MA, USA*

GUSTAVO LOPERA, MD, *Division of Cardiology, University of Miami/Miller School of Medicine and the Veterans Affairs Medical Center, Miami, FL, USA*

PEEM LORVIDHAYA, MD, *Department of Medicine, The Warren Alpert Medical School of Brown University, Providence, RI, USA*

JOSEPH E. MARINE, MD, *Department of Cardiology, The Johns Hopkins Hospital, Baltimore, MD, USA,*

ROBERT J. MYERBURG, MD, *Division of Cardiology, University of Miami/Miller School of Medicine and the Veterans Affairs Medical Center, Miami, FL, USA*

GERALD V. NACCARELLI, MD, *Division of Cardiology, Penn State Hershey Heart and Vascular Institute, Penn State Milton S. Hershey Medical Center, Hershey, PA, USA*

BRIAN OLSHANSKY, MD, *Department of Medicine, University of Iowa Hospitals, Iowa City, IA, USA*

RICHARD L. PAGE, MD, *Department of Medicine, University of Wisconsin School of Medicine & Public Health, Madison, WI, USA*

CHINMAY PATEL, MD, *Lankenau Institute for Medical Research, Main Line Health Heart Center, Wynnewood, PA, USA*

KRISTEN K. PATTON, MD, *Division of Cardiology, Department of Medicine, University of Washington School of Medicine, Seattle, WA, USA*

ERNEST MATTHEW QUIN, MD, *Division of Cardiology, Medical University of South Carolina, Charleston, SC, USA*

JAMES A. REIFFEL, MD, *Department of Medicine, Columbia University Medical Center, NY, USA*

STEVEN A. ROTHMAN, MD, *Division of Cardiology, Lankenau Hospital, Main Line Health Heart Center, Wynnewood, PA, USA*

SHANE B. ROWAN, MD, *Department of Medicine, Vanderbilt University School of Medicine, Nashville, TN, USA*

DEEPAK SALUJA, MD, *Cardiac Care Unit, UMDNJ-Robert Wood Johnson Medical School, New Brunswick, NJ, USA*

MELVIN M. SCHEINMAN, MD, *Department of Medicine, Division of Cardiology, University of California, San Francisco, CA, USA*

RENEE M. SULLIVAN, MD, *Department of Medicine, University of Iowa Hospitals, Iowa City, IA, USA*

KAREN E. THOMAS, MD, *Department of Medicine, Division of Cardiovascular Medicine, Beth Israel Deaconess Medical Center, Harvard Medical School, Boston, MA, USA*

BHAVYA TRIVEDI, MD, PHD, *Pediatric Cardiology and Electrophysiology, Pediatrix Medical Group/Pediatric Cardiology Associates, Tampa, FL, USA*

J. MARCUS WHARTON, MD, *Department of Medicine, Medical University of South Carolina, Charleston, SC, USA*

GAN-XIN YAN, MD, PHD, *Main Line Health Heart Center and Lankenau Institute for Medical Research, Wynnewood, PA, USA; Division of Cardiovascular Diseases, Jefferson Medical College, Philadelphia, PA, USA; Xi'an Jiaotong University, Xi'an, China*

YANFEI YANG, MD, *Department of Medicine, Division of Cardiology, University of California, San Francisco, San Francisco, CA, USA*

PETER J. ZIMETBAUM, MD, *Department of Medicine, Division of Cardiology, Beth Israel Deaconess Medical Center, Harvard Medical School, Boston, MA, USA*

I INTRODUCTION

1

Management of Ventricular Arrhythmias: An Historical Perspective

David J. Callans and Mark E. Josephson

Contents

Abstract

The treatment of ventricular arrhythmias has undergone vibrant change in the last 40 years, evolving from a largely intellectual exercise to an evidence-based, guideline-supported set of patient care strategies. This progress have been fueled by basic and clinical science and by the initial application of randomized clinical trials to the study of electrophysiology. Along the way, several strongly held beliefs were reconsidered, most notably the use of programmed stimulation or serial Holter montoring to guide pharmacologic therapy for ventricular tachycardia. Although antiarrhythmic drugs are still considered useful in reducing the frequency of recurrent VT episodes, our loss of confidence in guided drug therapy led to the development of device, surgical ablation, and catheter ablation therapies, which form the mainstay of treatment today.

Key Words: Ventricular tachycardia; ventricular fibrillation; premature ventricular complexes; electrophysiologic study; implantable cardioverter defibrillators (ICD); antitachycardia pacing; catheter ablation; SCD-HeFT; Multicenter Automatic Defibrillator Trial; pace mapping.

> *A few hours before his death he told me . . . he did not feel any bodily ailments, and . . . without any sign of anything amiss, he passed away from this life.*
>
> *. . . through failure of the artery that feeds the heart . . . which I found to be very parched and shrunk and withered.*
>
> – Leonardo DaVinci

Interest in the management of ventricular arrhythmias developed with the understanding that ventricular tachyarrhythmias were responsible for sudden cardiac arrest (Table 1). Although sudden death has been recognized for many centuries, true sudden cardiac arrest was probably initially described by Leonardo DaVinci (see quote above). It was not until the second half of the twentieth century and the development of electrocardiographic monitoring that physicians recognized the initiation of ventricular fibrillation by premature ventricular complexes (PVCs), particularly in the early post-infarction period (Fig. 1) *(1)*. With the advent of Holter monitoring, several studies demonstrated that the risk of sudden death and cardiac mortality increased as PVC frequency increased (particularly at a

From: *Contemporary Cardiology: Management of Cardiac Arrhythmias*
Edited by: Gan-Xin Yan, Peter R. Kowey, DOI 10.1007/978-1-60761-161-5_1
© Springer Science+Business Media, LLC 2011

Table 1
Strategies for Treatment of VT/VF

Pharmacologic
  Empiric
  Holter-guided
  EPS-guided
  Combination
Non-phamacologic
  Antitachycardia pacing
  Implantable cardioverter defibrillator (ICD)
  Surgical ablation
  Catheter ablation

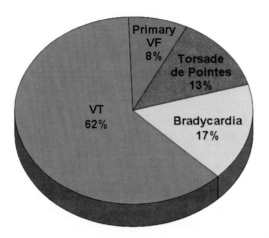

Fig. 1. Holter monitoring study demonstrating the rhythm recorded at the time of cardiac arrest in ambulatory patients. The vast majority of sudden death in this study was caused by ventricular tachyarrhythmias, with ventricular tachycardia (at least as this initial arrhythmia) being the most common. Adapted from Ref. *(1)*.

"threshold" of greater than 10 PVCs per hour) and/or the complexity of the PVCs increased *(2, 3)*. In fact, PVC grading systems were developed by Lown that attempted to signify an increasing risk of sudden death with more malignant ventricular ectopic beats *(4)*. This led to the PVC hypothesis that treating spontaneous ventricular arrhythmias would prevent the induction of sustained ventricular arrhythmias, resulting in a reduction of sudden death risk. Initially, therapy was empiric use of antiarrhythmic agents, particularly sodium channel blocking agents since these agents stabilized membranes and reduced the frequency of PVCs (Table 2). Unfortunately, as later trials would eventually demonstrate, none of these agents prevented sudden cardiac death, particularly in the post-infarction setting. Empiric use of beta-blockers, however, seemed to decrease mortality, both total and sudden in the Beta Blocker Heart Attack Study (BHAT) *(5)*. Because of the failure of empiric use of antiarrhythmic agents, Holter guided therapy was attempted. It was clearly realized, however, that Holter monitoring itself had many limitations. First of all, the frequency and complexity of arrhythmias could vary from hour to hour and day to day. The longer one was monitored, the more frequent arrhythmias were noted. This became even more evident when Holter monitoring was performed during the administration of antiarrhythmic drugs. Many studies showed that the frequency of spontaneous arrhythmias bore no relationship to the spontaneous episodes of sustained ventricular arrhythmias (Fig. 2). Thus, the following basic assumptions of Holter guided therapy were shown to be in error.

Table 2
Pharmacologic Therapy for Treatment of VT/VF

Advantages:
- Noninvasive
- No surgical morbidity or mortality
- Inexpensive in short run
- May be appropriate for certain subgroups:
  - Refused ICD
  - Multisystem disease
  - Poor overall prognosis

Disadvantages:
- Often empiric, even if EP-guided, since not all drugs can be serially tested due to expense
- Often associated with intolerable side effects, organ toxicity, and non-compliance
- Even if EP-guided, many patients remain non-suppressible and have a poor prognosis

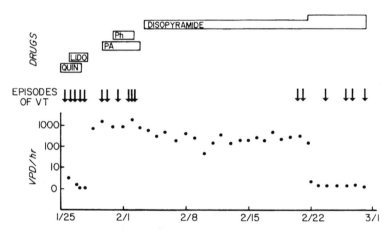

Fig. 2. The lack of ventricular ectopy and spontaneous episodes of sustained VT is one of the limitations of managing antiarrhythmic therapy guided by Holter monitoring. In this example, multiple antiarrhythmic drugs were used and treatment efficacy was assessed with monitoring. Despite a marked reduction of ventricular ectopy during quinidine and subsequently diisopyramide therapy, frequent episodes of sustained VT were observed. (From Ref. *(38)*).

1. Frequent and complex ectopy are specifically and causally related to VT/VF.
2. Holter monitoring reliably identifies these arrhythmias.
3. Elimination of PVCs prevents sudden death

   This led to the demise of the use of Holter monitoring as a mode of prevention of lethal arrhythmias. Moreover, the Cardiac Arrhythmia Suppression Trial (CAST) demonstrated that in patients with coronary artery disease, moderately reduced injection fractions and chronic stable angina, use of 1C agents was associated with an increase in mortality *(6)*. The conclusions from CAST were that treatment of asymptomatic or mildly symptomatic arrhythmias with Class IC agents in such patients was associated with excess mortality and no benefit. Proarrhythmia caused by these sodium channel blocking agents may occur late and elimination of ventricular ectopy did not provide protection against sudden cardiac death. It was the CAST Study that put an end to pharmacologic-directed therapy for the treatment of spontaneous ectopy.

In the early 1970s, clinical electrophysiology began to develop as a tool to investigate the mechanisms of arrhythmias. Wellens in 1972 first demonstrated that sustained ventricular tachycardia could be initiated by programmed electrical stimulation (Fig. 3) *(7)*. Shortly thereafter, Josephson and his colleagues from the University of Pennsylvania demonstrated that using aggressive stimulation protocols, sustained ventricular tachycardia and coronary artery disease could be reproducibly initiated in the vast majority of patients with healed myocardial infarction who presented with VT. Furthermore, VT could be reproducibly induced in patients who had more rapid arrhythmias, clinical arrhythmias associated with cardiac arrest and even those nonsustained ventricular arrhythmias, albeit in a much lower percentage of cases (Fig. 4) *(8)*. The sensitivity and specificity of programmed stimulation were validated in a number of centers. As a result, the concept of electrophysiologic testing of VT induction as a way to evaluate therapy was advanced *(9)*. In this philosophy, one considered that there needed to be a substrate in which spontaneous or stimulated extra beats could initiate lethal arrhythmias. Studies from Horowitz, Fisher, Mason and others demonstrated that one could use the response to programmed electrical stimulation to evaluate whether or not drugs could prevent spontaneous events *(9–11)*. In Fig. 5, a series of drugs was administered and the response to programmed stimulation evaluated. A variety of antiarrhythmic drugs were tested and it was established that the class 1A agents more frequently prevented induction than other agents. Moreover, noninducibility of arrhythmia was associated with

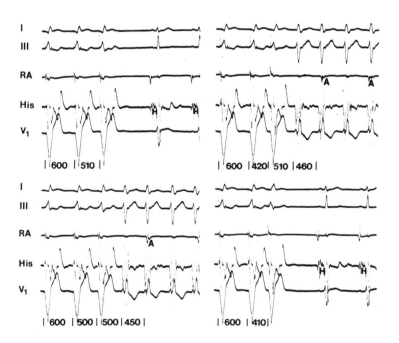

Fig. 3. Programmed ventricular stimulation for the induction of VT in one of Dr. Wellens' original patients. Following a drive train at 600 msec, an extrastimulus at 510 msec does not induce VT (*upper left*). When the extrastimulus coupling interval is decreased to 500, VT is induced and the interval to the first tachycardia beat is 500 msec (*lower left*). When the coupling interval is decreased to 420 msec (*upper right*), VT is induced and the interval to the first VT beat increases to 510 msec. Finally, when the coupling interval is decreased to 410 msec, VT is no longer induced. The observations of an extrastimulus coupling interval "window" which results in VT induction, and a reciprocal relationship between the extrastimulus coupling interval and the timing of the first tachycardia beat provide evidence for a reentrant mechanism for VT in the setting of healed infarction.

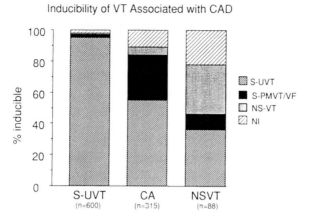

Fig. 4. The ability to reproducibly induce VT in patients with healed infarction varies according to their clinical presentation. In patients who present with tolerated sustained VT, VT is induced in over 95%. The frequency of VT induction is less in patients who present with cardiac arrest or nonsustained VT; in addition, the frequency is less in patients with non-infarct-related forms of structural heart disease. Reproduced from Ref. *(8)* with permission.

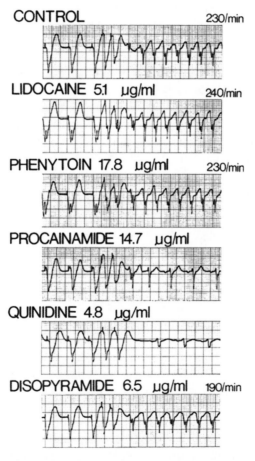

Fig. 5. The use of programmed stimulation to predict the efficacy of antiarrhythmic agents. A collection of separate electrophysiologic study data from the same patient being treated with different drug regimens is shown. Ventricular stimulation resulted in VT induction in the baseline state, which was not prevented by treatment with lidocaine, phenytoin or disopyramide, but was prevented by procainamide and quinidine. (From Ref. *(39)*).

freedom of events with a predictive accuracy of approximately 80% in a 2-year follow-up. Unfortunately, VT inducibility on a given antiarrhythmic regimen did not always predict recurrence. This was particularly true with amiodarone. Despite this limitation, it was also noted that these sodium channel blocking drugs could frequently slow VT, resulting in well-tolerated recurrent events as opposed to syncope or cardiac arrest (12). Thus, such agents not only could prevent arrhythmia but could make it tolerated so that elective cardioversion or other stimulation techniques could be used to terminate the arrhythmia. While these findings applied to patients with VT in the setting of prior myocardial infarction, the ability to use programmed stimulation to predict successful antiarrhythmic therapy for nonischemic cardiomyopathy was unsuccessful. In such patients, reproducible initiation was less often noted, and response to drug therapy was not predictive of freedom from sudden cardiac death (13).

The use of electrophysiologic guided therapy had limitations aside from the inability to use it in cardiomyopathy, however. First, none of the studies which demonstrated favorable outcomes were randomized. Secondly, most results were actually a combination of prospective and retrospective data (i.e., prior clinical drug failure associated with inducible VT and EP studies). Finally, the follow-up of all of these studies was short, somewhere between 1 and 2 years. Nonetheless, all studies showed a higher occurrence rate and/or mortality in those patients with persistently inducible VT.

The use of electrophysiologically guided antiarrhythmic drug therapy came to an abrupt halt with the Electrophysiologic Study versus Electrocardiographic Monitoring (ESVEM) Study. This was the first prospective randomized trial to evaluate the role of antiarrhythmic therapy guided by the results of programmed stimulation versus Holter monitoring. This was a highly selected patient population of patients with sustained VT (15 beats or more), cardiac arrest (less than 15% of patients) and syncope (15%). In addition, the inclusion criteria required patients to have both >10 PVCs per hour on Holter monitoring and inducible VT with programmed stimulation. The results of ESVEM Study showed that both methodologies, as applied, were not useful to predict drug efficacy; recurrence was frequent independent of which strategy was used (14). Sotalol was a well-tolerated, moderately successful drug in patients with reasonable ventricular function who had not failed prior antiarrhythmic therapy. However, these results did not permit relative drug efficacy comparisons in untreated patients, since those effectively treated were excluded from the ESVEM trial. These results are also not applicable to cardiac arrest patients with VT in clinical settings besides healed infarction, as these patients were not well represented in this study. There were many limitations to the ESVEM Study. There was no placebo armed to access mortality of untreated patients. Because of the known risks of many of the antiarrhythmic agents that were used, it is not inconceivable that a placebo group may even have faired better. The data may apply to only 15% of patients who present with frequent ectopy and/or nonsustained VT on Holter who have inducible VT on EPS. There is a bias against EPS and a bias against type 1 agents, because patients with VT who were successfully treated with class 1 agents were excluded and patients with VT failing drug therapy (particularly class 1 agents) were included. This latter limitation is extremely important, since prior study suggested that failure of one or more class 1 agents (typically procainamide) predicted failure of any antiarrhythmic agent as assessed by programmed stimulation. In total, 2/3 of the patients had failed standard drugs. In our opinion, there were other limitations that prohibit generalization of the ESVEM trial. First, the stimulation protocol was inadequate and not uniform. The number of extrastimuli was never more aggressive than during stimulation in the baseline state; if three extrastimuli were not delivered at baseline, three extrastimuli would never be delivered in interpreting the efficacy of a drug regimen. Thus, what was considered successful may not have been. Second, the ability for a patient to tolerate sotalol, particularly with regard to absence of severe LV dysfunction, may have biased the apparent response to sotalol. Many patients had already failed class 1 agents, but none were included who had been successfully treated, a significant bias against class 1 agents. There is a very high recurrence rate despite "best" therapy, probably due to the prior failure of class I agents in many subjects (which predicts failure of other drugs, as discussed above). Finally, amiodarone was not included in this trial. Regardless of these limitations which we believe

Table 3
History of the Development of Nonpharmacologic Therapy for VT

- 1977–1985 – anti-tachycardia pacing for VT
- 1978–1985 – development of surgery for VT
- 1980–1999 – development and refinement of the implantable defibrillator
- 1984–1993 – refinement of mapping techniques and development of catheter ablation for monomorphic VT; change from direct current ablation (fulguration) to radiofrequency energy.
- 1998–2002 – application of catheter-based identification of the arrhythmia substrate to treat untolerated VTs by RF ablation

significant and biased against EP studies, the use of EP-guided pharmacologic therapy virtually ended following completion of the ESVEM study. The recognition of significant pro-arrhythmia also shifted the approach towards nonpharmacologic therapy (Table 3).

NONPHARMACOLOGIC MANAGEMENT OF VT/VF

The nonpharmacologic modalities that have been developed to treat VT/VF include:

1. antitachycardia pacing
2. antiarrhythmic surgery
3. implantable cardioverter defibrillators (ICDs)
4. catheter ablation

The concept of antitachycardia pacing was obvious at the time of the initial studies of programmed stimulation for ventricular tachycardia by Wellens and Josephson *(15, 16)*. Both labs demonstrated that reproducible termination of arrhythmias was possible in patients whose tachycardia could be reproducibly initiated. The group from The University of Pennsylvania demonstrated that the rate of tachycardia influenced the ability to terminate by programmed stimulation. The success of programmed stimulation (in the form of burst pacing, programmed stimuli or autodecremental pacing) was high at rates <200 beats per minute or less; for more rapid VT, antitachycardia pacing was still successful in at least 50% VTs, but acceleration to ventricular fibrillation was more common. Furthermore, antiarrhythmic drug therapy, which consistently slows VT rate, also has a favorable influence on termination with overdrive pacing. Although there was a period of time in which specific antitachycardia pacing devices were used, the possibility of accelerating the tachycardia or producing ventricular fibrillation led to abandonment of this modality of therapy as a stand alone therapy.

Three forms of therapy eventually evolved. The earliest was antiarrhythmic surgery. Surgical procedures evolved initially in the mid-1970s and continued to the early 1990s. Catheter endocardial mapping was developed in the mid-1970s and demonstrated for the first time that the majority of arrhythmias in coronary artery disease originated on or near the endocardium *(17)*. Intra-operative mapping of the endocardium and epicardium confirmed these findings in coronary artery disease *(18)*. In addition, Cassidy et al. demonstrated that the substrate in which the tachycardia arose could be defined by abnormal electograms, those of low amplitude, broad width, fractionation and those which were late (i.e., recorded beyond the termination of the QRS complex) *(19)*. Studies by Kienzle in the operating room confirmed these findings *(20)*. Mapping in the catheterization lab could identify exit sites of early activation of the ventricular myocardium giving rise to specific QRS morphologies. These data were confirmed by mapping in the operating room. As a result of these mapping studies, the group at the University of Pennsylvania developed the subendocardial resection to remove the arrhythmogenic substrate responsible for ventricular tachycardia and ventricular fibrillation (Fig. 6)

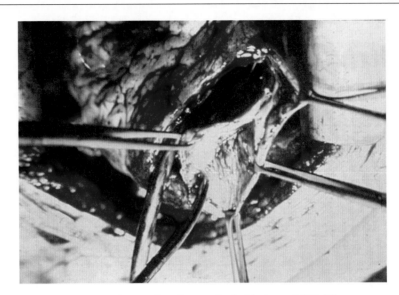

Fig. 6. The technique of subendocardial resection for surgical ablation of VT. The aneursymal segment of the left ventricle was opened, and after endocardial mapping, the subendocardial VT substrate was "peeled" from the surviving epicardial tissue. Ventricular stimulation was repeated, and if residual VT morphologies existed outside of the dense infarct, they were typically treated with focal cryoablation.

(21). These investigations demonstrated that map-guided endocardial resections could successfully prevent sudden cardiac death (4% in 5 years) or recurrent VT (8% in 5 years) *(8).* The surgical procedure was successful in patients with recent or remote myocardial infarction. Other non-map-guided procedures such as encircling subendocardial resection or encircling cryoablation were developed by Guiraudon as a method to facilitate surgical procedures without the complexity of mapping equipment *(22).* When map-guided and non-map-guided therapies were compared at the University of Pennsylvania, map-guided therapy appeared to have significantly better outcomes. While surgical therapy was successful for patients with coronary artery disease, there was a lesser experience and lower success rate in patients with cardiomyopathies. These patients appeared to have a lesser amount of endocardial electrical abnormalities and origins of VT and a greater amount of epicardial abnormalities. Not enough data were available to surgically address patients with cardiomyopathies and VT, and they continued to be considered nonsurgical candidates. Because of relatively high operative mortality (10–15%) and requirement for "a surgical electrophysiological team" the procedure was used minimally with the development of the ICD.

The implantable defibrillator was developed initially by Mirowski and colleagues despite initial deridement by many in the field *(23).* Mirowski's persistence, however, led to the development of an implantable cardioverter defibrillator, which was initially improved in 1985 (Fig. 7). The initial devices required thoracotomy for the placement of epicardial patches. Since that time, the ICD has been miniaturized (20–25 cc) and has added an increasingly greater complexity in terms of number of leads (dual chamber or biventricular) or pacing (for rate support and antitachycardia pacing) as well as additional leads to assure adequate defibrillation thresholds (subcutaneous or dual coil leads in the SVC). The ability to implant these devices as simply as a pacemaker with transvenous leads led to the widespread application of this form of therapy throughout the world. The growth of ICD implantations has become exponential, such that more than 200,000 ICDs are implanted yearly in the United States alone. The Antiarrhythmic Versus Implantable Defibrillator (AVID) Study was the first to demonstrate that the ICD was superior to antiarrhythmic drugs (primarily amiodarone) in patients who had experienced a

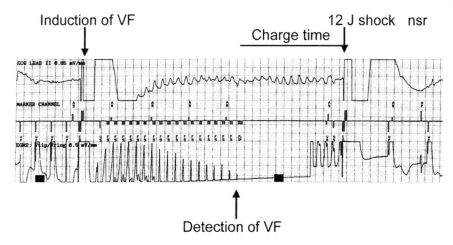

Fig. 7. Demonstration of efficacy in defibrillation during ICD testing. Surface ECG lead II, the electrogram recorded from the ICD lead and ICD sensing markers are recorded via the device. A low energy shock delivered at the crest of the T wave results in induction of ventricular fibrillation. This is promptly detected by the device, and sinus rhythm is restored with the delivery of a 12 joule shock.

cardiac arrest or untolerated VT *(24)*. The increase in survival was not impressive, but was diluted by cross over from initial treatment assignment. It was not very cost-effective ($125,000 per year life saved). Nevertheless, guidelines were established that suggested ICDs should be implanted in patients suffering from a hemodynamically untolerated VT or a cardiac arrest who had ejection fractions of less than 40%. Although limited data are available, ICD therapy has not been demonstrated to be effective (in terms of saving lives) in patients with ejection fractions of greater than 40% (except in specific clinical situations, such as long QT syndrome or hypertrophic cardiomyopathy). This demonstrates the inherent limitation of basing guideline recommendations on even well-constructed randomized controlled trials. Clearly, young patients without structural heart disease and high-risk channelopathies, whose only possible cause for death would be arrhythmic, require an ICD; however, these patients were underrepresented in the trials to make that point. In addition, the guidelines suggest that patients with well-tolerated VT also should receive devices because they had the same mortality as the untreated patients with poorly tolerated VT/VF. This conclusion is invalid since there has never been a trial assessing other strategies (pharmacologic, ablation) versus ICD therapy for tolerated VT. This is further attested to by the fact that surgical therapy for VT/VF was more effective than any ICD, yet the mortality was 50% at 5 years. As such, using total mortality as the primary endpoint, as was done in AVID as well as most contemporary randomized trials, carries with it significant limitations, particularly in patients with advanced structural heart disease. It is not reasonable to expect that ICD therapy would have any effect on mortality aside from sudden death mortality, and competing causes of death remain high, even with contemporary pharmacologic therapy for heart failure. Finally, an additional limitation of the AVID trial was that the control group received far less beta blockade than the ICD group. In fact, given the known benefit of beta-blockers in preventing both sudden and total mortality, it is conceivable that this difference could have been responsible for a majority of the difference in survival between groups.

More recently, the use of ICDs for primary prevention has been championed. Several studies evaluating ICDs alone versus paired with pharmacologic therapy or ICDs versus EP-guided therapy have demonstrated in patients with low injection fractions (less than 30%) and coronary artery disease (Multicenter Automatic Defibrillator Trial – MADIT II) *(25)*, less than 40% in coronary artery disease with nonsustained VT and inducible VTs (Multicenter Unsustained Tachycardia Trial – MUSTT) *(26)*, less than 35% in coronary artery disease with nonsustained VT and failure to respond to intravenous procainamide (Multicenter Automatic Defibrillator Trial MADIT I) *(27)* and those patients with injection fractions of less than 35% who have class 2 or 3 heart failure (Sudden Cardiac Death in Heart Failure Trial -SCD-HeFT) *(28)* all demonstrated some benefit from ICD therapy. MUSTT and MADIT I, trials that by design enriched the arrhythmic risk in the studied population prior to enrollment by prior EP studies and the presence of spontaneous nonsustained VT, had a significant mortality reduction and good cost-effectiveness with number of needed to treat from three to fourpatients per life saved. However, MADIT II and SCD-HeFT had poorer number needed to treat parameters and lower absolute benefit. In fact in SCD-HeFT, the mortality benefit was 1.4% per year over 5 years. When one compares the noncoronary artery patients as a subgroup of SCD-HeFT as well as the noncoronary artery patients seen in the Defibrillators in Nonischemic Cardiomyopathy Treatment Evaluation (DEF-INITE) *(29)* trial and the Amiodarone Versus Implantable Cardioverter-defibrillator (AMIOVIRT) *(30)* trial, there has been no consistent benefit in survival from primary prevention ICD therapy. This was recently re-evaluated by Tung et al. and raises the prospect of potential overuse of the device in such patients. Of note is the fact that in Europe, the use of ICDs for primary prevention of cardiomyopathy patients is a class 2 indication, whereas it is a class 1 in the United States. Viewing the lack of striking benefit from the device as well as potential complications (which have been recently summarized by Josephson and coworkers) *(31)* many in the United States have reassessed device usage.

With the reduction of the use of surgery, and the simultaneous development of newer mapping tools, the possibility of catheter ablation to cure VT or abolish the substrate of arrhythmias has become a possibility. This is particularly true in the case of scar-related VT due to healed infarction but with the development of epicardial approaches, ablation for control of VT for patients with cardiomyopathy and in whom the substrate appears to be primarily epicardial or subepicardial. In addition, many other forms of ventricular arrhythmias which are highly symptomatic (RVOT and idiopathic LV tachycardia) and which can lead to cardiomyopathy can be cured by catheter ablation. Many of the mapping techniques established to localize critical areas of re-entrance circuits of scar-related VT were established in the mid-1970s and early 1980s by a group at the University of Pennsylvania. Resetting and entrainment were further designed by Almendal, Josephson, Morady, and Stevenson et al. in the 1980s to allow precise localization of critical components of re-entry circuits of scar-related VT that could be destroyed, eliminating the arrhythmia *(32–35)*. The findings during entrainment or resetting of VT which identify a critical isthmus through which an impulse must travel and is bordered by anatomic and/or functional barriers and is ideal for ablation and termination of VT include the following:

1. A paced QRS morphology which is identical to VT (concealed entrainment) which identifies that the paced site is in, attached to or just proximal to a protected isthmus
2. The stimulus to QRS is approximately equal to the electogram to the QRS during VT, which means that the paced LV site is not a dead end pathway attached to the circuit.
3. The return cycle measured at the pacing site is equal to the VT cycle length, which means that the site of pacing is within the tachycardia circuit.

These observations require pacing at rates not significantly faster than the VT cycle, to prevent slowing of conduction or using very premature stimuli to reset the tachycardia. In addition, it requires that the current used may not be too high to capture more distant tissues. An example of a perfect entrainment map with successful ablation is shown (Fig. 8). Failure to terminate a tachycardia, even when the entrainment map is apparently good may be related to a sub-epicardial location of the circuit, a wide isthmus or endocardial thrombus. Although dealing with insultating thrombus may be extremely difficult, the sub-epicardial location can be dealt with an epicardial approach and a wide isthmus can be dealt with by defining those sites which meet characteristics for an isthmus and ablating over a larger area.

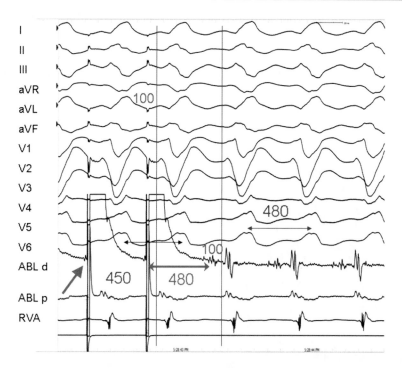

Fig. 8. Entrainment mapping for well-tolerated uniform VT. Surface leads and intracardiac recordings from the ablation catheter (ABL distal and proximal) and the right ventricle (RVA) are shown. Pacing is performed during an episode of VT. The following characteristics suggest that the ablation catheter is within a protected isthmus of the VT circuit: (1) pacing from the catheter results in a perfect match in all surface ECG leads, (2) the stimulus to QRS onset during pacing equals the electrogram to QRS onset during VT (100 msec) and (3) the return cycle (the first spontaneous VT beat after pacing) measured at the pacing site is equal to the VT cycle length (480 msec).

Although use of entrainment or reset mapping is useful for tolerated ventricular tachycardia, the majority of tachycardias occurring today are untolerated and cannot be mapped in detail by using these techniques. A different approach to those tachycardias is needed. Such an approach requires an understanding of the pathophysiological substrate of the arrhythmia. While the basic principles of substrate mapping were established in the mid-1980s by Cassidy et al., it was a development of electroanatomic mapping that allowed one to localize these electrograms in three-dimensional space and record them automatically, which allowed for the potential of ablating components of the substrate that were arrhythmogenic *(36)*. The approach to mapping and ablating the substrate involved finding potential channels of activation, which could form critical isthmuses responsible for arrhythmias within the scar *(37)*. The methods which are used include:

1. Pace mapping at a border zone to identify exit sites and isthmuses (long stimulus to QRS with the same morphology as the pacing is moved deeper into the scar).
2. Redefining voltage windows to find potential channels of viability within scar initially in scar defined by a voltage of 0.5 millivolts.
3. Pacing at high voltage to identify inexcitable tissue that could form barriers through which viable tissue is identified.
4. Identification of split potentials to define potential barriers of an isthmus

5. Define late potentials in order to identify critical isthmus sites leading to isolated mid-diastolic potentials.

Examples of pace mapping to define an exit site and an isthmus are shown in Fig. 9. Once these exit sites or channels have been identified, ablation perpendicular to the channel and into the channel can be used to prevent that channel from being used as an arrhythmia. Identifying channels of viable tissue either by changing the voltage definitions or by looking for an excitable tissue surrounding excitable pathways can identify channels that can also be ablated. Finally, ablating all late potentials is another potential methodology, but is much more difficult given the lack of ability for precisely identifying and ablating all existing late potentials.

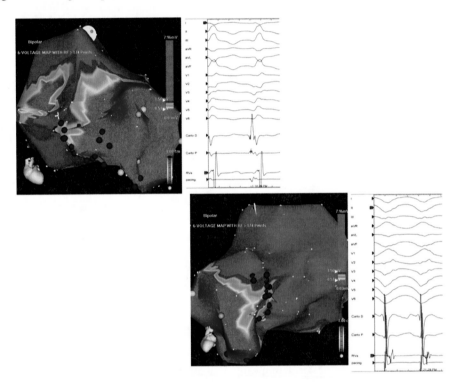

Fig. 9. Voltage mapping during sinus rhythm using electroanatomic mapping. A "shell" of the LV is made during sinus rhythm – each mapped point is assigned a location in three dimensional space, and information about the electrophysiologic characteristics of that point, in this case bipolar electrogram voltage, is presented in color coding: purple corresponds to normal, red to dense infarct (electrograms $\leq$ 0.5 mV) and the intervening colors to the intervening voltages. A large apical infarction is demonstrated, and two VT morphologies are mapped and ablated with substrate-based techniques. A right bundle right inferior axis VT (*top panel*) is mapped to the septal aspect of the infarct border, and linear ablation is performed perpendicularly to the presumed exit site (each *red icon* corresponds to a single ablation lesion), which was established as the site with the closest pacemap. A right bundle right superior axis VT is similarly mapped and ablated to the lateral aspect of the infarct (*bottom panel*).

There are limitations to all of these techniques that involve both false positive and false negative results. Many of these are related to using high current outputs at the pacing site, which leads to capture across circuit barriers, and effects more tissue than can be ablated with a single lesion. Despite these limitations, a recent randomized trial using a substrate-based ablation strategy in patients with prior ICD implantations for cardiac arrest or documented syncope with inducible VT demonstrated that this ablation strategy could reduce ICD therapies by nearly 70% in a 2-year follow-up period *(40)*.

Further work is necessary to demonstrate whether this is a valid approach with the implantation of devices for both secondary and primary prevention. However, since this ablation carries a risk, this strategy needs to be compared to standard antiarrhythmic therapies, beta-blockers and ace inhibitors, before widespread use is accepted.

CONCLUSIONS

The history of EP therapy has been one of continuous evolution for understanding of the mechanism and underlying physiological substrate of arrhythmias. The development of new technology to allow precise identification of arrhythmogenic sites has aided measurably to our ability to use catheter-based ablative procedures to treat these arrhythmias. It is our hope that with greater understanding of all the processes involved in development of the substrate may lead to improved antiarrhythmic agents which are less toxic and more targeted as well as better based techniques to treat these arrhythmias. Moreover, the role of surgery, which deals with the arrhythmogenic substrate of VT/VF, coronary artery disease, and adverse ventricular remodeling resulting in heart failure, needs to be reevaluated. Clearly, prevention of developing the physiological substrate by preventing infarction is the prime consideration. Regardless of the therapeutic modality used, it is important to treat every patient as an individual; since all trials have inherent limitations and biases, and one must recognize that one bullet does not fit all guns.

REFERENCES

1. Bayes de Luna A, Coumel P, Leclerq JF (1989) Ambulatory sudden cardiac death: mechanisms of production of fatal arrhythmia on the basis of data from 157 cases. Am Heart J 117:151–159
2. Bigger JT Jr, Fleiss JL, Kleiger R et al (1984) The relationships among ventricular arrhythmias, left ventricular dysfunction, and mortality in the 2 years after myocardial infarction. Circulation 69:250–258
3. Ruberman W, Weinblatt E, Goldberg JD et al (1981) Ventricular premature complexes and sudden death after myocardial infarction. Circulation 64:297–305
4. Lown B (1979) Sudden cardiac death – 1978. Circulation 60:1593–1599
5. The Beta Blocker Heart Attack Study Group (1981) The beta-blocker heart attack trial. JAMA 246:2073–2074
6. Echt DS, Liebson PR, Mitchell LB et al (1991) Mortality and morbidity in patients receiving encainide, flecainide, or placebo. The cardiac arrhythmia suppression trial. N Engl J Med 324:781–788
7. Wellens HJ, Schuilenburg RM, Durrer D (1972) Electrical stimulation of the heart in patients with ventricular tachycardia. Circulation 46:216–226
8. Josephson M (2008) Clinical cardiac electrophysiology: techniques and interpretations, 4th edn. Lippincott Williams & Wilkins, Philadelphia
9. Horowitz LN, Josephson ME, Farshidi A et al (1978) Recurrent sustained ventricular tachycardia 3. Role of the electrophysiologic study in selection of antiarrhythmic regimens. Circulation 58:986–997
10. Mason JW, Winkle RA (1978) Electrode-catheter arrhythmia induction in the selection and assessment of antiarrhythmic drug therapy for recurrent ventricular tachycardia. Circulation 58:971–985
11. Waspe LE, Seinfeld D, Ferrick A et al (1985) Prediction of sudden death and spontaneous ventricular tachycardia in survivors of complicated myocardial infarction: value of the response to programmed stimulation using a maximum of three ventricular extrastimuli. J Am Coll Cardiol 5:1292–1301
12. Waller TJ, Kay HR, Spielman SR et al (1987) Reduction in sudden death and total mortality by antiarrhythmic therapy evaluated by electrophysiologic drug testing: criteria of efficacy in patients with sustained ventricular tachycardia. J Am Coll Cardiol 10:83–89
13. Poll DS, Marchlinski FE, Buxton AE et al (1984) Sustained ventricular tachycardia in patients with idiopathic dilated cardiomyopathy: electrophysiologic testing and lack of response to antiarrhythmic drug therapy. Circulation 70:451–456
14. Investigators E (1989) The ESVEM trial. Electrophysiologic study versus electrocardiographic monitoring for selection of antiarrhythmic therapy of ventricular tachyarrhythmias. Circulation 79:1354–1360
15. Wellens HJ, Bar FW, Farre J et al (1980) Initiation and termination of ventricular tachycardia by supraventricular stimuli. Incidence and electrophysiologic determinants as observed during programmed stimulation of the heart. Am J Cardiol 46:576–582

16. Roy D, Waxman HL, Buxton AE et al (1982) Termination of ventricular tachycardia: role of tachycardia cycle length. Am J Cardiol 50:1346–1350

17. Josephson ME, Horowitz LN, Farshidi A et al (1978) Recurrent sustained ventricular tachycardia. 2. Endocardial mapping. Circulation 57:440–447

18. Josephson ME, Horowitz LN, Spielman SR et al (1980) Comparison of endocardial catheter mapping with intraoperative mapping of ventricular tachycardia. Circulation 61:395–404

19. Cassidy DM, Vassallo JA, Miller JM et al (1986) Endocardial catheter mapping in patients in sinus rhythm: relationship to underlying heart disease and ventricular arrhythmias. Circulation 73:645–652

20. Kienzle MG, Miller J, Falcone RA et al (1984) Intraoperative endocardial mapping during sinus rhythm: relationship to site of origin of ventricular tachycardia. Circulation 70:957–965

21. Guiraudon G, Fontaine G, Frank R et al (1978) Encircling endocardial ventriculotomy: a new surgical treatment for life-threatening ventricular tachycardias resistant to medical treatment following myocardial infarction. Ann Thoracic Surg 26:438–444

22. Mirowski M, Mower MM, Reid PR et al (1982) The automatic implantable defibrillator. New modality for treatment of life-threatening ventricular arrhythmias. Pacing Clin Electrophysiol 5:384–401

23. AVID (1997) A comparison of antiarrhythmic-drug therapy with implantable defibrillators in patients resuscitated from near-fatal ventricular arrhythmias. The antiarrhythmics versus implantable defibrillators (AVID) investigators. N Engl J Med 337:1576–1583

24. Moss AJ, Zareba W, Hall WJ (2002) Prophylactic implantation of a defibrillator in patients with myocardial infarction and reduced ejection fraction. N Engl J Med 348:1882–1890

25. Buxton AE, Lee KL, DiCarlo L et al (2000) Electrophysiologic testing to identify patients with coronary artery disease who are at risk for sudden death. Multicenter unsustained tachycardia trial investigators. N Engl J Med 342:1937–1945

26. Moss AJ, Zareba W, Hall WJ et al (2002) Prophylactic implantation of a defibrillator in patients with myocardial infarction and reduced ejection fraction. N Engl J Med 346:877–883

27. Bardy GH, Lee KL, Mark DB et al (2005) Amiodarone or an implantable cardioverter-defibrillator for congestive heart failure. 352:225–237

28. Kadish A, Quigg R, Schaechter A et al (2000) Defibrillators in nonischemic cardiomyopathy treatment evaluation. Pacing Clin Electrophysiol 23:338–343

29. Strickberger SA, Hummel JD, Bartlett TG et al (2003) Amiodarone versus implantable cardioverter-defibrillator: randomized trial in patients with nonischemic dilated cardiomyopathy and asymptomatic nonsustained ventricular tachycardia AMIOVIRT. J Am Coll Cardiol 41:1707–1712

30. Tung R, Zimetbaum P, Josephson ME (2008) A critical appraisal of implantable cardioverter-defibrillator therapy for prevention of sudden cardiac death. J Am Coll Cardiol 52:1111–1121

31. Almendral JM, Stamato NJ, Rosenthal ME et al (1986) Resetting response patterns during sustained ventricular tachycardia: relationship to the excitable gap. Circulation 74:722–730

32. Almendral JM, Gottlieb CD, Rosenthal ME et al (1988) Entrainment of ventricular tachycardia: explanation for surface electrocardiographic phenomena by analysis of electrograms recorded within the tachycardia circuit. Circulation 77:569–580

33. Morady F, Kadish AH, Rosenheck S et al (1991) Concealed entrainment as a guide for catheter ablation of ventricular tachycardia in patients with prior myocardial infarction. J Am Coll Cardiol 17:678–689

34. Stevenson W, Khan H, Sager P et al (1993) Identification of reentry circuit sites during catheter mapping and radiofrequency ablation of ventricular tachycardia late after myocardial infarction. Circulation 88:1647–1670

35. Marchlinski FE, Callans DJ, Gottlieb CD et al (2000) Linear ablation lesions for control of unmappable ventricular tachycardia in patients with ischemic and nonischemic cardiomyopathy. Circulation 101:1288–1296

36. Arenal A, del Castillo S, Gonzalez-Torrecilla E et al (2004) Tachycardia related channel in the scar tissue in patients with sustained monomorphic ventricular tachycardias. Influence of the voltage scar definition. Circulation 110:2568–2574

37. Reddy VY, Reynolds MR, Neuzil P et al (2007) Prophylactic catheter ablation for the prevention of defibrillator therapy. N Engl J Med 357:2657–2665

38. Horowitz LN, Josephson ME, Kastor JA (1980) Intracardiac electrophysiologic studies as a method for the optimization of drug therapy in chronic ventricular arrhythmia. Prog Cardiovasc Dis 23:81–98

39. Kastor JA, Horowitz LN, Harken AH et al (1981) Clinical electrophysiology of ventricular tachycardia. N Engl J Med 304:1004

40. Stevenson WG, Wilber DJ, Natale A, et al (2008) Irrigated radiofrequency catheter ablation guided by electroanatomic mapping for recurrent ventricular tachycardia after myocardial infarction: the multicenter thermocool ventricular tachycardia ablation trial. Circulation 118:2773–2782

2 History of Supraventricular Tachycardia

Yanfei Yang, Edmund C. Keung,
and Melvin M. Scheinman

CONTENTS

INTRODUCTION
ATRIOVENTRICULAR NODAL REENTRY
WOLFF–PARKINSON–WHITE SYNDROME
ATRIAL FLUTTER
ATRIAL FIBRILLATION
REFERENCES

Abstract

In this chapter, we will discuss the history of supraventricular tachycardia (SVT) that includes four sections: atrioventricular (AV) nodal reentry, AV reentry, atrial flutter (AFL), and atrial fibrillation (AF). We will focus on the historical evolution of the electrophysiologic study of the mechanism and the development of surgical and catheter ablation of these SVTs. We will also discuss potentially newer therapeutic approaches for these arrhythmias.

Key Words: Supraventricular tachycardia; atrioventricular (AV) nodal reentry; AV node; pre-excitation; accessory pathways; Wolf–Parkinson–White syndrome; atrial flutter; cavotricuspid isthmus-dependent atrial flutter; atypical atrial flutter; atrial fibrillation; catheter ablation; cardiac electrosurgery.

INTRODUCTION

We have divided the history of supraventricular tachycardia (SVT) into four sections: atrioventricular (AV) nodal reentry, AV reentry, atrial flutter (AFL), and atrial fibrillation (AF).

ATRIOVENTRICULAR NODAL REENTRY

The debate about precise anatomic boundaries of AV nodal reentry has been lasting for more than 60 years, since the first proposal that various mechanisms of SVT involve the region of the AV node *(1)*. This debate continues even though the vast majority of these patients are cured by standard ablative maneuvers.

From: *Contemporary Cardiology: Management of Cardiac Arrhythmias*
Edited by: Gan-Xin Yan, Peter R. Kowey, DOI 10.1007/978-1-60761-161-5_2
© Springer Science+Business Media, LLC 2011

Anatomy of AV Nodal and AV Junction

The works by His (2) and Tawara (3) firmly established the electrical connection between the atrium and ventricle. The AV node consists of closely packed nodal cells in open contact with atrial muscle at its proximal end (4). Its distal end is linked to the AV bundle which is normally completely insulated by the central fibrous body (5). The AV bundle links with the specialized ventricular conduction system (Purkinje) which is likewise insulated from ventricular myocardium. The proximal portion of the compact node is coated with layers of transitional cells. These morphologically distinct cells have histologic features of both nodal and ordinary atrial myocardial cells. Of potentially great importance is the recent rediscovery of posterior extensions of the AV node (6). These extensions may play a vital role in nodal reentrant circuits. One set of posterior extensions is covered by transitional cells over the left margin of the node in contact with the left atrial (LA) myocardium. More elaborate and extensive posterior extensions extend postero-inferiorly toward the area between the coronary sinus (CS) and tricuspid annulus (TA).

Strong evidence has been marshaled to place doubt on the existence of specialized atrial tracts (7). Instead, input into the AV node is thought to consist of an anterior input from the septal atrial musculature and a posterior input emanating from the crista terminalis (CT) and skirting the inferior vena cava (IVC) to proceed into the region between the CS and TA (slow pathway area) (8). The actual slow pathway may, in fact, be the nodal extension described above.

In a series of observations Moe and colleagues (9, 10) deduced evidence for dual AV nodal conduction in dogs and rabbits by using microelectrode recordings within the AV node. A critically timed premature beat was shown to block in one pathway (fast or beta pathway) but allowed for depolarization of a separate region (slow or alpha pathway). The latter was associated with slower conduction allowing for retrograde reciprocation into the beta pathway and producing an atrial echo (Fig. 1). These important concepts were rapidly assimilated into human studies and established the basis of our current understanding of AV nodal reentry in humans.

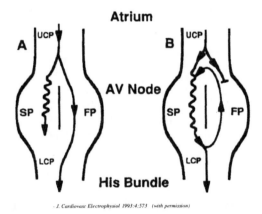

J. Cardiovasc Electrophysiol 1993;4:573 (with permission)

Fig. 1. "Classical" model of AVNRT. The AV node is "longitudinally dissociated" into a slow pathway (SP) and a fast pathway (FP). During sinus rhythm (**panel A**), impulses are conducted over the FP; in **panel B**, an atrial premature beat finds the FP refractory and is conducted over the SP. The conduction delay in the SP allows the FP to recover excitability; therefore, the impulse can conduct retrogradely via the FP and excite the upper end of the SP and initiate sustained reentry. Upper (UCP) and lower (LCP) common pathways of AV nodal tissue are present above and below the reentrant circuit. (Figure from J Cardiovasc Electrophysiol 1993; 4:573, with permission).

McGuire and colleagues (11) showed strong evidence that "AV junctional cells in the posterior AV nodal approaches appear to participate in slow pathway conduction." A later important study by Medkour et al. (12) described a combined anatomic and electrophysiologic examination of the

RAO view

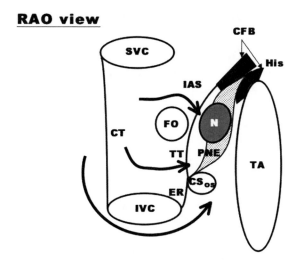

Fig. 2. A schema showing anterior (septal – 2 *upper arrows*) inputs into the AV node (N) and posterior inputs (*lower arrow*) into the node. SVC = superior vena cava; IVC = inferior vena cava; CT = crista terminalis; ER = eustachian ridge; TT = tendon of Todaro: FO = foramen ovale; IAS = interatrial septum; CS os = ostium of coronary sinus; PNE = posterior nodal extension; CFB = central fibrous body; His = His bundle; TA = tricuspid annulus.

posterior nodal extension (PNE) in the rabbit heart. As shown in Fig. 2, anatomically the extension appeared as a bundle of specialized tissues between the CS and compact node. They found no distinct separation between the compact node, lower nodal cell bundle, and the PNE. However, they found distinct differences in electrophysiologic properties between the PNE and compact node. The PNE showed cycle length-dependent slow conduction with its refractory period shorter than that of the node. Critically timed premature atrial depolorizations that blocked in the transitional cells could propagate in the PNE and thus explain the discontinuities in nodal conduction as well as in atrial echo beats (Fig. 3a and b). This study accumulated convincing evidence that the PNE provides substrate for slow pathway conduction.

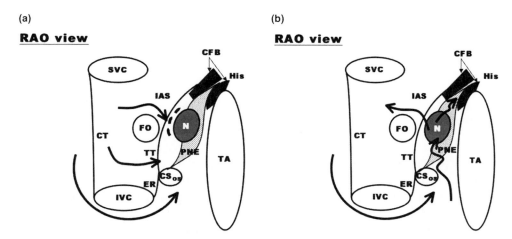

(a)
RAO view

(b)
RAO view

Fig. 3. (a) A schema showing a premature atrial complex that is blocked in the transitional cells surrounding the septal inputs to the node and the PNE as well as the node are engaged over the inferior inputs. **(b)** The pathogenesis of an echo beat. The impulse blocked in the septal inputs proceeds over the inferior input and activates the node via the PNE and is able to turn around in the node and reactivate the atrium.

Human Electrophysiologic Studies

As mentioned above, early observations by Moe and Menedez *(9, 10)* on reciprocal beats in rabbits were rapidly applied to humans. These seminal findings were introduced just as the field of clinical invasive electrophysiology began to emerge. Early invasive electrophysiologic studies *(13–16)* attributed AV nodal reentry as cause of paroxysmal SVT. Of particular note was the work of Dr. Ken Rosen and colleagues *(15)* who demonstrated evidence for dual AV nodal physiology manifest by an abruptly increase in AV nodal conduction time in response to critically timed atrial premature depolarizations. These data served as an excellent supportive compliment to the original observations of Moe and Menendez.

By the end of the 1970s, the concept of dual AV nodal conduction in humans had been well established.

However, the precise anatomic components of the AV nodal reentrant circuit remained controversial. Josephson and colleagues *(17)* showed impressive evidence that the circuit was intranodal and this concept was contested by Jackman et al. *(18)* and McGuire et al. *(19, 20)*. The newer anatomic understanding of the node has made this debate largely moot. If one accepts the concept that the posterior nodal extensions as well as the transitional cells are part of the node *(12)* then the debate is largely resolved. Current understanding suggests that most subjects with AV nodal reentry have a final common pathway within the AV node and an upper pathway involving the fast and slow pathways surrounding the compact node.

In 1993 McGuire et al. *(19, 20)* nicely summarized the available information and proposed various models for tachycardia mechanisms which involve right-sided atrial inputs. Lately Jackman and colleagues have expanded on various subforms of AV nodal reentrant tachycardia (AVNRT) *(21)*. These include slow–fast form (antegrade conduction over the slow pathway and retrograde conduction over the fast pathway) (81.4%), slow–slow form (both antegrade and retrograde conduction over the slow pathway) (13.7%), and fast–slow forms (antegrade conduction over the fast and retrograde conduction over the slow pathway) (4.9%). The differentiation among these subforms is made based on the location of earliest atrial activation. The slow pathway retrograde conduction is manifest over the CS ostium region while fast retro conduction occurs over the antero-septal area just superior to the His bundle-recording site. In addition, Jackman et al. *(22)* have suggested left-sided inputs as part of the AV nodal reentrant circuit. Recently Gonzalez et al. *(23)* proved the existence of LA input to the AV node in humans with structurally normal hearts.

In addition, there are several case reports that documented the need to ablate AVNRT from the left annulus or left posteroseptal area *(24–26)*. One source of LA input is via the left-sided posterior nodal extension. The hypothetical left-sided inputs to the AV node and possible tachycardia circuits are illustrated in Fig. 4.

Surgical Ablation of AVNRT

Ross et al. *(27)* first introduced a non-pharmacologic therapy of AVNRT that involved surgical dissection in Koch's triangle, of which the results were confirmed by a number of surgical groups *(28–30)*. This technique also led to a better understanding of this tachycardia. For example, high-resolution mapping of Koch's triangle showed two distinct types of atrionodal connections in patients with "typical" slow–fast AVNRT. In most patients the retrograde fast pathway (either during tachycardia or ventricular pacing) showed earliest atrial activation over the apex of Koch's triangle while in the minority earliest atrial activation occurred near the CS. This would nicely compliment the current designation of AVNRT subforms *(21)*.

LAO View

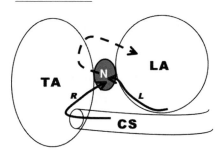

Fig. 4. Hypothesis of left-sided inputs to the AV node. In one iteration the coronary sinus musculature is involved with input into the region of the PNE. Ablation either within the coronary sinus or over the traditional slow pathway region (R) would be expected to ablate the circuit. Alternatively, the circuit may involve activation of the left atrium (LA) (shown by the *broken arrow*) either via the septum or Bachmann's bundle. Activation toward the AV node is through the tracts (L) along the mitral annulus. In the latter instance ablation over the putative left-sided inputs (L) will be required for arrhythmia cure.

Catheter Ablation of AVNRT

Catheter ablation of the AV junction using high-energy direct current (DC) shocks for control of drug-refractory SVT was first introduced in 1981 *(31)*. In 1989, two groups *(32, 33)* almost simultaneously reported success using high-energy discharge in the region of slow pathway. The subsequent use of radiofrequency (RF) energy completely revolutionized catheter cure of AVNRT. The initial attempts targeted the fast pathway by applying RF energy superior and posterior to the His bundle region until the prolongation of AV nodal conduction occurred. Initial studies *(32–36)* showed a success rate of 80–90%, but the risk of AV block was up to 21%. Jackman et al. *(37)* first introduced the technique of ablation of the slow pathway for AVNRT. Among experienced centers the current acute success rate for this procedure is 99% with a recurrence rate of 1.3% and a 0.4% incidence of AV block *(38)* requiring a pacemaker.

Ablation of the slow pathway is achieved by applying RF energy at the posterior–inferior septum in the region of the CS. This technique can be guided by either via discrete potentials *(37, 39)* or via an anatomic approach *(40)*; both have equal success rate. Radiofrequency energy is applied until junctional ectopics appear but at times successful slow pathway ablation may result without eliciting the junctional ectopic complexes. Final testing involves proof that either the slow pathway has been eliminated or no more than one AV nodal echo is present *(37, 41)*.

More recently cryoenergy has been used for the slow pathway ablation *(42, 43)*. The potential advantage of cryoenergy is the fact that the catheter sticks to adjacent endocardium during application of energy; hence, inadvertent catheter displacement and damage to the node are not possible. In addition, regions closer to the node may be explored since injury during the test procedure is reversible.

WOLFF–PARKINSON–WHITE SYNDROME

The Story of Wolff–Parkinson–White (WPW) Syndrome

The WPW syndrome holds particular interest not only for clinical cardiologists but also for anatomists, surgeons as well as clinical and experimental electrophysiologists. The definition of this syndrome was dependant upon a clear knowledge of both the normal conducting system and mechanism of reentrant arrhythmias.

The first complete description of the syndrome by Drs. Wolff, Parkinson, and White was published in the American Heart Journal in August 1930 *(44)*. They described 11 patients without structural cardiac disease who had a short P–R interval and "bundle branch block (BBB)" (Fig. 5) and paroxysmal SVT and/or AF. They made particular note of the fact that use of atropine or exercise would tend to normalize the ECG in sinus rhythm, while increases in vagal tone had the opposite effect. They felt that the arrhythmias were due to "associated nervous control of the heart." In their report they also credited Dr. F.N. Wilson (1915) and Dr. Wedd (1921) who described the pattern in case reports *(45, 46)*.

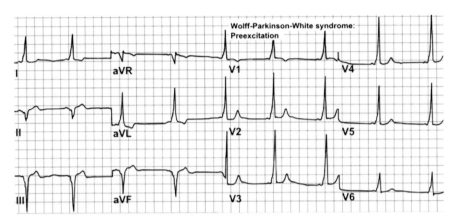

Fig. 5. Surface 12-lead ECG in a patient with WPW syndrome. The ECG showed ventricular pre-excitation in sinus rhythm with the presentation of short P–R interval and delta waves in 12 leads. The polarity of delta wave in 12 leads indicated that the atrioventricular accessory pathway was located at left posterior free wall.

Anatomic Studies of Atrioventricular (AV) Connections

At the time of the initial observations it was appreciated that the atrium and ventricles were electrically linked via the AV node and His bundle. Also, the bundle branches and Purkinje system had already been described and the electrocardiographic pattern of BBB had been identified *(47–49)*. It is, therefore, clear why the early clinicians categorized ventricular pre-excitation as BBB.

We now need to digress a bit and discuss the work of the anatomists in the late nineteenth and early twentieth century. It was appreciated that electrical connections bridged the atrium and ventricles in mammalian hearts *(50, 51)* and the nature of these connections were of great interest. Stanley Kent *(52)* in 1893 described lateral AV connections and thought that these constituted the normal AV conduction system in man. This work proved controversial and was, in fact, rejected by Sir Thomas Lewis as well as by Drs. Keith and Flack. In contrast the work of His *(53)* and Tawara *(54)* clearly defined the normal AV conducting system. Of interest, there was a later study by Kent, describing a lateral AV connection and a node-like structure within the connection *(55)*. While some have interpreted this finding as the first description of a right atriofascicular tract, but it should be appreciated that Kent felt that this structure was part of the normal AV conduction system. It is indeed odd that Kent is given credit for first describing accessory extranodal AV pathways since that credit clearly belongs to others, neither should he be properly credited with the first description of atriofascicular pathways.

In contrast, the persons who deserve credit are Wood et al. *(56)* for first describing a right-sided extranodal accessory pathway (1943) and Öhnell *(57)* for first reporting a left lateral pathway (1944). Other important contributions included the work of Mahaim *(58)* who described connections between the AV node or His bundle, to the fascicles or ventricular muscle. It was Lev who found that Mahaim

(59) tracts could produce a pattern of pre-excitation and nicely consolidated our modern understanding of the normal conduction system *(60)*. In a landmark study Lev and Lerner presented detailed anatomic studies of 33 fetal and neonatal hearts *(60)*. They concluded that no accessory pathways existed outside the AV conduction system; and that in fetal or neonatal hearts there were sparse development of collagen and hence there was close proximity but no communication between the atrium and ventricle.

Historical Evolution of Ventricular Pre-excitation and Circus-Movement Tachycardia

The early clinicians were focused on the "vagal" effects on the pre-excitation pattern and invoked vague neuro-cardiac mechanisms to explain associated arrhythmias. The concept of reciprocal rhythms was well established and Mines, who in fact, postulated a reciprocal rhythm involving the AV node and accessory pathway *(61)*. According to TN James *(62)*, Holzmann and Scherf *(63)* in 1932 were the first to describe pre-excitation as being due to an extranodal accessory pathway. Similar descriptions were made by Wolferth and Wood *(64)* who labeled this pathway as "bundle of Kent."

However, there were controversies regarding these findings at the time, and it leads to a profusion of alternative ideas. For example, Hunter et al. *(65)* suggested that the syndrome was due to a fusion of pacemakers (sinus conducted complexes and a pacemaker from the bundle branches). Printzmetal *(66)* attributed the findings to accelerated AV conduction with pathways around the node. Sodi-Pallares (1952) invoked "hyperexcitability of the right side of the septum" *(67)*.

The work by Butterworth and Poindexter *(68)* in 1942 clearly demonstrated that an artificial connection between the atrium and ventricle could mimic classic pre-excitation and led to the acceptance of an extranodal pathway as the cause for pre-excitation. The understanding of this syndrome was enhanced by the observation of Pick, Langendorf, and Katz *(69–71)*. They noted some 60 theories used to explain pre-excitation but felt that only the presence of extranodal accessory pathway could explain all their findings. By detailed and painstaking deductive analyses of literally thousands of ECGs, they amazingly described variations in the nodal vs. pathway refractoriness as a mechanism for initiation and sustaining paroxysmal SVT. They studied the relationship between tachycardia and AF and distinguished extranodal from AV nodal pathways. Their incredible insights heavily influenced subsequent human cardiac electrophysiologic studies.

Clinical Electrophysiologic Study

Drs. Durrer and Wellens *(72, 73)* were the first to use programmed electrical stimulation of the heart in order to better define the mechanism(s) of arrhythmias. It should be emphasized that their observation antedated the recording of His bundle activity in humans *(74)*. They showed that reciprocating tachycardia could be induced by premature atrial or ventricular stimulation and could be either orthodromic or antidromic; they also defined the relationship of the accessory pathway refractory period to the ventricular response during AF. These workers provided the framework for use of intracardiac electrophysiological studies to define the location (Fig. 6) and electrophysiology of these atrioventricular accessory pathways *(75, 76)*.

Cardiac-Surgical Contribution

Prior to the era of catheter ablation, patients with SVT that were refractory to medical therapy underwent direct surgical ablation of the AV junction *(77, 78)*. This approach, however, is not appropriate for the management of the patient with AF with rapid conduction over a bypass tract. Durrer and Roos *(79)* were the first to perform intraoperative mapping and cooling to locate a right free wall accessory pathway. Burchell et al. *(80)* used intraoperative mapping to locate a right-sided pathway and showed

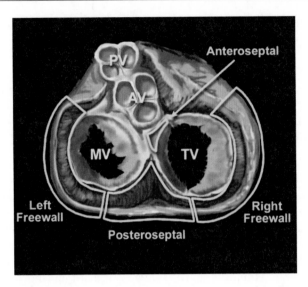

Fig. 6. Anatomic locations of atrioventricular accessory pathway in a superior view of the cross-sectional plane at the level of atrioventricular annulus. PV = pulmonary valve; AV = aortic valve; MV = mitral valve; TV = tricuspid valve.

that pre-excitation could be abolished by injection of procainamide (1967). A limited surgical incision over this area resulted in only transient loss of pre-excitation. Sealy *(81)* and the Duke team were the first to successfully ablate a right free wall pathway (1968). They initially used an epicardial approach. Their subsequent amazing results conclusively showed that a vast majority of WPW patients could be cured by either direct surgical or cryoablation *(82)* of these pathways. Iwa from Japan concurrently demonstrated the effectiveness of cardiac electrosurgery for these patients *(83)*. He is credited with being the first to use an endocardial approach for pathway ablation. The endocardial approach was subsequently independently used by the Duke team of Sealy and Cox. Only later was the "closed" epicardial approach reintroduced by Guiraudon.

Catheter Ablation

The technique of catheter ablation of the AV junction was introduced by Scheinman et al. in 1981 *(31)*. The initial attempts used high-energy DC countershocks to destroy cardiac tissue, but expansion of its use to other arrhythmias was limited due to its high risk of causing diffuse damage from barotrauma. Fisher et al. *(84)* also attempted to ablate left-sided accessory pathways through the CS by using the DC energy. This technique was eventually abandoned due to its limited efficacy and a high incidence of cardiac tamponade. Morady and Scheinman *(85)* introduced a catheter technique for disruption of posteroseptal accessory pathways. This was associated with a 65% efficacy and cardiac tamponade could be avoided by shock delivery just outside the CS *(86)*. Warin et al. described successful ablation of non-septal pathways *(87)*.

The introduction of RF energy in the late 1980s *(88, 89)* completely altered catheter ablative procedures. The salient advances in addition to RF energy included much better catheter design, together with the demonstration that pathway localization could be facilitated by direct recording of the pathway potential (Fig. 7). The remarkable work of Jackman et al. *(89)*, Kuck et al. *(90)*, and Calkins *(91)* ushered in the modern era of ablative therapy for patients with accessory pathways in all locations.

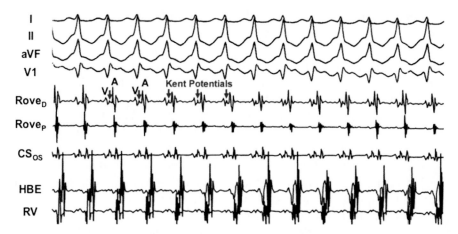

Fig. 7. Atrioventricular reentrant tachycardia in a patient with WPW syndrome. The accessory pathway potentials (Kent potentials, as marked by *arrows*) were recorded at the distal of mapping catheter (Rove$_D$). Rove$_P$ = proximal of mapping catheter; CS$_{OS}$ = ostium of coronary sinus; HBE = His bundle electrogram; RV = right ventricle; V = ventricular signal; A = atrial signal.

Moreover, a variety of registry and prospective studies have documented the safety and efficacy of ablative procedures for these patients *(92, 93)*.

The Future

At present time, catheter ablation procedures are approaching the apogee of its success and while future developments in catheter design, alternative energy sources (i.e., cryoablation), and advanced imaging will likely lead to improvements. These advances will be largely incremental. Clearly the future major advances belong in the realm of better understanding of the molecular genetics and basic pathophysiologic processes that produce this syndrome. Recently Gollob et al. *(94)* successfully identified a gene responsible for the WPW syndrome. They identified two separate families with the same genetic abnormality. Of interest were the unusual clinical features which included an approximately 40% incidence of AF and/or AFL, a high incidence of pathways with decremental conduction, ventricular hypertrophy, sinus node abnormalities, and sudden death. They identified a missense mutation in the gene that encodes the gamma 2 regulatory subunit of AMP-activated protein kinase. Protein kinase is involved in phosphorylation of many downstream substrates. The link between the genetic abnormality and pre-excitation is known to be due to development of cardiac glycogen storage disease leading to apposition of atrial and ventricular muscles *(95)*. How this and other genes control cardiac morphogenesis is a great challenge for future understanding of the development of these aberrant pathways.

ATRIAL FLUTTER

Historical Studies of AFL

The term of flutter was first used by MacWilliam *(96)*, who referred it to as visual observations of a rapid, seemingly regular excitation of the atrium. Atrial flutter was clearly differentiated from AF in man by Jolly and Ritchie *(97)*. Lead II and III inscribed by these authors are clearly compatible with counterclockwise (CCW) cavotriscupid isthmus (CTI)-dependent flutter.

The most important early contributions related to the mechanism of AFL come from the brilliant work of Sir Thomas Lewis and associates *(98)*. With induction of sustained flutter in dogs, mapping was obtained by direct recordings from the atrial epicardial surface together with surface ECG recordings. They showed that there was an orderly sequence of atrial activation, and the absence of a true diastole which explained the surface pattern. They concluded that in most experiments the excitation wave was reentrant and appeared to involve both vena cava. The circulating wave front was inscribed either in a caudo-cranial or in a cranial–caudal fashion in the right atrium (RA). It was felt that the circulating wave front could also involve the left atrium (LA). Incredibly, they suspected rotation around the AV valves in several experiments. It should be emphasized that their observations were not universally accepted. Others (e.g., Scherf and Schott) *(99)* favored enhanced automaticity as a mechanism.

Induction of AFL was uncommon in normal canines and stable mappable flutter was even less frequent. Rosenblueth and Garcia Ramos created a canine model of sustained flutter by introduction of a crush lesion between the cavae *(100)* and found that the flutter wave front rotated around the crush lesion using epicardial mapping. Of interest, they also noted that in some animals, an additional lesion that "was made starting at the lower edge of the orifice of the IVC and extending the limit ... toward the AV groove" could make the flutter disappear without re-inducibility. The latter is the identical lesion currently used to ablate CTI-dependent flutter.

We are indebted to Waldo and his colleagues for their seminal observations explaining the physiology of AFL. He and his colleagues studied patients with postoperative flutter by means of fixed atrial electrodes *(101, 102)*. They confirmed that the AFL cycle length was remarkably consistent with mean variations of less than 4 ms. Moreover, Waldo and colleagues taught us the importance of using entrainment both for detection of reentrant circuits and for discerning whether a given region is critical for tachycardia maintenance *(102)*. They also found an interesting relationship between AF and AFL in those patients in whom the onset of AFL was recorded that the transition to AFL was preceded by short episodes of rapid transitional rhythm (or AF) *(103)*.

Another major advance relates to the studies by Frame et al. *(104, 105)*. They introduced a canine model with the intercaval lesion extended into the RA free wall *(104)*. In this model, instead of the "expected" circuit around the "Y" lesion, mapping revealed evidence of electrical activation around the tricuspid orifice. In a further study *(105)*, they proved the reentrant circuit around the annulus by entrainment pacing and showed the presence of an excitable gap. This study established the need for barriers for tachycardia initiation and perpetuation. Further observations supporting the reentrant nature of AFL were provided by the studies of Boineau et al. (colony of dogs with spontaneous flutter) *(106)*, Hayden and Rytand *(107)*, Kimura et al. *(108)*, and Kato et al. *(109)*.

Another notable contribution came from Klein and Guiraudon *(110)* who mapped two patients with AFL in the operating room. They found evidence of a large RA reentrant circuit and the narrowest part of the circuit lay between the TA and the IVC. They successfully treated the flutter by using cryoablation around the CS and surrounding atrium.

Following the report of Klein et al. *(110)*, there appeared several studies using high-energy shocks in an attempt to cure AFL *(111, 112))*.

Subsequently both Drs. Feld and Cosio almost simultaneously described using RF energy for disruption of CTI conduction in order to cure patients with AFL. Feld et al. *(113)* contributed an elegant study using endocardial mapping techniques and entrainment pacing to prove that the area posterior or inferior to the CS was a critical part of the flutter circuit and application of RF energy to this site terminated AFL. Cosio et al. used similar techniques but placed the ablative lesion at the area between the TA and IVC *(114)*. The latter technique forms the basis for current ablation of CTI-dependent flutter.

Terminology of AFL

Rapid regular single macroreentrant atrial arrhythmias with little or no isoelectric interval are termed AFL. Historically, AFL was defined as being typical, reverse typical, or atypical. With increased

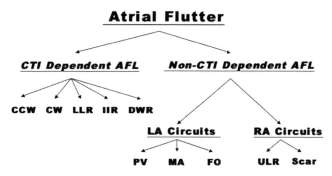

Fig. 8. Nomenclature of atrial flutter (AFL). CTI = cavotricuspid isthmus; CCW = counterclockwise AFL around the tricuspid annulus (TA); CW = clockwise AFL around the TA; LLR = lower loop reentry around inferior vena cava; IIR = intra-isthmus reentry; DWR = double-wave reentry around the TA; LA = left atrium; RA = right atrium; PV = reentrant circuit around the pulmonary vein (s) with or without scar(s) in the LA; MA = reentrant circuit around mitral annulus; FO = reentrant circuit around the fossa ovalis; ULR = upper loop reentry in the RA.

knowledge a new terminology appears to be appropriate. As shown in Fig. 8, we have recently proposed a revised nomenclature of AFL.

CAVOTRICUSPID ISTHMUS-DEPENDENT AFL

In the majority of the RA flutter, the CTI is a critical part of the reentrant circuit, which is also the target for AFL ablation.

Counterclockwise or clockwise (CW) AFL: These are macroreentrant circuits around the TA *(115–120)*. The CW or CCW designation is made on the basis of wave front activation in the left anterior oblique (LAO) projection. Counterclockwise AFL is the most common and the surface ECG shows continuous sawtooth-like flutter wave dominantly negative in the inferior leads (II, III, and aVF) and positive in V1; whereas CW flutter shows positive waves in the inferior leads and negative waves in V1 (Fig. 9). These types of AFL may be seen both in patients with or without congenital heart disease or cardiac surgery.

Double-wave reentry (DWR): Flutter circuits have an excitable gap. A critical timed premature beat is able to invade the circuit and if that impulse experiences antidromic block but yet is able to propagate orthodromically, then two wave fronts may occupy the circuit simultaneously *(121)*. This arrhythmia is manifest by acceleration of the tachycardia rate but with identical surface and intracardiac electrogram morphology. Double-wave reentry is usually produced by extrastimuli and is usually short lived, but may serve as a trigger for AFib *(122)*.

Lower loop reentry (LLR): Lower loop reentry is a form of CTI-dependent flutter with a reentrant circuit around the IVC, therefore, it is confined to the lower part of the RA *(123–125)*. It often co-exists with typical CCW or CW flutter and involves posterior breakthrough(s) across the CT. Since the CTI is still a necessary part of the circuit, LLR is amenable to CTI ablation as is true of patients with CCW or CW flutter. The surface morphology of LLR usually is very similar to that of CCW or CW flutter *(126)*.

Intra-isthmus reentry (IIR): We have recently reported a novel reentrant circuit within the region of the septal (medial) CTI and CS ostium *(127, 128)*. In the initial report of this flutter form, entrainment pacing from the antero-inferior (lateral) CTI shows post-pacing interval (PPI) > tachycardia cycle length (TCL), indicating the lateral CTI is out of the reentrant circuit; whereas, pacing from the region of septal isthmus or CS ostium shows concealed entrainment with PPI = TCL. Fractionated or double

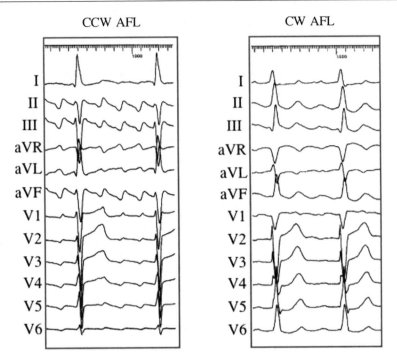

CCW AFL   CW AFL

Fig. 9. Surface ECG of CTI-dependent AFL. *Left panel* shows the simultaneous 12-lead ECG in a patient with counterclockwise (CCW) AFL; *Right panel* shows the surface ECG in a patient with clockwise (CW) AFL.

potentials usually can be recorded in this area and can be entrained. Applying RF energy at the site of maximal fractionated potentials can always abolish the tachycardia.

NON-CTI-DEPENDENT AFL

Right Atrial Flutter Circuits. *Scar-related RA macroreentrant tachycardia*: Previous studies have shown that macroreentrant tachycardia can occur in patients with or without atriotomy or congenital heart disease *(124, 129, 130)*. In these patients, electroanatomic voltage maps from the RA often show "scar" or low-voltage area(s) which acts as the central obstacle or channels for the reentrant circuit. The morphology of surface ECG may vary depending on where the scar(s) and low-voltage area(s) are and how the wave fronts exit the circuits.

Upper loop reentry (ULR): This is a type of atypical AFL involving the upper portion of RA with transverse conduction over the CT and wave front collision occurring at lower part of RA or within the CTI *(124, 131)*. Therefore, this tachycardia is a non-CTI-dependent flutter and the CTI is found to be outside of the circuit by entrainment pacing. Upper loop reentry was initially felt to involve a reentrant circuit using the channel between the superior vena cava (SVC), fossa ovalis (FO), and CT *(124)*. A study by Tai et al. using non-contact mapping technique showed that this form of AFL was a macroreentrant tachycardia in the RA free wall with the CT as its functional central obstacle *(131)*. They successfully abolished ULR by linear ablation of the gap in the CT. Like LLR, ULR also can occur in conjunction with typical CW and/or CCW flutter, as well as LLR.

Left Atrial Flutter Circuits. Left AFL circuits are often related to AF. In recent years, these circuits have been better defined by use of electroanatomic or non-contact mapping techniques *(132)*. Cardiac surgery involving the LA or atrial septum can produce different left flutter circuits. But, left AFL circuits also can be found in patients without a history of atriotomy. Electroanatomic maps in these patients often show low-voltage or scar areas in the LA, which act as either a central obstacle or a barrier in the circuit. The surface ECG of left AFLs are variable due to different reentrant circuits. However, several sub-groups have been identified (Fig. 8).

Mitral annular (MA) AFL: This flutter circuit involves reentry around the MA either in a CCW or in a CW fashion. This arrhythmia is more common in patients with structural heart disease. However, it has been described in patients without obvious structural heart disease *(126, 132)*, but in these patients, electroanatomic voltage map often shows scar or low-voltage area(s) on the posterior wall of LA as a posterior boundary of this circuit. The surface ECG of MA flutter can mimic CTI-dependent CCW or CW flutter, but usually shows low flutter wave amplitude in most of the 12 leads *(126)*.

Pulmonary vein(s) (PVs) with or without LA scar circuits: Various left AFL circuits involve the PVs, especially in those patients with AF or mitral valve disease. Reentry can circle around one or more PVs and/or posterior scar or low-voltage area(s) *(126, 132)*. In order to cure these complex circuits, electroanatomic mapping is required to reveal the circuit and guide ablation (Fig. 10). Since these circuits are related to low-voltage or scar area(s), the surface ECG usually shows low-amplitude or flat flutter waves.

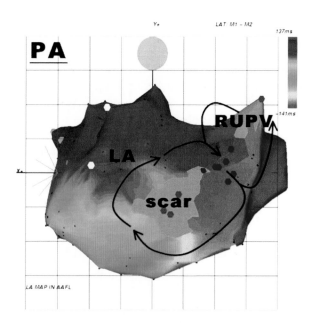

Fig. 10. Electroanatomic activation map in a patient with left atrial (LA) flutter with posterior–anterior (PA) project view. The activation map demonstrates a reentrant circuit (figure of eight) around the right upper pulmonary vein (RUPV) and scar on the LA posterior wall, as shown by the *arrows*.

ATRIAL FIBRILLATION

The history of AF has been described in a number of excellent articles *(133–135)*. It is not clear who first described AF. The legendary Chinese Yellow Emperor (Huangdi), who ruled China from 2497 to 2398 BC, reportedly described irregular and weak pulses in the Yellow Emperor's Classic of Internal Medicine *(133)*. Circa 1187, Moses Maimondides described irregular pulses suggesting AF *(134)*. Hanon, Shapiro, and Schweitzer published a very detailed account of the original investigations and evolving theories of this important arrhythmia in more modern times *(135)*. Irregular pulses in the presence of mitral stenosis were first described by de Senac in the eighteenth century and later by Robert Adams in 1827 *(133, 136)*. Stokes described irregular pulses in 1854 and Wenckebach in 1904 *(137, 138)*. Rothberger and Winterberg described AF in two patients with *arrhythmia perpetua* in 1909 *(139)*. Irregular pulse tracings showing discrepancies between simultaneously recorded apical and radial pulses were published by Etienne Marey (1863), Heinrich Hering (1903), James Mackenzie (1907), and Thomas Lewis (1909) *(135)*. Willem Einthoven and Thomas Lewis first recorded AF with electrocardiograhy in 1909. In 1910, Lewis published a landmark treatise on AF and established the term auricular fibrillation, which he defined as "a condition in which normal impulse formation in the auricle is replaced by stimulus production at multiple auricular foci. Co-ordinate contraction is lost; the normal and regular impulses transmitted to the ventricle are absent, while rapid and haphazard impulses produced in the auricle take their place and produces gross irregularity of the ventricular action" *(140)*.

Mechanisms of AF

Competing models for mechanism underlying AF were reviewed by Garrey in 1924 *(141)*. Spontaneous rapidly discharging atrial foci and a single reentry circuit with fibrillatory conduction were the first two mechanisms proposed for AF. Scherf developed the first animal model of AF by applying aconitine on an atrial site causing rapid firing *(142)*. Moe and his colleagues in 1964 proposed that AF was due to random reentry of multiple, simultaneously circulating reentrant wavelets *(143)*. It was further developed by Allessie and his colleagues in the 1970s *(144)*. It hypothesized that AF was due to multiple randomly propagating reentrant waves in the atrium and AF required at least six to eight circular reentrant wave fronts and a critical atrial mass *(145)*. It had been accepted as the mechanism until the recent discovery of spontaneous electrical activity in pulmonary vein, first in isolated guinea pig pulmonary vein and later in humans during electrophysiologic study, clearly indicating a spontaneous rapidly discharging atrial focus can be the underlying mechanism for AF *(146, 147)*. Nattel reviewed the mechanisms of AF at the tissue and cellular levels and how our treatment approaches are modified and guided by our understanding of the underlying mechanisms *(148, 149)*.

Clinical Implications of AF

Epidemiology of AF: In 1965, a study reported that the incidence of AF was 4.3 per 1000 when routine ECGs were recorded in one community with 5179 adults *(150)*. Katz and Pick reported that in 50,000 consecutive patients with suspected heart disease 3.1% had paroxysmal AF and 8.6% had chronic AF *(151)*. Most of our knowledge of the epidemiology of AF came from studies published in the late 1970s–2000. And the Framingham Heart Study provided a majority of the data. The increased prevalence of AF with age was clearly demonstrated in a number of epidemiology studies *(152, 153)*. The Framingham Heart Study first established that AF increased mortality in older men and women (55–94 years of age) even after adjustment for the pre-existing cardiovascular conditions *(154)*. The effect appears more prominent in women – 1.5-fold in men and 1.9-fold in women. Both heart failure and stroke contributed to the excessive mortality.

Thromboembolism and Anticoagulation: The role of nonrheumatic AF as a precursor of stroke and higher stroke events at the onset of AF was first identified in the Framingham Heart Study in 1978 *(155, 156)*. The risks factors for stroke and the efficacy of warfarin in decreasing stroke were established in five randomized trials published between 1989 and 1992 (AF, Aspirin, Anticoagulation Study from Copenhagen, Denmark (AFASAK), the Stroke Prevention in Atrial Fibrillation (SPAF) study, the Boston Area Anticoagulation Trial in Atrial Fibrillation (BAATAF), the Canadian Atrial Fibrillation Anticoagulation (CAFA) study, and the Veterans Affairs Stroke Prevention in Nonrheumatic Atrial

Fibrillation (SPINAF) study) *(157–162)*. In patients with AF for whom warfarin was unsuitable, the addition of clopidogrel to aspirin reduced the stroke risk *(163)*. In the 1980s, transesophageal echocardiography (TEE) was introduced as a sensitive and specific diagnostic tool to identify high-risk patients by detecting thrombus in the LA appendage *(164)*. In 1993, Manning and his coworkers introduced TEE-guided strategy for elective cardioversion without prolonged anticoagulation *(165)*.

Therapy

Pharmacological Therapy: The treatment of AF had been limited to restoring normal sinus rhythm with either DC shock or pharmacologic agents and maintenance of normal sinus rhythm with long-term drug treatment. In the case of chronic AF, rate control was the alternative. For many years, quinidine and procaineamide were the only drugs available for chemical cardioversion and rhythm maintenance. Flecainide, propafenone, amiodarone, ibutilide, and dofetilide were introduced in the past 30 years. Their efficacy in maintaining normal sinus rhythm has not been satisfactory and their pro-rhythmic risk well documented. In two randomized studies, the rate of recurrence ranged from about 35% for amiodarone to about 60% for sotalol and propafenone *(166, 167)*. For controlling of rate only, the oldest drug is digitalis, which was first used by Jean Baptiste Bouilland in 1835 *(133)*. Because of its ineffectiveness, it has been replaced with beta-blockers and calcium channel blockers. For years, conversion to and maintenance of normal sinus rhythm have always been the main goal of AF therapy; rate control was attempted only if repeated attempts in rhythm control failed. Two large randomized prospective clinical trials compared rate vs. rhythm control in AF therapy in elderly patients *(168, 169)*. In the AFFIRM trial, rate control lowered 5-year overall mortality rate (21.3% in rate vs. 23.8% in rhythm control, but without significant statistic difference). In the RACE trial, rate control increased 3-year event-free survival (17.2 in rate vs. 22.6% in rhythm control). Events included cardiovascular death, heart failure, thromboembolism, bleeding, pacemaker implantation, and anti-arrhythmic drug side effects. Embolization occurs with equal frequency in both trials. More importantly, despite successful cardioversion, recurrence rate of AF was high and many AF episodes were asymptomatic. Accordingly, anticoagulation consideration is dependent on stroke risks and not on rate or rhythm control management strategy.

Non-pharmacological Therapy: DC trans-thoracic defibrillation with synchronization was first introduced by Lown and his coworkers in 1962 *(170)*. This method remains the most effective method for acute conversion of AF to normal sinus rhythm. Surgical interventions were designed to prevent random reentry. These include reduction and fragmentation of atrial surface area, exclusion of the fibrillating atrium, and creation of one-dimensional conduction with multiple surgical incisions *(171)*. The best known surgical ablation of AF was the MAZE procedure first performed by Cox in 1987 *(172)*. Because of the complexity and morbidity surgical ablation quickly gave way to catheter ablation. Catheter ablation of the AV node with implantation of a permanent pacemaker was first used to achieve rate control in AF with rapid ventricular response *(31, 173)*. Since John F. Swartz introduced the procedure, curative catheter ablation therapy has been the major focus of electrophysiologists since the early 1990s. Spragg and Caulkins recently published an overview of the development catheter-based AF therapy and the relative merits of the different techniques *(174)*. Major contributors to the innovation and advancement of AF ablation include groups led by Michel Haissaguerre, Andrea Natale, Carlo Pappone, Morady, and Shih-Ann Chen. The first attempt entailed creation of linear lesions in the RA only or in combination with the LA (including the PVs) *(175–177)*. This was met with little success. But the experience allowed Haissaguerre to discover that focal atrial triggers (predominantly located in the PVs) are frequently responsible for initiation of AF *(178)*. However, ablation of focal PV trigger sites carries risk of PV stenosis and high recurrence rate because the focus cannot be consistently triggered during the procedure and precisely localized. Segmental ostial and circumferential PV isolation techniques were introduced to electrically isolate these triggering foci from the body of the LA by eliminate conduction between the pulmonary triggers and the atrial myocardium, thereby preventing initiation of AF *(179, 180)*.

Future

The last 30 years have seen enormous and rapid growth in our knowledge of AF. We learned the epidemiology of AF, the stroke risks, the importance of anticoagulation, the use of echocardiographic techniques, especially TEE in managing AF, the merits of rate and rhythm management, and finally, catheter-based curative ablation. On the other hand, we may have not reached the end of the ascending portion of our knowledge curve. It has been 10 years since catheter ablation of AF was first used clinically, but we still do not have a standard ablation approach *(181)*. The successful cure rates for paroxysmal, persistent, and chronic AF have not been significantly improved in the past few years. The success rates may be limited by our one-size-fit-all approach to a disease with diverse underlying mechanisms. Our curative success in other tachyarrhythmias has largely been driven by our knowledge of their underlying mechanisms. Similarly, higher success rate in AF ablation will be achieved largely by improving our knowledge of its mechanisms and pathophysiology. Meanwhile, improvement in mapping techniques and equipment such as three-dimensional electroanatomical mapping system, CT, MRI and robotic navigation, catheter designs, and ablation energy sources will help to further reduce operation time and possible the need for repeat procedures. The importance of anticoagulation in AF even after apparent successful cardioversion cannot be overemphasized. There is an obvious need for newer anticoagulation agents with a better safety profile and less monitoring. Left atrial appendage plug in prevention of clot formation has shown very promising results in clinical trial (PROTECT-AF). Lastly, insights into genetic determinants will help us to further understand the mechanisms of AF.

REFERENCES

1. Barker PS, Wilson FN, Johnston FD (1943) The mechanism of auricular paroxysmal tachycardia. Am Heart J 26: 435–445
2. His W Jr (1893) Die Tatigkeit des embryonalen Herzens und deren bedeutung fur de Lehre von de Herzbewegung beim Erwachsenen. Arbeiten aus der Medizinischen Klinik zu Leipzig 1:14–49
3. Tawara S (1906) Das Reizleitungssystem des Saugetirherzens: Eine anatomisch-histologische Studie uber das Atrioventrikularbundel und die Purkinjeschen Faden. Jena, gustav Fischer, Germany, pp 9–70, 114–156
4. Ho SY, Kilpatrick L, Kanai T et al (1995) The architecture of the atrioventricular conduction axis in dog compared to man: its significance to ablation of the atrioventricular nodal approaches. J Cardiovasc Electrophysiol 6:26–39
5. Anderson RH, Ho SY, Becker AE (2000) Anatomy of the human atrioventricular junctions revisited. Anat Rec 260: 81–91
6. Waki K, Kim JS, Becker AE (2000) Morphology of the human atrioventricular node is age-dependent: a feature of potential clinical significance. J Cardiovasc Electrophysiol 11:1144–1151
7. Mazgalev TN, Ho SY, Anderson RH (2001) Anatomic-electrophysiological correlations concerning the pathways for atrioventricular conduction. Circulation 103:2660–2667
8. Anderson RH, Becker AE, Brechenmacher C et al (1975) The human antrioventricular junctional area. A morphological study of the AV node and bundle. Eur J Cardiol 3:11–25
9. Moe GK, Preston JB, Burlington H (1956) Physiologic evidence for a dual A-V transmission system. Circ Res 4: 357–375
10. Mendez C, Moe GK (1966) Demonstration of a dual A-V nodal conduction system in the isolated rabbit heart. Circ Res 19:378–393
11. McGuire MA, Robotin M, Yip AS et al (1994) Electrophysiologic and histologic effects of dissection of the connections between the atrium and posterior part of the atrioventricular node. J Am Coll Cardiol 23:693–701
12. Medkour D, Becker AE, Khalife K, Billette J (1998) Anatomic and functional characteristics of a slow posterior AV nodal pathway: role in dual-pathway physiology and reentry. Circulation 98:164–174
13. Goldreyer BN, Bigger JT (1971) The site of reentry in paroxysmal supraventricular tachycardia in man. Circulation 43:15–26

14. Goldreyer BN, Damato AN (1971) The essential role of atrioventricular conduction delay in the initiation of paroxysmal supraventricular tachycardia. Circulation 43:679–687

15. Denes P, Wu D, Dhingra RC et al (1973) Demonstration of dual A-V nodal pathways in patients with paroxysmal supraventricular tachycardia. Circulation 48:549–555

16. Schuilenburg RM, Durrer D (1968) Atrial echo beats in the human heart elicited by induced atrial premature beats. Circulation 37:680–693

17. Josephson ME, Kastor JA (1976) Paroxysmal supraventircular tachycardia. Is the atrium a necessary link? Circulation 54:430–435

18. Jackman WM (1991) Participation of atrial myocardium (posterior septum) in AV nodal reentrant tachycardia: evidence from resetting by atrial extrastimuli. Pacing Clin Electrophysiol 14:646

19. Janse MJ, Anderson RH, McGuire MA et al (1993) "AV nodal" reentry: part I: "AV nodal" reentry revisited. J Cardiovasc Electrophysiol 4:561–572

20. McGuire MA, Janse MJ, Ross DL (1993) "AV Nodal" reentry: part II: AV nodal, AV junctional, or atrionodal reentry? J Cardiovasc Electrophysiol 4:573–586

21. Heidbüchel H, Jackman WM (2004) Characterization of subforms of AV nodal reentrant tachycardia. Europace 6: 316–29

22. Otomo K, Wang Z, Lazarra R, Jackman WM (1999) Atrioventricular nodal reentrant tachycardia: electrophysiological characteristics of four forms and implications for the reentrant circuit. In: Zipes DP, Jalife J (eds) Cardiac electrophysiology: from cell to bedside, 3rd edn. W.B. Saunders Company, Philadelphia, PA, pp 504–521

23. Gonzalez MD, Contreras LJ, Cardona F et al (2002) Demonstration of a left atrial input to the atrioventricular node in humans. Circulation 106:2930–2934

24. Jais P, Haissaguerre M, Shah DC et al (1999) Successful radiofrequency ablation of a slow atrioventricular nodal pathway on the left posterior atrial septum. Pacing Clin Electrophysiol 22:525–527

25. Tondo C, Otomo K, McClelland J et al (1996) Atrioventricular nodal reentrant tachycardia: is the reentrant circuit always confined in the right atrium? (abstract) J Am Coll Cardiol 27:159A

26. Sousa J, El-Atassi R, Rosenheck S et al (1991) Radiofrequency catheter ablation of the atrioventricular junction from the left ventricle. Circulation 84:567–571

27. Ross D, Johnson D, Denniss A et al (1985) Curative surgery for atrioventricular junctional ("AV nodal") reentrant tachycardia. J Am Coll Cardiol 6:1383–1392

28. Cox J, Holman W, Cain M (1987) Cryosurgical treatment of atrioventricular node reentrant tachycardia. Circulation 76:1329–1336

29. Guiraudon GM, Klein GJ, van Hemel N et al (1990) Anatomically guided surgery to the AV node. AV nodal skeletonization: experience in 26 patients with AV nodal reentrant tachycardia. Eur J Cardiothorac Surg 4:464–465

30. Ruder MA, Mead RH, Smith NA et al (1990) Comparison of pre- and postoperative conduction patterns in patients surgically cured of atrioventricular node reentrant tachycardia. J Am Coll Cardiol 17:397–402

31. Scheinman MM, Morady F, Hess DS, Gonzalez R (1982) Catheter-induced ablation of the atrioventricular junction to control refractory supraventricular arrhythmias. JAMA 248:851–855

32. Haissaguerre M, Warin J, Lemetayer P et al (1989) Closed-chest ablation of retrograde conduction in patients with atrioventricular nodal reentrant tachycardia. N Engl J Med 320:426–433

33. Epstein LM, Scheinman MM, Langberg JJ et al (1989) Percutaneous catheter modification of the atrioventricular node: a potential cure for atrioventricular nodal tachycardia. Circulation 80:757–768

34. Lee MA, Morady F, Kadish A et al (1991) Catheter modification of the atrioventricular junction with radiofrequency energy for control of atrioventricular nodal reentry tachycardia. Circulation 83:827–835

35. Jazayeri MR, Hempe SL, Sra JS et al (1992) Selective transcatheter ablation of the fast and slow pathways using radiofrequency energy in patients with atrioventricular nodal reentrant tachycardia. Circulation 85:1318–1328

36. Langberg JJ, Leon A, Borganelli M et al (1993) A randomized, prospective comparison of anterior and posterior approaches to radiofrequency catheter ablation of atrioventricular nodal reentry tachycardia. Circulation 87:1551–1556

37. Jackman WM, Beckman KJ, McClelland JH et al (1992) Treatment of supraventricular tachycardia due to atrioventricular nodal reentry, by radiofrequency catheter ablation of slow-pathway conduction. N Engl J Med 327: 313–318

38. Morady F (2004) Catheter ablation of supraventricular tachycardia: state of the art. J Cardiovasc Electrophysiol 15:124–139

39. Haissaguerre M, Gaita F, Fischer B et al (1992) Elimination of atrioventricular nodal reentrant tachycardia using discrete slow potentials to guide application of radiofrequency energy. Circulation 85:2162–2175

40. Kalbfleisch SJ, Strickberger SA, Williamson B et al (1994) Randomized comparison of anatomic and electrogram mapping approaches to ablation of the slow pathway of atrioventricular node reentrant tachycardia. J Am Coll Cardiol 23:716–723

41. Hummel JD, Strickberger SA, Williamson BD et al (1995) Effect of residual slow pathway function on the time course of recurrences of atrioventricular nodal reentrant tachycardia after radiofrequency ablation of the slow pathway. Am J Cardiol 75:628–630

42. Skanes AC, Dubuc M, Klein GJ et al (2000) Cryothermal ablation of the slow pathway for the elimination of atrioventricular nodal reentrant tachycardia. Circulation 102:2856–2860

43. Rodriguez LM, Geller JC, Tse HF et al (2002) Acute results of transvenous cryoablation of supraventricular tachycardia (atrial fibrillation, atrial flutter, Wolff-Parkinson-White syndrome, atrioventricular nodal reentry tachycardia). J Cardiovasc Electrophysiol 13:1082–1089

44. Wolff L, Parkinson J, White PD (1930) Bundle-branch block with short P-R interval in healthy young people prone to paroxysmal tachycardia. Am Heart J 5:685–704

45. Wilson FN (1915) A case in which the vagus influenced the form of the ventricular complex of the electrocardiogram. Arch Intern Med 16:1008–1027

46. Wedd AM (1921) Paroxysmal tachycardia, with reference to nomotropic tachycardia and the role of the extrinsic cardiac nerves. Arch Intern Med 27:571–590

47. Eppinger H, Rothberger J (1909) Zur analyse des elektrokardiogramms. Wien Klin Wehnsehr 22:1091

48. Eppinger H, Rothberger J (1910) Ueber die folgen der durchschneidung der Tawaraschen schenkel des reizleitungssystems. Zeitschr Klin Med 70:1–20

49. Eppinger H, Stoerk O (1910) Zur klinik des elektrokardiogramms. Zeitschr Klin Med 71:157

50. Paladino G (1876) Contribuzione all anatomia, istologia e fisiologia del cuore. Movemento Napoli 8:428

51. Gaskell WH (1883–1884) On the innervation of the heart. with especial reference to the heart of the tortoise. J Physiol 4:43

52. Kent AFS (1893) Researches on the structure and function of the mammalian heart. J Physiol 14:233

53. His W (1893) die thatigkeit des embryonalen herzens unde deren bedeutung fur die lehre von de herzbewegung beim erwachsenen. Med Klinik in Leipzig I:14

54. Tawara S (1906) Des reizleitungsystem des Saugetierherzens. Eine anatomischhistologische studie uder das atrioventrikularbundle under die Purkinjeschen faden. Jena, Germany, Verlag von Gustav Fischer, p 200

55. Kent AFS (1914) A conducting path between the right auricle and the external wall of the right ventricle in the heart of the mammal. J Physiol 48:57

56. Wood FC, Wolferth CC, Geckeler GD (1943) Histologic demonstration of accessory muscular connections between auricle and ventricle in a case of short P-R interval and prolonged QRS complex. Am Heart J 25:454–462

57. Öhnell RF (1944) Pre-excitation, cardiac abnormality, pathophysiological, patho-anatomical and clinical studies of excitatory spread phenomenon bearing upon the problem of the WPW (Wolff, Parkinson, and White) electrocardiogram and paroxysmal tachycardia. Acta Med Scand 152:1–167

58. Mahaim I, Benatt A (1937) Nouvelles recherches sur les connexions superieures de la branche gauche du faisceau de His-Tawara avec la cloison interventriculaire, Cardiologia 1:61–73

59. Lev M, Leffler WB, Langendorf R, Pick A (1966) Anatomic findings in a case of ventricular pre-excitation (WPW) terminating in complete atrioventricular block. Circulation 34:718–733

60. Lev M, Lerner R (1955) The theory of Kent. A histologic study of the normal atrioventricular communications of the human heart. Circulation 12:176–184

61. Mines GR (1914) On circulating excitations in heart muscles and their possible relationship to tachycardia and fibrillation. Proc Trans R Soc Can 8:43–52

62. James TN (1970) The Wolff-Parkinson-white syndrome: evolving concepts of its parthogenesis. Progr Cardiovasc Dis XIII(2): 159–189

63. Holzmann M, Scherf D (1932) Uber elektrokardiogramme mit verkurzter Vorhof-Kammer Distanz und positiven P. Zacken Z Klin Med 121:404–410

64. Wolferth CC, Wood FC (1933) This mechanism of production of short P-R intervals and prolonged QRS complexes in patients with presumably undamaged hearts: hypothesis of an accessory pathway of auriculo-ventricular conduction (bundle of Kent). Am Heart J 8:297–311

65. Hunter A, Papp C, Parkinson J (1940) The syndrome of short P-R interval, apparent bundle branch block, and associated paroxysmal tachycardia. Brit Heart J 2:107

66. Prinzmetal M et al (1952) Accelerated conduction: the Wolff-Parkinson-White syndrome and related conditions. Grune & Stratton, New York

67. Sodi-Pallares D, Cisneros F, Medrano GA et al (1963) Electrocardiographic diagnosis of myocardial infarction in the presence of bundle branch block (right and left), ventricular premature beats and Wolff-Parkinson-white syndrome. Progr Cardiovasc Dis 6:107–136

68. Butterworth JS, Poindexter CA (1942) Short PR interval associated with a prolonged QRS complex. Arch Intern Med 69:437–445

69. Pick A, Katz LN (1955) Disturbances of impulse formation and conduction in the pre-excitation (WPW) syndrome – their bearing on its mechanism. Am J Med 19:759–772

70. Pick A, Langendorf R (1968) Recent advances in the differential diagnosis of A-V junctional arrhythmias. Am Heart J 76:553–575

71. Katz LN, Pick A (1956) Clinical electrocardiography: part I. The arrhythmias: with an atlas of electrocardiograms, vol 43. Lea & Febiger, Philadelphia, pp 679–708

72. Durrer D, Schoo L, Schuilenburg RM, Wellens HJ (1967) The role of premature beats in the initiation and the termination of supraventricular tachycardia in the Wolff-Parkinson-White syndrome. Circulation 36:644–662

73. Wellens HJ, Schuilenburg RM, Durrer D (1971) Electrical stimulation of the heart in patients with Wolff-Parkinson-White syndrome, type A. Circulation 43:99–114

74. Scherlag BJ, Lau SH, Helfant RH et al (1969) Catheter technique for recording His bundle activity in man. Circulation 39:13–18

75. Gallagher JJ, Pritchett ELC, Sealy WC et al (1976) The preexcitation syndrome. Circulation 54:571–591

76. Jackman WM, Friday KJ, Scherlag BJ et al (1983) Direct endocardial recording from an accessory atrioventricular pathway, localization of the site of block effect of antiarrhythmic drugs and attempt at nonsurgical ablation. Circulation 68:906–916

77. Dreifus LS, Nichols H, Morse D et al (1968) Control of recurrent tachycardia of Wolff-Parkinson-White syndrome by surgical ligature of the A-V bundle. Circulation 38:1030–1036

78. Edmunds JH, Ellison RG, Crews TL (1969) Surgically induced atrio-ventricular block as treatment for recurrent atrial tachycardia in Wolff-Parkinson-White syndrome. Circulation 39(Suppl):105–111

79. Durrer D, Roos JP (1967) Epicardial excitation of ventricles in patient with Wolff-Parkinson-White syndrome (type B). Circulation 35:15–21

80. Burchell HB, Frye RL, Anderson MW, McGoon DC (1967) Atrioventricular and ventriculoatrial excitation in Wolff-Parkinson-White syndrome (type B). Circulation 36:663–669

81. Cobb FR, Blumenschein SD, Sealy WC, et al (1968) Successful surgical interruption of the bundle of Kent in a patient with Wolff-Parkinson-White syndrome. Circulation 38:1018–1029

82. Cox JL (2004) NASPE history: Cardiac surgery for arrhythmias. Pacing Clin Electrophysiol 27:266–282

83. Iwa T, Kazui T, Sugii S, Wada J (1970) Surgical treatment of Wolff-Parkinson-White syndrom. Kyobu Geka 23:513–8

84. Fisher JD, Brodman R, Kim SG et al (1984) Attempted nonsurgical electrical ablation of accessory pathways via the coronary sinus in the Wolff-Parkinson-White syndrome. J Am Coll Cardiol 4:685–694

85. Morady F, Scheinman MM (1984) Transvenous catheter ablation of a posteroseptal accessory pathway in a patient with the Wolff-Parkinson-White syndrome. N Engl J Med 310:705–707

86. Morady F, Scheinman MM, Kou WH et al (1989) Long-term results of catheter ablation of a posteroseptal accessory atrioventricular connection in 48 patients. Circulation 79:1160–1170

87. Warin JF, Haissaguerre M, Lemetayer P et al (1988) Catheter ablation of accessory pathways with a direct approach. Results in 35 patients. Circulation 78:800–815

88. Borggrefe M, Budde T, Podczeck A, Breithardt G (1987) High frequency alternating current ablation of an accessory pathway in humans. J Am Coll Cardiol 10:576–582

89. Jackman WM, Wang XZ, Friday KJ et al (1991) Catheter ablation of accessory atrioventricular pathways (Wolff-Parkinson-White syndrome) by radiofrequency current. N Engl J Med 334:1605–1611

90. Kuck KH, Schlüter M, Geiger M et al (1991) Radiofrequency current catheter ablation of accessory atrioventricular pathways. Lancet 337:1557–1561

91. Calkins H, Sousa J el Atassi R et al (1991) Diagnosis and cure of the Wolff-Parkinson-white syndrome or paroxysmal supraventricular tachycardias during a single electrophysiologic test. N Engl J Med 324:1612–1618

92. Scheinman MM (1995) NASPE survey on catheter ablation. Pacing Clin Electrophysiol 18:1474–1478

93. Hindricks G (1993) The multicentre European radiofrequency survey (MERFS) investigators of the work group on arrhythmias of the European society of cardiology. The multicentre European radiofrequency survey (MERFS): complications of radiofrequency catheter ablation of arrhythmias. Eur Heart J 14:1644–1653

94. Gollob MH, Green MS, Tang AS et al (2001) Identification of a gene responsible for familial Wolff-Parkinson-White syndrome. N Engl J Med 344:1823–1831

95. Wolf CM, Arad M, Ahmad F et al (2008) Reversibility of PRKAG2 glycogen-storage cardiomyopathy and electrophysiological manifestations. Circulation 117:144–154

96. McWilliam JA (1886) Fibrillar contraction of the heart. J Physiol 8:296

97. Jolly WA, Ritchie TW (1911) Auricular flutter and fibrillation. Heart 3:177–221

98. Lewis T, Feil HS, Stroud WD (1920) Observations upon flutter and fibrillation: part II: the nature of auricular flutter and Part III: some effects of rhythmic stimulation of the auricle. Heart 7:191–292

99. Scherf D, Schott A (1973) Extrasystoles and allied arrhythmias. Year Book Medical, Chicago, pp 402–420

100. Rosenblueth A, Garcia Ramos J (1947) Studies on flutter and fibrillation II. The influence of artificial obstacles on experimental auricular flutter. Am Heart J 33:677–684

101. Wells JL, MacLean WA, James TN et al (1979) Characterization of atrial flutter. Studies in man after open heart surgery using fixed atrial electrodes. Circulation 60:665–673

102. Waldo AL, MacLean WAH, Karp RB et al (1977) Entrainment and interruption of atrial flutter with atrial pacing. Studies in man following open heart surgery. Circulation 56:737–745
103. Waldo AL, Cooper TB (1996) Spontaneous onset of type I atrial flutter in patients. J Am Coll Cardiol 28:707–712
104. Frame LH, Page RL, Hoffman BF (1986) Atrial reentry around an anatomic barrier with a partially refractory excitable gap. A canine model for atrial flutter. Circ Res 58:495–511
105. Frame LH, Page RL, Boyden PA et al (1987) Circus movement in the canine atrium around the tricuspid ring during experimental atrial flutter and during reentry in vitro. Circulation 76:1155–1175
106. Boineau JP, Mooney CR, Hudson RD et al (1977) Observations on re-entrant excitation pathways and refractory period distributions in spontaneous and experimental atrial flutter in the dog. In: Kulbertus HE (ed) Re-entrant arrhythmias – mechanisms and treatment. University Park, Baltimore, p 72
107. Hayden WG, Hurley EJ, Rytand DA (1967) The mechanism of canine atrial flutter. Circ Res 20:496–505
108. Kimura E, Kato K, Murao S et al (1954) Experimental studies on the mechanism of the auricular flutter. Tohoku J Exptl Med 60:197
109. Kato K, Sato M, Harumi K et al (1957) Studies on auricular flutter. Observations upon F wave. Resp Circ (Tokyo) 5:837
110. Klein GJ, Guiraudon GM, Sharma AD et al (1986) Demonstration of macroreentry and feasibility of operative therapy in the common type of atrial flutter. Am J Cardiol 57:587–591
111. Saoudi N, Atallah G, Kirkorian G et al (1990) Catheter ablation of the atrial myocardium in human type I atrial flutter. Circulation 81:762–771
112. Chauvin M, Brechenmacher C (1989) A clinical study of the application of endocardial fulguration in the treatment of recurrent atrial flutter. Pacing Clin Electrophysiol 12:219–224
113. Feld GK, Fleck RP, Chen PS et al (1992) Radiofrequency catheter ablation for the treatment of human type 1 atrial flutter: identification of a critical zone in the reentrant circuit by endocardial mapping techniques. Circulation 86: 1233–1240
114. Cosio FG, Lopez-Gil M, Goicolea A et al (1993) Radiofrequency ablation of the inferior vena cava-tricuspid valve isthmus in common atrial flutter. Am J Cardiol 71:705–709
115. Cosio FG, Arribas F, Barbero JM et al (1988) Validation of double spike electrograms as markers of conduction delay or block in atrial flutter. Am J Cardiol 61:775–780
116. Olshansky B, Okumura K, Hess PG et al (1990) Demonstration of an area of slow conduction in human atrial flutter. J Am Coll Cardiol 15:833–841
117. Olgin JE, Kalman JM, Fitzpatrick AP et al (1995) Role of right atrial structures as barriers to conduction during human type I atrial flutter. Activation and entrainment mapping guided by intracardiac echocardiography. Circulation 92:1839–1848
118. Nakagawa H, Lazzara R, Khastgir T et al (1996) Role of the tricuspid annulus and the eustacian valve/ridge on atrial flutter: relevance to catheter ablation of the septal isthmus and a new technique for rapid identification of ablation success. Circulation 94:407–424
119. Kalman J, Olgin J, Saxon L et al (1996) Activation and entrainment mapping defines the tricuspid annulus as the anterior barrier in typical atrial flutter. Circulation 94:398–406
120. Friedman PA, Luria D, Fenton AM et al (2000) Global right atrial mapping of human atrial flutter: the presence of posteromedial (sinus venosa region) functional block and double potentials: a study in biplane fluoroscopy and intracardiac echocardiography. Circulation 101:1568–1577
121. Cheng J, Scheinman MM (1998) Acceleration of typical atrial flutter due to double-wave reentry induced by programmed electrical stimulation. Circulation 97:1589–1596
122. Yang Y, Mangat I, Glatter KA et al (2003) Mechanism of conversion of atypical right atrial flutter to atrial fibrillation. Am J Cardiol 91:46–52
123. Cheng J, Cabeen WR, Scheinman MM (1999) Right atrial flutter due to lower loop reentry; mechanism and anatomic substrates. Circulation 99:1700–1705
124. Yang Y, Cheng J, Bochoeyer A et al (2001) Atypical right atrial flutter patterns. Circulation 103:3092–3098
125. Zhang S, Younis G, Hariharan R et al (2004) Lower loop reentry as a mechanism of clockwise right atrial flutter. Circulation 109:1630–1635
126. Bochoeyer A, Yang Y, Cheng J et al (2003) Surface electrocardiographic characteristics of right and left atrial flutter. Circulation 108:60–66
127. Yang Y, Varma N, Scheinman MM (2003) Reentry within the cavotricuspid isthmus: a novel isthmus dependent circuit. (abstract) J Am Coll Cardiol 41:119A
128. Yang Y, Varma N, Keung EC et al (2005) Reentry within the cavotricuspid isthmus: an isthmus dependent circuit. PACE 28:808–818
129. Kall JG, Rubenstein DS, Kopp DE et al (2000) Atypical atrial flutter originating in the right atrial free wall. Circulation 101:270–279

130. Nakagawa H, Shah N, Matsudaira K et al (2001) Characterization of reentrant circuit in macroreentrant right atrial tachycardia after surgical repair of congenital heart disease: isolated channels between scars allow "focal" ablation. Circulation 103:699–709

131. Tai CT, Huang JL, Lin YK et al (2002) Noncontact three-dimensional mapping and ablation of upper loop re-entry originating in the right atrium. J Am Coll Cardiol 40:746–753

132. Jais P, Shah DC, Haissaguerre M et al (2000) Mapping and ablation of left atrial flutters. Circulation 101:2928–2934

133. Lip GYH, Beevers DG (1995) ABC of atrial fibrillation: history, epidemiology, and importance of atrial fibrillation. BMJ 311:1361

134. Prystowsky EN (2008) The history of atrial fibrillation: the last 100 years. J Cardiovsasc Electrophysiol 19:575–582

135. Hanon S, Shapiro M, Schweitzer P (2005) A troubled beginning: evolving concepts of an old arrhythmia. J Electrocardiol 38:213–217

136. McMichael J (1982) History of atrial fibrillation 1628–1819. Harvey-de Senac-Laennec. Br Heart J 48:1973–197

137. Stokes W (1854) The disease of the heart and the aorta. Hodges and Smith, Dublin

138. Wenckebach KF (1904) Arrhythmia of the heart. A physiological and clinical study. William Green and Sons, Edinburgh

139. Rothberger CJ, Winterberg H (1909) Vorhofflimmenern und arrhythmia perpetua. Wein Klin Woschenschr 22:839

140. Lewis T (1921) Auricular fibrillation. In: Clinical disorder of the heartbeat. Shaw & Son, London, pp 71–91

141. Garrey WE (1924) Auricular fibrillation. Physiol Rev 4:215–250

142. Sherf D (1947) Studies on auricular tachycardia caused by aconitine administration. Proc Exp Biol Med 64: 233–239

143. Moe GK, Rheinboldt WC, Abildskov JA (1964) A computer model of atrial fibrillation. Am Heart J 67:200–220

144. Allessie MA, Bonke FI, Schopman FJ (1977) Circus movement in rabbit atrial muscle as a mechanism of tachycardia. III. The "leading circle" concept: a new model of circus movement in cardiac tissue without the involvement of an anatomical obstacle. Circ Res 41:9–18

145. Allessie MA, Lammers WJEP, Smeets J et al (1982) Tital mapping of atrial excitation during acetylcholine-induced atrial flutter and fibrillation in the isolated canine heart. In: Kulbertus HE, Olsson SB, Schlepper M (eds) Atrial fibrillation. A.B. Hassell, Molndal, Sweden, pp 44–59

146. Cheung DW (1981) Electrical activity of the pulmonary vein and its interaction with the right atrium in the guinea-pig. J Physiol 314:445–456

147. Haissaguerre M, Jais P, Shah DC et al (1998) Spontaneous initiation of atrial fibrillation by ectopic beats originating from the pulmonary veins. N Engl J Med 339:659–666

148. Nattel S (2002) New ideas about atrial fibrillation 50 years on. Nature 415:219–226

149. Nattel S (2003) Atrial electrophysiology and mechanisms of atrial fibrillation. J Cardiovasc Pharmacol Therapeut 8(Suppl):S5–S11

150. Ostrander LD, Brandt RL, Kjelsberg MO et al (1965) Electrocardiographic findings among the adult population of a total natural community, Tecumsch, Michigan. Circulation 31:888–898

151. Katz LN, Pick A (1956) Clinical electrocardiography. Part I. The arrhythmias. Lea & Febiger, Philadelphia, PA

152. Wolf PA, Abbott RD, Kannel WB (1987) Atrial fibrillation: a major contributor to stroke in the elderly. The Framingham study. Arch Intern Med 147:1561–1564

153. Go AS, Hylek EM, Phillips KA et al (2001) Prevalence of diagnosed atrial fibrillation in adults: national implications for rhythm management and stroke prevention: the AnTicoagulation and Risk Factors in Atrial Fibrillation (ATRIA) Study. JAMA 285:2370–2375

154. Benjamin EJ, Wolf PA, D'Agostino RB et al (1998) Impact of atrial fibrillation on the risk of death: the Framingham heart study. Circulation 98:946–952

155. Wolf PA, Dawber TR, Thomas HE et al (1978) Epidemiologic assessment of chronic atrial fibrillation and risk of stroke: The Framingham study. Neurology 28:973–977

156. Wolf PA, Kannel WB, McGee DL et al (1983) Duration of atrial fibrillation and imminence of stroke: the Framingham study. Stroke 14:664–667

157. Petersen P, Boysen G, Godtfredsen J et al (1989) Placebo-controlled, randomized trial of warfarin and aspirin for prevention of thromboembolic complications in chronic atrial fibrillation: the Copenhagen AFASAK study. Lancet 1:175–178

158. Stroke Prevention in Atrial Fibrillation Investigators (1991) Stroke prevention in atrial Fibrillation study: final results. Circulation 84:527–539

159. The Boston Area Anticoagulation Trial for Atrial Fibrillation Investigators (1990) The effect of low-dose warfarin on the risk of stroke in patients with nonrheumatic atrial fibrillation. N Engl J Med 323:1505–1511

160. Connolly SJ, Laupacis A, Gent M et al (1991) Canadian atrial fibrillation anticoagulation (CAFA) study. J Am Coll Cardiol 18:349–355

161. Ezekowitz MD, Bridgers SL, James KE et al (1992) Warfarin in the prevention of stroke associated with nonrheumatic atrial fibrillation. N Engl J Med 327:1406–1412

162. Risk factors for stroke and efficacy of antithrombotic therapy in atrial fibrillation (1994) Analysis of pooled data from five randomized controlled trials. Arch Intern Med 154:1449–1457

163. The ACTIVE Investigators (2009) Effect of clopedogrel added to aspirin in patients with atrial fibrillation. N Engl J Med 360:2066–2078

164. Aschenberg W, Schluter M, Kremer P et al (1986) Transesophageal two-dimensional echocardiography for the detection of left atrial appendage thrombus. J Am Coll Cardiol 7:163– 166

165. Manning WJ, Silverman DI, Gordon SP et al (1993) Cardioversion from atrial fibrillation without prolonged anticoagulation with use of transesophageal echocardiography to exclude the presence of atrial thrombi. N Engl J Med 328:750–755

166. Roy D, Talajic M, Dorian P et al (2000) Amiodarone to prevent recurrence of atrial fibrillation. Canadian trial of atrial fibrillation investigators. N Engl J Med 342:913–920

167. Singh BN, Singh SN, Reda DJ et al (2005) Amiodarone versus sotalol for atrial fibrillation. N Engl J Med 352:1861–1872

168. The Atrial Fibrillation Follow-up Investigation for Rhythm Management (AFFIRM) Investigators (2002) A comparison of rate control and rhythm control in patients with atrial fibrillation. N Engl J Med 347:1825–1833

169. Van Gelder IC, Hagens VE, Bosker HA et al (2002) A comparison of rate control and rhythm control in patients with recurrent persistent atrial fibrillation. N Engl J Med 347:1834–1840

170. Lown B, Amarasingham R, Neuman J, Berkovits BV (1962) New method for terminating cardiac arrhythmias. JAMA 182:548–555

171. Guiraudon GM, Guiraudon CM, Klein GJ et al (1998) Atrial fibrillation: functional anatomy and surgical rationales. In: Farre J, Moro C (eds) Ten years of radiofrequency catheter ablation. Futura, Armonk, NY, pp 289–310

172. Cox JL, Boineau JP, Schuessler RB et al (1995) Electrophysiologic basis, surgical development and clinical results of the Maze procedure for atrial flutter and fibrillation. In: Karp RB, Wechsler AS (eds) Advances in cardiac surgery, vol 6. Mosby-Year Book, St. Louis, MO, pp 1–67

173. Gallagher JJ, Swenson RH, Kasell JH et al (1982) Catheter technique for closed-chest ablation of the atrioventricular conduction system. N Engl J Med 266:1976–1980

174. Spragg DD, Calkins H (2008) Nonpharmacological therapy for atrial fibrillation. In: Calkins H, Jais P, Steinberg JS (eds) A practical approach to catheter ablation of atrial fibrillation. Wolters Kluwer, Lippincott Williams & Wilkins, Philadelphia, PA, pp 11–24

175. Haissaguerre M, Gencel L, Fischer B et al (1994) Successful catheter ablation of atrial fibrillation. J Cardiovasc Electrophysiol 5:1045–1052

176. Haissaguerre M, Jais P, Shah DC et al (1996) Right and left atrial radiofrequency catheter therapy of paroxysmal atrial fibrillation. J Cardiovasc Electrophysiol 7:1132–1144

177. Jais P, Shah DC, Haissaguerre M et al (1999) Efficacy and safety of septal and left-atrial linear ablation for atrial fibrillation. Am J Cardiol 84:139–146

178. Haisssaguerre M, Jais P, Shah DC et al (1998) Spontaneous initiation of atrial fibrillation by ectopic beats originated from the pulmonary veins. N Engl J Med 339:659–666

179. Haissaguerre M, Shah DC, Jais P et al (2000) Electrophysiological breakthroughs from the left atrium to the pulmonary veins. Circulation 102:2463–2465

180. Pappone C, Oreto G, Lamberti F et al (1999) Catheter ablation of paroxysmal atrial fibrillation using a 3D mapping system. Circulation 100:1203–1208

181. Calkins H, Brugada J, Packer DL et al (2007) HRS/EHRA/ECAS expert consensus statement on catheter and surgical ablation of atrial fibrillation: recommendations for personnel, policy, procedures, and follow-up. Heart Rhythm 4:816–861

II CARDIAC ELECTROPHYSIOLOGY

3

Ionic and Cellular Basis for Arrhythmogenesis

Charles Antzelevitch and Gan-Xin Yan

CONTENTS

Abstract

Recent years have witnessed important advances in our appreciation of the mechanisms underlying the development of cardiac arrhythmias. Our understanding of these phenomena has been fueled by innovative advances in the genetic, ionic, and cellular basis for electrical disturbances of the heart. This chapter focuses on our present understanding of ionic and cellular mechanisms responsible for common cardiac arrhythmias. The mechanisms responsible for cardiac arrhythmias are divided into two major categories: (1) enhanced or abnormal impulse formation and (2) reentry, which occurs when a propagating impulse fails to die out after normal activation of the heart and persists to re-excite the heart after expiration of the refractory period.

Key Words: Arrhythmias; automaticity; triggered activity; reentry; early afterdepolarization (EAD); delayed afterdepolarization (DAD); late-phase 3 EAD; M cells; transient outward current (I_{to}); hyperpolarization-activated inward current (I_f); I_{Ks}; I_{Kr}; late sodium current ($I_{Na,L}$); L-type calcium current ($I_{Ca,L}$); figure of eight model; reflection; spiral wave and rotor; leading circle model; monomorphic ventricular tachycardia; ventricular fibrillation; phase 2 reentry; Brugada syndrome; J wave; J wave syndromes; transmural dispersion of repolarization; T_{p-e} interval; T_{p-e}/QT ratio; Torsade de Pointes.

Cardiac arrhythmias occur in approximately 5.3% of the population and contribute substantially to morbidity and mortality. Recent years have witnessed important advances in our understanding of the molecular and electrophysiologic mechanisms underlying the development of a variety of cardiac arrhythmias (Table 1). Our understanding of these phenomena has been fueled by innovative advances in our understanding of the genetic, ionic, and cellular basis for electrical disturbances of the heart. This chapter focuses our present understanding on ionic and cellular mechanisms responsible for common cardiac arrhythmias. The molecular mechanisms for arrhythmogenesis are discussed in Chapter 4.

The mechanisms responsible for cardiac arrhythmias are generally divided into two major categories: (1) enhanced or abnormal impulse formation and (2) reentry, i.e., circus movement (Fig. 1). Reentry occurs when a propagating impulse fails to die out after normal activation of the heart and persists to re-excite the heart after expiration of the refractory period. Evidence implicating reentry as a mechanism of cardiac arrhythmias stems back to the turn of century *(1–4)*. Phase 2 reentry

From: *Contemporary Cardiology: Management of Cardiac Arrhythmias*
Edited by: Gan-Xin Yan, Peter R. Kowey, DOI 10.1007/978-1-60761-161-5_3
© Springer Science+Business Media, LLC 2011

Table 1
Characteristics and Presumed Mechanisms of Cardiac Arrhythmias

Tachycardia	Mechanism	Origin	Rate range, bpm	AV or VA conduction
Sinus node reentry	Reentry	Sinus node and right atrium	? 110–180	1:1 or variable
Atrial fibrillation	Reentry, fibrillatory conduction, triggered activity	Atria, pulmonary veins, SVC	>350	Variable
Atrial flutter	Reentry	Right atrium, left atrium (infrequent)	240–350, usually 300 ± 20	2:1 or variable
Atrial tachycardia	Reentry, automatic, triggered activity	Atria	150–240	1:1, 2:1, or variable
AV nodal reentry tachycardia	Reentry	AV node with dual pathways	120–250, usually 150–220	1:1, very rarely 2:1
AV reentry (WPW or concealed accessory AV connection)	Reentry	Circuit includes accessory AV connection, atria, AV node, His–Purkinje system, ventricles	140–250, usually 150–220	1:1
Accelerated AV junctional tachycardia	Automatic	AV junction (AV node and His bundle)	61–200, usually 80–130	1:1 or variable
Accelerated idioventricular rhythm	Abnormal automaticity	Purkinje fibers	>60–?	Variable, 1:1, or AV dissociation
Ventricular tachycardia	Reentry, automatic, triggered	Ventricles	120–300, usually 140–240	AV dissociation, variable
Bundle branch reentrant tachycardia	Reentry	Bundle branches and ventricular septum	160–250, usually 195–240	AV dissociation, variable, or 1:1
Right ventricular outflow tract	Automatic, triggered activity	Right ventricular outflow tract	120–200	AV dissociation, variable, or 1:1
Torsade de Pointes tachycardia	Triggered, but maintaining via reentry	Ventricles (but more likely in left ventricle)	>200	AV dissociation

AV atrioventricular, *DAD* delayed afterdepolarization, *WPW* Wolff–Parkinson–White syndrome, *EAD* early afterdepolarization, *bpm* beats per minute, *SVC* superior vena cava (modified from Waldo and Wit-Hurst 11th edition, with permission)

(5–8) and fibrillatory conduction *(9, 10)* are interesting new concepts of reentrant activity advanced to explain the development of extrasystolic activity and atrial as well as ventricular fibrillation, respectively. Mechanisms responsible for abnormal impulse formation include enhanced automaticity and triggered activity. The triggered activity is consisting of (1) early afterdepolarizations (EADs) and (2) delayed afterdepolarizations (DADs). Recent studies have identified a novel mechanism, termed late-phase 3 EAD, representing a hybrid between those responsible for EAD and DAD activity *(11–13)*. The underlying mechanisms for common cardiac arrhythmias are summarized in Table 1.

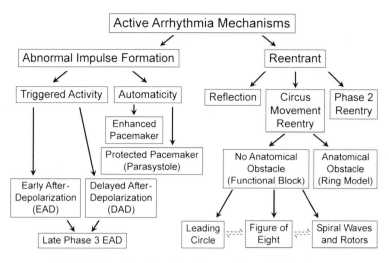

Fig. 1. Classification of active cardiac arrhythmias.

ABNORMAL IMPULSE FORMATION

Normal Automaticity

Automaticity is the property of cardiac cells to generate spontaneous action potentials. Spontaneous activity is the result of diastolic depolarization caused by a net inward current flowing during phase 4 of the action potential, which progressively brings the membrane potential to threshold for excitation. The sino-atrial (SA) node normally displays the highest intrinsic rate and is the primary pacemaker in the normal heart. All other pacemakers are referred to as subsidiary or latent pacemakers including atrioventricular (AV) node and Purkinje system, since they take over the function of initiating excitation of the heart only when the SA node is unable to generate impulses or when these impulses fail to exit SA. The automaticity of all subsidiary pacemakers within the heart is inhibited when they are overdrive paced *(14)*. This inhibition is called *overdrive suppression*. Under normal condition all subsidiary pacemakers are overdrive-suppressed by SA nodal activity. Overdrive suppression is largely mediated by intracellular accumulation of Na$^+$ leading to enhanced activity of the sodium pump (Na$^+$–K$^+$ ATPase), which generates a hyperpolarizing electrogenic current that opposes phase 4 depolarization *(15, 16)*. The faster the overdrive rate or the longer the duration of overdrive, the greater the enhancement of sodium pump activity, so that the period of quiescence after cessation of overdrive is directly related to the rate and duration of overdrive.

The ionic mechanism underlying normal SA and AV nodes and Purkinje system automaticity includes (1) a hyperpolarization-activated inward current (I_f) *(17, 18)* and/or (2) decay of outward potassium current (I_K) *(19, 20)*. The rate at which pacemaking cells initiate impulses is determined by the interplay of the following three factors: (1) maximum diastolic potential, (2) threshold potential, and (3) slope of phase 4 depolarization. Parasympathetic and sympathetic influences can alter one or more of these three parameters and thus modulate the intrinsic rate of discharge of biological pacemakers. In general, β-adrenergic receptor stimulation increases, whereas muscarinic receptor stimulation reduces the rate of phase 4 depolarization. Parasympathetic agonists such as acetylcholine also hyperpolarize the cell leading to an increase in maximum diastolic potential. Acetylcholine exerts these actions by activating a K current, $I_{K–ACh}$ *(21)*, reducing inward Ca^{2+} current (I_{Ca}) as well as reducing the pacemaker current (I_f) *(22)*. Vagal-induced hyperpolarization and slowing of phase 4 depolarization act in concert to reduce sinus rate and are the principal causes of sinus bradycardia.

Abnormal Automaticity

Abnormal automaticity can be enhanced activities in normal and/or subsidiary pacemakers or acquired automaticity in those cells like atrial and ventricular myocardial cells that do not display spontaneous diastolic depolarization under normal conditions (Fig. 1).

Enhanced automaticity like inappropriate sinus tachycardia and accelerated junctional rhythm may be due to an enhanced sympathetic nerve activity or the flow of injury current between partially depolarized myocardium due to ischemia or acute stretch and normally polarized latent pacemaker cells (23). This mechanism is also thought to be responsible for ectopic beats that arise at the borders of ischemic zones (24). Other causes of enhanced pacemaker activity include a decease in the extracellular potassium and enhanced hyperpolarization-activated I_f current. Recent data have shown that blockade of I_f current with ivabradine is a promising treatment option for patients with inappropriate sinus tachycardia (25). It is noteworthy that myocytes isolated from failing and hypertrophied animal and human hearts have been shown to manifest diastolic depolarization (26, 27) and to possess enhanced I_f pacemaker current (28, 29) suggesting that these mechanisms contribute to extrasystolic and tachyarrhythmias arising with these pathologies.

Atrial and ventricular myocardial cells do not display spontaneous diastolic depolarization under normal conditions, but may develop repetitive impulse initiation under conditions of reduced resting membrane potential, such as ischemia, stretch, or injury during heart surgery. This phenomenon is termed *depolarization-induced automaticity*. The membrane potential at which abnormal automaticity develops ranges between –70 and –30 mV (30).

The rate of abnormal automaticity is substantially higher than that of normal automaticity and is a sensitive function of resting membrane potential (i.e., the more depolarized resting potential the faster the rate). Similar to normal automaticity, abnormal automaticity is enhanced by β-adrenergic agonists and by reduction of external potassium (31). Compared to normal automaticity, abnormal automaticity in Purkinje fibers or ventricular and atrial myocardium is more readily suppressed by calcium channel blockers and shows little to no overdrive suppression (31, 32).

The ionic basis for diastolic depolarization in abnormal automaticity may be similar to that of normal automaticity, consisting of a time-dependent activation of sodium current (33) and pacemaker current I_f, as well as decay of I_K (34, 35). Action potential upstrokes of associated with abnormal automaticity may be mediated either by sodium channel current (I_{Na}) or by I_{Ca}, depending on the takeoff potential. In the range of takeoff potentials between approximately –70 and –50 mV, repetitive activity is dependent on I_{Na} and may be depressed or abolished by sodium channel blockers. In a takeoff potential range of –50 to –30 mV, repetitive activity depends on I_{Ca} and may be abolished by calcium channel blockers.

Although abnormal automaticity is not responsible for most rapid tachyarrhythmias, it can precipitate or trigger reentrant arrhythmias. Haissaguerre and co-workers have shown that atrial fibrillation can be triggered by rapid automaticity arising in the pulmonary veins (36). It is noteworthy that atrial tissues isolated from patients with atrial fibrillation exhibit increased I_f mRNA levels (37).

Triggered Activities

Oscillatory depolarizations that attend or follow the cardiac action potential and depend on preceding transmembrane activity for their manifestation are referred to as afterdepolarizations. Two subclasses traditionally recognized: (1) early and (2) delayed. Early afterdepolarizations (EAD) interrupt or retard repolarization during phase 2 and/or phase 3 of the cardiac action potential, whereas delayed afterdepolarizations (DAD) arise after full repolarization. When EAD in cells with longer action potential duration (APD) is able to initiate a new action potential in cells with relatively shorter APD (38) or DAD amplitude suffices to bring the membrane to its threshold potential, a spontaneous action potential referred to as a triggered response is the result. These triggered events may be responsible for extrasystoles and tachyarrhythmias that develop under conditions predisposing to the development of afterdepolarizations.

EARLY AFTERDEPOLARIZATION-INDUCED TRIGGERED ACTIVITIES

EADs are observed in isolated cardiac tissues exposed to altered electrolytes, hypoxia, acidosis *(39)*, catecholamines *(40, 41)*, and QT-prolonging agents *(42)* (Fig. 2). Ventricular hypertrophy and heart failure also predispose to the development of EADs *(43, 44)*. EAD-induced triggered activity is a sensitive function of stimulation rate. Agents with Class III action generally induce EAD activity at slow stimulation rates and totally suppress EADs at rapid rates *(45, 46)*. In contrast, β-adrenergic agonist-induced EADs are fast rate dependent *(40, 41)*.

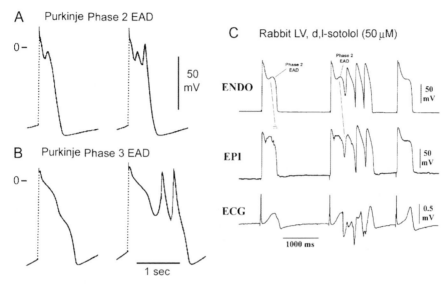

Fig. 2. Early afterdepolarizations (EAD) and triggered activity. Each panel shows intracellular activity simultaneously recorded from the two ends of a Purkinje preparation pretreated with quinidine. *Left panels* depict responses displaying only EADs; *right panels* show responses manifesting triggered activity. (**a**) EAD and triggered activity occurring at the plateau level (phase 2). (**b**) EAD and triggered activity occurring during phase 3. Modified from Ref. *(46)* with permission. (**c**) I_{Kr} blocker prolonged action potential and caused phase 2 EAD in the endocardium (ENDO) of the rabbit left ventricle (LV). Phase 2 EAD in the endocardium was able to produce a new action potential in the epicardium (EPI), manifesting an R-on-T extrasystole capable of initiating a short run of polymorphic VT.

Our early understanding of the basis for the EAD was largely based studies involving Purkinje fiber preparations (Fig. 2). Recent studies have demonstrated that among three myocardial cell types, i.e., epicardium, midmyocardium (M cells), and endocardium, M cells readily develop EAD activity when exposed to QT-prolonging agents *(47)*. Failure of epicardial tissues to develop EADs has been ascribed to the presence of a strong I_{Ks} in these cells *(48)*. M cells have a weak I_{Ks} *(48)*, predisposing them to the development of EADs in the presence of I_{Kr} block. In the presence of chromanol 293B to block I_{Ks}, I_{Kr} blockers such as E-4031 or sotalol induce EAD activity in canine-isolated epicardial and endocardial tissues as well as in M cells *(49)*. The predisposition of cardiac cells to the development of EADs depends principally on the reduced availability of I_{Kr} and I_{Ks} or increased late sodium current ($I_{Na,L}$) as occurs in many forms of cardiomyopathy *(50–52)*. Under these conditions, EADs can appear in any part of the ventricular myocardium. While EAD-induced extrasystoles are capable of triggering TdP, the arrhythmia is considered by many, but not all, to be maintained by a reentrant mechanism *(38, 53, 54)*.

An EAD occurs when the balance of current active during phase 2 or 3 of the action potential shifts in the inward direction due to either a reduction in outward currents or an increase in inward currents or a combination of both. The upstroke of the EAD is generally carried by calcium current from reactivation of $I_{Ca,L}$ during action potential phases 2 and 3 *(10, 55)*. Since $I_{Ca,L}$ recovery is time as well as voltage dependent, pure I_{Kr} blocker, which may not only delay action potential repolarization but also produce action potential triangulation in phases 2 and 3, facilitates $I_{Ca,L}$ recovery, leading to development of EADs *(56)*. It is noteworthy that drug-induced action potential triangulation itself should not be treated as an arrhythmogenic parameter because its risk of arrhythmogenesis is dependent on how the triangulatis is produced. Although drugs that inhibit both outward currents and inward currents like amiodarone may also produce action potential triangulation *(57)*, their potential to produce EADs are low *(42)*.

EAD-induced triggered activity plays a major role in the development of Torsade de Pointes under condition of congenital and acquired long QT syndromes *(38, 54)* (Fig. 2). EAD activity may also be involved in the genesis of cardiac arrhythmias in cases of hypertrophy and heart failure which are commonly associated with prolongation of the ventricular action potential *(27, 43, 44)*.

It is noteworthy that EADs developing in select transmural subtypes (such as M cells) can exaggerate transmural dispersion of repolarization (TDR), thus setting the stage for reentry. As will be discussed in more detail below, transmural dispersion of repolarization is thought to be an reentrant substrate for maintenance of TdP *(38, 58, 59)*.

DELAYED AFTERDEPOLARIZATION-INDUCED TRIGGERED ACTIVITY

Oscillations of transmembrane activity that occur after full repolarization of the action potential and depend on previous activation of the cell for their manifestation are referred to as delayed afterdepolarizations (DAD) (Fig. 3). When DADs reach the threshold potential, they give rise to spontaneous action potentials generally referred to as triggered activity. Delayed afterdepolarizations and accompa-

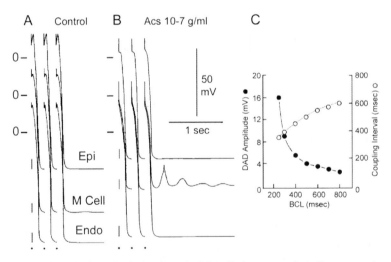

Fig. 3. Digitalis-induced delayed afterdepolarizations in M cells but not epicardium or endocardium. Effects of acetylstrophanthidin (AcS) on transmembrane activity of an epicardial (Epi), endocardial (Endo), and M cell preparation. $[K^+]_o = 4$ mM. (**a**) Control. (**b**) Recorded after 90 min of exposure to 10^{-7} g/ml AcS. Each panel shows the last 3 beats of a train of 10 basic beats elicited at a basic cycle length (BCL) of 250 msec. Each train is followed by a 3 s pause. AcS induced prominent delayed afterdepolarizations (DADs) in the M cell preparation but not in epicardium or endocardium. (**c**) Rate dependence of coupling interval and amplitude of the AcS-induced DADs. Measured is the first DAD recorded from the M cell. From Ref. *(47)* with permission.

nying aftercontractions are caused by spontaneous release of calcium from the sarcoplasmic reticulum (SR) under calcium overload conditions. The afterdepolarization is believed to be induced by a transient inward current (I_{ti}) generated either by: (1) a non-selective cationic current (I_{ns}) *(60, 61)*, (2) the activation of an electrogenic Na/Ca exchanger *(60, 62–64)*, or (3) calcium-activated Cl⁻ current *(63, 64)*. All are secondary to the release of Ca from the overloaded SR.

The overloaded SR and associated DAD-induced triggered activity are observed under conditions of exposure to toxic levels of cardiac glycosides (digitalis) (Fig. 3) or catecholamines, in hypertrophied and failing hearts *(26, 65)* and in Purkinje fibers surviving myocardial infarction *(66)*. Intervention capable of altering intracellular calcium, either by modifying transsarcolemmal calcium current or by inhibiting sarcoplasmic reticulum storage or release of calcium, can affect the manifestation of the DAD. DADs can also be modified by interventions capable of directly inhibiting or enhancing the transient inward current, I_{ti}. DADs are modified by extracellular K⁺, Ca²⁺, lysophosphoglycerides, and the metabolic factors such as ATP, hypoxia, and pH. Lowering extracellular K⁺ (<4 mM) promotes DADs, while increasing K⁺ attenuates or totally suppresses DADs. Lysophosphatidylcholine, in concentrations similar to those that accumulate in ischemic myocardium, has been shown to induce DAD activity *(67)*. Elevating extracellular Ca²⁺ promotes DADs and an increase of extracellular ATP potentiates isoproterenol-induced DAD *(68)*. In contrast to EADs, DADs are always induced at relatively rapid rates.

Pharmacological agents that affect the release and re-uptake of calcium by the SR, including caffeine and ryanodine, can also influence the manifestation of DADs and triggered activity. Low concentrations of caffeine facilitate Ca release from the SR and thus contribute to augmentation of DAD and triggered activity. High concentration of caffeine prevents Ca uptake by the SR and thus abolish I_{ti}, DADs, aftercontractions, and triggered activity. Doxorubicin, an anthracycline antibiotic, has been shown to be effective in suppressing digitalis-induced DADs, possibly through inhibition of the Na–Ca exchange mechanism *(69)*. Potassium channel activators, like pinacidil, can also suppress DAD and triggered activity by activating ATP-regulated potassium current ($I_{K–ATP}$) *(70)*. Flunarizine is another agent shown to suppress DAD and triggered activity, in part through inhibition of both L-type and T-type calcium current *(71, 72)*. Ranolazine, an antianginal agent with potent late sodium channel blocking action, has also been shown to reduce the amplitude of delayed afterdepolarizations (DADs) induced by isoproterenol, forskolin, or ouabain *(73–75)*.

Although a wide variety of studies performed in isolated tissues and cells suggest an important role for DAD-induced triggered activity in the genesis of cardiac arrhythmias, especially bigeminal rhythms and tachyarrhythmias observed in the setting of digitalis toxicity, little direct evidence of DAD-induced triggered activity is available in vivo. Consequently, even when triggered activity appears a likely mechanism, it is often impossible to completely rule out other mechanisms (e.g., reentry, enhanced automaticity).

Clinical arrhythmias suggested to be caused by DAD-induced triggered activity include (1) *idiopathic ventricular tachyarrhythmias (55, 76–78)*, (2) *idioventricular rhythms* – accelerated A–V junctional escape rhythms that occur as a result of digitalis toxicity or in a setting of myocardial infarction. Other possible "DAD-mediated" arrhythmias include exercise-induced adenosine-sensitive ventricular tachycardia as described by Lerman et al. *(79)*, repetitive monomorphic ventricular tachycardia caused presumably cAMP-mediated triggered activity *(80)*, supraventricular tachycardias, including arrhythmias originating in the coronary sinus, and some heart failure-related arrhythmias *(81)*.

DADs are thought to play a prominent role in catecholaminergic or familial polymorphic ventricular tachycardia, a rare, autosomal dominant inherited disorder, predominantly affecting children or adolescents with structurally normal hearts. It is characterized by bidirectional ventricular tachycardia (BVT), polymorphic VT (PVT), and a high risk of sudden cardiac death (30–50% by the age of 20–30 years) *(82, 83)*. Recent molecular genetic studies have identified mutations in genes encoding for the cardiac ryanodine receptor 2 (RyR2) or calsequestrin 2 (CASQ2) in patients with this phenotype *(84–86)*. Several lines of evidence point to delayed afterdepolarization (DAD)-induced triggered activity (TA) as the mechanism underlying monomorphic or bidirectional VT in these patients. These include the identification of genetic mutations involving Ca^{2+} regulatory proteins, a similarity of the ECG features to those associated with digitalis toxicity, and the precipitation by adrenergic stimulation. A recent model of catecholaminergic polymorphic ventricular tachycardia (CPVT) developed using the left ventricular coronary-perfused wedge preparation was shown to recapitulate the electrocardiographic and arrhythmic manifestations of the disease, most of which were secondary to DAD-induced triggered activity *(87)*. DAD-induced extrasystolic activity arising from epicardium was also shown to provide the substrate for the development of reentrant tachyarrhythmias due to reversal of the direction of activation of the ventricular wall *(87)*.

LATE-PHASE 3 EARLY AFTERDEPOLARIZATIONS (EAD) AND THEIR ROLE IN INITIATION OF ATRIAL FIBRILLATION (AF)

Recent studies have uncovered a novel mechanism giving rise to triggered activity, termed "late-phase 3 EAD," which combines properties of both EAD and DAD, but has its own unique character. Late-phase 3 EAD-induced triggered extrasystoles represent a new concept of arrhythmogenesis in which abbreviated repolarization permits "normal SR calcium release" to induce an EAD-mediated closely coupled triggered response, particularly under conditions permitting intracellular calcium loading *(11, 12)*. These EADs are distinguished by the fact that they interrupt the final phase of repolarization of the action potential (late-phase 3). In contrast to previously described DAD or Ca_i-depended EAD, it is *normal*, not spontaneous SR calcium release that is responsible for the generation of the DAD. Late-phase 3 EADs are observed only when APD is markedly abbreviated as with acetylcholine (Fig. 4) *(11)*. Based on the time-course of contraction, levels of intracellular calcium (Ca_i) would be expected to peak during the plateau of the action potential (membrane potential of approximately –5 mV) under control conditions control, but during the late phase of repolarization (membrane poten-

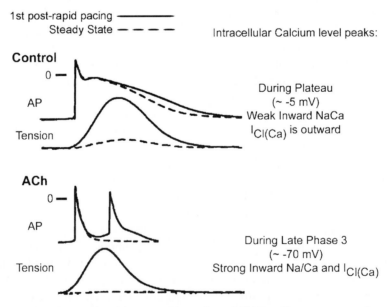

Fig. 4. Proposed mechanism for the development of late-phase 3 EADs. Shown are superimposed action potential (AP) and phasic tension recordings obtained under steady-state conditions and during the first regular post-rapid pacing beat in control and in the presence of acetylcholine. See text for further discussion (reproduced with permission from Ref. *(11)*).

tial of approximately – 70 mV) in the presence of acetylcholine. As a consequence, the two principal calcium-mediated currents, I_{Na-Ca} and $I_{Cl(Ca)}$, would be expected to be weakly inward or even outward ($I_{Cl(Ca)}$) when APD is normal (control), but strongly inward when APD is very short (acetylcholine). Thus, abbreviation of the atrial APD allows for a much stronger recruitment of both I_{Na-Ca} and $I_{Cl(Ca)}$ in the generation of a late-phase 3 EADs. It is noteworthy that the proposed mechanism is similar to that thought to underlie the development of DADs and conventional Ca_i-dependent EAD (64, 88). The principal difference is that in the case of these DADs/EADs, I_{Na-Ca} and $I_{Cl(Ca)}$ are recruited secondary to a *spontaneous* release of calcium from the SR, whereas in the case of late-phase 3 EADs, these currents are accentuated as a consequence of the *normal* SR release mechanisms.

In the isolated canine atria, late-phase 3 EAD-induced extrasystoles have been shown to initiate AF, particularly following spontaneous termination of the arrhythmia (11). The appearance of late-phase 3 EAD immediately following termination of AF or rapid pacing has been recently reported by in the canine atria in vivo (12). Patterson et al. (89) recently described "tachycardia-pause"-induced EAD in isolated superfused canine pulmonary vein muscular sleeve preparations in the presence of both simultaneous parasympathetic (to abbreviate APD) and sympathetic (to augment Ca_i) nerve stimulation. This Patterson also appears during late-phase 3 of the action potential and a similar mechanism has been proposed (89). A similar mechanism has recently been invoked to explain catecholamine-induced afterdepolarizations and ventricular tachycardia in mice (90).

REENTRANT ARRHYTHMIAS

Circus Movement Reentry

The circuitous propagation of an impulse around an anatomical or functional obstacle leading to re-excitation of the heart describes a circus movement reentry. Four distinct models of this form of reentry have been described: (1) the ring model; (2) the leading circle model; (3) the figure of eight model; and (4) the spiral wave model. The ring model of reentry differs from the other three in that an anatomical obstacle is required. The leading circle, figure of eight, and spiral wave models of reentry require only a functional obstacle.

RING MODEL (ANATOMICAL REENTRY)

The ring model is the simplest form of reentry in which an anatomical obstacle with a relative fixed pathway is present. Mines was the first to develop the concept of circus movement reentry as a mechanism responsible for cardiac arrhythmias (1). The criteria developed by Mines for identification of circus movement reentry remains in use today: (1) an area of unidirectional block must exist; (2) the excitatory wave progresses along a distinct pathway, returning to its point of origin and then following the same path again; and (3) interruption of the reentrant circuit at any point along its path should terminate the circus movement.

Schmitt and Erlanger in 1928 suggested that coupled ventricular extrasystoles in mammalian hearts could arise as a consequence of circus movement reentry within loops composed of terminal Purkinje fibers and ventricular muscle. Using a theoretical model consisting of a Purkinje bundle that divides into two branches which insert distally into ventricular muscle (Fig. 5), they suggested that a region of depression within one of the terminal Purkinje branches could provide for unidirectional block and conduction slow enough to permit successful re-excitation within a loop of limited size (91).

It was recognized that successful reentry could occur only when the impulse was sufficiently delayed in an alternate pathway to allow for expiration of the refractory period in the tissue proximal to the site of unidirectional block. Both conduction velocity and refractoriness determine the success or failure of reentry and the general rule is that the length of the circuit (*pathlength*) must exceed that of the

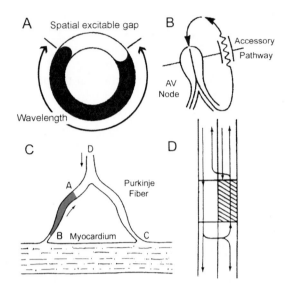

Fig. 5. Ring models of reentry. (**a**) Schematic of a ring model of reentry. (**b**) Mechanism of reentry in the Wolff–Parkinson–White syndrome involving the AV node and an atrioventricular accessory pathway (AP). (**c**) A mechanism for reentry in a Purkinje-muscle loop proposed by Schmitt and Erlanger. The diagram shows a Purkinje bundle (D) that divides into two branches, both connected distally to ventricular muscle. Circus movement was considered possible if the stippled segment, A → B, showed unidirectional block. An impulse advancing from D would be blocked at A, but would reach and stimulate the ventricular muscle at C by way of the other terminal branch. The wavefront would then reenter the Purkinje system at B traversing the depressed region slowly so as to arrive at A following expiration of refractoriness. (**d**) Schematic representation of circus movement reentry in a linear bundle of tissue as proposed by Schmitt and Erlanger. The upper pathway contains a depressed zone (*shaded*) serves as a site of unidirectional block and slow conduction. Anterograde conduction of the impulse is blocked in the upper pathway but succeeds along the lower pathway. Once beyond the zone of depression, the impulse crosses over through lateral connections and reenters through the upper pathway (panels c and d are from Schmitt and Erlanger *(91)*).

wavelength that is defined as the product of the conduction velocity and the refractory period. The openings of the vena cava in the right atrium, an aneurysm or a scar secondary to myocardial infarction in the ventricles, the presence of bypass tracts between atria and ventricles (Kent bundle), or dual AV node pathways can form a ring-like path for the development of reentrant arrhythmias like atrial flutter, some forms of monomorphic ventricular tachycardia and supraventricular tachycardia via use of an AV accessory pathway or dual AV node pathways.

Slowed or delayed conduction of the impulse can facilitate the development of reentrant arrhythmias by reducing the wavelength (conduction velocity × action potential refractory period) of the reentry wavefront so that it can be accommodated by the available path length. There are several causes for slow conduction capable of leading to reentry: (1) slow or discontinuous conduction that may be a normal property of some regions of the heart, such as the sinus and AV node, (2) depressed fast responses or discontinuities of conduction caused by pathophysiological conditions like ischemia, heart failure, and use of sodium channel blockers like class Ic antiarrhythmic drugs, and (3) anisotropy, i.e., intracellular or extracellular resistance to the flow of current within the heart can result in differences in longitudinal vs. transverse conduction velocities *(92)*.

On the other hand, any agent that prolongs the wavelength of the reentry wavefront interrupts the circus movement. Class III antiarrhythmic drugs like sotalol, amiodarone, and dofetilide that prolong action potential duration and refractory period suppress not only anatomically reentrant arrhythmias like atrial flutter and monomorphic VT using an anatomical obstacle, but also some forms of functional reentry like atrial fibrillation.

FUNCTIONAL REENTRY

Leading circle model. In 1970s, Allessie and co-workers *(93, 94)* performed experiments in which they induced a tachycardia in isolated preparations of rabbit left atria by applying properly timed premature extrastimuli. Using multiple intracellular electrodes, they showed that although the basic beats elicited by stimuli applied near the center of the tissue spread normally throughout the preparation, premature impulses propagate only in the direction of shorter refractory periods. An arc of block thus develops around which the impulse is able to circulate and re-excite the tissue. Recordings near the center of the circus movement showed only subthreshold responses. Thus arose the concept of the leading circle *(94)*, a form of circus movement reentry occurring in structurally uniform myocardium, requiring no anatomic obstacle (Fig. 6). The functionally refractory region that develops at the vortex of the circulating wavefront prevents the centripetal waves from short circuiting the circus movement and thus serves to maintain the reentry. Since the head of the circulating wavefront usually travels on relatively refractory tissue, a fully excitable gap of tissue may not be present; unlike other forms of reentry the leading circle model may not be readily influenced by extraneous impulses initiated in areas outside the reentrant circuit and thus may not be easily entrained.

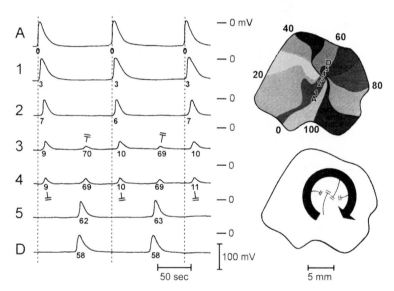

Fig. 6. Leading circle model of reentry. Activation maps during steady-state tachycardia induced by a premature stimulus in an isolated rabbit atrium (*upper right*). On the *left* are transmembrane potentials recorded from seven fibers located on a *straight line* through the center of the circus movement. Note that the central area is activated by centripetal wavelets and that the fibers in the central area show double responses of subnormal amplitude. Both responses are unable to propagate beyond the center, thus preventing the impulse from short-cutting the circuit. *Lower right*: the activation pattern is schematically represented, showing the leading circuit and the converging centripetal wavelets. Block is indicated by *double bars* (from Allessie et al. *(94)* with permission).

Figure of eight model. The figure of eight model of reentry was first described by El-Sherif and co-workers in the surviving epicardial layer overlying infarction produced by occlusion of the left anterior descending artery in canine hearts in the late 1980s *(95)*. In the figure of eight model, the reentrant beat produces a wavefront that circulates in both directions around a long line of functional

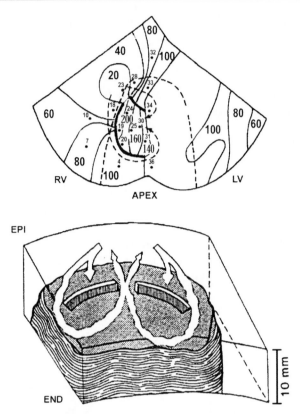

Fig. 7. Figure of eight model of reentry. Isochronal activation map during monomorphic reentrant ventricular tachycardia occurring in the surviving epicardial layer overlying an infarction. Recordings were obtained from the epicardial surface of a canine heart 4 days after ligation of the left anterior descending coronary artery. Activation isochrones are drawn at 20 msec intervals. The reentrant circuit has a characteristic figure eight activation pattern. Two circulating wavefronts advance in clockwise and counterclockwise directions, respectively, around two zones (arcs) of conduction block (represented by *heavy solid lines*). The epicardial surface is depicted as if the ventricles were unfolded following a cut from the crux to the apex. A three-dimensional diagrammatic illustration of the ventricular activation pattern during the reentrant tachycardia is shown in the lower panel. RV, right ventricle; LV, left ventricle; EPI, epicardium; END, endocardium (from Ref. *(95)*, with permission).

conduction block (Fig. 7) rejoining on the distal side of the block. The wavefront then breaks through the arc of block to re-excite the tissue proximal to the block. The single arc of block is thus divided into two and the reentrant activation continues as two circulating wavefronts that travel in clockwise and counterclockwise directions around the two arcs in a pretzel-like configuration. The diameter of the reentrant circuit in the ventricle may be as small as a few millimeters or as large as a several centimeters. In 1999, Lin and co-workers *(96)* described a novel quatrefoil-shaped reentry induced by delivering long stimuli during the vulnerable phase in rabbit ventricular myocardium. This pattern, a variant of figure of eight reentry, consists of two pairs of opposing rotors with all four circuits converging in the center.

Spiral waves and rotors. Originally used to describe reentry around an anatomical obstacle, the term spiral wave reentry was later adopted to describe circulating waves in the absence of an anatomical obstacle *(97, 98)*, similar to the circulating waves of the leading circle mechanism. Spiral wave theory has advanced our understanding of the mechanisms responsible for the functional form of reentry. Although leading circle and spiral wave reentry are considered by some to be similar, a number of distinctions have been suggested *(99–101)*. The curvature of the spiral wave is the key to the formation of the core *(101)*. The curvature of the wave forms a region of high impedance mismatch (sink–source mismatch), where the current provided by the reentering wavefront (source) is insufficient to charge the capacity and thus excite larger volume of tissue ahead (sink). A prominent curvature of the spiral

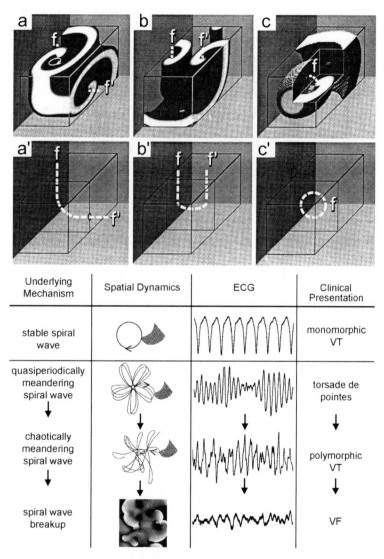

Fig. 8. Schematic representation of basic scroll-type reentry in three-dimensional and spiral wave phenotypes with their possible clinical manifestations. *Upper panel*: Basic configurations of vortex-like reentry in three dimensions: **a** and **a'**, L-shaped scroll wave and filament, respectively. The scroll rotates in a clockwise direction (*on the top*) about the L-shaped filament (**f, f'**) shown in (**a'**, **b**, and **b'**), U-shaped scroll wave and filament, respectively. **c** and **c'**, O-shaped wave and filament, respectively (from Ref *(128)* with permission). *Bottom panel*: Four types of spiral wave phenotypes and associated clinical manifestations. A stable spiral wave mechanism gives rise to monomorphic ventricular tachycardia (VT) on the ECG. A quasi-periodic meandering spiral wave is responsible for Torsade de Pointes, whereas a chaotically meandering spiral wave is revealed as polymorphic VT. A ventricular fibrillation (VF) pattern is caused by spiral wave breakup. Second column, spiral waves are shown in *gray*; the path of their tip is shown as *solid lines* (from Ref. *(129)* with permission).

wave is generally encountered following a wave break, a situation in which a planar wave encounters an obstacle and breaks up into two or more daughter waves. Because it has the greatest curvature, the broken end of the wave moves most slowly. As curvature decreases along the more distal parts of the spiral, propagation speed increases. Another difference between the leading circle and spiral wave is the state of the core; in former it is kept permanently refractory, whereas in the latter the core is excitable but not excited. The term spiral wave is usually used to describe reentrant activity in two dimensions. The center of the spiral wave is called the core and the distribution of the core in three dimensions is referred to as the filament (Fig. 8).

The functional reentrant mechanisms can underlie many forms of tachyarrhythmias in ischemic or /infarcted hearts *(102)* and in structurally normal ventricles, as in the short QT (Chapter 20), long QT (Chapter 19), and J wave syndromes (Chapter 21). While the leading circle and spiral wave models have some conceptual differences (discussed above), it is difficult to determine which of these is more likely to underlie a given functional reentrant arrhythmias in the heart. Spiral wave activity has been used to explain the electrocardiographic patterns observed during monomorphic and polymorphic cardiac arrhythmias as well as during fibrillation *(98, 103, 104)*. Monomorphic ventricular tachycardia (VT) results when the spiral wave is anchored and not able to drift within the ventricular myocardium. In contrast, a polymorphic VT and ventricular fibrillation (VF) such as that encountered with short QT, LQTS, and the J wave syndromes is due to a meandering or drifting spiral wave. Similarly, spiral waves are responsible for the development of atrial fibrillation (AF).

Reflection

Direct evidence in support of reflection as a mechanism of arrhythmogenesis was first provided by Antzelevitch and co-workers in the early 1980s *(105, 106)*. In a model with use of "ion-free" isotonic sucrose solution to create a narrow (1.5–2 mm) central inexcitable zone (gap) in unbranched Purkinje fibers (Fig. 9), stimulation of the proximal (P) segment elicits an action potential that propagates to the proximal border of the sucrose gap *(105)*. Active propagation across the sucrose gap is not possible because of the ion-depleted extracellular milieu, but local circuit current continues to flow through the intercellular low-resistance pathways (a Ag/AgCl extracellular shunt pathway is provided). This local circuit or electrotonic current, very much reduced upon emerging from the gap, gradually discharges the capacity of the distal (D) tissue thus giving rise to a depolarization that manifests as either a subthreshold response (last distal response) or a foot potential that brings the distal excitable tissue to its threshold potential.(Fig. 9b). Active impulse propagation stops and then resumes after a delay that can be as long as several hundred milliseconds. When anterograde (P to D) transmission time is sufficiently delayed to permit recovery of refractoriness at the proximal end, electrotonic transmission of the impulse in the retrograde direction is able to re-excite the proximal tissue, thus generating a closely coupled reflected reentry. Reflection therefore results from the to and fro electrotonically mediated transmission of the impulse across the same inexcitable segment; neither longitudinal dissociation nor circus movement need be invoked to explain the phenomenon.

Success or failure of reflection depends on the degree to which conduction is delayed in both directions across the functionally inexcitable zone. These transmission delays in turn depend on the width of the inexcitable segment, the intracellular and extracellular resistance to the flow of local circuit current across the inexcitable zone, and the excitability of the distal active site (sink). Because the excitability of cardiac tissues continues to recover for hundreds of milliseconds after an action potential, impulse transmission across the inexcitable zone is a sensitive function of frequency *(105, 107, 108)*. Because reflection can occur within areas of tissue of limited size (as small as 1–2 mm^2), it is likely to appear as focal in origin. Its identification as a mechanism of arrhythmia may be difficult even with very high spatial resolution mapping of the electrical activity of discrete sites. The delineation of delayed impulse conduction mechanisms at discrete sites generally requires the use of intracellular microelectrode techniques in conjunction with high-resolution extracellular mapping techniques.

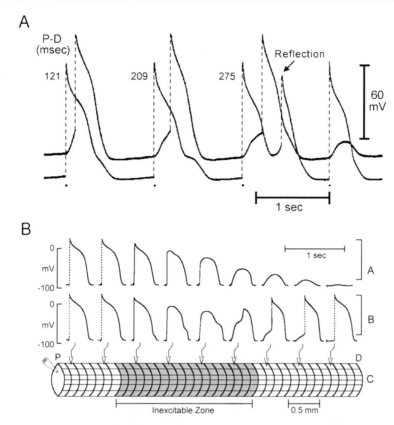

Fig. 9. (a) Delayed transmission and reflection across an inexcitable gap created by superfusion of the central segment of a Purkinje fiber with an "ion-free" isotonic sucrose solution. The two traces were recorded from proximal (P) and distal (D) active segments. P–D conduction time (indicated in the *upper* portion of the figure, in msec) increased progressively with a 4:3 Wenckebach periodicity. The third stimulated proximal response was followed by a reflection (from Antzelevitch *(130)*, with permission). **(b)** Discontinuous conduction (B) and conduction block (A) in a Purkinje strand with a central inexcitable zone (C). The schematic illustration is based on transmembrane recordings obtained from canine Purkinje fiber-sucrose gap preparations. An action potential elicited by stimulation of the proximal (P) side of the preparation conducts normally up to the border of the inexcitable zone. Active propagation of the impulse stops at this point, but local circuit current generated by the proximal segment continues to flow through the preparation encountering a cumulative resistance (successive gap junctions). Transmembrane recordings from the first few inexcitable cells show a response not very different from the action potentials recorded in the neighboring excitable cells, in spite of the fact that no ions may be moving across the membrane of these cells. The responses recorded in the inexcitable region are the electrotonic images of activity generated in the proximal excitable segment. The resistive–capacitive properties of the tissue lead to an exponential decline in the amplitude of the transmembrane potential recorded along the length of the inexcitable segment and to a slowing of the rate of change of voltage as a function of time. If, as in panel b, the electrotonic current is sufficient to bring the distal excitable tissue to its threshold potential, an action potential is generated after a step delay imposed by the slow discharge of the capacity of the distal (D) membrane by the electrotonic current (foot-potential). Active conduction of the impulse therefore stops at the proximal border of the inexcitable zone and resumes at the distal border after a step delay that may range from a few to tens or hundreds of milliseconds. Modified from Ref. *(131)* with permission.

These limitations considered, reflection has been suggested as the mechanism underlying reentrant extrasystolic activity in ventricular tissues excised from a one-day-old infarcted canine heart *(109)* and in a clinical case of incessant ventricular bigeminy in a young patient with no evidence of organic heart disease *(110)*.

Phase 2 Reentry

Another reentrant mechanism that can appear to be of focal origin is phase 2 reentry. Phase 2 reentry occurs when the I_{to}-mediated dome of the action potential, most commonly in the epicardium, propagates from sites at which it is maintained to sites at which it is abolished, causing local re-excitation of the epicardium and the generation of a closely coupled extrasystole. The closely coupled extrasystole via Phase 2 reentry can serve as a trigger to initiate polymorphic VT and VF (Fig. 10). Phase 2 reentry is a key mechanism responsible for arrhythmogenesis in J wave syndromes *(111)* and is discussed in more detail in Chapter 21.

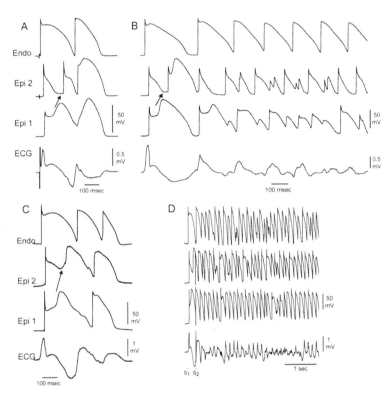

Fig. 10. Spontaneous and programmed electrical stimulation-induced polymorphic VT in RV wedge preparations pretreated with terfenadine (5–10 μM). (**a**) Phase 2 reentry in epicardium gives rise to a closely coupled extrasystole. (**b**) Phase 2 reentrant extrasystole triggers a brief episode of polymorphic VT. (**c**) Phase 2 reentry followed by a single circus movement reentry in epicardium gives rise to a couplet. (**d**) Extrastimulus (S1–S2 = 250 msec) applied to epicardium triggers a polymorphic VT (modified from Ref. *(132)*, with permission).

Reentry due to Spatial Dispersion of Repolarization

Studies conducted overt the past 15 years have established that ventricular myocardium is not homogeneous, as previously thought, but is comprised of at least three electrophysiologically and functionally distinct cell types: epicardial, M, and endocardial cells *(112, 113)*. These three principal ventricular myocardial cell types differ with respect to phase 1 and phase 3 repolarization characteristics (Fig. 11). Ventricular epicardial and M, but not endocardial, cells generally display a prominent phase 1, due to a large 4-aminopyridine (4-AP)-sensitive transient outward current (I_{to}), giving the action potential a spike and dome or notched configuration. Differences in the magnitude of the action potential notch and corresponding differences in I_{to} have also been described between right and left

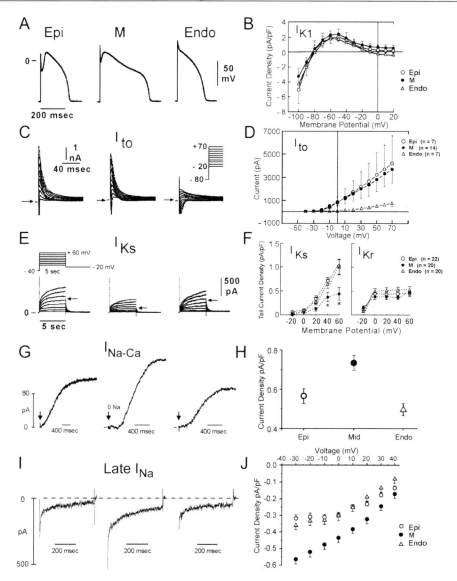

Fig. 11. Ionic distinctions among epicardial, M, and endocardial cells. (**a**) Action potentials recorded from myocytes isolated from the epicardial, endocardial, and M regions of the canine left ventricle. (**b**) I–V relations for I_{K1} in epicardial, endocardial, and M region myocytes. Values are mean ± S.D. (**c**) Transient outward current (I_{to}) recorded from the three cell types (current traces recorded during depolarizing steps from a holding potential of –80 mV to test potentials ranging between –20 and +70 mV (**d**) The average peak current–voltage relationship for I_{to} for each of the three cell types. Values are mean ± S.D. (**e**) Voltage-dependent activation of the slowly activating component of the delayed rectifier K^+ current (I_{Ks}) (currents were elicited by the voltage pulse protocol shown in the inset; Na^+-, K^+-, and Ca^{2+}-free solution). (**f**) Voltage dependence of I_{Ks} (current remaining after exposure to E-4031) and I_{Kr} (E-4031-sensitive current). Values are mean ± S.E. *$p < 0.05$ compared with Epi or Endo (from Refs. *(48, 117, 133)* with permission). (**g**) Reverse-mode sodium–calcium exchange currents recorded in potassium- and chloride-free solutions at a voltage of –80 mV. $I_{Na–Ca}$ was maximally activated by switching to sodium-free external solution at the time indicated by the *arrow*. (**h**) Midmyocardial sodium–calcium exchanger density is 30% greater than endocardial density, calculated as the peak outward $I_{Na–Ca}$ normalized by cell capacitance. Endocardial and epicardial densities were not significantly different. (**i**) TTX-sensitive late sodium current. Cells were held at –80 mV and briefly pulsed to –45 mV to inactivate fast sodium current before stepping to –10 mV. (**j**) Normalized late sodium current measured 300 msec into the test pulse was plotted as a function of test pulse potential (modified from Ref. *(117)* with permission).

ventricular epicardium *(114)*. Similar interventricular differences in I_{to} have also been described for canine ventricular M cells *(115)*.

Between the surface epicardial and endocardial layers are transitional and M cells. M cells are distinguished by the ability of their action potential to prolong disproportionately relative to the action potential of other ventricular myocardial cells in response to a slowing of rate and/or in response to action potential duration (APD)-prolonging agents *(47, 112)*. In the dog, the ionic basis for these features of the M cell includes the presence of a smaller slowly activating delayed rectifier current (I_{Ks}) *(48)*, a larger late sodium current (late I_{Na}) *(116)*, and a larger Na–Ca exchange current (I_{Na-Ca}) *(117)*. In the canine heart, the rapidly activating delayed rectifier (I_{Kr}) and inward rectifier (I_{K1}) currents are similar in the three transmural cell types. Histologically M cells are similar to epicardial and endocardial cells. Electrophysiologically and pharmacologically, they appear to be a hybrid between Purkinje and ventricular cells. Like Purkinje fibers, M cells show a prominent APD prolongation and develop early afterdepolarizations (EAD) in response to I_{Kr} blockers, whereas epicardium and endocardium do not. Like Purkinje fibers, M cells develop delayed afterdepolarizations (DAD) in response to agents that calcium load or overload the cardiac cell; epicardium and endocardium do not.

Distribution of M cells within the ventricular wall has been investigated in greatest detail in the left ventricle of the canine heart. Although transitional cells are found throughout the wall in the canine left ventricle, M cells displaying the longest action potentials (at BCLs $\geq$ 2000 msec) are often localized in the deep subendocardium to midmyocardium in the anterior wall *(118)* and throughout the wall in the region of the right ventricular (RV) outflow tracts *(113)*. M cells are also present in the deep cell layers of endocardial structures, including papillary muscles, trabeculae, and the interventricular septum *(119)*. Unlike Purkinje fibers, M cells are not found in discrete bundles or islets *(119, 120)*, although there is evidence that they may be localized in discrete muscle layers. Cells with the characteristics of M cells have been described in the canine, guinea pig, pig, and human ventricles *(113)*. Amplification of pre-existed transmural dispersion of repolarization may serve as a reentrant substrate for functional reentry. In the temporal window when some cells have completed their repolarization while others are still in their repolarization phases 2 and 3, any trigger that occurs within this window can potentially initiate functional reentry, leading to polymorphic VT or VF.

Repolarization of M cells and its interaction with that of the epicardial and endocardial layers contribute important to the genesis of T wave and determine QT interval under physiological conditions *(10, 118)*. On the ECG, the time interval from the T wave peak to the end (T_{p-e}) has been shown to provide an index of transmural dispersion of repolarization *(10, 42, 113, 121)*. The available data suggest that T_{p-e} measurements are generally limited to precordial leads (V1–V6) since these leads more accurately reflect transmural dispersion of repolarization. While the clinical applicability of these concepts remains to be carefully validated, significant progress toward validation of the T_{p-e} interval as an index of transmural dispersion has been achieved. Lubinski et al. *(122)* demonstrated that this interval is increased in patients with congenital long QT syndrome. Recent studies suggest that the T_{p-e} interval may be a useful index of transmural dispersion and thus may be prognostic of arrhythmic risk under a variety of conditions *(123–126)*.

It also appears that T_{p-e} interval is proportional to QT interval under physiological conditions across a variety of species *(10)*. In other words, the ratio of T_{p-e}/QT remains relatively constant among different species despite the fact that their QTc intervals are significantly different. In addition, the T_{p-e}/QT also remains relatively constant in physiological heart rates in normal human individuals *(121)*. In drug-induced QT prolongation, the T_{p-e}/QT increases markedly prior to the onset of Torsade de Pointes *(42, 127)*. Amplification of transmural heterogeneities is observed in a variety of arrhythmias associated with channelopathies, including J wave syndromes (Chapter 21), long QT syndrome (Chapter 19) and short QT syndrome (Chapter 20) as well as catecholaminergic VT. Interestingly, the T_{p-e}/QT is increased in these arrhythmias (Fig. 12) *(121)*.

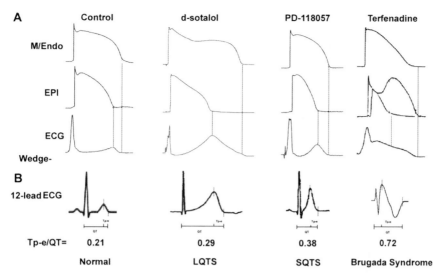

Fig. 12. Recordings from experiments involving canine left ventricular wedge preparations demonstrating cellular basis of ECG phenotype in long QT syndrome (LQTS), short QT syndrome (SQTS), and Brugada syndrome. In LQTS, preferential prolongation of action potential of M cells leads to amplification of T_{p-e} interval (TDR at cellular level). In SQTS, preferential abbreviation of epicardium leads to amplification of T_{p-e} interval. In case of Brugada syndrome, all or none repolarization in epicardium at the end of phase 1 leads to increase in T_{p-e} interval. (**b**) Body surface ECG of the patients with corresponding disease closely resembles the pseudo-ECG. Epi, Epicardium; M, M cell; Endo, Endocardium; LQTS, long QT syndrome; SQTS, short QT syndrome. Note that the time scale of the figure is not absolutely correct due to reproduction from multiple references and use of different experiments (modified and reproduced with permission from references *(134–136)*.

REFERENCES

1. Mines GR (1914) Further experiments on the action of the vagus on the electrogram of the frog's heart. J Physiol 47(6):419–430
2. Moe GK (1975) Evidence for reentry as a mechanism of cardiac arrhythmias. Rev Physiol Biochem Pharmacol 72: 55–81
3. Hoffman BF, Dangman KH (1987) Mechanisms for cardiac arrhythmias. Experientia 43(10):1049–1056
4. Lazzara R (1988) Electrophysiological mechanisms for ventricular arrhythmias. Clin Cardiol 11(3 Suppl 2):II1–II4
5. Lukas A, Antzelevitch C (1996) Phase 2 reentry as a mechanism of initiation of circus movement reentry in canine epicardium exposed to simulated ischemia. Cardiovasc Res 32(3):593–603
6. Yan GX, Antzelevitch C (1999) Cellular basis for the Brugada syndrome and other mechanisms of arrhythmogenesis associated with ST-segment elevation. Circulation 100(15):1660–1666
7. Antzelevitch C (2005) In vivo human demonstration of phase 2 reentry. Heart Rhythm 2(8):804–806
8. Yan GX, Joshi A, Guo D, Hlaing T, Martin J, Xu X et al (2004) Phase 2 reentry as a trigger to initiate ventricular fibrillation during early acute myocardial ischemia. Circulation 110(9):1036–1041
9. Jalife J (2003) Rotors and spiral waves in atrial fibrillation. J Cardiovasc Electrophysiol 14(7):776–780
10. Guo D, Zhou J, Zhao X, Gupta P, Kowey PR, Martin J et al (2008) L-type calcium current recovery versus ventricular repolarization: preserved membrane-stabilizing mechanism for different QT intervals across species. Heart Rhythm 5(2):271–279
11. Burashnikov A, Antzelevitch C (2003) Reinduction of atrial fibrillation immediately after termination of the arrhythmia is mediated by late phase 3 early afterdepolarization-induced triggered activity. Circulation 107(18):2355–2360
12. Burashnikov A, Antzelevitch C (2006) Late-phase 3 EAD. A unique mechanism contributing to initiation of atrial fibrillation. Pacing Clin Electrophysiol 29(3):290–295
13. Patterson E, Lazzara R, Szabo B, Liu H, Tang D, Li YH et al (2006) Sodium-calcium exchange initiated by the Ca^{2+} transient: an arrhythmia trigger within pulmonary veins. J Am Coll Cardiol 47(6):1196–1206
14. Vassalle M (1977) Cardiac automaticity and its control. Am J Physiol 233(6):H625–H634
15. Glitsch HG (1979) Characteristics of active Na transport in intact cardiac cells. Am J Physiol 236(2):H189–H199

16. Gadsby DC, Cranefield PF (1979) Direct measurement of changes in sodium pump current in canine cardiac Purkinje fibers. Proc Natl Acad Sci USA 76(4):1783–1787

17. DiFrancesco D (1985) The cardiac hyperpolarizing-activated current, if. Origins and developments. Prog Biophys Mol Biol 46(3):163–183

18. DiFrancesco D (1995) The pacemaker current (I(f)) plays an important role in regulating SA node pacemaker activity. Cardiovasc Res 30(2):307–308

19. Satoh H, Hashimoto K (1984) Effect of 3, 4-dihydro-6-[4-(3,4-dimethoxybenzoyl)-1-piperazinyl]-2(1H)-qu inolinone (OPC-8212) on the membrane currents of rabbit sino-atrial node cells. Arzneimittelforschung 34(3A):376–380

20. Vassalle M, Yu H, Cohen IS (1995) The pacemaker current in cardiac Purkinje myocytes. J Gen Physiol 106(3): 559–578

21. Soejima M, Noma A (1984) Mode of regulation of the ACh-sensitive K-channel by the muscarinic receptor in rabbit atrial cells. Pflugers Arch 400(4):424–431

22. DiFrancesco D, Tromba C (1988) Inhibition of the hyperpolarization-activated current (if) induced by acetylcholine in rabbit sino-atrial node myocytes. J Physiol 405:477–491

23. Katzung BG, Hondeghem LM, Grant AO (1975) Letter: cardiac ventricular automaticity induced by current of injury. Pflugers Arch 360(2):193–197

24. Janse MJ, Wilms-Schopman F (1982) Effect of changes in perfusion pressure on the position of the electrophysiologic border zone in acute regional ischemia in isolated perfused dog and pig hearts. Am J Cardiol 50(1):74–82

25. Winum PF, Cayla G, Rubini M, Beck L, Messner-Pellenc P (2009) A case of cardiomyopathy induced by inappropriate sinus tachycardia and cured by ivabradine. Pacing Clin Electrophysiol 32(7):942–944

26. Vermeulen JT, McGuire MA, Opthof T, Coronel R, de Bakker JM, Klopping C et al (1994) Triggered activity and automaticity in ventricular trabeculae of failing human and rabbit hearts. Cardiovasc Res 28(10):1547–1554

27. Nuss HB, Kaab S, Kass DA, Tomaselli GF, Marban E (1999) Cellular basis of ventricular arrhythmias and abnormal automaticity in heart failure. Am J Physiol 277(1 Pt 2):H80–H91

28. Hoppe UC, Jansen E, Sudkamp M, Beuckelmann DJ (1998) Hyperpolarization-activated inward current in ventricular myocytes from normal and failing human hearts. Circulation 97(1):55–65

29. Cerbai E, Barbieri M, Mugelli A (1996) Occurrence and properties of the hyperpolarization-activated current If in ventricular myocytes from normotensive and hypertensive rats during aging. Circulation 94(7):1674–1681

30. Hauswirth O, Noble D, Tsien RW (1969) The mechanism of oscillatory activity at low membrane potentials in cardiac Purkinje fibres. J Physiol 200(1):255–265

31. Imanishi S, Surawicz B (1976) Automatic activity in depolarized guinea pig ventricular myocardium. Characteristics and mechanisms. Circ Res 39(6):751–759

32. Dangman KH, Hoffman BF (1983) Antiarrhythmic effects of ethmozin in cardiac Purkinje fibers: suppression of automaticity and abolition of triggering. J Pharmacol Exp Ther 227(3):578–586

33. Rota M, Vassalle M (2003) Patch-clamp analysis in canine cardiac Purkinje cells of a novel sodium component in the pacemaker range. J Physiol 548(Pt 1):147–165

34. Katzung BG, Morgenstern JA (1977) Effects of extracellular potassium on ventricular automaticity and evidence for a pacemaker current in mammalian ventricular myocardium. Circ Res 40(1):105–111

35. Pappano AJ, Carmeliet EE (1979) Epinephrine and the pacemaking mechanism at plateau potentials in sheep cardiac Purkinje fibers. Pflugers Arch 382(1):17–26

36. Haissaguerre M, Jais P, Shah DC, Takahashi A, Hocini M, Quiniou G et al (1998) Spontaneous initiation of atrial fibrillation by ectopic beats originating in the pulmonary veins. N Engl J Med 339(10):659–666

37. Lai LP, Su MJ, Lin JL, Tsai CH, Lin FY, Chen YS et al (1999) Measurement of funny current (I(f)) channel mRNA in human atrial tissue: correlation with left atrial filling pressure and atrial fibrillation. J Cardiovasc Electrophysiol 10(7):947–953

38. Yan GX, Wu Y, Liu T, Wang J, Marinchak RA, Kowey PR (2001) Phase 2 early afterdepolarization as a trigger of polymorphic ventricular tachycardia in acquired long-QT syndrome : direct evidence from intracellular recordings in the intact left ventricular wall. Circulation 103(23):2851–2856

39. Adamantidis MM, Caron JF, Dupuis BA (1986) Triggered activity induced by combined mild hypoxia and acidosis in guinea-pig Purkinje fibers. J Mol Cell Cardiol 18(12):1287–1299

40. Priori SG, Corr PB (1990) Mechanisms underlying early and delayed afterdepolarizations induced by catecholamines. Am J Physiol 258(6 Pt 2):H1796–H1805

41. Volders PG, Kulcsar A, Vos MA, Sipido KR, Wellens HJ, Lazzara R et al (1997) Similarities between early and delayed afterdepolarizations induced by isoproterenol in canine ventricular myocytes. Cardiovasc Res 34(2): 348–359

42. Liu T, Brown BS, Wu Y, Antzelevitch C, Kowey PR, Yan GX (2006) Blinded validation of the isolated arterially perfused rabbit ventricular wedge in preclinical assessment of drug-induced proarrhythmias. Heart Rhythm 3(8): 948–956

43. Volders PG, Sipido KR, Vos MA, Kulcsar A, Verduyn SC, Wellens HJ (1998) Cellular basis of biventricular hypertrophy and arrhythmogenesis in dogs with chronic complete atrioventricular block and acquired Torsade de Pointes. Circulation 98(11):1136–1147

44. Yan GX, Rials SJ, Wu Y, Liu T, Xu X, Marinchak RA et al (2001) Ventricular hypertrophy amplifies transmural repolarization dispersion and induces early afterdepolarization. Am J Physiol Heart Circ Physiol 281(5):H1968–H1975

45. Roden DM (1986) Pharmacologic information required for design of programmed electrical stimulation protocols. Circulation 73(2 Pt 2):II39–II44

46. Davidenko JM, Cohen L, Goodrow R, Antzelevitch C (1989) Quinidine-induced action potential prolongation, early afterdepolarizations, and triggered activity in canine Purkinje fibers. Effects of stimulation rate, potassium, and magnesium. Circulation 79(3):674–686

47. Sicouri S, Antzelevitch C (1991) Afterdepolarizations and triggered activity develop in a select population of cells (M cells) in canine ventricular myocardium: the effects of acetylstrophanthidin and Bay K 8644. Pacing Clin Electrophysiol 14(11 Pt 2):1714–1720

48. Liu DW, Antzelevitch C (1995) Characteristics of the delayed rectifier current (IKr and IKs) in canine ventricular epicardial, midmyocardial, and endocardial myocytes. A weaker IKs contributes to the longer action potential of the M cell. Circ Res 76(3):351–365

49. Burashnikov A, Antzelevitch C (2002) Prominent I(Ks) in epicardium and endocardium contributes to development of transmural dispersion of repolarization but protects against development of early afterdepolarizations. J Cardiovasc Electrophysiol 13(2):172–177

50. Yan GX, Rials SJ, Wu Y, Liu T, Xu X, Marinchak RA et al (2001) Ventricular hypertrophy amplifies transmural repolarization dispersion and induces early afterdepolarization. Am J Physiol Heart Circ Physiol 281(5):H1968–H1975

51. Xu X, Rials SJ, Wu Y, Salata JJ, Liu T, Bharucha DB et al (2001) Left ventricular hypertrophy decreases slowly but not rapidly activating delayed rectifier potassium currents of epicardial and endocardial myocytes in rabbits. Circulation 103(11):1585–1590

52. Valdivia CR, Chu WW, Pu J, Foell JD, Haworth RA, Wolff MR et al (2005) Increased late sodium current in myocytes from a canine heart failure model and from failing human heart. J Mol Cell Cardiol 38(3):475–483

53. Belardinelli L, Antzelevitch C, Vos MA (2003) Assessing predictors of drug-induced Torsade de Pointes. Trends Pharmacol Sci 24(12):619–625

54. Lankipalli RS, Zhu T, Guo D, Yan GX (2005) Mechanisms underlying arrhythmogenesis in long QT syndrome. J Electrocardiol 38(4 Suppl):69–73

55. Viswanathan PC, Rudy Y (1999) Pause induced early afterdepolarizations in the long QT syndrome: a simulation study. Cardiovasc Res 42(2):530–542

56. Guo D, Zhao X, Wu Y, Liu T, Kowey PR, Yan GX (2007) L-type calcium current reactivation contributes to arrhythmogenesis associated with action potential triangulation. J Cardiovasc Electrophysiol 18(2):196–203

57. Hondeghem LM, Lu HR, van Rossem K, De Clerck F (2003) Detection of proarrhythmia in the female rabbit heart: blinded validation. J Cardiovasc Electrophysiol 14(3):287–294

58. Antzelevitch C, Sun ZQ, Zhang ZQ, Yan GX (1996) Cellular and ionic mechanisms underlying erythromycin-induced long QT intervals and Torsade de Pointes. J Am Coll Cardiol 28(7):1836–1848

59. Antzelevitch C, Belardinelli L (2006) The role of sodium channel current in modulating transmural dispersion of repolarization and arrhythmogenesis. J Cardiovasc Electrophysiol 17(Suppl 1):S79–S85

60. Kass RS, Tsien RW, Weingart R (1978) Ionic basis of transient inward current induced by strophanthidin in cardiac Purkinje fibres. J Physiol 281:209–226

61. Cannell MB, Lederer WJ (1986) The arrhythmogenic current ITI in the absence of electrogenic sodium-calcium exchange in sheep cardiac Purkinje fibres. J Physiol 374:201–219

62. Fedida D, Noble D, Shimoni Y, Spindler AJ (1987) Inward current related to contraction in guinea-pig ventricular myocytes. J Physiol 385:565–589

63. Laflamme MA, Becker PL (1996) Ca^{2+}-induced current oscillations in rabbit ventricular myocytes. Circ Res 78(4):707–716

64. Zygmunt AC, Goodrow RJ, Weigel CM (1998) INaCa and ICl(Ca) contribute to isoproterenol-induced delayed after depolarizations in midmyocardial cells. Am J Physiol 275(6 Pt 2):H1979–H1992

65. Aronson RS (1981) Afterpotentials and triggered activity in hypertrophied myocardium from rats with renal hypertension. Circ Res 48(5):720–727

66. Lazzara R, el Sherif N, Scherlag BJ (1973) Electrophysiological properties of canine Purkinje cells in one-day-old myocardial infarction. Circ Res 33(6):722–734

67. Pogwizd SM, Onufer JR, Kramer JB, Sobel BE, Corr PB (1986) Induction of delayed afterdepolarizations and triggered activity in canine Purkinje fibers by lysophosphoglycerides. Circ Res 59(4):416–426

68. Song Y, Belardinelli L (1994) ATP promotes development of afterdepolarizations and triggered activity in cardiac myocytes. Am J Physiol 267(5 Pt 2):H2005–H2011

69. Caroni P, Villani F, Carafoli E (1981) The cardiotoxic antibiotic doxorubicin inhibits the Na^+/Ca^{2+} exchange of dog heart sarcolemmal vesicles. FEBS Lett 130(2):184–186

70. Spinelli W, Sorota S, Siegal M, Hoffman BF (1991) Antiarrhythmic actions of the ATP-regulated K^+ current activated by pinacidil. Circ Res 68(4):1127–1137

71. So HS, Park C, Kim HJ, Lee JH, Park SY, Lee JH et al (2005) Protective effect of T-type calcium channel blocker flunarizine on cisplatin-induced death of auditory cells. Hear Res 204(1–2):127–139

72. Chattipakorn N, Ideker RE (2003) Delayed afterdepolarization inhibitor: a potential pharmacologic intervention to improve defibrillation efficacy. J Cardiovasc Electrophysiol 14(1):72–75

73. Letienne R, Vie B, Puech A, Vieu S, Le Grand B, John GW (2001) Evidence that ranolazine behaves as a weak beta1- and beta2-adrenoceptor antagonist in the cat cardiovascular system. Naunyn Schmiedebergs Arch Pharmacol 363(4):464–471

74. Antzelevitch C, Belardinelli L, Zygmunt AC, Burashnikov A, Di Diego JM, Fish JM et al (2004) Electrophysiological effects of ranolazine, a novel antianginal agent with antiarrhythmic properties. Circulation 110(8):904–910

75. Song Y, Shryock JC, Wu L, Belardinelli L (2004) Antagonism by ranolazine of the pro-arrhythmic effects of increasing late INa in guinea pig ventricular myocytes. J Cardiovasc Pharmacol 44(2):192–199

76. Ritchie AH, Kerr CR, Qi A, Yeung-Lai-Wah JA (1989) Nonsustained ventricular tachycardia arising from the right ventricular outflow tract. Am J Cardiol 64(10):594–598

77. Wilber DJ, Davis MJ, Rosenbaum M, Ruskin JN, Garan H (1987) Incidence and determinants of multiple morphologically distinct sustained ventricular tachycardias. J Am Coll Cardiol 10(3):583–591

78. Cardinal R, Scherlag BJ, Vermeulen M, Armour JA (1992) Distinct activation patterns of idioventricular rhythms and sympathetically-induced ventricular tachycardias in dogs with atrioventricular block. Pacing Clin Electrophysiol 15(9):1300–1316

79. Lerman BB, Belardinelli L, West GA, Berne RM, DiMarco JP (1986) Adenosine-sensitive ventricular tachycardia: evidence suggesting cyclic AMP-mediated triggered activity. Circulation 74(2):270–280

80. Lerman BB, Stein K, Engelstein ED, Battleman DS, Lippman N, Bei D et al (1995) Mechanism of repetitive monomorphic ventricular tachycardia. Circulation 92(3):421–429

81. Pogwizd SM, McKenzie JP, Cain ME (1998) Mechanisms underlying spontaneous and induced ventricular arrhythmias in patients with idiopathic dilated cardiomyopathy. Circulation 98(22):2404–2414

82. Leenhardt A, Thomas O, Cauchemez B, Maison-Blanche P, Denjoy I, de Jode P et al (1995) Value of the exercise test in the study of arrhythmia. Arch Mal Coeur Vaiss 88(Spec No 1):59–66

83. Swan H, Piippo K, Viitasalo M, Heikkila P, Paavonen T, Kainulainen K et al (1999) Arrhythmic disorder mapped to chromosome 1q42–q43 causes malignant polymorphic ventricular tachycardia in structurally normal hearts. J Am Coll Cardiol 34(7):2035–2042

84. Priori SG, Napolitano C (2002) Genetic defects of cardiac ion channels. The hidden substrate for Torsades de Pointes. Cardiovasc Drugs Ther 16(2):89–92

85. Priori SG, Napolitano C, Tiso N, Memmi M, Vignati G, Bloise R et al (2001) Mutations in the cardiac ryanodine receptor gene (hRyR2) underlie catecholaminergic polymorphic ventricular tachycardia. Circulation 103(2):196–200

86. Laitinen PJ, Brown KM, Piippo K, Swan H, Devaney JM, Brahmbhatt B et al (2001) Mutations of the cardiac ryanodine receptor (RyR2) gene in familial polymorphic ventricular tachycardia. Circulation 103(4):485–490

87. Nam GB, Burashnikov A, Antzelevitch C (2005) Cellular mechanisms underlying the development of catecholaminergic ventricular tachycardia. Circulation 111(21):2727–2733

88. Volders PG, Vos MA, Szabo B, Sipido KR, de Groot SH, Gorgels AP et al (2000) Progress in the understanding of cardiac early afterdepolarizations and Torsades de Pointes: time to revise current concepts. Cardiovasc Res 46(3):376–392

89. Patterson E, Po SS, Scherlag BJ, Lazzara R (2005) Triggered firing in pulmonary veins initiated by in vitro autonomic nerve stimulation. Heart Rhythm 2(6):624–631

90. Kirchhof P, Klimas J, Fabritz L, Zwiener M, Jones LR, Schafers M et al (2007) Stress and high heart rate provoke ventricular tachycardia in mice expressing triadin. J Mol Cell Cardiol 42(5):962–971

91. Schmitt FO, Erlanger J (1928) directional differences in the conduction of the impulse through heart muscle and their possible relation to extrasystolic and fibrillary contractions. Am J Physiol 87:326–341

92. Spach MS (1999) Anisotropy of cardiac tissue: a major determinant of conduction? J Cardiovasc Electrophysiol 10(6):887–890

93. Allessie MA, Bonke FI, Schopman FJ (1976) Circus movement in rabbit atrial muscle as a mechanism of tachycardia. II. The role of nonuniform recovery of excitability in the occurrence of unidirectional block, as studied with multiple microelectrodes. Circ Res 39(2):168–177

94. Allessie MA, Bonke FI, Schopman FJ (1977) Circus movement in rabbit atrial muscle as a mechanism of tachycardia. III. The "leading circle" concept: a new model of circus movement in cardiac tissue without the involvement of an anatomical obstacle. Circ Res 41(1):9–18

95. el Sherif N (1988) Reentry revisited. Pacing Clin Electrophysiol 11(9):1358–1368
96. Lin SF, Roth BJ, Wikswo JP Jr (1999) Quatrefoil reentry in myocardium: an optical imaging study of the induction mechanism. J Cardiovasc Electrophysiol 10(4):574–586
97. Davidenko JM, Kent PF, Chialvo DR, Michaels DC, Jalife J (1990) Sustained vortex-like waves in normal isolated ventricular muscle. Proc Natl Acad Sci USA 87(22):8785–8789
98. Pertsov AM, Davidenko JM, Salomonsz R, Baxter WT, Jalife J (1993) Spiral waves of excitation underlie reentrant activity in isolated cardiac muscle. Circ Res 72(3):631–650
99. Anumonwo JM, Delmar M, Vinet A, Michaels DC, Jalife J (1991) Phase resetting and entrainment of pacemaker activity in single sinus nodal cells. Circ Res 68(4):1138–1153
100. Athill CA, Ikeda T, Kim YH, Wu TJ, Fishbein MC, Karagueuzian HS et al (1998) Transmembrane potential properties at the core of functional reentrant wave fronts in isolated canine right atria. Circulation 98(15):1556–1567
101. Vaidya D, Morley GE, Samie FH, Jalife J (1999) Reentry and fibrillation in the mouse heart. A challenge to the critical mass hypothesis. Circ Res 85(2):174–181
102. Waldecker B, Coromilas J, Saltman AE, Dillon SM, Wit AL (1993) Overdrive stimulation of functional reentrant circuits causing ventricular tachycardia in the infarcted canine heart. Resetting and entrainment. Circulation 87(4): 1286–1305
103. Davidenko JM (1993) Spiral wave activity: a possible common mechanism for polymorphic and monomorphic ventricular tachycardias. J Cardiovasc Electrophysiol 4(6):730–746
104. Qu Z, Weiss JN, Garfinkel A (1999) Cardiac electrical restitution properties and stability of reentrant spiral waves: a simulation study. Am J Physiol 276(1 Pt 2):H269–H283
105. Antzelevitch C, Jalife J, Moe GK (1980) Characteristics of reflection as a mechanism of reentrant arrhythmias and its relationship to parasystole. Circulation 61(1):182–191
106. Antzelevitch C, Moe GK (1981) Electrotonically mediated delayed conduction and reentry in relation to "slow responses" in mammalian ventricular conducting tissue. Circ Res 49(5):1129–1139
107. Antzelevitch C, Bernstein MJ, Feldman HN, Moe GK (1983) Parasystole, reentry, and tachycardia: a canine preparation of cardiac arrhythmias occurring across inexcitable segments of tissue. Circulation 68(5):1101–1115
108. Delmar M, Michaels DC, Jalife J (1989) Slow recovery of excitability and the Wenckebach phenomenon in the single guinea pig ventricular myocyte. Circ Res 65(3):761–774
109. Rosenthal JE (1988) Reflected reentry in depolarized foci with variable conduction impairment in 1 day old infarcted canine cardiac tissue. J Am Coll Cardiol 12(2):404–411
110. Van Hemel NM, Swenne CA, de Bakker JM, Defauw JJ, Guiraudon GM (1988) Epicardial reflection as a cause of incessant ventricular bigeminy. Pacing Clin Electrophysiol 11(7):1036–1044
111. Antzelevitch C, Yan GX (2010) J Wave Syndromes. Heart Rhythm 7(4):549–558
112. Antzelevitch C, Sicouri S, Litovsky SH, Lukas A, Krishnan SC, Di Diego JM et al (1991) Heterogeneity within the ventricular wall. Electrophysiology and pharmacology of epicardial, endocardial, and M cells. Circ Res 69(6): 1427–1449
113. Antzelevitch C, Shimizu W, Yan GX, Sicouri S, Weissenburger J, Nesterenko VV et al (1999) The M cell: its contribution to the ECG and to normal and abnormal electrical function of the heart. J Cardiovasc Electrophysiol 10(8): 1124–1152
114. Di Diego JM, Sun ZQ, Antzelevitch C (1996) I(to) and action potential notch are smaller in left vs. right canine ventricular epicardium. Am J Physiol 271(2 Pt 2):H548–H561
115. Volders PG, Sipido KR, Vos MA, Spatjens RL, Leunissen JD, Carmeliet E et al (1999) Downregulation of delayed rectifier K(+) currents in dogs with chronic complete atrioventricular block and acquired Torsades de Pointes. Circulation 100(24):2455–2461
116. Zygmunt AC, Eddlestone GT, Thomas GP, Nesterenko VV, Antzelevitch C (2001) Larger late sodium conductance in M cells contributes to electrical heterogeneity in canine ventricle. Am J Physiol Heart Circ Physiol 281(2): H689–H697
117. Zygmunt AC, Goodrow RJ, Antzelevitch C (2000) I(NaCa) contributes to electrical heterogeneity within the canine ventricle. Am J Physiol Heart Circ Physiol 278(5):H1671–H1678
118. Yan GX, Shimizu W, Antzelevitch C (1998) Characteristics and distribution of M cells in arterially perfused canine left ventricular wedge preparations. Circulation 98(18):1921–1927
119. Sicouri S, Antzelevitch C (1993) Drug-induced afterdepolarizations and triggered activity occur in a discrete subpopulation of ventricular muscle cells (M cells) in the canine heart: quinidine and digitalis. J Cardiovasc Electrophysiol 4(1):48–58
120. Sicouri S, Fish J, Antzelevitch C (1994) Distribution of M cells in the canine ventricle. J Cardiovasc Electrophysiol 5(10):824–837
121. Gupta P, Patel C, Patel H, Narayanaswamy S, Malhotra B, Green JT et al (2008) T(p-e)/QT ratio as an index of arrhythmogenesis. J Electrocardiol 41(6):567–574

122. Lubinski A, Lewicka-Nowak E, Kempa M, Baczynska AM, Romanowska I, Swiatecka G (1998) New insight into repolarization abnormalities in patients with congenital long QT syndrome: the increased transmural dispersion of repolarization. Pacing Clin Electrophysiol 21(1 Pt 2):172–175

123. Wolk R, Mazurek T, Lusawa T, Wasek W, Rezler J (2001) Left ventricular hypertrophy increases transepicardial dispersion of repolarisation in hypertensive patients: a differential effect on QTpeak and QTend dispersion. Eur J Clin Invest 31(7):563–569

124. Tanabe Y, Inagaki M, Kurita T, Nagaya N, Taguchi A, Suyama K et al (2001) Sympathetic stimulation produces a greater increase in both transmural and spatial dispersion of repolarization in LQT1 than LQT2 forms of congenital long QT syndrome. J Am Coll Cardiol 37(3):911–919

125. Yamaguchi M, Shimizu M, Ino H, Terai H, Uchiyama K, Oe K et al (2003) T wave peak-to-end interval and QT dispersion in acquired long QT syndrome: a new index for arrhythmogenicity. Clin Sci (Lond) 105(6):671–676

126. Takenaka K, Ai T, Shimizu W, Kobori A, Ninomiya T, Otani H et al (2003) Exercise stress test amplifies genotype-phenotype correlation in the LQT1 and LQT2 forms of the long-QT syndrome. Circulation 107(6):838–844

127. Wang D, Patel C, Cui C, Yan GX (2008) Preclinical assessment of drug-induced proarrhythmias: role of the arterially perfused rabbit left ventricular wedge preparation. Pharmacol Ther 119(2):141–151

128. Pertsov AM, Jalife J (1995) Three-dimensional vortex-like reentry. In: Zipes DP, Jalife J (eds) Cardiac electrophysiology: from cell to bedside. W.B. Saunders, Philadelphia, pp 403–410

129. Qu Z, Garfinkel A (2004) Nonlinear dynamics of excitation and propagation in cardiac muscle. In: Zipes DP, Jalife J (eds) Cardiac electrophysiology: from cell to bedside. W.B. Saunders, Philadelphia, pp 327–335

130. Antzelevitch C (1983) Clinical application of new concepts of parasystole, reflection, and tachycardia. Cardiol Clin 1(1):39–50

131. Antzelevitch C (1990) Electrotonus and reflection. In: Rosen MR, Janse MJ, Wit AL (eds) Cardiac electrophysiology: a textbook. Futura, Mount Kisco, NY, pp 491–516

132. Fish JM, Antzelevitch C (2004) Role of sodium and calcium channel block in unmasking the Brugada syndrome. Heart Rhythm 1(2):210–217

133. Liu DW, Gintant GA, Antzelevitch C (1993) Ionic bases for electrophysiological distinctions among epicardial, mid-myocardial, and endocardial myocytes from the free wall of the canine left ventricle. Circ Res 72(3):671–687

134. Yan GX, Antzelevitch C (1998) Cellular basis for the normal T wave and the electrocardiographic manifestations of the long-QT syndrome. Circulation 98(18):1928–1936

135. Antzelevitch C (2006) Brugada syndrome. Pacing Clin Electrophysiol 29(10):1130–1159

136. Patel C, Antzelevitch C (2008) Cellular basis for arrhythmogenesis in an experimental model of the SQT1 form of the short QT syndrome. Heart Rhythm 5(4):585–590

4 Genetic and Molecular Basis of Arrhythmias

Shane B. Rowan and Dawood Darbar

CONTENTS

Abstract

In recent years, the identification of gene defects in a vast array of monogenic disorders has revolutionized our understanding of the basic mechanisms underlying many disease processes. Mutations in cardiac ion channels have been identified as the basis of a wide range of inherited arrhythmia syndromes, including the long QT syndrome (LQTS), catecholaminergic polymorphic ventricular tachycardia (CPVT), Brugada syndrome, short QT syndrome (SQTS), Andersen–Tawil syndrome (ATS), progressive cardiac conduction disease, familial atrial fibrillation (AF), and idiopathic ventricular fibrillation (VF). More recently, it has been observed that not only transmembrane cardiac ion channels cause cardiac arrhythmias, but also intracellular channel and non-ion conduction proteins that may be pathophysiologically linked to inherited arrhythmias. The identification of genes underlying the inherited arrhythmia syndromes has greatly contributed to our understanding of the substrates for arrhythmia development. Although the fundamental pathogenic mechanisms responsible for many inherited arrhythmia syndromes have been partially elucidated, it is apparent that there is marked clinical and genetic heterogeneity, i.e., several genes and allelic variants can be responsible for disease pathogenesis. Hundreds of disease-causing or contributing mutations at the single nucleotide level have been identified in nearly 20 channelopathy-susceptibility genes: 12 LQTS genes; 3 SQTS genes, 3 CPVT genes, and 6 susceptibility genes associated with the Brugada

From: *Contemporary Cardiology: Management of Cardiac Arrhythmias*
Edited by: Gan-Xin Yan, Peter R. Kowey, DOI 10.1007/978-1-60761-161-5_4
© Springer Science+Business Media, LLC 2011

syndrome. Most represent primary pathogenic disease-causing mutations only identified in disease cohorts, but others represent common or rare polymorphisms identified not only in disease but also in health that might confer an increased risk for arrhythmias under certain settings.

Key Words: Arrhythmias; genetics; molecular; mechanisms; long QT syndrome; Brugada syndrome; atrial fibrillation; catecholaminergic polymorphic ventricular tachycardia.

INTRODUCTION

Although we have witnessed significant strides in our understanding of the genetic basis of inherited arrhythmia syndromes in the past decade, many challenging issues still need to be addressed. Developments are likely to come from studies using new model systems that assess the function of mutant proteins in preparations that are more closely allied to the physiological environment in which these proteins are distributed. These more physiological expression systems will be useful not only to characterize individual mutations or polymorphisms, but also to elucidate the effects of mutations on the complex physiology of cardiac cells. In this chapter we summarize our present understanding of the molecular basis for cardiac arrhythmias using the congenital LQTS as a case study in monogenic diseases.

BASIC GENETIC PRINCIPLES

Hereditary information is encoded as a series of bases – adenine, guanine, cytosine, and thymine – on a backbone of sugar and phosphate groups, referred to as deoxyribonucleic acid (DNA). A matched pair of strands of DNA is called a chromosome. The normal human complement of chromosomes comprises 23 pairs (22 autosomal pairs, 1 sex chromosome pair). One member of each pair is inherited from each parent. Sequences of base pairs along a chromosome that encode proteins are referred to as genes. There are an estimated 30,000–35,000 genes in the human genome, each of which exists at a specific location, or locus. The sequence of a particular gene can vary in a population (or between chromosomes in an individual); when such variation exists, there are said to be multiple possible forms, or alleles, of a gene. Classically, genes are thought to serve as a code for protein manufacture within the cell. In this model, the sequence of base pairs is transcribed via a specialized enzyme apparatus into messenger ribonucleic acid (mRNA). These mRNA molecules are then translated in the cytoplasm into strings of amino acids, or proteins. After translation of mRNA into a protein, additional modifications to the protein can be made via post-translational processing. Proteins destined for the cell surface must then be shuttled via intracellular transport systems to their ultimate destination.

The transmission of genetic information between generations and the translation of the genetic code into proteins are both highly regulated processes with error-reducing safeguards; nonetheless, mistakes can occur. Mistakes in the transmission of DNA cause mutations and polymorphisms, or rare and common alterations in the sequence of base pairs on a chromosome, respectively. It is the study of these genetic changes that has increased our understanding of the molecular basis of arrhythmias.

Classically, genetics revolved around the study of monogenic disorders caused by chromosomal rearrangement or point mutation. Chromosomal rearrangements include duplication, insertion, and translocation. Point mutations are changes, additions, or deletions of single base pairs. While some of these changes may be silent (i.e., they do not change the amino acid sequence of a protein), others have profound consequences for protein structure. Such changes may be broadly categorized as missense, nonsense, and frameshift mutations. Missense mutations result in substitution of one amino acid for another. Nonsense mutations result in premature truncation of a protein. Frameshift mutations alter all of the succeeding information downstream from the site of mutation.

Because each person inherits two copies of the genetic code for autosomal proteins, they may be heterozygous (having only one copy) or homozygous (having two copies) for a particular mutation. This allows further classification of mutations into dominant (a single mutant copy is sufficient for expression of the clinical phenotype), recessive (a single copy does not change the phenotype from wild type; two mutant copies are required for clinical expression), incompletely dominant (a single copy causes a phenotype between homozygous wild-type and mutant phenotypes), and co-dominant (both the mutant copy and the wild-type copy are expressed).

Although it was initially assumed that all carriers of pathogenic mutations would manifest the corresponding phenotype, it soon became apparent that the clinical consequences of genetic defects are far more variable than expected. Some of this variability is related to incomplete penetrance and variable expressivity. The penetrance of a monogenic disease is defined as the percentage of individuals with a mutant allele who develop the phenotype of the related disease and it can vary from 10 to 100%. The expressivity of a disease is defined as the different phenotypical manifestations that can be observed among carriers of the same genetic defect. Consequently, the combination of variable penetrance and expressivity dictates that carriers of a DNA mutation may manifest either no clinical phenotype or phenotypes that are not the classical "textbook" type. Thus genotyping patients affected by "simple" monogenic diseases is more complicated than initially envisioned.

In contrast to the classical study of monogenic disorders, attention in the last several years has focused on genome-wide association studies (GWAS). In these studies, a phenotype of interest is correlated with the incidence of common genetic variants. For example, recent papers have identified loci on chromosome 4q25 and 16q22 that confer a predisposition to developing AF *(1, 2)*. GWAS differ significantly from classical genetic association studies, and a discussion of these details is beyond the scope of this chapter. However, it is important to recognize that such association studies do not, by themselves, inform us about the mechanism of an arrhythmia. The genetic loci that are described are markers for areas of the chromosome, and it is presumably a gene or gene modifier in that area that causes the studied effect. Thus, while genetic association studies can provide valuable guidance when searching for mechanisms, they do not, by themselves, describe a mechanism or cause.

THE MOLECULAR BASIS OF ARRHYTHMIAS

The cardiac action potential is mediated by a well-orchestrated activity of a diversity of ion channels (Fig. 1). The cardiac ion channels are proteins located in the sarcolemma of cardiomyocytes which, via highly regulated opening and closing (gating), conduct a selective and rapid flow of ions through a central pore. Spatial heterogeneity of ion channel expression underlies the different action potential morphology of the different parts of the heart which in turn ensure coordinated contraction. Abnormalities in ion channels function can have dramatic consequences that manifest themselves not only as electrocardiographic (ECG) abnormalities but also as arrhythmias. These disorders of ion channels, commonly referred to as "cardiac channelopathies," have been brought into focus in recent years as mutation in genes coding for specific ion channels was shown to underlie specific forms of heritable arrhythmogenic disorders occurring in the structurally normal heart. There include the long QT syndrome (LQTS), short QT syndrome (SQTS), Brugada syndrome, catecholaminergic polymorphic ventricular tachycardia (CPVT), familial atrial fibrillation (AF), and idiopathic ventricular fibrillation (VF).

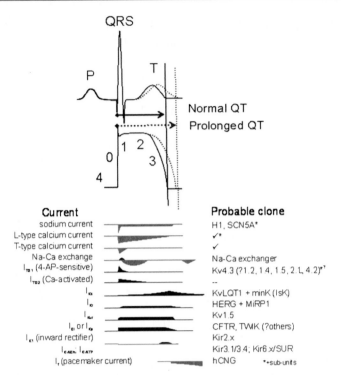

Fig. 1. The relationship between ionic currents and the duration of cardiac repolarization recorded from the ECG and the myocardial action potential. The *upper panels* show an idealized ECG recording aligned with a schematized ventricular myocyte action potential. Repolarization is controlled by a balance between inward (*red*) and outward (*black*) currents and repolarization is driven to completion by a relative increase of outward over inward currents. The action potential is initiated by inward sodium current (phase 0) and proceeds through early (phases 1 and 2) and late (phase 3) stages of repolarization. Increases in net inward current prolong repolarization. The "plateau" phases (2 and 3) are vulnerable to minor increases in net inward current, which can initiate early after-depolarizations that are one likely cause of Torsades de Pointes in LQTS.

When considering the molecular causes of arrhythmia, it is vital to recall that each gene and the protein or proteins that it encodes are but one step in a biological pathway. Therefore, multiple different mutations can result in similar phenotypes if they occur at distinct steps in the pathway or if they affect one step in different ways. For example, an inherited arrhythmia syndrome may be caused by one of several mutations in an ion channel protein, a mutation in another ion channel opposed to first, a protein involved in calcium handling within the cell, or a protein involved in cell-to-cell connections. This concept, that mutations in various genes can give rise to a common phenotype, is referred to as "genetic heterogeneity."

Cardiac arrhythmias generally result from abnormalities in four classes of protein: (1) ion channels, exchangers, and their modulators (primary electrical disease); (2) cell-to-cell junction proteins, such as those responsible for arrhythmogenic right ventricular cardiomyopathy (ARVC); (3) contractile sarcomeric proteins, such as those responsible for hypertrophic cardiomyopathy (HCM); and (4) cytoskeletal proteins, which are responsible for dilated cardiomyopathy (DCM). Tables 1 and 2 present a list of known atrial and ventricular inherited arrhythmia syndromes based on phenotypic characteristics.

Table 1
Atrial Arrhythmias Due to Monogenic Disorders

Phenotype	Rhythm	Inheritance	Locus	Ion channel/protein	Gene
AF	AF	AD	10q22–24	–	–
			11p15	I_{Ks}	KCNQ1
			6q14–16	–	–
			5p15	–	–
			21q22	I_{Ks}	KCNE2
			17q23	I_{K1}	KCNJ2
			12p13	I_{Kur}	KCNA5
			21q22	I_{Kr}	KCNH2
			1q21.1	Connexin 40	GJA5
			1p35–36	ANP	NPPA
		AR	5p13	Nucleoporin	NUP155
SND	Sinus brady-cardia, AF	AD		HCN4	HCN4
Atrial standstill	SND, AF	AD	3q21	I_{Na}	SCN5A
WPW syndrome	AVRT	AD			PRKAG2
Progressive conduction disease	AVB	AD	19q13 3q21	I_{Na}	SCN5A

AD autosomal dominant, AF atrial fibrillation, ANP atrial natriuretic peptide, AR autosomal recessive, AVRT atrioventricular reentrant tachycardia, AVB atrio-ventricular block, SND sinus node dysfunction, WPW Wolff–Parkinson–White

Table 2
Genetic Arrhythmia Syndromes Associated with Ventricular Arrhythmias

Syndrome	Inheritance	Locus	Ion channel/protein	Gene
LQT syndrome (RW)				
LQT1	AD	11p15.5	I_{Ks}	KCNQ1
LQT2		7q35–q36	I_{Kr}	KCNH2
LQT3		3p21	I_{Na}	SCN5A
LQT4		4q25–q27	Ankyrin-B	ANK2
LQT5		21q22.1q22.2	I_{Ks}	KCNE1
LQT6		21q22.1	I_{Kr}	KCNE2
LQT7		17q23.1–q24.2	I_{K1}	KCNJ2
LQT8		12p13.3	I_{Ca-L}	CACNA1C
LQT9		3p25	Caveolin-3	CAV3
LQT10		11q23.3	$NaV_{1.5}\ \beta4$	SCN4B
LQT11		7q21–q22	Yotiao	AKAP9
LQT12		20q11.2	A1-syntrophin	SNTA1
JLN1	AR	11p15	I_{Ks}	KCNQ1
JLN2	AR	21q22	I_{Kr}	KCNE1
Catecholaminergic polymorphic VT	AD	1q42		RYR2
	AR	1p13-p11		CASQ2
		7p14-p22		

(Continued)

Table 2
(Continued)

Syndrome	Inheritance	Locus	Ion channel/protein	Gene
Brugada syndrome	AD	3p21	I_{Na}	SCN5A
		3p22–25	I_{Na}	GPDL-1
		12p13.3	$Ca_v\beta1.2$	CACNA1C
		10p12.33	$Ca_v\beta2$	CACNB2
		19q13.1	$Na_v\beta$	SCN1B
		11q13–q14	MiRP2	KCNE3
		11q23.3	$Na_v\beta3$	SCN3B
Short QT syndrome	AD	21q22	I_{Kr}	KCNH2
		21q22	I_{Ks}	KCNQ1
		17q23	I_{K1}	KCNJ2
ARVC				
ARVC1	AD	14q23–24	TGFβ-3	
ARVC2		1q42	Ryanodine Receptor 2	RYR2
ARVC3		14q11–q12		
ARVC4		2q32		
ARVC5		3p23	Transmembrane protein 43	
ARVC6		10p12–p14		
ARVC7		10q22		
ARVC8		6p28	Desmoplakin	DSP
ARVC9		12p11	Plakophilin-2	PKP2
ARVC10	AR	18q12	Desmoglein-2	DSG2
ARVC11		18q12.1	Desmocollin-2	DSC2
Naxos disease		17q21	Plakoglobin	JUP

ARVC arrhythmogenic right ventricular cardiomyopathy, *JLN* Jervell and Lange-Nielsen, *LQT* long QT, *RV* right ventricular, *RW* Romano-Ward, *TGF-β* transforming growth factor – beta, *VT* ventricular tachycardia. See Table 1 for remaining abbreviations

THE CONGENITAL LONG QT SYNDROME – A CASE STUDY OF MONOGENIC ARRHYTHMIA SYNDROMES

Since the initial description of congenital deafness, prolongation of the QT interval, and sudden cardiac death (SCD) by Jervell and Lange-Nielsen in 1957 *(3)*, our understanding of the molecular and genetic basis of the congenital LQTS has progressed significantly. Shortly after the autosomal recessive Jervell–Lange-Nielsen syndrome was described, Romano and Ward each independently described an "autosomal dominant" form without congenital deafness *(4, 5)*. The findings that the QT interval could be prolonged by right stellectomy and the successful treatment of a medically refractory young patient with LQTS by left stellectomy led to the hypothesis that the disease was primarily a disorder of cardiac sympathetic innervation *(6)*. Although we now know that this is not the primary cause of LQTS, the importance of these early observations is evident in that autonomic modulation remains an important therapeutic approach in LQTS patients *(7)*.

The subsequent theory that the underlying cause of LQTS was an alteration of one of the repolarizing potassium currents was proposed nearly 10 years prior to the identification of the first LQTS genes in 1995 *(8–11)*. Indeed, four forms of LQTS, and the two most common forms (LQT1 and LQT2) are caused by mutations in genes that encode proteins that form repolarizing potassium channels. In the late 1990s the first five LQTS genes were identified (Table 2), all of which encoded proteins that form ion channels that underlie the cardiac action potential (Fig. 1). The most commonly identified genes, KCNQ1 and KCNH2, encode proteins that form the α-subunits of two major repolarizing potassium currents, I_{Ks} and I_{Kr}. Two other LQTS genes encode for the corresponding β-subunits (KCNE1 and KCNE2). The other major LQTS gene, SCN5A, encodes the α-subunit of the cardiac sodium channel. Either "loss-of-function" mutations in potassium channel genes, or "gain-of-function" mutations in the cardiac sodium or calcium channels lead to prolongation of ventricular repolarization, and therefore, a prolonged QT interval. Furthermore, we now know that the Jervell–Lange-Nielsen syndrome is simply a more severe form of LQTS, as patients with "Romano-Ward syndrome" carry a single mutation, while it is now accepted that homozygous mutations of KCNQ1 or KCNE1 cause Jervell–Lange-Nielsen syndrome *(12, 13)*. The extracardiac finding of congenital deafness requires the presence of two mutant alleles and results from lack of functioning I_{Ks} in the inner ear *(14)*. Jervell–Lange-Nielsen syndrome patients are also thought to be highly susceptible to arrhythmias; thus, arrhythmia risk seems partly dependent on "gene dosage." These first five forms of LQTS represent classic LQTS, in that single mutations in ion channel genes resulted in action potential prolongation and prolonged QT intervals with an increased risk for Torsades de Pointes and SCD with no significant extracardiac manifestations.

With the finding of ANK2 mutations underlying LQT4 *(15)*, we find that the spectrum of LQTS genes are not limited to genes that encode ion channel proteins. ANK2 encodes ankyrin-B, one isoform of a ubiquitously expressed family of proteins originally identified in the erythrocyte as a link between membrane proteins. Cardiomyocytes heterozygous for a null mutation in ankyrin-B display reduced expression and abnormal localization of the Na/Ca exchanger, Na/K ATPase, and InsP3 receptor, but normal expression and localization of other cardiac proteins, including the L-type Ca^{2+} channel and the cardiac Na^+ channel *(16)*. Action potential duration is normal, but myocytes display abnormalities in calcium homeostasis leading to early and delayed after-depolarizations. Further clinical characterization of patients with ANK2 mutations reveals that these patients, while at risk for sudden death, do not uniformly display prolonged QT intervals *(16)*, suggesting that ankyrin-B diseases are distinct from LQTS *(17)*. Andersen–Tawil syndrome (ATS), termed by some as LQT7 *(18)* is due to mutations in KCNJ2 and is associated with significant extracardiac findings, including periodic paralysis, hypertelorism, and clinodactyly *(19)*. As many patients with ATS have mild or no prolongation of the QT interval, and as the clinical manifestations, ECG characteristics, and outcomes are quite different from LQTS, it seems that ATS is not a subtype of long QT syndrome, and it has been recommended that the annotation of KCNJ2-positive ATS individuals should be ATS1 rather than LQT7 *(20)*. Recently, mutations in the gene encoding the L-type calcium channel have been found to underlie Timothy Syndrome, a rare multisystem disorder characterized by QT prolongation as well as syndactyly, autism, and immune deficiencies *(21)*. This has been termed LQT8 and does cause a "gain of function" of I_{Ca} due to slowed inactivation, which directly prolongs the QT interval (Fig. 1), similar to the other forms of LQTS. However, the first described case of Timothy syndrome differs from classic forms of LQTS in that it is associated with significant extracardiac manifestations. More recently, other Ca^{2+} channel gene (CACNA1C) mutations have been identified that increased QT interval but result in less severe extracardiac manifestations *(22)*.

Even when limited to "classic" forms of LQTS, important clinical differences among affected patients depending on the specific gene (and in some cases the specific mutation) have been observed – so called genotype–phenotype correlation. Much of the clinical information in large numbers of genotyped patients is possible primarily because of the international LQTS registry *(23)*. As the majority (>90%) of genotyped LQTS patients have LQT1, LQT2, or LQT3 *(24)*, most of the differences are observed among these genotypes. Important differences among LQTS types 1–3 include different ECG T-wave patterns *(25)*, clinical course *(26)*, triggers of cardiac events *(27)*, response to sympathetic stimulation *(28, 29)*, and effectiveness and limitations of β-blocker therapy *(30)*. These clinical observations, combined with an improved understanding of the molecular mechanisms underlying the various forms of LQTS, have allowed a framework for developing some genotype-specific therapies. Since beta-adrenergically mediated increases in I_{Ks} are the predominant mechanism of QT shortening with adrenergic stimulation *(31)*, patients with defective I_{Ks} (LQT1 and LQT5) are most sensitive to autonomic influences, and beta-blockers and left cardiac sympathetic denervation seem most effective for these LQTS types. Increased extracellular potassium paradoxically increases I_{Kr} *(32)*; therefore, supplemental, potassium seems most appropriate for patients with defective I_{Kr} (LQT2 and LQT6) and has been shown to shorten QT interval in patients with LQT2, both acutely and chronically *(33, 34)*. Patients with augmented I_{Na} (LQT3) would be expected to improve with sodium channel blockers and have been shown to shorten QT intervals with mexilitene *(35)*. LQT3 patients also display bradycardia and shorten their QT interval with increases in heart rate, leading to the recommendation for treatment with pacemakers.

Despite genotype-specific mechanisms, many therapies have beneficial effects on patients with any form of LQTS. Beta-blockers are recommended for all patients with LQTS, and mexiletine may have beneficial effects in LQT1 and LQT2 *(36, 37)*. This is consistent with the concept of "reduced repolarization reserve" *(38)*; multiple redundant mechanisms contribute to normal repolarization, and when one or more of these cause a net increase in inward current during repolarization it manifests as QT prolongation with increased risk for Torsades de Pointes. A specific therapy may target the underlying defect as when a sodium channel blocker normalizes the QT interval in a LQT3 patient with abnormally augmented sodium current. Alternatively, a therapy may enhance a normal mechanism and thereby offset the diseased one. For example, a patient with LQT1 with reduced I_{Ks} may benefit from supplemental potassium, which augments normal I_{Kr} and thereby helps restore the balance of repolarization.

Important clinical distinctions can be made amongst the different forms of long QT syndrome. In some cases, it also appears that disease "hot spots" may confer enhanced proarrhythmic risk. For example, among patients with LQT2, increased risk has been associated with mutations located in the pore region of the protein, compared to mutations in other locations *(39)*. In patients with LQT1, transmembrane domain mutations were associated with more frequent events, as well as longer QTc and longer peak to end of QT interval than those with C-terminal mutations *(40)*. Understanding the protein structure–function underpinnings of disease severity will require improved cellular models. Despite these findings and the hope for genotype-guided therapy, there is tremendous clinical variability even within families with a single specific mutation, with variable penetrance and expression, likely due to modifier genes which alter the phenotype *(41)*. Multiple genes may influence cardiac repolarization and alter the phenotype in patients with the same LQTS mutation.

The identification of LQTS disease genes represents a crucial first step in developing an understanding of the molecular basis for normal cardiac repolarization. This information will be important not only for identifying new therapies in LQTS, but also for further understanding arrhythmias, and their potential therapies, in situations such as heart failure, cardiac hypertrophy, myocardial infarction, or sudden infant death syndrome, where abnormal repolarization has been linked to sudden death *(42)*. The congenital LQTS thus represents a paradigm for studying monogenic arrhythmia syndromes, but the revealed complexities have highlighted the need for more integrated systems-based approaches to understanding, modeling, and predicting arrhythmia risk in patients. The congenital LQTS also shares similarities with proarrhythmic "electrical remodeling" that occurs in common forms of structural heart disease. The action potential duration is prolonged in human heart failure due to a variety of causes, including myocardial infarction, hypertension, and genetic mutations. It now seems likely that arrhythmia mechanisms identified in models of LQTS, such as after-depolarizations and transmural dispersion of repolarization, are also operative and contribute to SCD in patients with common forms of structural heart disease. Thus, genetically defined arrhythmias may reveal important insights into mechanisms of arrhythmias that impact large numbers of people and represent a significant public health challenge.

FAMILIAL ATRIAL FIBRILLATION (AF)

AF has not previously been considered one of the classical inherited arrhythmia syndromes, although inherited forms of the disease have been recognized for decades. Recently, new genetic approaches have become powerful enough to elucidate the mutations that cause some forms of familial AF. These discoveries have, in turn, informed our understanding of the molecular and electrical events that give rise to AF.

Monogenic familial AF was first reported in 1943 *(43)*, and while it may be uncommon, there has been no attempt to determine the overall prevalence of familial AF. Recent analysis of the Framingham data, however, has shown genetic susceptibility to AF; in this cohort, parental AF increased the risk of the arrhythmia in the offspring *(44)*. Furthermore, studies indicate that 5% of the patients with typical AF and up to 15% of the individuals with lone AF may have a familial form of the disease *(45)*. This suggests that familial AF may have a higher prevalence than previously suspected. A gene locus for AF was first reported in 1997, based on genetic mapping studies in three families from Spain who appeared to share common ancestry *(46)*. However, the gene responsible for AF in this kindred has not yet been identified, but resides within a relatively large chromosomal region spanning 14 centi-Morgans. In addition, three other loci on chromosomes 6q14–16 *(47)*, 5p13 *(48)*, and 10p11–q21 *(49)* have been reported, with no defective genes yet identified. Recently, a novel AF locus on chromosome 5p15 was identified by genome-wide linkage analysis of a four-generation kindred *(50)*. Importantly, this study established an abnormally prolonged P wave (>155 ms) determined by signal-averaged ECG analysis as an "endophenotype" that improved statistical power of the linkage study in this family. Taken together, these reports support the idea that familial AF is a genetically heterogeneous disease much like many other inherited arrhythmia syndromes.

Since these initial chromosomal studies, the first genes for AF have been identified, providing a link between ion channelopathies and the disease. In a single four-generation Chinese family in which the LQT syndrome and early-onset AF co-segregate, a mutation (S140G) in *KCNQ1* gene on chromosome 11p15.5 has been reported *(51)*. The *KCNQ1* gene encodes the pore-forming α subunit of the cardiac I_{Ks} (*KCNQ1/KCNE1*), the *KCNQ1/KCNE2*, and the *KCNQ1/KCNE3* potassium channels. Functional analysis of the S140G mutant revealed a gain-of-function effect in the *KCNQ1/KCNE1* and *KCNQ1/KCNE2* currents, which contrasts with the dominant negative or loss-of-function effects of the *KCNQ1* mutations previously identified with LQTS. The gain-of-function mutation is a logical explanation for the shortening of the action potential duration and effective refractory period that is linked to the mechanism of AF but is at odds with the loss-of-function mechanism thought to underlie the LQTS phenotype. More recently, also from the same group in China, a link between *KCNE2* and AF has been provided with the identification of the same mutation in two families with AF *(52)*. The mutation R27C caused a gain of function when co-expressed with *KCNQ1* but had no effect when expressed with *HERG*.

Another study linking potassium channel mutations to AF identified mutations in *KCNA5*, a gene that encodes Kv1.5, a potassium channel in human atria. The mutation studied caused loss of function of the encoded protein and a decrease in I_{Kur}, the ultrarapid delayed rectifier current that participates in atrial repolarization. In contrast to the potassium channel mutations previously discussed, this mutation prolonged action potential duration; however, it resulted in an increase in triggered activity, particularly with adrenergic stimulation *(53)*. Triggered atrial activity such as this is the target of many current ablative procedures for AF. We recently identified a novel KCNA5 variant in a kindred with early-onset lone familial AF (Fig. 2) *(54)*. This variant disrupts a proline-rich motif involved in tyrosine kinase modulation of I_{Kur}, reduces wild-type current but renders the channel kinase-resistant (Fig. 3). These data implicate abnormal atrial potential control due to abnormal tyrosine kinase signaling as a mechanism in this familial form of AF, and thereby suggest a role for modulation of this pathway in AF and its treatment. These studies clearly establish several potential mechanisms by which cardiac potassium ion channel abnormalities may cause AF.

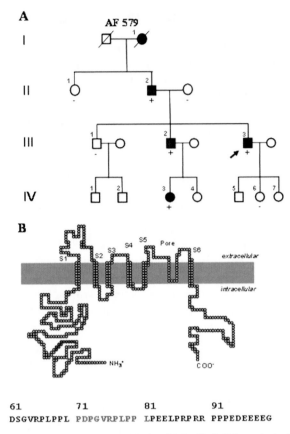

Fig. 2. (a) A KCNA5 mutation identified in family with familial AF. *Solid symbols* denote AF, and *open symbols* individuals without a documented history of AF. Male subjects are shown as squares and female subjects as *circles*. The proband (*arrow*) and the presence (+) or absence (–) of the KCNA5 71–81deletion (del) are indicated. **(b)** The location of the del in the KCNA5 protein and a portion of the KCNA5 N-terminus amino acid showing the indel mutant sequence in *red*.

In addition to the evidence linking cardiac potassium channels to AF, there is also research implicating the cardiac sodium channel. Olson et al. *(55)* identified mutations in *SCN5A*, the gene encoding the cardiac sodium channel, in a group of patients with dilated cardiomyopathy. Mutations in this group also predisposed to AF. AF in the incident kindred often preceded the development of cardiomyopathy. Since this publication, multiple other mutations in *SCN5A* and related proteins have been associated with AF *(56–58)*. Both gain-of-function *(58)* and loss-of-function *(57)* mutations have been described. Paralleling developments in potassium channel research, mechanisms invoking decreased refractory periods and increased excitability have also been proposed.

Non-ion channel mutations associated with AF have also been identified. As might be expected in an electrical syncytium such as the human atrium, abnormalities in cell-to-cell connections have also been associated with AF. Gollob et al. *(59)* showed that a mutation in connexin-40 affected intracellular transport of the mutant protein and affected cell surface gap junction formation. A recent study demonstrated a unique association between a frameshift mutation in *NPPA*, the gene that encodes atrial natriuretic peptide (ANP), and AF *(60)*. The frameshift disrupts the protein's usual stop codon and creates an elongated version of ANP. In a whole-heart model, the mutant protein caused shortening of the action potential and effective refractory period. A particularly novel aspect of this study was that it is the first to identify a mutation in a circulating protein that predisposes to AF.

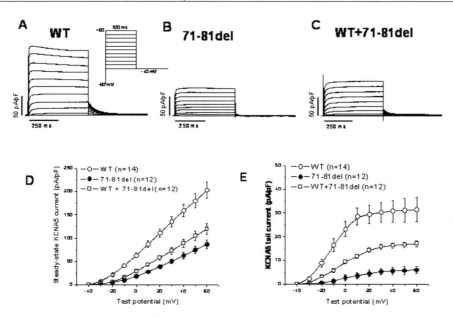

Fig. 3. The 71–81del in the N-terminus of KCNA5 expressed a reduced current. **Panels A, B,** and **C** show wild-type (WT), 71–81del and the WT+71–81del currents, respectively, with a dominant negative effect. **Panels D** and **E** summarize both steady-state and tail currents in the three groups.

Although mutations in multiple genes have been implicated in familial AF, the underlying mechanisms, and thus implications for therapy, remain ill-defined. Recently, we identified a novel mutation in KCNQ1 and separately a mutation in the NPPA gene, both segregating with early-onset lone AF in different kindreds (Figs. 4 and 5) *(61)*. The functional effects of these mutations yielded strikingly similar I_{Ks} "gain of function." In Chinese Hamster Ovary (CHO) cells, coexpression of mutant KCNQ1 with its ancillary subunit KCNE1 generated ~3-fold larger currents that activated much faster than wild-type (WT)-I_{Ks}. Application of the WT NPPA peptide fragment produced similar changes in WT-I_{Ks}, and these were exaggerated with the mutant NPPA S64R peptide fragment. Anantin, a competitive ANP receptor antagonist, completely inhibited the changes in I_{Ks} gating observed with NPPA-S64R. Computational simulations identified accelerated transitions into open states as the mechanism for variant I_{Ks} gating. Incorporating these I_{Ks} changes into computed human atrial action potentials resulted in 37% shortening (120 vs. 192 ms at 300 ms cycle length), reflecting loss of the phase II dome which is dependent on L-type calcium channel current. This study found striking functional similarities due to mutations in *KCNQ1* and *NPPA* genes which led to I_{Ks} "gain of function," atrial action potential shortening, and consequent altered calcium current as a common mechanism between diverse familial AF syndromes.

The classical paradigm for AF was that of multiple sites of functional reentry causing rapid, colliding, and chaotic wavefronts of atrial conduction that gave rise to the characteristic electrocardiographic appearance of AF. More recently, this concept has been challenged by the clinical observations that the pulmonary veins are sites of active foci that appear to give rise to AF and that electrical isolation of the pulmonary veins from the atrium may cure AF. Knowledge of the mutations that have been associated with AF to date fits well with this model; increased excitability and triggered activity in the pulmonary veins combined with shortened atrial refractory periods would provide the substrate to initiate and sustain AF.

In 2007, a genome-wide association study (GWAS) in Icelanders identified a locus on chromosome 4q25 associated with AF in subjects of all ages *(1)*. Within this locus, two non-coding single nucleotide

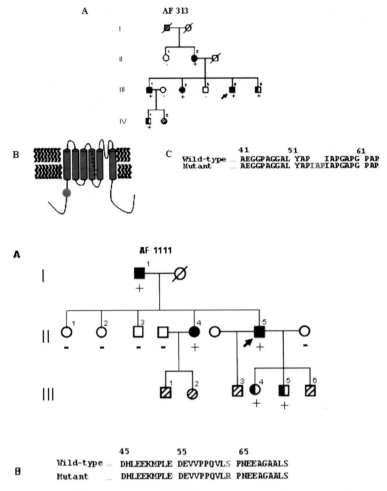

Fig. 4. A KCNQ1 mutation identified in a kindred with familial AF. (**a**) The family pedigree. The proband (*arrow*) and the presence (+) or absence (–) of the KCNQ1-IAP54–56 indel are indicated. (**b**) The location of the variant in the KCNQ1 protein. (**c**) The portion of the KCNQ1 N-terminus amino acid WT and mutant sequence. *Symbols* as in Fig. 2.

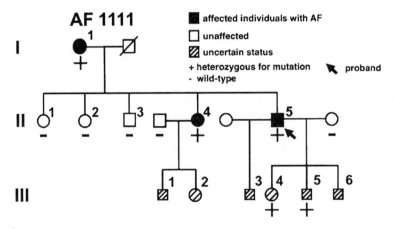

Fig. 5. *NPPA* mutation identified in a kindred with familial AF. Shown is the family pedigree (AF 1111). Symbols as in Fig. 2.

polymorphisms (SNPs) were independently associated with AF, and these findings were replicated in two populations of European descent and one of Asian descent. The SNP most strongly associated with AF, rs2200733, conferred a 1.71-fold increased odds of AF while the other SNP, rs10033464, conferred a 1.42-fold increased odds of AF. Kaab et al. *(62)* replicated this association in a study of four large populations with ambulatory AF, and most recently a study has also shown that this association holds in post-cardiac surgery AF, a setting thought to be related to inflammation *(63)*.

Although the potential mechanism of action of the chromosome 4q25 locus identified by the two non-coding SNPs is unknown and may be mediated through effects of distant genes, it is interesting to note that the closest gene, located approximately 90 kb centromeric, is the paired-like homeodomain transcription factor 2 (*PITX2*). Mouse *PITX2* knockouts have demonstrated a critical role for one isoform, *PITX2c*, in left–right asymmetry, specifically the development of the left atrium *(64)*. Loss of *PITX2c* leads to right atrial isomerization and a failure to suppress a default pathway for sinus node development of the pulmonary myocardium, or the sleeve of cardiomyocytes extending from the left atrium into the initial portion of the pulmonary vein *(65)*. Importantly, this area has been implicated as a source for the ectopic atrial activity necessary for the initiation and propagation of AF *(66)*. Furthermore, recent data also strongly implicate *PITX2* as the causative gene. In a recent GWAS, conducted by Chung et al. *(67)*, a single SNP (rs4611994) in the same LD block on 4q25 met genome-wide significance and was again genotyped in 46 left atrial appendage tissue samples, with *PITX2* expression levels also obtained. This analysis demonstrated a significant association of rs4611994 genotype with the C isoform of *PITX2* *(67)*.

BRUGADA SYNDROME

The Brugada syndrome – a characteristic pattern of "right bundle branch block", ST segment elevation, and SCD – was initially described as a clinical entity in 1992 and is an archetypical example of an arrhythmia syndrome arising from ion channel dysfunction (Fig. 6) *(68)*. Consideration of this syndrome illustrates several important points touched upon in the previous section. First, multiple mutations in a protein can yield similar or highly variable phenotypes depending on how they affect the function of the protein. Second, knowledge of the genetic cause of a disease can be helpful in determining the molecular mechanism. Third, mutations in multiple proteins can cause similar clinical phenotypes.

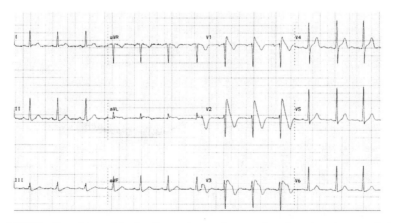

Fig. 6. Twelve-lead ECG of patient with the Brugada syndrome showing the characteristic coved-type ST-segment elevation in leads V_1 and V_2. This is a 12-lead ECG showing sinus rhythm with marked ST-segment elevation that is characteristic of some patients with Brugada syndrome.

The genetic basis for the syndrome was first identified several years after the description of the syndrome itself *(69)*. Researchers identified three genetic mutations leading to alterations in the α-subunit of the cardiac sodium channel (SCN5A). The first was a missense mutation, the second was a splice-donor mutation (a mutation that occurs at the site of joining of two exons after elimination of an intron), and the third was a frameshift mutation caused by the deletion of a single codon.

As mentioned in the previous section, multiple mutations within a single protein can yield a similar phenotype. In this fashion, the three distinct alterations in the *SCN5A* gene described in this chapter lead to alterations in the function of the sodium channel protein. These alterations lead, in turn, to the clinical phenotype of Brugada syndrome. Since this original description of *SCN5A* mutations, investigators have identified over 90 other mutations in this gene in patients with the Brugada syndrome. The mutations described to date have in common that they cause loss of function of the sodium channel. The mechanisms by which the mutations cause this loss of function vary. For example, mutations have been described that produce a non-functioning protein product, change time constants of inactivation or recovery of inactivation of the sodium channel, abolish sodium current in the cells, and affect intracellular trafficking of the sodium channel *(70–72)*. Notably, mutations in *SCN5A* do not always cause the Brugada syndrome. Mutations at residues or near residues associated with the Brugada syndrome have been associated with the LQTS3. In the case of LQT3, rather than causing loss of function, mutations have been associated with gain of function *(70)*.

The identification of SCN5A mutations associated with the Brugada syndrome led to further exploration of the mechanism of this syndrome. Yan and Antzelevitch were able to reproduce the electrocardiographic findings of Brugada syndrome in a canine model *(73)*. Pharmacologic manipulation led to the loss of the normal action potential dome in regions of the epicardium with preservation of the dome in the endocardium. This variation led to a transmural voltage gradient, giving rise to the characteristic ST elevation of the Brugada syndrome. Additionally, they noted dispersion of repolarization on the epicardial surface and phase 2 reentry. Thus, they recapitulated the electrocardiographic findings of Brugada syndrome and described a potential mechanism for the induction of the characteristic ventricular arrhythmias. As they noted in their discussion, the dependence of their findings on the loss of the action potential dome points to the loss of currents that balance I_{to}. One such current that they specifically cite is I_{Na}, the current carried by the sodium channel *(74)*.

While this elegant experiment used genetic information to generate a model that was consistent with the putative molecular mechanism, other research invokes selective heterogeneous slowing of conduction in the right ventricle to explain the electrical manifestations of Brugada syndrome *(75)*.

Not only can several mutations within one gene cause the same clinical phenotype, but mutations in distinct genes can also do so. For example, mutations in two other genes that encode proteins that affect sodium channel function have recently been implicated in Brugada syndrome. In one case, a mutation in *GPD1-L* is hypothesized to alter sodium channel trafficking within the cell, leading to an effective loss of function at the cell membrane *(76)*. In the second, mutations in *SCN1B*, the gene encoding the β-subunit of the cardiac sodium channel, were identified in patients with the Brugada syndrome *(77)*. The β-subunit modifies the function of the sodium channel; these mutations again caused loss of function of the channel.

There have also been mutations identified that do not appear to affect sodium channel function that cause the Brugada syndrome phenotype. Antzelevitch et al. *(78)* described mutations in the L-type calcium channel genes *CACNA1C* and *CACNB2b*. Despite the large number of identified causative mutations in *SCN5A* and other genes, in the majority of patients with Brugada syndrome a genetic mutation has not been identified. This fact emphasizes the concept that the initiation and propagation of the action potential are events that involve cellular and signaling pathways; therefore, similar phenotypes may arise as a consequence of defects at multiple steps along these pathways. It is likely that further research will uncover additional mutations in these and other pathways and allow further explanation of the cause of the Brugada syndrome.

As might be predicted with so many mutations, the degree of loss of function of the sodium channel can vary as can the expression of the clinical phenotype. A genetic mutation may be necessary to allow abnormal function of the sodium channel but may be, by itself, insufficient to cause overt Brugada syndrome. Physiologic and pharmacologic stressors can alter sodium channel function sufficiently to expose subclinical abnormalities in the sodium channel. For example, fever has been associated with ventricular fibrillation and worsened sodium channel function *(79, 80)*. Likewise, procainamide and other sodium channel blockers are used clinically to provoke electrocardiographic changes in patients in whom Brugada syndrome is suspected but who do not have diagnostic findings at baseline *(81)*.

In summary, the Brugada syndrome is an arrhythmic disease characterized primarily by mutations that result in loss of normal cardiac sodium channels. The mutations that cause this disorder may be in the sodium channel itself, or they may arise in genes that modify the function or intracellular handling of the sodium channel. The mutations vary in degree of effect on sodium channel function; this variance, in combination with environmental factors, affects phenotypic expression of a genetic disorder.

CATECHOLAMINERGIC POLYMORPHIC VENTRICULAR TACHYCARDIA (CPVT)

CPVT also is a classic example of an inherited arrhythmia syndrome. Unlike Brugada syndrome, a disease of sodium channel dysfunction, CPVT is primarily a disorder of cytoplasmic proteins involved with intracellular calcium handling. First described in 1975 and clinically characterized as a distinct entity in 1999, CPVT is a malignant arrhythmia syndrome characterized by stress (exercise or emotional)-induced bidirectional ventricular tachycardia, polymorphic ventricular tachycardia, and ventricular fibrillation in the absence of apparent structural heart disease *(82, 83)*. More than 25 years after the initial description of CPVT in a pediatric patient, Priori et al. identified missense mutations in the ryanodine receptor gene *(hRyR2)* in several patients with CPVT *(84)*. In a follow-up paper a year later, Priori et al. showed that *hRyR2* mutations were present in ~50% of patients with CPVT *(84)*. The ryanodine receptor is the largest protein of the calcium release channel, a protein complex that connects the cytosolic and luminal portions of the sarcoplasmic reticulum. During a normal cardiac cycle, small amounts of calcium that enter the cell through L-type calcium channels stimulate the release of large amounts of calcium from the sarcoplasmic reticulum (SR) through the calcium release channel. As the concentration of calcium in the SR decreases, calcium movement through the calcium release channel is inhibited. Knowledge of the location of the mutations in the ryanodine receptor that cause CPVT led to the hypothesis that these mutations alter the sensitivity of the protein to intraluminal calcium and cause additional calcium release. This, in turn, leads to delayed after-depolarizations and arrhythmia *(85)*. Importantly, in addition to providing valuable insights about the mechanism of the disease, the work by Priori et al. also showed another aspect of genetic research into arrhythmias. In their paper, patients with a mutation in *hRyR2* had a distinctly worsened prognosis when compared with those patients without a described mutation. Knowledge of the genetic basis of arrhythmia may sometimes be helpful for risk prediction and therapeutic recommendations.

Recent research has shown that the ryanodine receptor is not the lone culprit in CPVT. As was the case with Brugada syndrome, other proteins involved in the same pathway, in this case, calcium handling, have also been implicated. Mutations in *CASQ2*, the gene that encodes the cardiac form of calsequestrin, have also been demonstrated in patients with CPVT. These have included both missense and, in more severe forms, nonsense mutations *(86, 87)*. The mechanism by which *CASQ2* mutations cause CPVT appears to be tied intimately to the ryanodine receptor. CASQ2 is located in the SR and serves as a calcium sensor that helps inhibit the ryanodine receptor when intra-SR calcium levels decrease. Mutations in CASQ2 affect its ability to sense calcium levels or to inhibit the ryanodine receptor. In either case, this leads again to increased cytosolic calcium influx and delayed after-depolarizations *(85)*.

Knowledge of the mechanism of increased intracellular calcium release and spontaneous delayed after-depolarizations paved the way for recent work showing that a sodium channel blocker, flecainide, can achieve a remarkable reduction in ventricular tachycardia burden in patients with medically refractory CPVT *(88)*. The story of CPVT demonstrates how a clinical description of a syndrome can lead to genetic insight, which in turn can lead to information on a molecular mechanism. Therapy directed at the molecular mechanism can then close the circle and lead to effective treatments in humans. Leenhardt et al.'s *(83)* insight in their 1999 description of the entity that "This ECG pattern is most commonly described in digitalis toxicity. . ." led researchers to focus on characterization of genes involved in calcium handling. Knowledge of the genes involved in calcium homeostasis permitted the creation of murine models which then allowed elucidation of the underlying electrophysiologic mechanisms of the disorder. Armed with this knowledge, researchers were then able to pursue a mechanism-based approach to treat this life-threatening syndrome.

ARRHYTHMOGENIC RIGHT VENTRICULAR CARDIOMYOPATHY (ARVC)

In contrast to Brugada syndrome and CPVT, most cases of ARVC do not arise from ion channel or cytoplasmic protein dysfunction; instead, ARVC commonly arises from problems with the desmosome, an integral component of cell-to-cell connections. ARVC is a genetic cardiomyopathy characterized by ventricular arrhythmias and structural abnormalities of the right ventricle, resulting from progressive fibrofatty infiltration of right ventricular myocardium *(89)*. It may be a relatively common cause of ventricular tachycardia in young patients with previously unrecognized heart disease, and accounts for up to 10% of unexpected SCD *(90)*, though its prevalence may vary by geographic location *(91)*. The diagnosis of ARVC is based on clinical criteria including structural abnormalities, tissue characterization, abnormalities in depolarization or repolarization, arrhythmias, and family history *(92)*. These criteria are often subjective, and may be too stringent, especially for family members of patients with known ARVC *(93)*. Familial occurrence of ARVC is well recognized, most commonly with autosomal dominant inheritance.

To date, five genes have been identified in autosomal dominant ARVC: the cardiac ryanodine receptor *(RYR2)* in ARVC2 *(94)*, desmoplakin *(DSP)* in ARVC8 *(95)*, plakophilin-2 *(PKP2)* in ARVC9 *(96)*, desmoglein-2 *(DSG2)* *(97)*, and desmocollin-2 *(DSC2)* *(98)*. ARVC2 is a rare and atypical form, with only mild structural abnormalities and a characteristic bidirectional ventricular tachycardia very similar to CPVT. It is still unclear whether such patients fulfill the diagnostic criteria for ARVC. Mutations in the non-coding region of the transforming growth factor β3 have been identified in one kindred with ARVC1 *(99)*. One form of ARVC, inherited in an autosomal recessive fashion, is associated with wooly hair and palmoplantar keratoderma (Naxos disease) and caused by mutations in plakoglobin (JUP) *(100)*. Five of the seven identified genes encode key components of the desmosome–protein complexes which provide structural and functional integrity to adjacent cells, suggesting that ARVC is a disease of the desmosome.

Although mutations in desmosomal proteins have been clearly implicated in ARVC, the mechanisms by which disruption in the normal function of the desmosome translates into the clinicopathologic disease are uncertain. Hypotheses about simple structural changes, disruption of WNT-β (beta)-catenin signaling, increased apoptosis, and remodeling of the gap junction are currently active areas of research *(101)*. For example, a 2007 study identified a mutation in the gene encoding plakoglobin with in vitro studies of this mutation demonstrating increased ubiquitinization of the mutant protein, leading to increased turnover in the cell *(102)*. A biopsy specimen from a patient with this mutation showed decreased localization of plakoglobin and other desmosomal components to intercalated disks, suggesting that the mutant protein interfered with these cell-to-cell junctions. Similarly, a separate study identified missense mutations in *PKP2,* the gene that encodes plakophilin-2, that were associated with abnormalities of cell-to-cell junctions. Garcia-gras and colleagues showed in cellular and murine models that inhibition of expression of desmoplakin (encoded by *Dsp*) leads to inhibition of WNT-β(beta)-catenin signaling (involved in the regulation of adipogenesis) and caused increased myocardial adipocytes, fibrosis, and arrhythmias. Finally, cellular work in rat myocytes shows that silencing of *PKP2* that encodes plakophilin leads to effects on Cx43 gap junctions. Gap junctions are an integral component of electrical communication between cells; an abnormality in these structures provides a plausible structural mechanism for the arrhythmias characteristic of ARVC. Whatever the mechanism, the presence of structural heart disease differentiates this disease from primary electrical diseases such as Brugada syndrome and CPVT. The zones of fibrofatty tissue that replace normal myocardium in the right ventricle serve as zones of scar that allow reentry and ventricular arrhythmias.

While the mechanism by which desmosomal abnormalities cause the disease remains uncertain, knowledge of desmosomal involvement underpins a recent study that looked at a novel diagnostic test for ARVC. In this study, immunohistochemical labeling of plakoglobin proved to be a sensitive and specific method of differentiating ARVC from other cardiomyopathies *(103)*. If this result is confirmed in further study, this will be an invaluable tool for the notoriously difficult diagnosis of this disease.

CONCLUSIONS

Over the last decade, we have witnessed remarkable advances in our understanding of cardiac arrhythmia syndromes. These advances have stemmed from the discovery of mutations, primarily in ion channel genes, underlying inherited arrhythmia syndromes such as LQTS, Brugada syndrome, and familial AF. The recognition of the genetic substrate underlying these syndromes has provided remarkable insight into the molecular basis of arrhythmias.

Based on current knowledge, it is clear that many arrhythmia syndromes arise from abnormalities in the protein systems used by the heart to initiate and propagate the cardiac action potential. Until recently, much research has focused on abnormalities of ion channels that are intimately involved in depolarization and repolarization of the cell; however, proteins that affect intracellular ion storage and intercellular communication have now also been implicated in arrhythmogenesis. Importantly, even in the well-described inherited arrhythmia syndromes reviewed in this chapter, many patients with the disease phenotype do not have an identified mutation. This suggests that other basic genetic causes and cellular mechanisms remain obscure, and that, as demonstrated in the case of ANP and AF, further research may well identify novel pathways essential for the normal electrical function of the heart. While traditional candidate gene association studies have provided much of the knowledge of the genetic causes of arrhythmias to date, the recent availability of high-throughput resequencing and GWASs will likely identify novel genes and pathways. GWAS, by virtue of being inherently "agnostic," or free of any preconceived notions about mechanism, offer this possibility.

With greater understanding of the genetic and molecular mechanisms of arrhythmias comes the hope that we will then be better able to diagnose, counsel, and treat patients with these arrhythmia syndromes.

GENETICS GLOSSARY

Allele: Alternate form of a gene.
Alternative splicing: A regulatory mechanism by which variations in the incorporation of a gene's exons, or coding regions, into mRNA lead to the production of more than one related protein, or isoform.
Codon: A three-base sequence of DNA or RNA that specifies a single amino acid.

Conservative mutation: A change in a DNA or RNA sequence that leads to the replacement of one amino acid with a biochemically similar one.

Complex disease: Combining the effects of several gene(s) and environment; also referred to as multifactorial or polygenic.

Compound heterozygote: Carrying two different mutations for one gene, each provided by a different parent.

Exon: A region of a gene that codes for a protein.

Frameshift mutation: The addition or deletion of a number of DNA bases that is not a multiple of three, thus causing a shift in the reading frame of the gene. This shift leads to a change in the reading frame of all parts of the gene that are downstream from the mutation, often leading to a premature stop codon and ultimately, to a truncated protein.

Gain-of-function mutation: A mutation that produces a protein that takes on a new or enhanced function.

Gene dose effect: A relationship between the number of diseased alleles and phenotype severity.

Genomics: The study of functions and interactions of all the genes in the genome, including their interactions with environmental factors.

Genotype: The genetic makeup of an individual; it also refers to the alleles at a given locus.

Genetic heterogeneity: Mutations in several genes causing similar phenotype.

Haplotype: A group of nearby alleles that are inherited together.

Heterozygous: Carrying two different alleles of a given gene.

Homozygous: Carrying two identical alleles of a given gene.

Intron: A region of a gene that does not code for a protein.

Loss-of-function mutation: A mutation that decreases the production or function of a protein (or does both).

Locus: Location of a gene on a chromosome.

Missense mutation: Substitution of a single DNA base that results in a codon that specifies an alternative amino acid.

Monogenic: Caused by a mutation in a single gene.

Modifier gene: Genes that are not primarily responsible for a trait but alters a trait's expression or severity.

Nonsense mutation: Substitution of a single DNA base that results in a stop codon, thus leading to truncation of a protein.

Penetrance: The likelihood that a person carrying a particular mutant gene will have an altered phenotype.

ACKNOWLEDGEMENTS

Supported in part by grants from the United States Public Health Service (HL085690, HL092217, and U01 HL65962) and the AHA 0940116 N.

REFERENCES

1. Gudbjartsson DF, Arnar DO, Helgadottir A et al (2007) Variants conferring risk of atrial fibrillation on chromosome 4q25. Nature 488:353–357

2. Gudbjartsson DF, Holm H, Gretarsdottir S et al (2009) A sequence variant in ZFHX3 on 16q22 associates with atrial fibrillation and ischemic stroke. Nat Genet published online 13 July 2009

3. Jervell A, Lange-Nielsen F (1957) Congenital deaf-mutism, functional heart disease with prolongation of the Q-T interval and sudden death. Am Heart J 54:59–68

4. Romano C, Gemme G, Pongiglione R (1963) Rare cardiac arrhythmias of the pediatric age. Ii. Syncopal attacks due to paroxysmal ventricular fibrillation. Presentation of 1st case in Italian pediatric literature. Clin Pediatr (Bologna) 45:656–683

5. Ward OC (1964) A new familial cardiac syndrome in children. J Ir Med Assoc 54:103–106

6. Schwartz PJ, Periti M, Malliani A (1975) The long Q-T syndrome. Am Heart J 89:378–390

7. Schwartz PJ (2009) Cutting nerves and saving lives. Heart Rhythm 6:760–763

8. Moss AJ (1986) Prolonged QT-interval syndromes. JAMA 256:2985–2987

9. Wang Q, Shen J, Splawski I et al (1995) SCN5A mutations associated with an inherited cardiac arrhythmia, long QT syndrome. Cell 80:805–811

10. Curran ME, Splawski I, Timothy KW et al (1995) A molecular basis for cardiac arrhythmia: HERG mutations cause long QT syndrome. Cell 80:795–803

11. Wang Q, Curran ME, Splawski I et al (1996) Positional cloning of a novel potassium channel gene: KVLQT1 mutations cause cardiac arrhythmias. Nat Genet 12:17–23

12. Schulze-Bahr E, Wang Q, Wedekind H et al (1997) KCNE1 mutations cause Jervell and Lange-Nielsen syndrome. Nat Genet 17:267–268

13. Tyson J, Tranebjaerg L, Bellman S et al (1997) IsK and KvLQT1: mutation in either of the two subunits of the slow component of the delayed rectifier potassium channel can cause Jervell and Lange-Nielsen syndrome. Hum Mol Genet 6:2179–2185

14. Neyroud N, Tesson F, Denjoy I et al (1997) A novel mutation in the potassium channel gene KVLQT1 causes the Jervell and Lange-Nielsen cardioauditory syndrome. Nat Genet 15:186–189

15. Mohler PJ, Schott JJ, Gramolini AO et al (2003) Ankyrin-B mutation causes type 4 long-QT cardiac arrhythmia and sudden cardiac death. Nature 421:634–639

16. Mohler PJ, Splawski I, Napolitano C et al (2004) A cardiac arrhythmia syndrome caused by loss of ankyrin-B function. Proc Natl Acad Sci USA 101:9137–9142

17. Mohler PJ, Bennett V (2005) Ankyrin-based cardiac arrhythmias: a new class of channelopathies due to loss of cellular targeting. Curr Opin Cardiol 20:189–193

18. Tristani-Firouzi M, Jensen JL, Donaldson MR et al (2002) Functional and clinical characterization of KCNJ2 mutations associated with LQT7 (Andersen syndrome). J Clin Invest 110:381–388

19. Plaster NM, Tawil R, Tristani-Firouzi M et al (2001) Mutations in Kir2.1 cause the developmental and episodic electrical phenotypes of Andersen's syndrome. Cell 105:511–519

20. Zhang L, Benson DW, Tristani-Firouzi M et al (2005) Electrocardiographic features in Andersen-Tawil syndrome patients with KCNJ2 mutations: characteristic T-U-wave patterns predict the KCNJ2 genotype. Circulation 111:2720–2726

21. Splawski I, Timothy KW, Sharpe LM et al (2004) Ca(V)1.2 calcium channel dysfunction causes a multisystem disorder including arrhythmia and autism. Cell 119:19–31

22. Splawski I, Timothy KW, Decher N et al (2005) Severe arrhythmia disorder caused by cardiac L-type calcium channel mutations. Proc Natl Acad Sci USA 102:8089–8968

23. Moss AJ, Schwartz PJ (2005) 25th anniversary of the international long-QT syndrome registry: an ongoing quest to uncover the secrets of long-QT syndrome. Circulation 111:1199–1201

24. Splawski I, Shen J, Timothy KW et al (2000) Spectrum of mutations in long-QT syndrome genes. KVLQT1, HERG, SCN5A, KCNE1, and KCNE2. Circulation 102:1178–1185

25. Moss AJ, Zareba W, Benhorin J et al (1995) ECG T-wave patterns in genetically distinct forms of the hereditary long QT syndrome. Circulation 92:2929–2934

26. Zareba W, Moss AJ, Schwartz PJ et al (1998) Influence of genotype on the clinical course of the long-QT syndrome. International long-QT syndrome registry research group. N Engl J Med 339:960–965

27. Schwartz PJ, Priori SG, Spazzolini C et al (2001) Genotype-phenotype correlation in the long-QT syndrome: gene-specific triggers for life-threatening arrhythmias. Circulation 103:89–95

28. Shimizu W, Noda T, Takaki H et al (2004) Diagnostic value of epinephrine test for genotyping LQT1, LQT2, and LQT3 forms of congenital long QT syndrome. Heart Rhythm 276–283

29. Noda T, Takaki H, Kurita T et al (2002) Gene-specific response of dynamic ventricular repolarization to sympathetic stimulation in LQT1, LQT2 and LQT3 forms of congenital long QT syndrome. Eur Heart J 23:975–983

30. Moss AJ, Zareba W, Hall WJ et al (2000) Effectiveness and limitations of beta-blocker therapy in congenital long-QT syndrome. Circulation 101:616–623

31. Marx SO, Kurokawa J, Reiken S et al (2002) Requirement of a macromolecular signaling complex for beta adrenergic receptor modulation of the KCNQ1-KCNE1 potassium channel. Science 295:496–499

32. Sanguinetti MC, Jurkiewicz NK (1992) Role of external Ca^{2+} and K^+ in gating of cardiac delayed rectifier K^+ currents. Pflugers Arch 420:180–186

33. Compton SJ, Lux RL, Ramsey MR et al (1996) Genetically defined therapy of inherited long-QT syndrome. Correction of abnormal repolarization by potassium. Circulation 94:1018–1022

34. Etheridge SP, Compton SJ, Tristani-Firouzi M et al (2003) A new oral therapy for long QT syndrome: long-term oral potassium improves repolarization in patients with HERG mutations. J Am Coll Cardiol 42:1777–1782

35. Schwartz PJ, Priori SG, Locati EH et al (1995) Long QT syndrome patients with mutations of the SCN5A and HERG genes have differential responses to Na^+ channel blockade and to increases in heart rate. Implications for gene-specific therapy. Circulation 92:3381–3386

36. Shimizu W, Antzelevitch C (1997) Sodium channel block with mexiletine is effective in reducing dispersion of repolarization and preventing torsade des pointes in LQT2 and LQT3 models of the long-QT syndrome. Circulation 96:2038–2047

37. Shimizu W, Antzelevitch C (1998) Cellular basis for the ECG features of the LQT1 form of the long-QT syndrome: effects of beta-adrenergic agonists and antagonists and sodium channel blockers on transmural dispersion of repolarization and torsade de pointes. Circulation 98:2314–2322

38. Roden DM (1998) Taking the "idio" out of "idiosyncratic": predicting torsades de pointes. Pacing Clin Electrophysiol 21:1029–1034

39. Moss AJ, Zareba W, Kaufman ES et al (2002) Increased risk of arrhythmic events in long-QT syndrome with mutations in the pore region of the human ether-a-go-go-related gene potassium channel. Circulation 105:794–799

40. Shimizu W, Antzelevitch C (2000) Differential effects of beta-adrenergic agonists and antagonists in LQT1, LQT2 and LQT3 models of the long QT syndrome. J Am Coll Cardiol 35:778–786

41. Priori SG, Napolitano C, Schwartz PJ (1999) Low penetrance in the long-QT syndrome: clinical impact. Circulation 99:529–533

42. Schwartz PJ, Priori SG, Dumaine R et al (2000) A molecular link between the sudden infant death syndrome and the long-QT syndrome. N Engl J Med 343:262–267

43. Wolff L (1943) Familial auricular fibrillation. N England J Med 396–397

44. Fox CS, Parise H, D'Agostino RB Sr et al (2004) Parental atrial fibrillation as a risk factor for atrial fibrillation in offspring. JAMA 291:2851–2855

45. Darbar D, Herron KJ, Ballew JD et al (2003) Familial atrial fibrillation is a genetically heterogeneous disorder. J Am Coll Cardiol 41:2185–2192

46. Brugada R, Tapscott T, Czernuszewicz GZ et al (1997) Identification of a genetic locus for familial atrial fibrillation. N Engl J Med 336:905–911

47. Ellinor PT, Shin JT, Moore RK et al (2003) Locus for atrial fibrillation maps to chromosome 6q14–16. Circulation 107:2880–2883

48. Oberti C, Wang L, Li L et al (2004) Genome-wide linkage scan identifies a novel genetic locus on chromosome 5p13 for neonatal atrial fibrillation associated with sudden death and variable cardiomyopathy. Circulation 110: 3753–3759

49. Volders PG, Zhu Q, Timmermans C et al (2007) Mapping a novel locus for familial atrial fibrillation on chromosome 10p11-q21. Heart Rhythm 4:469–475

50. Darbar D, Hardy A, Haines JL et al (2008) Prolonged signal-averaged P-wave duration as an intermediate phenotype for familial atrial fibrillation. J Am Coll Cardiol 51:1083–1089

51. Chen YH, Xu SJ, Bendahhou S et al (2003) KCNQ1 gain-of-function mutation in familial atrial fibrillation. Science 299:251–254

52. Yang Y, Xia M, Jin Q et al (2004) Identification of a KCNE2 gain-of-function mutation in patients with familial atrial fibrillation. Am J Hum Genet 75:899–905

53. Olson TM, Alekseev AE, Liu XK et al (2006) Kv1.5 channelopathy due to KCNA5 loss-of-function mutation causes human atrial fibrillation. Hum Mol Genet 15:2185–2191

54. Darbar D, Yang T, Yang P et al (2006) KCNA5 loss-of-function implicates tyrosine kinase signaling in human atrial fibrillation. Circulation Res 99:3 (abstract)

55. Olson TM, Michels VV, Ballew JD et al (2005) Sodium channel mutations and susceptibility to heart failure and atrial fibrillation. JAMA 293:447–454

56. Darbar D, Kannankeril PJ, Donahue BS et al (2008) Cardiac sodium channel (SCN5A) variants associated with atrial fibrillation. Circulation 117:1927–1935

57. Ellinor PT, Nam EG, Shea MA et al (2008) Cardiac sodium channel mutation in atrial fibrillation. Heart Rhythm 5:99–105

58. Benito B, Brugada R, Perich RM et al (2008) A mutation in the sodium channel is responsible for the association of long QT syndrome and familial atrial fibrillation. Heart Rhythm 5:1434–1440

59. Gollob MH, Jones DL, Krahn AD et al (2006) Somatic mutations in the connexin 40 gene (GJA5) in atrial fibrillation. N Engl J Med 354:2677–2688

60. Hodgson-Zingman DM, Karst ML, Zingman LV et al (2008) Atrial natriuretic peptide frameshift mutation in familial atrial fibrillation. N Engl J Med 359:158–165

61. Abraham R, Yang T, Kucera G et al (2010) Augmented potassium current is associated with a shared phenotype across multiple genetic defects causing familial atrial fibrillation. J Mol Cell Cardiol 48:181–190

62. Kaab S, Darbar D, van Noord C et al (2009) Large scale replication and meta-analysis of variants on chromosome 4q25 associated with atrial fibrillation. Eur Heart J 30:813–819

63. Body S, Collard CD, Shernan KS et al (2009) Variation in the 4q25 Chromosomal Locus Predicts Atrial Fibrillation after Coronary Artery Bypass Graft Surgery. Circ Cardiovasc Genet 2:499–506

64. Tessari A, Pietrobon M, Notte A et al (2008) Myocardial Pitx2 differentially regulates the left atrial identity and ventricular asymmetric remodeling programs. Circ Res 102:813–822

65. Mommersteeg MT, Brown NA, Prall OW et al (2007) Pitx2c and Nkx2–5 are required for the formation and identity of the pulmonary myocardium. Circ Res 101:902–909

66. Haissaguerre M, Jais P, Shah DC et al (1998) Spontaneous initiation of atrial fibrillation by ectopic beats originating in the pulmonary veins. N Engl J Med 339:659–666

67. Chung MK, Van Wagoner DR, Smith JD et al (2008) Significant single nucleotide polymorphism associated with atrial fibrillation located on chromosome 4q25 in a whole genome association study and association with left atrial gene expression [abstract]. Circulation 118:S882

68. Brugada J, Brugada P, Brugada R (2002) The syndrome of right bundle branch block, ST segment elevation in V1 to V3 and sudden death. Cardiovasc Drugs Ther 16:25–27

69. Chen Q, Kirsch GE, Zhang D et al (1998) Genetic basis and molecular mechanism for idiopathic ventricular fibrillation. Nature 392:293–296

70. Deschenes I, Baroudi G, Berthet M et al (2000) Electrophysiological characterization of SCN5A mutations causing long QT (E1784K) and Brugada (R1512W and R1432G) syndromes. Cardiovasc Res 46:55–65

71. Valdivia CR, Tester DJ, Rok BA et al (2004) A trafficking defective, Brugada syndrome-causing SCN5A mutation rescued by drugs. Cardiovasc Res 62:53–62

72. Wang DW, Makita N, Kitabatake A et al (2000) Enhanced Na(+) channel intermediate inactivation in Brugada syndrome. Circ Res 87:E37–E43

73. Yan GX, Antzelevitch C (1999) Cellular basis for the Brugada syndrome and other mechanisms of arrhythmogenesis associated with ST-segment elevation. Circulation 100:1660–1666

74. Ruan Y, Liu N, Priori SG (2009) Sodium channel mutations and arrhythmias. Nat Rev Cardiol 6:337–348

75. Coronel R, Casini S, Koopmann TT et al (2005) Right ventricular fibrosis and conduction delay in a patient with clinical signs of Brugada syndrome: a combined electrophysiological, genetic, histopathologic, and computational study. Circulation 112:2769–2777

76. London B, Michalec M, Mehdi H et al (2007) Mutation in glycerol-3-phosphate dehydrogenase 1 like gene (GPD1-L) decreases cardiac Na$^+$ current and causes inherited arrhythmias. Circulation 116:2260–2268

77. Watanabe H, Koopmann TT, Le Scouarnec S et al (2008) Sodium channel beta1 subunit mutations associated with Brugada syndrome and cardiac conduction disease in humans. J Clin Invest 118:2260–2268

78. Antzelevitch C, Pollevick GD, Cordeiro JM et al (2007) Loss-of-function mutations in the cardiac calcium channel underlie a new clinical entity characterized by ST-segment elevation, short QT intervals, and sudden cardiac death. Circulation 115:442–449

79. Dumaine R, Towbin JA, Brugada P et al (1999) Ionic mechanisms responsible for the electrocardiographic phenotype of the Brugada syndrome are temperature dependent. Circ Res 85:803–809

80. Keller DI, Huang H, Zhao J et al (2006) A novel SCN5A mutation, F1344S, identified in a patient with Brugada syndrome and fever-induced ventricular fibrillation. Cardiovasc Res 70:521–529

81. Brugada R, Brugada J, Antzelevitch C et al (2000) Sodium channel blockers identify risk for sudden death in patients with ST-segment elevation and right bundle branch block but structurally normal hearts. Circulation 101:510–515

82. Reid DS, Tynan M, Braidwood L et al (1975) Bidirectional tachycardia in a child. A study using His bundle electrography. Br Heart J 37:339–344

83. Leenhardt A, Lucet V, Denjoy I et al (1995) Catecholaminergic polymorphic ventricular tachycardia in children. A 7-year follow-up of 21 patients. Circulation 91:1512–1519

84. Priori SG, Napolitano C, Tiso N, Memmi M, Vignati G, Bloise R, Sorrentino V, Danieli GA (2001) Mutations in the cardiac ryanodine receptor gene (hRyR2) underlie catecholaminergic polymorphic ventricular tachycardia. Circulation 103:196–200

85. Gyorke S (2009) Molecular basis of catecholaminergic polymorphic ventricular tachycardia. Heart Rhythm 6:123–129

86. Eldar M, Pras E, Lahat H (2002) A missense mutation in a highly conserved region of CASQ2 is associated with autosomal recessive catecholamine-induced polymorphic ventricular tachycardia in Bedouin families from Israel. Cold Spring Harb Symp Quant Biol 67:333–337

87. Postma AV, Denjoy I, Hoorntje TM et al (2002) Absence of calsequestrin 2 causes severe forms of catecholaminergic polymorphic ventricular tachycardia. Circ Res 91:e21–26

88. Watanabe H, Chopra N, Laver D et al (2009) Flecainide prevents catecholaminergic polymorphic ventricular tachycardia in mice and humans. Nat Med 15:380–383

89. Calkins H (2006) Arrhythmogenic right-ventricular dysplasia/cardiomyopathy. Curr Opin Cardiol 21:55–63

90. Tabib A, Loire R, Chalabreysse L et al (2003) Circumstances of death and gross and microscopic observations in a series of 200 cases of sudden death associated with arrhythmogenic right ventricular cardiomyopathy and/or dysplasia. Circulation 108:3000–3005

91. Corrado D, Basso C, Thiene G (2001) Sudden cardiac death in young people with apparently normal heart. Cardiovasc Res 50:399–408

92. McKenna WJ, Thiene G, Nava A et al (1994) Diagnosis of arrhythmogenic right ventricular dysplasia/cardiomyopathy. Task force of the working group myocardial and pericardial disease of the european society of cardiology and of the scientific council on cardiomyopathies of the international society and federation of cardiology. Br Heart J 71:215–218

93. Hamid MS, Norman M, Quraishi A et al (2002) Prospective evaluation of relatives for familial arrhythmogenic right ventricular cardiomyopathy/dysplasia reveals a need to broaden diagnostic criteria. J Am Coll Cardiol 40:1445–1450

94. Tiso N, Stephan DA, Nava A et al (2001) Identification of mutations in the cardiac ryanodine receptor gene in families affected with arrhythmogenic right ventricular cardiomyopathy type 2 (ARVD2). Hum Mol Genet 10:189–194

95. Rampazzo A, Nava A, Malacrida S et al (2002) Mutation in human desmoplakin domain binding to plakoglobin causes a dominant form of arrhythmogenic right ventricular cardiomyopathy. Am J Hum Genet 71:1200–1206

96. Gerull B, Heuser A, Wichter T et al (2004) Mutations in the desmosomal protein plakophilin-2 are common in arrhythmogenic right ventricular cardiomyopathy. Nat Genet 36:1162–1164

97. Pilichou K, Nava A, Basso C et al (2006) Mutations in desmoglein-2 gene are associated with arrhythmogenic right ventricular cardiomyopathy. Circulation 113:1171–1179

98. Heuser A, Plovie ER, Ellinor PT et al (2006) Mutant desmocollin-2 causes arrhythmogenic right ventricular cardiomyopathy. Am J Hum Genet 79:1081–1088

99. Beffagna G, Occhi G, Nava A et al (2005) Regulatory mutations in transforming growth factor-beta3 gene cause arrhythmogenic right ventricular cardiomyopathy type 1. Cardiovasc Res 65:366–373

100. McKoy G, Protonotarios N, Crosby A et al (2000) Identification of a deletion in plakoglobin in arrhythmogenic right ventricular cardiomyopathy with palmoplantar keratoderma and woolly hair (Naxos disease). Lancet 355:2119–2124

101. Awad MM, Calkins H, Judge DP (2008) Mechanisms of disease: molecular genetics of arrhythmogenic right ventricular dysplasia/cardiomyopathy. Nat Clin Pract Cardiovasc Med 5:258–267

102. Lahtinen AM, Lehtonen A, Kaartinen M et al (2008) Plakophilin-2 missense mutations in arrhythmogenic right ventricular cardiomyopathy. Int J Cardiol 126:92–100

103. Asimaki A, Tandri H, Huang H et al (2009) A new diagnostic test for arrhythmogenic right ventricular cardiomyopathy. N Engl J Med 360:1075–1084

III DIAGNOSTIC TESTING

5

Diagnosis of Arrhythmias
with Non-invasive Tools

*Renee M. Sullivan, Wei Wei Li, Arthur C. Kendig,
and Brian Olshansky*

CONTENTS

Abstract

Non-invasive tools play a crucial role in the diagnosis, evaluation, and management of virtually all patients suspected to have or who have had cardiac arrhythmias. These non-invasive tools can help determine the clinical significance and prognostic importance of the arrhythmia and can help assess risk of serious arrhythmic consequences including death. Based on a non-invasive assessment, the need for prophylactic and/or potentially interventional therapy can be better ascertained. We provide a comprehensive, yet, concise overview of non-invasive tools to address practical, important, and contemporaneous issues

From: *Contemporary Cardiology: Management of Cardiac Arrhythmias*
Edited by: Gan-Xin Yan, Peter R. Kowey, DOI 10.1007/978-1-60761-161-5_5
© Springer Science+Business Media, LLC 2011

with a focus on patient management. We emphasize strategies to approach challenging clinical scenarios and address how monitoring adds value in specific clinical situations.

Key Words: Non-invasive tools; non-invasive evaluation; history and physical; electrocardiography; in-hospital telemetry; Holter monitor; event recorder; minimally invasive implantable loop recorder; transtelephonic monitoring; exercise testing; signal averaged electrocardiogram; T-wave alternans; heart rate variability; baroreflex sensitivity; heart rate turbulence; arrhythmia; use of non-invasive tools in diagnosis; assessment; prognosis; surveillance; treatment/response to therapy; risk stratification.

INTRODUCTION

A number of early ideas have led to the concept of breaking away from the limitations of orthodox electrocardiography to solve the scientific problem of adequate sampling and the medical problem of obtaining electrocardiograms in situations other than the highly artificial and unrealistic situation of resting quietly on a comfortable pad after a good sleep, with no breakfast, and with calm confidence in one's physician.

— Norman J. Holter (1961) (1)

Written decades ago, the words of Norman J. Holter revolutionized medicine by bringing forth the idea of ambulatory non-invasive cardiac monitoring. What originally began as a method to monitor heart rhythm "giving the subject the greatest possible freedom of activity" *(1)* has lead to the development of various technologies to capture cardiac data for diagnostic and prognostic purposes. Still today, when it comes to arrhythmia management, establishing a diagnosis remains the critical first step before considering any therapy. Non-invasive recording tools continue to be the principal diagnostic agents, but little focus is given to their proper use. This curious disconnect reflects a basic assumption that the use of non-invasive techniques is well established and self-evident. Nothing could be further from the truth. Some of these tools are used with reckless and purposeless abandon, while others are almost never considered, even for appropriate purposes.

Guidelines *(2–8)* regarding arrhythmia management include recommendations for the use of non-invasive tools. Recent technological enhancements have emerged to expand and modify the armamentarium of available tools. The role of non-invasive tools is being redefined as evidence from clinical trials has emerged. Ironically, non-invasive assessment is often dictated by individual clinical conditions rather than consensus or controlled clinical trials. This chapter addresses available non-invasive tools for arrhythmia diagnosis and management and provides a framework for their use in the practical care of patients.

WHAT ARE NON-INVASIVE DIAGNOSTIC ARRHYTHMIA TOOLS?

Non-invasive tools record cardiac electrical activity from the body surface (Table 1). Data are obtained while patients are engaged in their usual activities, making cardiovascular evaluation possible under physical, psychological, and neurohumoral conditions typical for each patient. They remain the "gold standard" by which a definitive arrhythmia diagnosis is possible, as linking an arrhythmia to a symptom can be diagnostic.

The use of the tools does not end there. They can diagnose dangerous arrhythmias during which a patient may have no symptoms (Fig. 1). Also, they can provide prognostic information to help pinpoint an individual's risk of ventricular tachyarrhythmias, sudden cardiac death, arrhythmic death, and total mortality. Moreover, non-invasive monitoring can be used as a surveillance tool to identify problematic – but asymptomatic – arrhythmias (e.g., atrial fibrillation) that may be otherwise difficult to detect.

Non-invasive tools include the electrocardiogram and monitoring systems such as Holter monitors, event recorders, in-hospital telemetry, and the minimally invasive implantable loop recorder. Other novel approaches have been developed to assess and process subtle signals present on the electrocardiogram, namely the signal averaged electrocardiogram (SAECG) and T wave alternans (TWA). Provocative maneuvers, such as exercise testing, can be used to secure a diagnosis or predict prognosis. Further, recorded information can be processed and, based on specific algorithms, be used to better understand autonomic and other effects on the risk of arrhythmic or sudden cardiac death. These approaches include assessment of heart rate turbulence, heart rate variability (HRV), and baroreflex sensitivity (BRS).

Table 1
Advantages, Disadvantages, and Uses of Non-Invasive Tools for Diagnosis and Management of Arrhythmias

Tools	Advantages	Disadvantages	Uses
Electrocardiography	– Diagnosis of arrhythmia or evaluation of baseline EKG abnormalities – May determine focus of arrhythmia from 12 lead recording if captured during rhythm disturbance – Easily accessible, inexpensive, safe	– Short recording period making it possible to miss arrhythmia – Obscuration of electrical data from body surface (poor lead placement, body habitus) – Artifact is possible	– All cases of arrhythmia or potential arrhythmia
Telemetry	– Multi-channel, real-time, full disclosure monitoring – Data sent to central work station – Correlation of symptoms with arrhythmia – Technology allows patients to be ambulatory – Alarm systems alert to presence of arrhythmia – Heart rate, rhythm, and other trends may be reviewed	– Recordings may represent artifact – Recordings may not correlate with symptoms – It is possible to miss a true arrhythmia if alarm does not sound – Recordings require careful scrutiny by trained personnel	– Patients admitted for evaluation of arrhythmia or those with underlying conditions which may predispose to arrhythmia – Determination of heart rate and rhythm – Monitors pacemakers and ICDs
Holter monitor	– 24 or 48 h evaluation with timestamps and event markers – Records without patient activation – Multiple channels are recorded to decrease possibility of artifact – Recordings are analyzed automatically but require short period of over reading by personnel – Heart rate, PR interval, QT interval, QRS width, pacemaker function, and heart rate variability may be determined	– Spontaneous variability in rhythm may allow for arrhythmia to be missed during monitoring period – Recordings may represent artifact – Patient recorded diaries are essential in correlating symptoms with rhythm disturbance; hence patient must be cooperative	– Patients with symptoms that might represent arrhythmia which occur almost daily – Patients with pacemakers or ICDs to determine if programmed settings are adequate – Surveillance of asymptomatic arrhythmia after therapy initiated

(Continued)

Table 1
(Continued)

Tools	Advantages	Disadvantages	Uses
Event monitor	– Evaluation over a longer period than Holter monitor, usually 30 days – Looping monitors record by patient activation or auto-triggering by pre-determined parameters – Nonlooping recorders are beneficial in patients with infrequent symptoms who can activate the monitor quickly – Data is sent to central location and physician alerted if serious arrhythmia or symptoms	– Could potentially delay diagnosis given length of monitoring period – Patient triggering of events requires cooperative patient who is not abruptly incapacitated – Landline phone required to transmit data accurately	– Patients with symptoms that occur on at least a monthly basis – Surveillance of arrhythmia therapy
Minimally invasive monitor	– Evaluation for longer periods of time, often 1–2 years – Data may be sent transtelephonically	– Single lead recording may be fraught with artifact – Requires surgical implantation	– Patients with unexplained syncope thought due to arrhythmia
Transtelephonic monitoring of pacemakers and ICDs	– Takes advantage of already implanted devices to give information about arrhythmias or the device itself – Information may be obtained over the phone	– None	– Patients with pacemakers or ICDs, to assess symptoms, function of devices, or cause for defibrillation
Exercise testing	– Attempts to reproduce activity so that arrhythmia may be provoked in patients with symptoms upon exercise	– Not all arrhythmias may be reproduced in this manner; some are induced only by other forms of activity	– Patients with symptoms with activity

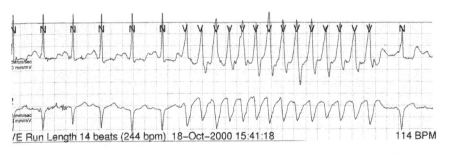

Fig. 1. Event monitor with ventricular tachycardia in a 58-year-old man with dilated cardiomyopathy and a left ventricular ejection fraction of 30% for the past 6 months. He reported intermittent dizziness prior to the monitor being placed but reported no symptoms with this arrhythmia.

Non-invasive approaches are moving in the direction of seamless integration with the electronic medical record. Transtelephonic transmission and internet data transfer can provide extensive and detailed rhythm information. This improves convenience for both the clinician and the patient, and with prompt data transfer in real time, can further enhance efficient delivery of therapy and safety for the patient.

Although their potential benefits are legion, non-invasive tools have drawbacks. For one, spontaneous variability may result in a non-diagnostic test even with prolonged recordings. Second, it is possible that an arrhythmia is either present but not linked to symptoms (and ultimately is of little clinical consequence) (Fig. 2), or is present during a symptom but is not its cause. The attempt to link an asymptomatic finding to a symptom is common and remains a concern because a presumptive diagnostic maneuver can be fraught with error. Even if a rhythm diagnosis is established, the mechanism of the symptom, assumed to be related to the arrhythmia, may not be clear (e.g., neurocardiogenic syncope and relative bradycardia). Third, in some instances, prolonged non-invasive outpatient monitoring may ultimately not be beneficial if the suspected arrhythmia is immediately life-threatening. Fourth, patient compliance is a factor that is difficult to control, even with implantable loop recorders (e.g., not recording symptoms). Finally, artifacts due to non-cardiac muscle potentials or motion may complicate diagnostic assessment. Risk assessment using non-invasive tools is far from foolproof.

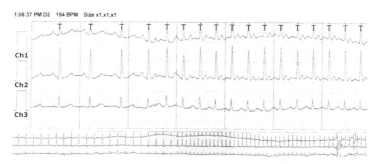

Fig. 2. Event monitor from a 48-year-old female with palpitations. Recording shows sinus rhythm with development of narrow complex tachycardia. The patient had no symptoms at the time of the recording.

Invasive evaluation and/or treatment may be necessary based on, or in lieu of, non-invasive results. Unlike an extended non-invasive approach, a primary invasive strategy can provide answers quickly, but the results may be "non-clinical" and of no clear significance. Provocative invasive arrhythmia induction by electrophysiological testing, for example, may not explain symptoms or even provide data of prognostic importance. Nonetheless, non-invasive and invasive strategies can have a synergistic role but should be used strategically, based upon an individual's clinical presentation.

Another important use of non-invasive tools is to evaluate the response to therapy and aid in better characterizing symptoms that occur after an apparent definitive therapy is delivered (e.g., palpitations after curative ablation). Non-invasive tools can also be used to determine the efficacy of a therapy even if the goals are not to reduce symptoms. For instance, if rate control is the treatment strategy for a patient with atrial fibrillation, an ambulatory monitor can evaluate the heart rate during routine activity and assess the need for further therapy to prevent the development of tachycardia-mediated cardiomyopathy or symptoms of heart failure (Fig. 3).

Likewise, non-invasive techniques may serve as surveillance tools in patients with asymptomatic arrhythmias *(9)*. For example, after atrial fibrillation ablation, a monitor can assess the subsequent

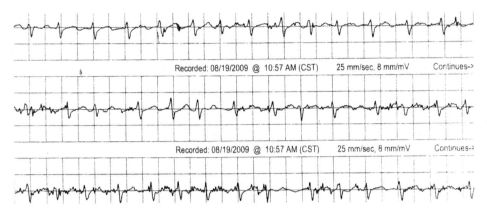

Fig. 3. Holter monitor recording from a 46-year-old female with atrial fibrillation, here with a rapid ventricular rate. The heart rate was 72 in the clinic, but a Holter monitor was placed to assess the quality of rate control. As a result of the Holter monitor, medications were adjusted.

Heart Rate Data						Ventricular Ectopy		
Total Beats	:	252002				Total VE Beats	:	37569 (14.9%)
Min HR	:	71 BPM at 10:54:00 PM				Vent Runs	:	7
Avg HR	:	88 BPM				Beats	:	34
Max HR	:	150 BPM at 12:46:12 PM				Longest	:	7 Beats at 8:21:52 AM
Heart Rate Variability						Fastest	:	156 BPM at 4:14:55 PM
						Triplets	:	245 Events
ASDNN 5	:	58.2 msec				Couplets	:	804 Events
SDANN 5	:	84.8 msec				Single/Interp PVC	:	14528/0
SDNN	:	132.3 msec				R on T	:	0
ST Episode Analysis						Single/Late VE's	:	223/29
		Ch1	Ch2	Ch3		Bi/Trigeminy	:	19263/1149 Beats
Min ST Level	:	-0.6	-3.7	-4.8		**Supraventricular Ectopy**		
Max ST Level	:	2.2	-0.1	-0.9		Total SVE Beats	:	692 (0.3%)
ST Episodes	:	0	0	6		Atrial Runs	:	0
Pacer Analysis						Beats	:	0
						Longest	:	0
Single Paced Beats	:	-				Fastest	:	0 BPM
Dual Paced Beats	:	-				Atrial Pairs	:	2 Events
Fusion Beats	:	-				Drop/Late	:	0/107
Atrial Fibrillation						Longest N-N	:	1.2 sec at 6:46:27 AM
						Single PAC's	:	36
AFib Beats	:	211053 (83.8%)				Bi/Trigeminy	:	545/0 Beats
AFib Duration	:	2436.3 min						

Fig. 4. Holter monitor recording in a 68-year-old male with asymptomatic atrial fibrillation after atrial fibrillation ablation. The monitor shows that 83.8% of total beats are atrial fibrillation, with a maximum rate of 150 beats per minute. Ventricular ectopy with ventricular tachycardia is also noted. The patient reported no symptoms during the monitoring period.

burden of atrial fibrillation as morbidity and mortality may be dependent on the continued presence of the arrhythmia despite lack of subsequent symptoms *(10)* (Fig. 4). Monitoring may also help plan strategies for concomitant therapy, such as anticoagulation *(11–13)*. Clinicians can also utilize the results of non-invasive tests for risk stratification and establishment of prognosis in patients with symptoms or with specific underlying conditions that predispose to arrhythmias.

INITIAL ARRHYTHMIA ASSESSMENT – HISTORY AND PHYSICAL EXAMINATION

A thorough history and physical examination are the pillars on which to build a solid evaluation. The information gathered may establish a diagnosis, determine the impact of symptoms on a patient's life and the need for further assessment, as well as target selection of the proper non-invasive diagnostic modality. The "H&P" also provides clues to a patient's compliance with diagnostic interventions and treatment.

The history should include a description of symptoms, including their frequency, severity, duration, and context *(14)*. If symptoms occur daily, for instance, short-term but continuous non-invasive monitoring such as a 24 or 48 h Holter monitor would be the best choice. Alternatively, if symptoms occur once a month, a 30-day event monitor would be more likely to document an episode.

Some modern monitoring devices can combine the capabilities of a Holter monitor with that of a long-term recorder. If the symptoms are long-lasting, a patient-activated short-term event recorder that requires only intermittent connection to the patient is the best option. For those who have an occasional difficult to record symptom, an automatically triggered or patient-activated endless loop recorder can be utilized. This is especially true for a patient with syncope who is unable to attach the recorder for any meaningful recording after the fact. Technology is evolving with mobile cardiac telemetry *(15–16)*.

If a patient reports incapacitating, dangerous, or potentially life-threatening symptoms, in-hospital evaluation is most appropriate. For such a patient, long-term non-invasive testing would not be initially recommended and an invasive strategy, if predictive and potentially diagnostic, would be preferable.

Careful characterization of symptoms, including a description of their onset and recovery, may provide important diagnostic clues that can help shape the subsequent evaluation. An irregular rhythm of sudden onset may represent atrial fibrillation or frequent ventricular ectopy. Episodic "skipped" beats are likely atrial or ventricular ectopy. A fast regular rhythm that includes a sensation of neck pounding is likely AV node reentry tachycardia *(17–18)*. A regular rapid rhythm without such pounding in the neck is more likely AV reentry, atrial, sinoatrial reentry, or ventricular tachycardia *(18)*.

An exhaustive past medical history may also provide clues, and patients should be queried to ascertain if co-morbid conditions that predispose to arrhythmia, such as a history of arrhythmias, structural heart disease (including coronary disease), cardiomyopathy, or cardiac transplant, are present, which can further help to focus the subsequent non-invasive assessment strategy. Medications used at the time of symptoms may predispose to an arrhythmia or affect its clinical presentation *(14)*. Furthermore, the family history can be crucial if there is a history of sudden cardiac death, Brugada syndrome, long QT interval syndrome, atrial fibrillation, or other such conditions that may explain a patient's symptoms and define risk. Data from prior assessments including careful analysis of old records (including those from other institutions and physicians) can assist the clinician in better understanding the complaints a patient may have in relation to symptoms.

Physical examination including properly determined vital signs (including an orthostatic assessment), presence or absence of a murmur and/or gallop and evidence for congestive heart failure based on neck veins, lower extremity edema, and lung sounds may better define the problem and further focus subsequent non-invasive assessment.

In summary, with a careful initial assessment similar to what is outlined here, non-invasive tools may then be used to correlate and better understand the link between a patient's symptoms and an arrhythmia.

ELECTROCARDIOGRAPHY

When an arrhythmia is suspected, a 12 lead surface electrocardiographic recording can facilitate diagnosis. Some arrhythmias are more evident during a 12 lead recording. A disadvantage of the 12 lead electrocardiogram (ECG) recording is that it represents only a small-time aliquot that may not be adequate to make a diagnosis. In addition, patient body habitus, artifact, and other factors may prove this evaluation difficult. An esophageal recording, although rarely used, may assist in determining atrial activity to better clarify an arrhythmia mechanism *(19, 20)*.

If the arrhythmia has ceased, additional clues may be evident (e.g., Wolff-Parkinson-White pattern, a long QT interval, a myocardial infarction, Brugada pattern, ventricular hypertrophy, or evidence for arrhythmogenic right ventricular cardiomyopathy). The presence of a myocardial infarction or a bundle branch block in a patient with syncope may indicate the presence of asystole, AV block, or ventricular tachycardia. Arrhythmias may persist in patients with prior symptoms. Reflex hemodynamic adjustments can transform syncopal ventricular tachycardia into a well-tolerated rhythm with resolution of symptoms.

Advanced electrocardiographic methods using body surface potential mapping provide a detailed method to analyze electrical activation. Utilizing up to 180 chest wall points, the location of an accessory pathway or the site of origin of a focal tachycardia can be mapped *(21)*. Perhaps such a method can ultimately facilitate curative and even non-invasive ablative procedures. Although such technology has been explored, no practical application for body surface potential mapping has yet emerged.

Twelve lead electrocardiography is an easily accessible, useful, safe and inexpensive initial study when an arrhythmia is suspected.

IN-HOSPITAL TELEMETRY

The advent of continuous electrocardiographic recording by hard-wired telemetry was the impetus that led to development of modern intensive care units *(22)*. It became evident that recognition and urgent treatment of life-threatening arrhythmias can improve outcomes, especially if monitors are watched *(23)*.

Since then, modern telemetry monitoring has transformed medical care by providing multi-channel, real-time, full-disclosure arrhythmia monitoring. Telemetry monitoring is possible from a central workstation where all signals are transmitted. Patients need not be hard-wired to a bedside monitor, but can be ambulatory. Modern equipment has noise reduction software and requires less policing as alarm systems triggered by pre-programmed and manually selected arrhythmia specifications are effective and generally reliable. Recordings can be stored for off-line playback and analysis. Efforts have been made to integrate this information into the electronic medical record.

Various telemetry monitoring systems exist. While a standard 12 lead electrocardiogram can provide detailed information about QRS morphology and AV relationships to help diagnose an arrhythmia, such continuous inpatient monitoring is simply not feasible. Inpatient monitoring systems instead rely on the use of a limited number of electrodes placed strategically on the chest. Many modern systems can derive a 12 lead ECG from the recorded data.

The simplest portable inpatient monitoring is a 3-electrode bipolar lead system that utilizes leads I, II, and III, or a modified chest lead (MCL1). While this allows for detection of heart rate and rhythm analysis, without a true V1 lead, this approach is less sensitive in diagnosing bundle branch block, confirming appropriate right ventricular pacing, and distinguishing supraventricular from ventricular tachycardia *(24)*.

The 5-electrode approach is the most common in telemetry monitoring. In this method, four limb leads and one precordial lead are used. This system has the advantage of easy accessibility to the chest for physical exam, x-rays, and cardiac resuscitation. The limb leads, moved to the torso, create fewer artifacts. While the exact position of the electrodes may differ, one validated method, the EASI™ system, is used commonly *(25)*. In this configuration, electrodes are placed at the upper sternum, lower sternum at the fifth intercostal space, the right and left midaxillary lines at the fifth intercostal space, and a "ground" lead anywhere on the chest. A derived 12 lead ECG can be generated from this arrangement.

In-hospital telemetry is an invaluable tool. It can be used to determine heart rate, diagnose arrhythmias, and record pacemaker or ICD activity or malfunction. Most importantly, it can record life-threatening arrhythmias and alert clinicians who then must respond in a timely manner to administer Advanced Cardiac Life Support (ACLS) when appropriate. Telemetry helps manage patients with arrhythmias by recording and highlighting arrhythmia events and by following trends in arrhythmia burden and heart rate. Careful review is possible during off-line assessment.

In many hospitals, telemetry monitoring is expected, and even mandated, in virtually every patient on a cardiovascular service (despite lack of indication in many cases). Monitoring may benefit those with recent onset heart failure, unstable cardiac conditions (hypotension, critical aortic stenosis, left main lesion), resuscitation from cardiac arrest, syncope of uncertain etiology, post-myocardial infarction, post-operative from cardiac surgery, diagnosed but uncontrolled arrhythmia (rapid rates in atrial fibrillation), recent arrhythmia with or without a pacemaker or ICD device, and post-catheter ablation. Patients admitted to other medical and surgical services may derive benefit if their primary issue is noncardiac but have cardiovascular complications or a significant history of life-threatening arrhythmias.

Overall, patients admitted with suspected arrhythmias or those who have risk for life-threatening problems are those most likely to benefit from inpatient monitoring. Recent recommendations have been published *(26)*. In terms of monitoring patients with an implanted pacemaker or ICD, indications include significant symptoms, arrhythmias, shocks, suspected malfunction, or other instability that requires continuous telemetry assessment. Ultimately, the decision to use monitoring is a clinical one as little hard data support outcomes benefits for many who are suspected of requiring telemetry monitoring.

All telemetry monitors were not created equal *(27)*, and monitoring itself can lead to potential harm. Arrhythmias recorded but not related to clinical events may be non-specific, confusing, or even dangerous as they can lead to inappropriate and unnecessary care. Artifacts can be mistaken for life-threatening ventricular arrhythmias, leading to inappropriate ICD implantation *(28)* (Fig. 5).

Although not commonly harmful, telemetry monitoring may not always be helpful. For instance, a given recording may be non-diagnostic, and if poorly tolerated arrhythmias are not detected, acted upon, and treated promptly, even the best system will have no impact. While technology has advanced,

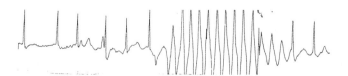

Fig. 5. A 52-year-old man was admitted to the hospital for evaluation of chest pain. In-hospital telemetry showed atrial fibrillation with the development of a wide complex tachycardia thought to be ventricular tachycardia. An electrophysiology consult was called for evaluation of ventricular tachycardia, but review of the strip showed atrial fibrillation with artifact. No further treatment for the heart rhythm was required.

it alone cannot manage the recorded arrhythmias; advanced technology is not necessarily coupled with improved implementation of advanced therapy.

In addition to potential harm or uselessness, telemetry monitoring can be a liability, can be ignored, and can be an unnecessary expense. Proper monitoring may not occur even if continuous recordings are made throughout the hospital stay. Problems with artifact *(29)*, signal loss, and issues of copious false alarms simply blending into the background noise of a hospital unit may lead to a lack of attention to specific alarms and increase the liability of missing true alarms. Often, telemetry is not carefully scrutinized by nurses or physicians. While immediate availability of resuscitation equipment is necessary on wards with telemetry monitoring, just being monitored and prepared does not necessarily change outcomes. A recent study of hospital variation in defibrillation times for in-hospital cardiac arrests showed there was often a delay in defibrillation (>2 min from onset of cardiac arrest). With the exception of the ICU setting, there was no significant difference in defibrillation time among patients on telemetry or non-telemetry units *(30)*. While not completely explained, this finding demonstrates the need for prompt arrhythmia recognition and subsequent treatment to improve outcomes (Fig. 6).

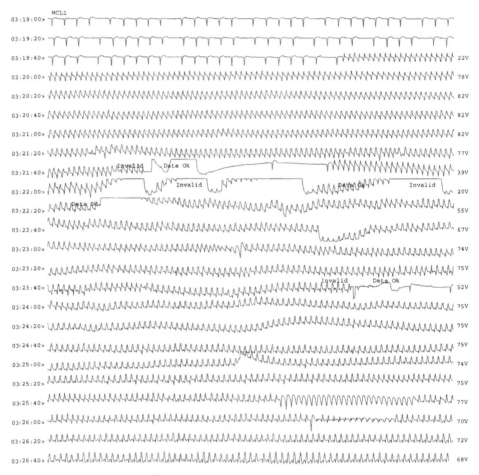

Fig. 6. In-hospital telemetry includes full disclosure recordings. This 75-year-old man was admitted for acute coronary syndrome. His heart rhythm changed from sinus rhythm with Mobitz I to ventricular tachycardia that goes unnoticed by staff for several minutes. The patient was asymptomatic, hemodynamically stable, and converted to sinus rhythm with lidocaine.

Table 2
Indications for In-Hospital Telemetry Monitoring for Arrhythmia Assessment *(24, 155)*

Class I indications: Patients at significant risk of immediate, life-threatening arrhythmia
- Post-resuscitation from cardiac arrest while cause is being determined and treatment is being initiated
- Minimum of 24 h after uncomplicated acute MI or for at least 24 h after complications have resolved
- Unstable angina or "rule out" myocardial infarction, until infarction is ruled out and patient is symptom free for 24 h
- Newly diagnosed left main or equivalent disease prior to revascularization
- After uncomplicated cardiac surgery for 48–72 h
- After coronary angioplasty or stenting for at least 24 h, especially if procedural complications
- Patients with intra-aortic balloon pump
- Until definitive therapy is initiated in patients requiring temporary transvenous or transcutaneous pacemakers
- After implantation of pacemaker or defibrillator for 12–24 h
- Mobitz II, advanced second degree AV block, complete heart block, or new onset bundle branch block
- Complete heart block or long sinus pauses with sick sinus syndrome as patients are predisposed to torsades de pointes
- Until definitive management in patients with arrhythmias exhibiting rapid antegrade conduction over accessory pathway
- Patients with long QT interval
- Patients receiving drugs which may prolong the QT interval (48–72 h for quinidine, procainamide, disopyramide, sotalol, dofetilide and 4–5 h for ibutilide)
- Patients admitted for drug overdose with proarrhythmic agent, until drug levels decrease and there is no prolonged QT or arrhythmia
- Patients with acute heart failure or pulmonary edema
- Indications for ICU management
- Patients undergoing conscious sedation
- Metabolic derangements which may predispose to arrhythmia

Class II indications: May be beneficial but not essential for all patients
- Patients with recent MI (monitoring > 48 h may help predict mortality if patient has arrhythmia at that time)
- Chest pain without ECG changes or elevated biomarkers
- Uncomplicated non-urgent coronary intervention (at least 6–8 h after stent and 12–24 h after angioplasty)
- Not pacemaker dependent with spontaneous rhythm in absence of pacing that does not cause hemodynamic instability (should monitor 12–24 h post procedure to assure pacing function and programming are appropriate)
- Uncomplicated arrhythmia ablation (12–24 h after prolonged rapid heart rates from incessant tachycardia and patients with organic heart disease who underwent VT ablation)
- Immediately after coronary angiography as vasovagal reaction possible
- Subacute heart failure while medications, device therapy, or both are being altered
- Patients with syncope when there is suspicion for arrhythmic cause or an EP disorder (monitor 24–48 h or until arrhythmic cause has been ruled out by invasive EP testing)
- Symptomatic palliative care patients, when adjustments in medications will increase comfort
- Patients with history of prolonged QT who require medications which may increase risk of torsades de pointes
- Patients with subarachnoid hemorrhage (predisposition to QT prolongation but rarely torsades)

Class III indications
- Post-operative patients at low risk of arrhythmia
- Obstetric patients without heart disease
- Permanent, rate controlled atrial fibrillation
- Hemodialysis
- Stable patients with chronic PVCs

In a time of austerity, the critical question of which patients require, and truly benefit from, telemetry monitoring has not yet been answered definitively. Despite this, consensus recommendations have emerged (Table 2). It is likely that important advances in telemetry monitoring may help provide enhanced continuous online recordings for more efficient and rapid diagnostic assessment followed by effective therapeutic intervention. For this to translate into better patient outcomes, clinicians adept at arrhythmia management must take responsibility for effective and rapid patient care. Perhaps, centralized telemetry control will be required.

HOLTER MONITORING

The first advance in diagnostic outpatient ambulatory electrocardiographic monitoring was the Holter monitor created by Norman "Jeff" Holter in 1961 (1). The original Holter monitor was bulky (85 pounds) and could only record a single electrocardiographic channel over 10 h on a reel-to-reel cassette tape. The evaluation and assessment was complex and time-consuming. Ambulatory monitors have since advanced to become more diminutive battery-operated digital devices that can record multiple electrocardiographic channels continuously over 24–48 h coupled with timestamps and event markers. Symptom diaries have been an integral part of the process of Holter monitor recordings, in that patients can press a button at the time they have symptoms and document what they experience to allow for arrhythmia/symptom correlation.

Holter monitors have also become less arduous to analyze. Digital data acquisition and storage has advanced with enhanced quality, length of recordings, accuracy, and reliability of interpretation. Automatic analysis of the full data set is performed, but a manual over read is generally completed from compressed data. A 24-h monitor can generally be reviewed manually in 20 min by an experienced clinician.

The present standard monitor analysis reports average, minimum, and maximum heart rate, in addition to the presence and morphology of atrial and ventricular ectopy, nonsustained atrial and ventricular arrhythmias (including atrial flutter and fibrillation), AV block, QT interval, and asystole/pauses. Holter monitors generally record three leads (lead II, V1, and V5, for example), but a 12 lead ECG can be derived from the recorded multichannel information (31).

Heart rate, PR and QT intervals, as well as QRS width and pacing can be assessed accurately. Thus, even individual beats of recorded arrhythmias can be classified by morphology, which then can be used to evaluate the approach to treatment. For instance, if ventricular premature complexes have a single morphology, their focus can potentially be targeted and ablated, if necessary (32) (Fig. 7). The information can also be used to derive heart rate variability and can signal average multiple beats. Ultimately, a Holter monitor may be used to assess T wave alternans or QT dispersion, but this requires high-resolution data acquisition (33).

There are several limitations to Holter monitoring. Recording of artifact, mostly related to motion and lead attachment, is a concern. Another limitation is missing an arrhythmia due to spontaneous variability within the limits of the Holter recording. As such, arrhythmias that occur frequently and reproducibly are most likely to be recorded.

The ambulatory monitor provides continuous recordings. It is best suited to evaluate short-lived arrhythmias frequent enough to be detected in the recorded time with the goal of linking the rhythm to the symptom and/or a specific diagnosis (Fig. 8). Recent developments in technology enhance recording time by coupling continuous Holter recording to subsequent event recordings if detection is not possible in a short-time window.

Findings from Holter monitoring may provide prognostic data, but there are limitations. For one, determination of risks from ventricular ectopy and nonsustained ventricular tachycardia are disease dependent. Frequent PVCs (>10/h) are a concern regarding risk for sudden death in post-myocardial

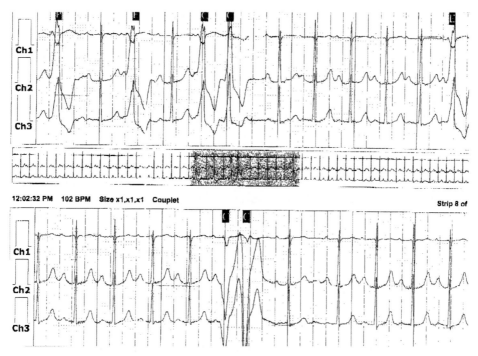

Fig. 7. Holter monitor recordings show two distinct morphologies of premature ventricular contractions (PVCs). The patient was referred to the electrophysiology clinic for evaluation of PVCs. He was asymptomatic at the time of these tracings, had a normal left ventricular ejection fraction and no structural heart disease by echocardiogram, and was treated with beta-blockers.

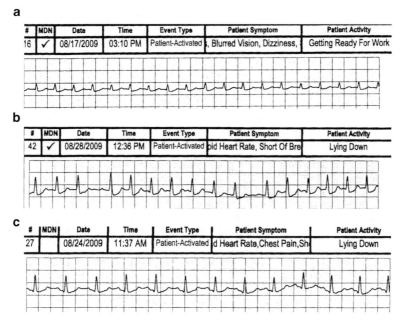

Fig. 8. Holter monitor recordings from a 19-year-old female reporting symptoms with tachycardia. Figure (**a**) shows narrow complex tachycardia consistent with AVNRT. Figure (**b**) depicts atrial tachycardia with AV block. Figure (**c**) demonstrates sinus tachycardia. She underwent ablation of AVNRT and atrial tachycardia and is currently symptom-free.

infarction patients, but may not be in other clinical scenarios *(34–36)*. Mortality is associated with frequency and "complexity" (couplets, triplets, non-sustained ventricular tachycardia) of PVCs especially in patients with ischemic heart disease and impaired left ventricular function *(37, 38)*. The reproducibility of abnormalities from one Holter monitor to another is low; and for a drug to show ventricular ectopy suppression, the reduction in frequency must be at least 90%. The assumption that suppression of ectopic beats would improve prognosis proved incorrect.

Ectopy serves as a marker of risk, but suppression by an antiarrhythmic drug did not improve, and, in fact, could substantially worsen survival *(39–42)*. As identification of ventricular ectopy lacks sensitivity and specificity to predict outcome, and as suppression of ectopy does not improve survival, interest in the prognostic utility of Holter monitoring has waned and remains low. Other prognostic information can be detected by ambulatory monitor recordings, such as heart rate variability and turbulence, but currently Holter recordings are rarely used for this purpose *(43)*.

Holter monitoring is generally utilized to detect the cause for symptoms and diagnose rhythm disturbances. Unfortunately, a Holter monitor is often either prescribed for the wrong condition (when yield is likely low to detect an arrhythmia) or when the chance to correlate a symptom to an arrhythmia is unlikely. An example is using Holter monitoring to diagnose the cause for syncope. The chance of making a diagnosis by Holter monitor is low (less than 3%, in some studies) depending on patient

Table 3
Indications for Ambulatory Electrocardiography in Assessment of Arrhythmia or Determination of Therapy Efficacy *(2)*

Class I
- Evaluation of pre-syncope, syncope, episodic dizziness in patients without obvious cause
- Evaluation of palpitations that are unexplained and recurrent
- Assessment of response to antiarrhythmic drug in patients with reproducible and frequent arrhythmia
- Evaluation of palpitations or other symptoms in patients with pacemakers to assess device function and to assist in programming rate responsive features and mode switching
- Assessment of potential device failure when interrogation of device is not sufficient
- Assessment of medication therapy in patients with devices

Class IIa
- Detection of proarrhythmic response to antiarrhythmic drugs in high-risk patients

Class IIb
- Unexplained episodic shortness of breath, chest pain, or fatigue
- Assessment of neurological events in patients with possible atrial fibrillation or flutter
- Patients with pre-syncope, syncope, or dizziness which continues despite treatment of another cause which is more likely than arrhythmia
- Assessment of rate control in atrial fibrillation
- Documentation of arrhythmia (symptomatic or asymptomatic) during outpatient treatment
- Post implantation evaluation in patients with pacemaker or ICD as alternative or adjunct to in-hospital telemetry
- Evaluation of supraventricular tachycardia rate in patients with ICDs

Class III
- Evaluation in patients with pre-syncope, syncope, dizziness, or palpitations with other identified causes
- Assessment of cerebrovascular events without other evidence for arrhythmia
- Assessment of device malfunction when underlying cause can be made by other means
- Follow up in asymptomatic patients

selection and the length of monitoring *(44–48)*. Nevertheless, non-invasive monitoring with Holter recordings can provide important clues about the cause of syncope *(49, 50)*. Loop recorders have a much higher diagnostic yield *(48)*.

Similarly, patients who have dizziness, lightheadedness, palpitations, weakness, fatigue, and other nonspecific symptoms potentially related to an arrhythmia rarely have a diagnosis secured by Holter unless the symptoms are frequent and occur during the recording. Further, an asymptomatic arrhythmia may have little clinical meaning. It is crucial to know that an arrhythmia is cause for a symptom; otherwise, therapy may fail to provide any benefit, may be unnecessary, and may even be dangerous.

Thus, Holter monitors are most useful for individuals who have frequent symptoms that are expected to occur within a 24 or 48-h monitoring period. Table 3 describes some potential reasons to use Holter monitoring to diagnose arrhythmias.

EVENT RECORDER

Similar to Holter monitors, event recorders can correlate symptoms to the presence or absence of an arrhythmia. They differ as they are utilized for a longer duration. The indications for these devices include diagnosis and management of palpitations, supraventricular tachycardias, and symptoms suspected to be directly caused by an arrhythmia (such as syncope, collapse, lightheadedness, dizziness, fatigue, and weakness) *(50)*. Event recorders are especially useful when symptoms occur less than every 24–48 h, the usual period for Holter monitoring, but are likely to happen within a 21–30 day period *(51)*. For infrequent episodes, they are also not very helpful *(52)*.

A small crossover study of patients with palpitations comparing diagnostic yield and cost-effectiveness of Holter monitoring versus event recorders showed that 67% of patients sent at least one interpretable recording while using an event recorder compared with only one third of the same patients wearing the Holter monitor *(53)*. The same study also showed that the diagnosis of a clinically significant arrhythmia was more likely with an event recorder (20%) versus a Holter monitor (0%). Other studies show similar utility of event recorders *(48, 54, 55)*.

There are several types of event recorders that are differentiated mainly by the presence or absence of "looping" during which the device can record information continuously but allow manual triggering to record an event after it occurs for subsequent playback and analysis. Such a device may also have the ability to record automatically depending on specific predetermined and preprogrammed parameters. Data from event recorders are usually transmitted from a patient transtelephonically to a central location for interpretation and dispersal. The data may then be sent via internet transmission or fax to the clinician (who may also be alerted if there is an urgent event), thereby improving the time from symptoms to diagnosis and treatment. An important caveat is that in rural practice areas where patients may not have a telephone, or landline (which anecdotally seems to transmit data more smoothly than mobile phones), rapid transmission of data may not be feasible.

Looping monitors record ECG data (possibly several electrocardiographic leads continuously) and store data lasting several minutes to an hour (depending upon the programming of the device) prior to a patient-triggered event recording. When the patient develops symptoms and activates the device, a recording of this time interval is saved. Looping monitors may also have an auto-trigger capability that allows for the detection of arrhythmias with predetermined parameters regardless of whether or not the patient is symptomatic or conscious during and/or after the event. This is especially useful for the diagnosis of profound bradycardias (including pauses) and tachycardias (Fig. 9). Auto-detection and triggering of atrial fibrillation, which may commonly be asymptomatic, are possible (LifeWatch, Inc., personal communication).

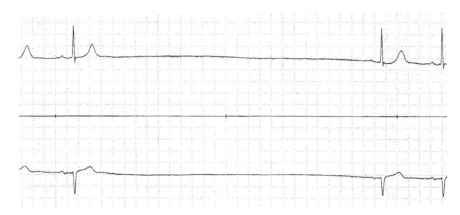

Fig. 9. Event monitor from an 80-year-old man with syncope shows sinus rhythm with sinus pause of 5.4 sec. Patient reported dizziness at the time of the pause. A pacemaker was placed and he is now doing well without symptoms.

Another indication for this type of device is surveillance in patients undergoing treatment or evaluation for an arrhythmia, especially in the asymptomatic patient. Patients with sudden incapacitation due to syncope or collapse may benefit from such algorithms as they do not have to trigger the device to record. Moreover, monitoring may also be useful to determine the presence of both asymptomatic and symptomatic atrial fibrillation *(11, 56)*. Newer devices can detect atrial fibrillation automatically and have demonstrated higher diagnostic yield and earlier diagnosis compared to memory loop recording alone *(57)*. The stepwise analysis involves measurement of RR variability. If irregular, an attempt is made to detect P waves. The sensitivity and specificity of detection algorithms have been touted as excellent by some and they may be improving; this is disputed. There are little hard data to support the accuracy of detecting atrial fibrillation at this time.

Non-looping recorders rely on patient-triggered recording and save data only during and after a symptomatic event in "real time" when the device is attached to the body. The duration of recordings is seconds to minutes and data can be stored for subsequent downloading. These recorders may not use attached electrodes, and are therefore ideal for use in patients with sensitivity or allergy to adhesives. This type of device is suitable for patients who have symptoms that last for at least several seconds so the recorder may be placed over the chest (or on the wrist) and information can be recorded. Given the technical aspects of this device, it is not practical for patients who have abrupt or severe symptoms that are transient as there may not be time to attach and trigger the device to record the event. Likewise, patients with physical or cognitive impairments may not be able to activate the device.

While event recorders have inherent advantages, there are drawbacks. For instance, most event recorders rely upon the patient to activate the device at the time of or directly after a given episode. As noted previously, patients with cognitive or physical impairments, including incapacitation at the time of symptoms, may not be good candidates for event recording. Similarly, patients without reliable access to a landline phone may not be able to transmit the recorded data for interpretation.

Newer capabilities include extended-term full disclosure ECG recording and remote monitoring in which devices are able to transmit heart rate trends, arrhythmia burden, and alert/high risk events on a daily basis or as needed. This type of data collection may improve arrhythmia management as well as morbidity and mortality. Ambulatory ECG monitoring may be enhanced by the features and capabilities of modern devices. According to the 1999 ACC/AHA guidelines for ambulatory ECG monitoring *(33)*, Class I indications include unexplained syncope, dizziness, or palpitations. Class IIb indications include unexplained chest pain or dyspnea, "neurological events" suspected to be arrhythmia-related, or syncope likely due to a non-arrhythmic cause that persists despite treatment. Class III indications (i.e., not indicated) are evaluation for occult arrhythmias as causes of stroke, or for syncope or dizziness due to a non-arrhythmic cause. Other uses include evaluation of antiarrhythmic drug efficacy, monitoring of pacemaker function, extended-term QT interval monitoring, diagnosis of long-QT syndrome, assessment of heart rate variability, surveillance for occult atrial flutter or fibrillation as a cause for stroke, home monitoring for sleep apnea, and even diagnosis of Brugada syndrome.

MINIMALLY INVASIVE IMPLANTABLE LOOP RECORDER

Implantable loop recorders (ILRs) have extended diagnostic capabilities beyond those of external loop recorders (58–64). They are generally indicated to diagnose the causes for syncope and associated symptoms and can be used to rule in or rule out an arrhythmic cause for symptoms (65). These small leadless devices are implanted subcutaneously and record local (single lead) electrocardiographic activity with P waves and QRS complexes generally being visible. The device can be programmed to record for a specific length of time and is dependent on the memory of the device. Typically, ILRs have a battery life of $1\frac{1}{2}$–2 years. Some monitors require interrogation by placing a programming head over the device while others allow transtelephonic transmission of data and events. All devices can be programmed to allow for manual and/or automatic recordings based on prespecified parameters.

The advantage of these devices is they can record longer episodes and the device is available for longer periods than an external loop recorder, allowing for better correlation of events with arrhythmias in patients with only occasional symptoms (66, 67). ILRs can record for and save data from long periods (up to 45 min). The average time to diagnosis for patients with syncope who have ILRs is generally 3–4 months, indicating a potential advantage over external loop recorders.

There are a few disadvantages of ILRs. Only one local chest lead is recorded. There can be noise and artifactual signals, sometimes related to patient position alone (68). Finally, the device requires surgical implantation with inherent associated risks.

For any arrhythmia monitor, including ILRs, the mechanism of events remains a critical issue. It can be difficult to know the role of arrhythmia as the cause for symptoms in some cases. For example, recording sinus tachycardia, bradycardia, or asystole, in a patient with syncope, does not necessarily indicate that the arrhythmia caused the problem. Sinus arrest due to sick sinus syndrome may be difficult to differentiate from asystole due to a neurocardiogenic cause. ILRs show that asystole occurs more often during a spontaneous episode of neurocardiogenic syncope compared to a tilt table test (69, 70).

Newer devices are designed for specific clinical conditions such as syncope or atrial fibrillation. They not only can be helpful in diagnosing an arrhythmic cause of symptoms but can be just as useful in determining that symptoms are not related to an arrhythmia. It is possible that newer devices will be developed that will be highly sensitive and specific for atrial fibrillation, whereas others may be better designed to assess syncope. Present indications for these devices have been published (50, 71).

TRANSTELEPHONIC RECORDING OF PACEMAKER AND DEFIBRILLATOR ACTIVITY

Pacemakers and implantable defibrillators can be monitored transtelephonically to help determine the cause of symptoms and aid in surveillance of arrhythmias (72). Although transtelephonic pacemaker monitoring technology has been evaluated and available since the 1970s (73), recent advances now allow detailed information to be downloaded and transmitted for physician interpretation (74, 75). It is now possible to understand better why a patient has syncope or ICD shocks via home monitoring (Fig. 10). This information can also be used to determine if there are problems with the leads or the device itself.

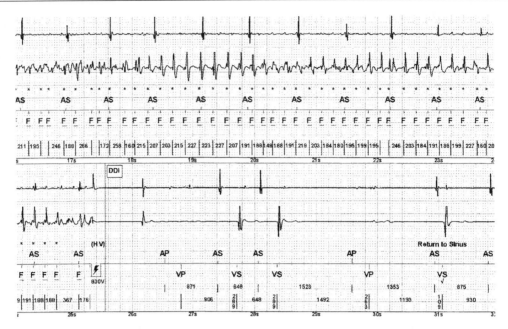

Fig. 10. Transtelephonic monitoring from a 72 year-old female who had an ICD shock while at home. The recording shows ventricular fibrillation, ICD shock, and then junctional escape with eventual return to sinus rhythm.

Typically, a patient has an interface device at home that communicates with the pacemaker or defibrillator. The external device can automatically download information from the implanted device and transmit it by telephone line where it is delivered via an internet site where electrograms and recorded events can be downloaded at a moment's notice. This new technology provides a methodology to diagnose rhythm disturbances rapidly.

All pacemaker and defibrillator companies have developed advanced means to interrogate these devices, determine the programming characteristics, and evaluate stored electrogram data from a distance *(72, 74)*. This can be extraordinarily helpful for a patient who has syncope, ICD shocks, or other symptoms that may be related to pacemaker or defibrillator failure. It can help assess the burden of atrial fibrillation. These devices can monitor changes in lead characteristics. This may be of crucial importance in patients who have recalled leads or recalled devices that have a low failure rate but are associated with the potential for catastrophic outcomes.

EXERCISE TESTING

Exercise testing can diagnose arrhythmias, particularly if symptoms due to a suspected arrhythmia occur with activity *(76–82)*. It can be useful for exercise-induced AV block, chronotropic incompetence, supraventricular tachycardia, and ventricular tachycardia, and has even been used to assess prognostic significance of the presence of an accessory pathway *(83)*. Exercise testing increases sympathetic activity and decreases parasympathetic activity. By increasing heart rate, cardiac output, and oxygen consumption, clinically important arrhythmias may be initiated.

While some forms of ventricular tachycardia are inducible with exercise (such as right ventricular outflow tract ventricular tachycardia in patients with normal hearts), some other forms are not. The utilization of treadmill testing in lieu of other forms of monitoring depends specifically on the type of

Table 4

Indications for Exercise Testing in Assessment of Heart Rhythm Disorders *(84)*

Class I
- Determination of appropriate settings for rate-adaptive pacemakers
- Evaluation of congenital complete heart block prior to increased activity or competitive sports

Class IIa
- Evaluation of patients with known or suspected exercise-induced arrhythmia
- Evaluation of medical, surgical, or ablative management in patients with exercise-induced arrhythmia

Class IIb
- Evaluation of ventricular ectopic beats in middle aged patients without evidence of coronary artery disease
- Evaluation of patients with first degree atrioventricular block or Mobitz I block, left or right bundle branch blocks, or isolated ectopic beats in young patients prior to participating in competitive sports

Class III
- Evaluation of ectopic beats in young patients

arrhythmia, the clinical circumstances under which the patient had the episodes, and the type of heart disease suspected. The ACC/AHA has established indications for exercise testing in the assessment of patients with possible cardiac arrhythmias *(84)* (Table 4).

Exercise testing can also be useful to determine prognosis with respect to arrhythmias. One study found that the 12-month mortality is three times greater in patients with exercise-induced ectopy compared to those with ectopy at rest only *(85)*. The mortality rate is higher for patients with complex ectopy compared to simple ectopy *(86)*. Class IC antiarrhythmic drugs can cause wide complex tachycardia due to 1:1 conduction of atrial tachycardia or slowed atrial flutter (Fig. 11). Treadmill testing may have a role to determine the presence of proarrhythmic effects from these drugs used to treat atrial flutter and atrial fibrillation, but the sensitivity and specificity of treadmill testing for this purpose is

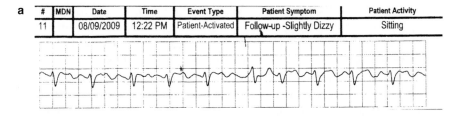

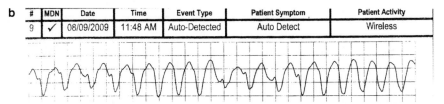

Fig. 11. A 50-year-old woman was started on propafenone for control of atrial fibrillation. While wearing a Holter monitor she developed symptomatic atrial flutter with variable conduction (**a**) and then a wide complex tachycardia consistent with atrial flutter with 1:1 conduction and aberrancy (**b**). She was asymptomatic during the episode.

low *(87)*. It has also been used in the past to assess antegrade conduction capabilities of the Kent bundle in patients with the Wolff-Parkinson-White syndrome *(88)*. Although exercise testing is a powerful tool to assess prognosis, it is rarely used in patients with arrhythmias for this purpose.

The exact role of treadmill testing in the assessment and management of arrhythmias remains somewhat uncertain as arrhythmias triggered by exercise are not necessarily reproducibly inducible. They may not occur with the type of exercise protocol that is typically performed in a monitored circumstance on a treadmill. For example, athletes may have specific and even life-threatening arrhythmias, but only during competition or playing a specific type of sport. In this instance, monitoring may provide additional data that could not be gleaned from routine treadmill testing (Fig. 12).

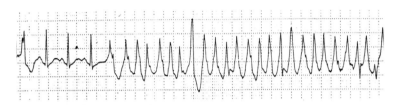

Fig. 12. A 24 year-old man reported dizziness and near syncope while playing hockey. He underwent a treadmill stress test during which he attained 100% maximum age predicted heart rate, had no ectopy, and remained free of symptoms. His symptoms were considered benign but he was given a monitor. Ventricular tachycardia was recorded while he was playing hockey.

PROGNOSIS

Numerous attempts have been made to characterize the individual at greatest risk for malignant ventricular arrhythmias and ultimately sudden and/or arrhythmic cardiac death. This issue is complicated by the fact that what appears to be sudden cardiac death due to an arrhythmia may in fact be sudden cardiac death, instead, with (or even without) an arrhythmia. Treating an arrhythmia may not prevent sudden death, and arrhythmic death is not necessarily equal to sudden cardiac death. Prevention of sudden cardiac death may not necessarily reduce total mortality, which is the ultimate goal. Any tool used to prognosticate has to be able to reduce the risk of total mortality and catastrophic events related to arrhythmia. To make this issue even more complex, tools used for prognostic purposes years ago may not necessarily apply to today's patients who are better treated with statins, beta-blockers, and ACE inhibitors, to name a few drugs. The mortality of patients with ischemic and non-ischemic cardiomyopathy and New York Heart Association (NYHA) Functional Class II–III congestive heart failure is lower now than it once was. Using any prognostic tool in the general population now would have to grapple with sensitivity and specificity issues and may not even be applicable.

The purpose of using a non-invasive prognostic tool must consider the potential benefits of knowing a patient's outcome. Presumably, there would be some therapeutic benefit since simply knowing which patient will die over time has little appeal. ICDs may offset the risk of an arrhythmic death and thereby reduce total mortality in select patients. A prognostic tool that can enhance the ability to determine which patients will benefit from an ICD, then, would have general appeal.

Prediction of life-threatening arrhythmias and total mortality often is based on historical features and determination of the severity of the underlying heart disease. The most commonly used clinical parameters of risk include the assessment of NYHA Functional Class and left ventricular ejection fraction (LVEF) in patients with ischemic and/or structural heart disease. The list of available clinical predictors involves parameters that cannot or will not be changed including gender, religious beliefs, alcohol use, and even geographic location.

Non-invasive tools have been evaluated regarding their ability to assess risk for arrhythmic death, sudden cardiac death, and total mortality. These techniques may help the clinician better understand which patient will derive the greatest benefit from a therapeutic intervention such as an ICD implant. These techniques may also help to better clarify the relationship between arrhythmias and some of their triggers (consider the relationship between autonomic tone as determined by heart rate variability measurements and arrhythmic death). Some of these tools use standalone technologies specifically designed to determine risk. Others attempt to glean information from routine monitoring systems using specific mathematical programs or algorithms. Risk stratification using these non-invasive tools involves the measurement of several unrelated parameters that represent different physiological parameters.

Important information can be obtained by careful study of not only the ECG and Holter monitoring but also by evaluating signal-averaged electrocardiography, T wave alternans, baroreceptor testing, heart rate variability, QT dispersion methodologies, spectral turbulence assessment, as well as a variety of clinical and historical features. These tools and techniques can provide insight into alterations in autonomic tone, repolarization and conduction that can be arrhythmogenic. Despite the potential predictive value of non-invasive modalities that measure these and other important parameters, they remain underutilized or not utilized at all. They have generally been relegated to obscurity in the dustbin of clinical management.

In 1991, Farrell (89) assessed the value of several non-invasive predictors to assess outcome in post-myocardial infarction patients. Heart rate variability, signal-averaged ECG, and frequent ventricular ectopy were highly predictive and significantly associated with outcomes (p value for each was 0.0000). In contrast, a LVEF <40% and Killip class, while predictive, were not as significant as predictors ($P<0.02$ for each). The combination of positive heart rate variability and positive signal-averaged electrocardiogram to predict arrhythmic events had a relative risk of 18.5. Despite these astounding results, the non-invasive predictors continue to be underutilized in comparison to other less powerful clinical predictors. The focus on LVEF and NYHA Functional Class continues.

Until this disconnect between practice and data is better understood, even the best non-invasive tools to predict outcomes may not be used. There are various potential reasons for this obvious dichotomy between evidence and practice. Part of the problem is that it is not entirely clear what risk of sudden death is too high and what proportion of deaths are due to arrhythmias and are sudden. When it comes to ICDs, Stevenson and Ridker (90) noted that the number needed to treat to prevent one death of a post-myocardial infarction patient with a LVEF <0.40 was 1 in 14. They asserted that the risk of sudden death in these patients was so low that "routine referral to arrhythmia specialist is not warranted". Using the concept of number needed to treat, preventing one death in 14 with an ICD is now considered an expected appropriate benefit.

The idea of "high risk" of sudden cardiac death and total mortality is a moving target. The actual definition of risk and benefit from therapy when it comes to ICDs still remains uncertain. When considering the use of a non-invasive risk predictor, the following issues need to be well defined: the absolute risk of mortality of a given patient, the relative risk of a positive test, the influence of confounding variables and comorbidities, the sensitivity and specificity of the test and the value of knowing the information regarding risk of arrhythmic death, sudden cardiac death, and total mortality. For example, even if a patient has a very high risk of arrhythmic death based on a variety of non-invasive predictors, other less specific predictors may be just as good at predicting time to total mortality, which is the real reason to assess risk. Even if non-invasive predictors could provide some evidence for increased risk, if that risk remains low despite evidence for benefit, it likely will not be used under any circumstance.

Recently, several novel predictors have been carefully evaluated. These include T wave alternans and spectral turbulence. Some non-linear algorithmic predictors may also be powerful predictors.

While these methodologies may have value in predicting outcomes, we suspect that these, and other non-invasive predictors, will suffer the same fate of underutilization despite potential compelling and cogent clinical information based on good trials. We suspect that non-invasive predictors, unless 100% reliable, will never see the light of day for routine screening use. Even if they are entirely reliable, altering therapy based on the test results would have to be shown to be beneficial in terms of long-term survival and not just mode of death.

Evaluation of non-invasive tools to attempt to predict risk of sudden arrhythmic and total mortality has generally fallen into disfavor despite the fact that some of the information is very provocative and persuasive. In fact, non-invasive tools can predict outcomes of patients fairly accurately. It remains puzzling why some of these tools have not been developed further and are not used clinically.

This section will address some of these tools in broad strokes but not deal with the details of measurements and analysis as these technologies have not yet been developed for widespread practical clinical purposes. While potentially highly valuable as predictors, the diverse group of tests, measuring a multiplicity of parameters, further drives home the point that there are many avenues to sudden, arrhythmic, and total mortality in patients with heart disease, with a genetic predisposition of arrhythmic death and even the population at large.

SIGNAL-AVERAGED ELECTROCARDIOGRAM

The signal-averaged electrocardiogram (SAECG) has been correlated with, and purportedly detects, slow ventricular and atrial conduction. Delayed ventricular activation, due to slowed ventricular conduction, caused by fibrosis or scar, is thought to be responsible for potentially life-threatening reentrant ventricular tachycardia. On the SAECG, high-frequency low-amplitude delayed signals ("late potentials") not seen on the standard electrocardiogram can be detected. Noise reduction, high-gain amplification, and proper filtering allow detection of these small amplitude signals at the end of the square root of the summation of the voltage of the squares of each of the X, Y, and Z leads *(91, 92)*. Interpretation is based upon the total QRS width and the voltage and length of the low-amplitude signal (Fig. 13).

SAECG abnormalities are associated with increased risk of ventricular arrhythmias in multiple clinical settings, including myocardial infarction, non-ischemic cardiomyopathy, and arrhythmogenic right ventricular cardiomyopathy *(93–96)*. The sensitivity and specificity are dependent on the underlying clinical condition. The test cannot be interpreted when the 12 lead QRS width exceeds 120 msec. The sensitivity may also depend on location of infarction (inferior vs. anterior).

In patients with ischemic heart disease, the SAECG is abnormal in more patients with history of ventricular tachycardia compared to those without ventricular tachycardia (prevalence of 93% and 18–33%, respectively) *(97–99)*. The SAECG has high negative predictive value for sudden cardiac death, ranging from 95% to 99% *(89, 100)*. However, the positive predictive value is low, ranging from 7% to 40% *(89, 100)*.

The relationship of the SAECG to arrhythmic events and total mortality is clear. It was assessed as a substudy of the Multicenter Unsustained Tachycardia Trial (MUSTT) where prolonged filtered SAECG QRS > 114 msec predicted significant increase in arrhythmic events (28% vs. 17%, $P = 0.0001$) and total mortality (43% vs. 35%, $P = 0.0001$) during 5 years of follow-up *(101)*. As a prelude to the CABG-Patch trial, patients with coronary artery disease and an abnormal SAECG were found to have a 28% 3-year mortality rate vs. 14% mortality in a similar group with a normal SAECG *(102)*.

SAECG abnormalities are lower in patients treated with thrombolytic therapy or angioplasty *(103, 104)*. The Late Assessment of Thrombolytic Efficiency (LATE) study investigators assessed the SAECG in patients who were administered thrombolytic therapy 6–24 h after myocardial

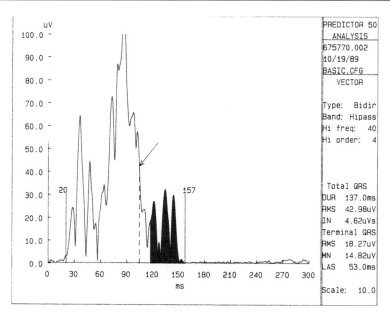

Fig. 13. Signal-averaged electrocardiogram showing late potential was obtained using a 40 Hz high-pass bidirectional filter. SAECG shows a filtered QRS duration of 137 msec, a signal of 18.27 μV in the terminal QRS, and voltage < 40 μV for 53 msec.

infarction *(105)*. SAECG abnormalities were 37% lower in those who received thrombolytic therapy vs. placebo. In another report, 9.3% who received primary reperfusion therapy had an abnormal SAECG, but these abnormalities did not correlate with cardiac death and arrhythmic events over a 34-month follow-up *(106)*. In separate studies, however, the SAECG is strongly associated with increased risk of arrhythmic events with a positive predictive accuracy of 11–25% *(103–104)*.

In one study, the predictive value of the SAECG, the LVEF, Holter monitor, and heart rate variability were tested in a cohort of patients after myocardial infarction *(107)*. In an univariate analysis, all four variables predicted arrhythmic and cardiac death, but in a multivariate analysis, only heart rate variability and nonsustained ventricular tachycardia were independent predictors of arrhythmic death. It appears that many of these non-invasive methods to assess arrhythmic outcomes lack sensitivity and specificity. The predictive value of any one non-invasive test may be low, but multiple non-invasive predictors can increase sensitivity to determine the risk of arrhythmic and total mortality *(108, 109)*.

Likewise, the value of SAECG in patients with non-ischemic cardiomyopathy remains speculative *(109–111)*. Among 114 patients with non-ischemic cardiomyopathy, those with abnormal SAECG had 39% 1-year event-free survival vs. 95% in patients with normal SAECG *(112)*. In a separate study of 131 patients with non-ischemic cardiomyopathy followed at 54 months, those with an abnormal SAECG had an increased incidence of all-cause mortality (relative risk 3.3) and arrhythmic events (relative risk 7.2) *(113)*. The negative and positive predictive accuracies for VT were 94–100% and 25–45%, respectively *(110, 111)*. In an advanced heart failure population, abnormal SAECG was not predictive of worse outcomes *(114)*.

Present use of the SAECG is limited. It is rarely used to define risk of arrhythmias or sudden death. It may have some diagnostic capabilities to detect ventricular tachycardia in select patients. Some scenarios in which the SAECG may be used include patients with an undiagnosed cause for syncope and evidence for mild to moderately impaired ventricular function. Patients with severe ventricular dysfunction, when severe symptoms are present, are likely to have an implantable defibrillator regardless of SAECG results. The SAECG may have some use to identify high-risk patients with arrhythmo-genic right ventricular cardiomyopathy *(115, 116)*, but the majority of such patients have an abnormal SAECG *(115)*.

The 2008 AHA/ACC/Heart Rhythm Society does not support the routine use of the SAECG as non-invasive risk stratification to identify patients at high risk for Sudden Cardier Death *(117)*. The 2006 AHA/ACC syncope guidelines also do not recommend using SAECG in the workup of syncope *(4)*.

T-WAVE ALTERNANS

T wave alternans (TWA) is defined as beat-to-beat alternation of the morphology and amplitude of the T wave on the ECG *(118, 119)*. Visible TWA has been linked to ventricular arrhythmias and sudden cardiac death. Contemporary TWA testing uses ECG signal processing and can detect TWA on the order of a few microvolts, termed MTWA *(120)*.

Evidence shows that alternans of intracardiac repolarization may be linked with MTWA *(121, 122)*. This could be due to spatial repolarization dispersion, in which regions of myocardium could have longer action potential duration and depolarize every other cycle. Alternatively, action potential duration may alternate at a single site (temporal dispersion) *(123, 124)*.

TWA is not generally present at rest and is rate related. Because of this, exercise testing or atrial pacing is used to increase the heart rate. Measurement at less than 109 beats per minute minimizes false positives *(125)*. Sequential ECG cycles are recorded and aligned to their QRS complexes. T wave amplitudes at a predefined point are measured. Computer algorithms are used to detect and quantify beat-to-beat amplitude variations. The most widely applied technique is the spectral analysis that considers TWA as a periodic signal superimposed on T waves at a frequency of half the heart rate *(126)*. The computer itself does the interpretation and there is little information to review. Therefore, this appears to be almost a black box or "divining rod" often based on interpretation using proprietary software. It appears that approximately 30% of individuals who have this test will have an indeterminate result. Indeterminate results appear to be associated with higher risk so that the lowest risk group includes only those who have a negative result.

TWA is linked to ventricular arrhythmias *(127, 128)* and it may be an important tool to predict the risk of ventricular arrhythmia in diverse populations, including those with ischemic and non-ischemic heart disease. In a large, prospective, multicenter study, Bloomfield *(128)* tested if TWA was associated with increased risk of death and arrhythmia events. Patients with LVEF <40% were enrolled, with half having ischemic cardiomyopathy. The all-cause mortality and sustained ventricular arrhythmia rate was 15% in the TWA-positive group vs. 2.5% in the TWA-negative group. TWA appeared to identify high-risk patients who may benefit from an ICD and low-risk patients unlikely to benefit from an ICD.

In patients with ischemic cardiomyopathy (LVEF ≤35%) and no prior history of ventricular arrhythmia, an abnormal TWA was associated with a higher risk of all-cause and arrhythmic mortality *(129)*. ICD therapy was associated with significantly lower all-cause mortality in TWA-positive patients but not in TWA-negative patients *(130)*.

The Alternans before Cardioverter Defibrillator (ABCD) Trial was the first trial to use TWA to guide prophylactic ICD insertion *(131)*. TWA and electrophysiology study were performed in 566 patients with ischemic cardiomyopathy and LVEF <40%. ICDs were implanted if either test was positive. During 1.9 years of follow-up, TWA had 1-year positive (9%) and negative (95%) predictive values that were comparable to electrophysiology study (11 and 95%, respectively). Positive TWA and positive electrophysiology study gave a hazard ratio of 2.1 and 2.4, respectively. A risk stratification strategy using non-invasive TWA was as effective as electrophysiology study in predicting VT events at 1 year in enrolled patients.

This trial confirmed findings from an earlier study, in which TWA had negative predictive value of 97% for 1-year arrhythmic mortality in patients with ischemic cardiomyopathy (LVEF 39% ± 18%) *(132)*. In patients with severely decreased LVEF (<30%), the effect of TWA was less clear. In a study of 144 patients with ischemic cardiomyopathy, TWA was a potent predictor of events in patients with LVEF 30–40%, but did not predict events in those with LVEF <30% (HR = 1.1, $P > 0.5$) *(133)*.

The predictive value of TWA is less in patients with prolonged QRS duration. Shalaby tested TWA to predict outcomes in patients with ischemic cardiomyopathy (LVEF <40%) who had bundle branch block or interventricular conduction delay or did not *(134)*. TWA predicted the combined endpoint of ventricular arrhythmia or death in patients with narrow QRS (HR = 1.64, $P = 0.04$) but not in those with prolonged QRS (HR = 1.04, $P = 0.91$). In multivariate analysis, QRS width and TWA, as well as QRS width and electrophysiology study, were independent predictors of events. Similarly, Rashba showed that TWA was a significant predictor of arrhythmic events and death in patients with normal QRS, but not among patients with prolonged QRS *(133)*.

The Microvolt T wave Alternans testing for Risk Stratification of Post-Myocardial Infarction Patients (MASTER) I trial included 654 patients who met the Multicenter Automatic Defibrillator Implantation Trial II (MADIT-II) indication for ICD implantation. After TWA testing, patients underwent ICD implant with programming to minimize risk of a non-life-threatening arrhythmia shock. TWA was negative in 214 patients (37%), positive in 293 patients (51%), and indeterminate in 68 patients (12%). The primary endpoint of life-threatening ventricular tachyarrhythmia events (assessed by ICD shocks) was not different between patients with negative and non-negative TWA tests, but the event rates in this population were much less than suspected *(135)*.

The T-wave Alternans in Patients with Heart Failure (ALPHA) study investigated TWA predictions in 446 patients with non-ischemic cardiomyopathy (LVEF <40%, NYHA FC II/III) who were followed 18–24 months. Primary endpoint (combination of cardiac death and life-threatening arrhythmias) event rates in patients with abnormal and normal MTWA tests were 6.5 and 1.6%, respectively *(136)*. The negative predictive value for TWA was >97%. Similar results were obtained from a previous trial of 547 patients with LVEF <40% and NYHA Functional Class II/III heart failure enrolled and followed for 2 years. In this non-ischemic cohort, patients with abnormal TWA had event rates (death and ventricular arrhythmia) of 13.3% vs. 0% in those with normal TWA *(128)*.

A substudy of 490 patients (average LVEF 25% and NYHA functional class II/III heart failure) from the Sudden Cardiac Death in Heart Failure Trial (SCD-HeFT) showed different results. The primary end point, sudden cardiac death, sustained VT, or appropriate ICD discharge, during 30-month follow-up was the same for TWA-positive and negative patients (HR = 1.24 for TWA, $P = 0.56$). TWA did not predict arrhythmic events or mortality *(137)*. Similarly, TWA did not predict ventricular arrhythmia or sudden cardiac death in the MArburg CArdiomyopathy Study (MACAS). Left ventricular ejection fraction was the only significant arrhythmia risk predictor *(138)*.

Such heterogeneous results may be due to the populations studied, the endpoints, and/or the methodology used. The underlying pathology of left ventricular dysfunction and the presence or absence of additional clinical risk factors may affect the pretest probability of ventricular arrhythmic events. Nevertheless, TWA has high negative predictive value in broad populations, and may provide important information in identifying a low-risk group with left ventricular dysfunction who is unlikely to benefit from prophylactic ICD. Thus, patients with negative TWA tests may not benefit from ICD implantation. TWA has a class IIa indication in the ACC/AHA/ESC 2006 guidelines *(4)*, but further studies are needed to better explore the technical features of the technologies used before it is incorporated into ICD implantation guidelines.

HEART RATE VARIABILITY

Heart rate variability is a marker of autonomic control. While the resting heartbeat in the normal heart is influenced mainly by parasympathetic innervation from the vagus, there is also sympathetic input as well. Heart rate variability evaluates variations in RR intervals and may be reported by time domain or frequency domain measures. Data have shown that patients with decreased heart rate variability are more susceptible to arrhythmias *(139)*.

Time domain measures assess the heart rate by recognizing and recording the intervals between QRS complexes. The NN interval (the interval between adjacent QRS complexes initiated by the sinus node) is determined. Other measures include mean heart rate, difference between NN intervals, and difference in day and night heart rate.

Frequency domain measures use power spectral analysis to determine the density of frequency bands. Recordings considered short term (2–5 min) can decipher very low-, low-, and high-frequency signals while long-term (24 h) recordings demonstrate ultra low-frequency components. While low- and high-frequency components comprise only 5% of the total analysis, they appear to be the most meaningful *(140)*. High-frequency bands represent vagal stimulation; low-frequency bands represent sympathetic activation *(140)*.

Heart rate variability may be useful in assessing patients after myocardial infarction, in patients with heart failure, or in those with diabetes. In post-myocardial infarction patients, decreased vagal activity, and hence decreased heart rate variability, represents an increase in sympathetic stimulation and possible electrical lability, independent of other risk factors *(140)*. In conjunction with other risk factors such as ejection fraction and presence of ectopic beats on 24 h monitoring, sensitivity is 25–75% *(140)*.

Another group reported that heart rate variability was more valuable in predicting arrhythmia than was a depressed ejection fraction after myocardial infarction *(141)*. It has also been reported that heart rate variability may be decreased after recent myocardial infarction, but may recover over time *(142)*. As such, it is recommended that HRV be evaluated 1 week after myocardial infarction *(140)*. Similar to patients after myocardial infarction, patients with left ventricular dysfunction demonstrate decreased heart rate variability, usually based upon sympathetic activation.

Heart rate variability measures that indicate increased sympathetic activation at rest and or decreased parasympathetic activation appear to be associated with increased risk for sudden cardiac death and total mortality. It appears that alterations in autonomic innervation *(143)* are associated with increased risk, but the mechanism by which this may occur is uncertain. It is unclear if sympathetic activation or lack of parasympathetic activation is the primary cause or if these just reflect the severity of underlying disease. Heart rate variability does not appear to be an independent predictor in all clinical circumstances. It seems to be a dynamic issue that may vary with severity of heart failure or heart disease. Various methodologies have incorporated the assessment of heart rate variability as a predictor of outcomes or worsening heart failure in patients, but it remains a rather non-specific entity and is therefore not yet used commonly to assess arrhythmia risk.

BAROREFLEX SENSITIVITY

The baroreflex affects autonomic input based on sensed pressure from the baroreptors. There are various methodologies by which to measure baroreflex sensitivity. In some instances, phenylephrine is given and alterations in blood pressure and heart rate are compared. This can give an indication of the sensitivity of the baroreflex *(144)*. During this reflex, the presence of bradycardia that occurs with transient increases in blood pressure is a result of sensitivity of the arterial baroreceptors. The interrelationships of blood pressure and heart rate are complex and may vary over time. Baroreflex sensitivity can be a potent marker of arrhythmic events and total mortality in a patient population with ischemic heart disease and/or cardiomyopathy *(145, 146)*. Alterations in the baroreflex are not necessarily fixed and abnormalities in baroreflex sensitivity may be due to many factors. Nevertheless, it is a reasonable predictor.

HEART RATE TURBULENCE

Heart rate turbulence (HRT) is the evaluation of heart rate following a premature ventricular contraction. Under normal circumstances, there is a short period of acceleration followed by deceleration of the pulse. This change in rate is thought to reflect baroreflex sensitivity, at least in part. Diminished turbulence slope has been shown to predict mortality and cardiac arrest in patients with myocardial infarction *(147, 148)*. The technology has also been used in patients to predict heart failure decompensation *(149)*. It has shown promise in evaluating patients with diabetes as many have autonomic dysfunction *(150)*. In addition, a future use may be to diagnose sleep apnea as HRT correlates with the apnea–hypopnea index *(151)*. HRT is a promising approach to predict risk in patients and it may be one of the best, if not the best, non-invasive predictor of outcomes for patients with structural heart disease.

OTHER PREDICTORS

The complexity of the relationship between non-invasive tools and arrhythmic outcomes is clear. This relates to the complexity of physiologic perturbations and outcomes in patients with various underlying cardiovascular conditions. Winfree has attempted to describe the dynamic and complex interplay mathematically *(152)*. He has considered that sudden cardiac death can be considered topologically and that arrhythmias are initiated by multiple interrelated factors. Based on the complexity of the variables involved and their interaction, it may be somewhat of a surprise that the heart has enough dynamic checks and balances to prevent sudden death with each heartbeat.

There are many algorithms used to assess the risk of sudden, arrhythmic, and total mortality. QT dispersion is one non-specific marker derived from the 12 lead ECG. A variety of nonlinear arrhythmia predictors including symbolic dynamics (every heart beat compared to a preceding beat), fractal dimension of the RR and QT intervals, QT variability, non-linear compression entropy, and joint symbolic dynamics (assessing systolic blood pressure respiration and heart rate in a moving window) have been used to associate the risk of death in cardiovascular events *(153, 154)*. The predictive values of these methodologies have not been tested rigorously.

A GLIMPSE AT THE FUTURE OF MONITORING

Modern ambulatory monitoring offers the possibility of multichannel real-time recording and instantaneous full disclosure transmission. It also offers the possibility of automatically, or by patient trigger, detecting, storing, and transmitting arrhythmia abnormalities for evaluation. Advancements in arrhythmia monitoring will provide improved diagnostic capabilities over longer periods to help secure diagnoses more accurately and for a broader range of conditions.

Determining a correlation between the heart rate, the rhythm, and symptoms is crucial. It is possible that a patient reports symptoms at the time of a tachycardia or bradycardia, but the symptoms are not a result of the arrhythmia itself. If monitors had an accelerometer, it would be possible to correlate heart rate with symptoms and specific activities to determine, for example, if sinus tachycardia is appropriate or not. Inappropriate increases in heart rate could be diagnosed while the patient is at rest or relatively inactive. If position and activity could be linked and recorded, the presence or absence of postural orthostatic tachycardia syndrome could also be documented. Chronotropic incompetence, difficult to diagnose but potentially ameliorated by a pacemaker, could be diagnosed by linking normal activities with heart rate rather than testing rate response artificially on a treadmill or by other means.

Monitoring may provide measurements of respiratory rate and minute ventilation which can then be linked to heart rate. The temporal relationship between these and a given activity may make it possible to determine the primary cause of a patient complaint or symptom. For example, it could be determined if the patient had worsening heart failure or if symptoms were due instead to an underlying lung condition that caused a change in heart rate. The diagnosis of functional disorders, such as anxiety or panic attacks, could also be made by linking respiratory rate with heart rate. Measurements including oxygen saturation, blood pressure, and pH may help determine relationships between respiratory rate and other clinical and physiological variables.

Blood pressure is an important variable to measure in addition to heart rate when it comes to symptoms such as syncope. Heart rate measurements alone do not necessarily indicate why a patient may lose consciousness, but knowing the heart rate in relation to blood pressure can help to identify the mechanism responsible for the episode. An asystolic or tachycardia episode associated with syncope does not mean that either is responsible for the problem. The temporal relationship between the blood pressure drop and/or change in heart rate may provide greater insight into the mechanism. For example, hypotension may precede bradycardia in patients with neurocardiogenic syncope and a pacemaker may not be useful. Alternatively, if asystole is the primary cause for the event, a pacemaker may be therapeutic.

Markers of autonomic pertubations such as skin conductance and heart rate variability may help better characterize the cause for symptoms. Transthoracic impedance can help diagnose congestive heart failure as it correlates with lung water. Sophisticated monitoring may also diagnose and aid in the treatment of sleep apnea.

Non-invasive monitors of the future will provide enhanced diagnostic and prognostic information. In order to do so, monitors must be capable of being worn for periods long enough to provide pertinent and definitive information concerning the relationship of symptoms to arrhythmias and arrhythmias to outcomes. Rapid advances are likely.

CONCLUSION

Non-invasive arrhythmia assessment is the critical first step to arrive at a definitive diagnosis. Technology has advanced rapidly, is highly refined, and can now provide important prognostic information. Despite evidence supporting the use of non-invasive tools to predict patient outcomes, these tools remain underutilized for this purpose.

Norman Holter dreamed of the day that, a then, "unorthodox" monitor would give patients greater freedom while providing clinicians with reliable information to secure an arrhythmia diagnosis. Use of these monitors now seems commonplace. Yet just as Holter saw beyond the realities of his day, visions of the future inspire today's pioneers to advance non-invasive technology.

There will always be room for improvement of the equipment, but, basically, "full freedom" means freedom to make long, continuous records of physiological phenomena as close as possible to the geographic site of occurrence. Thus the future – and this development may not be remote, in view of the present increasing interest in medical electronics – will see human beings and other animals "wired for research".

– Norman J. Holter (1961) *(1)*

REFERENCES

1. Holter NJ (1961) New method for heart studies. Science 134:1214–20
2. Crawford MH et al (1999) ACC/AHA guidelines for ambulatory electrocardiography. A report of the American College of Cardiology/American Heart Association Task Force on Practice Guidelines (committee to revise the guidelines for ambulatory electrocardiography). Developed in collaboration with the North American Society for Pacing and Electrophysiology. J Am Coll Cardiol 34(3):912–948
3. Lohman JE (1989) ACC/AHA task force report: guidelines for ambulatory electrocardiography. Circulation 80(4):1098–1100
4. Zipes DP et al (2006) ACC/AHA/ESC 2006 guidelines for management of patients with ventricular arrhythmias and the prevention of sudden cardiac death: a report of the American college of cardiology/American Heart Association Task Force and the European Society of Cardiology Committee for Practice Guidelines (writing committee to develop guidelines for management of patients with ventricular arrhythmias and the prevention of sudden cardiac death). J Am Coll Cardiol 48(5):e247–e346
5. Kadish AH et al (2001) ACC/AHA clinical competence statement on electrocardiography and ambulatory electrocardiography: a report of the ACC/AHA/ACP-ASIM task force on clinical competence (ACC/AHA committee to develop a clinical competence statement on electrocardiography and ambulatory electrocardiography) endorsed by the International Society for Holter and Noninvasive Electrocardiology. Circulation 104(25):3169–3178
6. Epstein AE et al (2008) ACC/AHA/HRS 2008 guidelines for device-based therapy of cardiac rhythm abnormalities: executive summary. Heart Rhythm 5(6):934–955
7. Fuster V et al (2006) ACC/AHA/ESC 2006 guidelines for the management of patients with atrial fibrillation: full text: a report of the American College of Cardiology/American Heart Association Task Force on Practice Guidelines and the European Society of Cardiology Committee for Practice Guidelines (writing committee to revise the 2001 guidelines for the management of patients with atrial fibrillation) developed in collaboration with the European heart rhythm association and the heart rhythm society. Europace 8(9):651–745
8. Blomstrom-Lundqvist C et al (2003) ACC/AHA/ESC guidelines for the management of patients with supraventricular arrhythmias – executive summary. a report of the American College of Cardiology/American Heart Association Task Force on Practice Guidelines and the European Society of Cardiology Committee for Practice Guidelines (writing committee to develop guidelines for the management of patients with supraventricular arrhythmias) developed in collaboration with NASPE-Heart Rhythm Society. J Am Coll Cardiol 42(8):1493–1531
9. Benjamin EJ et al (2009) Prevention of atrial fibrillation: report from a National Heart, Lung, and Blood Institute workshop. Circulation 119(4):606–618
10. Vasamreddy CR et al (2006) Symptomatic and asymptomatic atrial fibrillation in patients undergoing radiofrequency catheter ablation. J Cardiovasc Electrophysiol 17(2):134–139
11. Lickfett L et al (2008) Outcome of atrial fibrillation ablation: assessment of success. Minerva Cardioangiol 56(6): 635–641
12. Wiesel J, Wiesel DJ, Messineo FC (2007) Home monitoring with a modified automatic sphygmomanometer to detect recurrent atrial fibrillation. J Stroke Cerebrovasc Dis 16(1):8–13
13. Elijovich L et al (2009) Intermittent atrial fibrillation may account for a large proportion of otherwise cryptogenic stroke: a study of 30-day cardiac event monitors. J Stroke Cerebrovasc Dis 18(3):185–189
14. Buxton AE et al (2006) ACC/AHA/HRS 2006 key data elements and definitions for electrophysiological studies and procedures: a report of the American College of Cardiology/American Heart Association Task Force on Clinical Data Standards (ACC/AHA/HRS writing committee to develop data standards on electrophysiology). Circulation 114(23): 2534–2570
15. Rothman SA et al (2007) The diagnosis of cardiac arrhythmias: a prospective multi-center randomized study comparing mobile cardiac outpatient telemetry versus standard loop event monitoring. J Cardiovasc Electrophysiol 18(3): 241–247
16. Olson JA et al (2007) Utility of mobile cardiac outpatient telemetry for the diagnosis of palpitations, presyncope, syncope, and the assessment of therapy efficacy. J Cardiovasc Electrophysiol 18(5):473–477
17. Laurent G et al (2009) Influence of ventriculoatrial timing on hemodynamics and symptoms during supraventricular tachycardia. J Cardiovasc Electrophysiol 20(2):176–181
18. Gonzalez-Torrecilla E et al (2009) Combined evaluation of bedside clinical variables and the electrocardiogram for the differential diagnosis of paroxysmal atrioventricular reciprocating tachycardias in patients without pre-excitation. J Am Coll Cardiol 53(25):2353–2358
19. Li Y et al (2006) The combined use of esophageal electrocardiogram and multiple right parasternal chest leads in the diagnosis of PSVT and determination of accessory pathways involved: a new simple noninvasive approach. Int J Cardiol 113(3):311–319
20. Bagliani G et al (2003) Atrial activation analysis by surface P wave and multipolar esophageal recording after cardioversion of persistent atrial fibrillation. Pacing Clin Electrophysiol 26(5):1178–1188

21. Liebman J et al (1991) Electrocardiographic body surface potential mapping in the Wolff-Parkinson-White syndrome. Noninvasive determination of the ventricular insertion sites of accessory atrioventricular connections. Circulation 83(3):886–901

22. Julian DG (1987) The history of coronary care units. Br Heart J 57(6):497–502

23. Funk M et al (1997) Effect of dedicated monitor watchers on patients' outcomes. Am J Crit Care 6(4):318–323

24. Drew BJ et al (2005) AHA scientific statement: practice standards for electrocardiographic monitoring in hospital settings: an American Heart Association Scientific Statement from the Councils on Cardiovascular Nursing, Clinical Cardiology, and Cardiovascular Disease in the Young: endorsed by the International Society of Computerized Electrocardiology and the American Association of Critical-Care Nurses. J Cardiovasc Nurs 20(2):76–106

25. Drew BJ et al (1999) Accuracy of the EASI 12-lead electrocardiogram compared to the standard 12-lead electrocardiogram for diagnosing multiple cardiac abnormalities. J Electrocardiol 32(Suppl):38–47

26. Dhillon SK et al (2009) Telemetry monitoring guidelines for efficient and safe delivery of cardiac rhythm monitoring to noncritical hospital inpatients. Crit Pathw Cardiol 8(3):125–126

27. Brugada J, Brugada P, Brugada R (2000) Sudden death (VI). The Brugada syndrome and right myocardiopathies as a cause of sudden death. The differences and similarities. Rev Esp Cardiol 53(2):275–285

28. Knight BP et al (1999) Clinical consequences of electrocardiographic artifact mimicking ventricular tachycardia. N Engl J Med 341(17):1270–1274

29. Kumar SP, Yans J, Kwatra M (1979) Unusual artifacts in electrocardiographic monitoring. J Electrocardiol 12(3): 295–298

30. Chan PS et al (2009) Hospital variation in time to defibrillation after in-hospital cardiac arrest. Arch Intern Med 169(14):1265–1273

31. Nanke T et al (2004) New olter monitoring analysis system: a calculation of the lead vectors. Circ J 68(8): 751–756

32. Seidl K et al (1999) Radiofrequency catheter ablation of frequent monomorphic ventricular ectopic activity. J Cardiovasc Electrophysiol 10(7):924–934

33. Crawford MH et al (1999) ACC/AHA guidelines for ambulatory electrocardiography: executive summary and recommendations. A report of the American College of Cardiology/American Heart Association Task Force on Practice Guidelines (committee to revise the guidelines for ambulatory electrocardiography). Circulation 100(8):886–893

34. Hallstrom AP et al (1992) Prognostic significance of ventricular premature depolarizations measured 1 year after myocardial infarction in patients with early postinfarction asymptomatic ventricular arrhythmia. J Am Coll Cardiol 20(2):259–264

35. Bigger JT Jr (1983) Definition of benign versus malignant ventricular arrhythmias: targets for treatment. Am J Cardiol 52(6):47C–54C

36. Bigger JT Jr et al (1981) Prevalence, characteristics and significance of ventricular tachycardia (three or more complexes) detected with ambulatory electrocardiographic recording in the late hospital phase of acute myocardial infarction. Am J Cardiol 48(5):815–823

37. Odemuyiwa O et al (1992) Influence of age on the relation between heart rate variability, left ventricular ejection fraction, frequency of ventricular extrasystoles, and sudden death after myocardial infarction. Br Heart J 67(5): 387–391

38. Lown B (1982) Management of patients at high risk of sudden death. Am Heart J 103(4 Pt 2):689–697

39. Preliminary report: effect of encainide and flecainide on mortality in a randomized trial of arrhythmia suppression after myocardial infarction (1989) The Cardiac Arrhythmia Suppression Trial (CAST) investigators. N Engl J Med 321(6):406–412

40. Waldo AL et al (1996) Effect of d-sotalol on mortality in patients with left ventricular dysfunction after recent and remote myocardial infarction. The SWORD investigators. Survival with oral d-sotalol. Lancet 348(9019):7–12

41. International Mexiletine and Placebo Antiarrhythmic Coronary Trial: I. Report on arrhythmia and other findings (1984) Impact research group. J Am Coll Cardiol 4(6):1148–1163

42. Echt DS et al (1991) Mortality and morbidity in patients receiving encainide, flecainide, or placebo. The Cardiac Arrhythmia Suppression Trial. N Engl J Med 324(12):781–788

43. Koyama J et al (2002) Evaluation of heart-rate turbulence as a new prognostic marker in patients with chronic heart failure. Circ J 66(10):902–907

44. Gibson TC, Heitzman MR (1984) Diagnostic efficacy of 24-hour electrocardiographic monitoring for syncope. Am J Cardiol 53(8):1013–1017

45. Bass EB et al (1990) The duration of Holter monitoring in patients with syncope. Is 24 hours enough? Arch Intern Med 150(5):1073–1078

46. Lipski J et al (1976) Value of Holter monitoring in assessing cardiac arrhythmias in symptomatic patients. Am J Cardiol 37(1):102–107

47. Ayabakan C et al (2000) Analysis of 2017 Holter records in pediatric patients. Turk J Pediatr 42(4):286–293

48. Sivakumaran S et al (2003) A prospective randomized comparison of loop recorders versus Holter monitors in patients with syncope or presyncope. Am J Med 115(1):1–5

49. Gatzoulis KA et al (2009) Correlation of noninvasive electrocardiography with invasive electrophysiology in syncope of unknown origin: implications from a large syncope database. Ann Noninvasive Electrocardiol 14(2):119–127

50. Moya A et al (2009) Guidelines for the diagnosis and management of syncope (version 2009): the task force for the diagnosis and management of syncope of the European Society of cardiology (ESC). Eur Heart J 30(21):2631–2671

51. Gula LJ et al (2004) External loop recorders: determinants of diagnostic yield in patients with syncope. Am Heart J 147(4):644–648

52. Schuchert A et al (2003) Diagnostic yield of external electrocardiographic loop recorders in patients with recurrent syncope and negative tilt table test. Pacing Clin Electrophysiol 26(9):1837–1840

53. Kinlay S et al (1996) Cardiac event recorders yield more diagnoses and are more cost-effective than 48-hour Holter monitoring in patients with palpitations. A controlled clinical trial. Ann Intern Med 124(1 Pt 1):16–20

54. Grupi CJ et al (1998) The contribution of event monitor recorder to the diagnosis of symptoms. Arq Bras Cardiol 70(5):309–314

55. Linzer M et al (1990) Incremental diagnostic yield of loop electrocardiographic recorders in unexplained syncope. Am J Cardiol 66(2):214–219

56. Joshi S et al (2009) Prevalence, predictors, and prognosis of atrial fibrillation early after pulmonary vein isolation: findings from 3 months of continuous automatic ECG loop recordings. J Cardiovasc Electrophysiol 20(10):1089–1094

57. Reiffel JA et al (2005) Comparison of autotriggered memory loop recorders versus standard loop recorders versus 24-hour Holter monitors for arrhythmia detection. Am J Cardiol 95(9):1055–1059

58. Krahn AD et al (2004) The use of monitoring strategies in patients with unexplained syncope–role of the external and implantable loop recorder. Clin Auton Res 14(Suppl 1):55–61

59. Mason PK et al (2003) Usefulness of implantable loop recorders in office-based practice for evaluation of syncope in patients with and without structural heart disease. Am J Cardiol 92(9):1127–1129

60. Brignole M et al (2005) Proposed electrocardiographic classification of spontaneous syncope documented by an implantable loop recorder. Europace 7(1):14–18

61. Entem FR et al (2009) Utility of implantable loop recorders for diagnosing unexplained syncope in clinical practice. Clin Cardiol 32(1):28–31

62. Giada F et al (2007) Recurrent Unexplained Palpitations (RUP) study comparison of implantable loop recorder versus conventional diagnostic strategy. J Am Coll Cardiol 49(19):1951–1956

63. Simantirakis EN et al (2004) Severe bradyarrhythmias in patients with sleep apnoea: the effect of continuous positive airway pressure treatment: a long-term evaluation using an insertable loop recorder. Eur Heart J 25(12):1070–1076

64. Huikuri HV et al (2003) Cardiac Arrhythmias and Risk Stratification after MyocArdial infarction: results of the CARISMA pilot study. Pacing Clin Electrophysiol 26(1 Pt 2):416–419

65. Kabra R et al (2009) The dual role of implantable loop recorder in patients with potentially arrhythmic symptoms: a retrospective single-center study. Pacing Clin Electrophysiol 32(7):908–912

66. Nierop PR et al (2000) Heart rhythm during syncope and presyncope: results of implantable loop recorders. Pacing Clin Electrophysiol 23(10 Pt 1):1532–1538

67. Rossano J et al (2003) Efficacy of implantable loop recorders in establishing symptom-rhythm correlation in young patients with syncope and palpitations. Pediatrics 112(3 Pt 1):e228–e233

68. van Dam P et al (2009) Improving sensing and detection performance in subcutaneous monitors. J Electrocardiol 42(6):580–583

69. Brignole M (2009) Different electrocardiographic manifestations of the cardioinhibitory vasovagal reflex. Europace 11(2):144–146

70. Brignole M (2007) International Study on Syncope of Uncertain aEtiology 3 (ISSUE 3): pacemaker therapy for patients with asystolic neurally-mediated syncope: rationale and study design. Europace 9(1):25–30

71. Brignole M et al (2009) Indications for the use of diagnostic implantable and external ECG loop recorders. Europace 11(5):671–87

72. Chen J et al (2008) Design of the Pacemaker Remote Follow-up Evaluation and Review (PREFER) trial to assess the clinical value of the remote pacemaker interrogation in the management of pacemaker patients. Trials 9:18

73. Parsonnet V, Crawford CC, Bernstein AD (1984) The 1981 United States survey of cardiac pacing practices. J Am Coll Cardiol 3(5):1321–1332

74. Joseph GK et al (2004) Remote interrogation and monitoring of implantable cardioverter defibrillators. J Interv Card Electrophysiol 11(2):161–166

75. Gessman LJ et al (1995) Accuracy and clinical utility of transtelephonic pacemaker follow-up. Pacing Clin Electrophysiol 18(5 Pt 1):1032–1036

76. Hayashi M et al (2009) Incidence and risk factors of arrhythmic events in catecholaminergic polymorphic ventricular tachycardia. Circulation 119(18):2426–2434

77. Tan JH, Scheinman MM (2008) Exercise-induced polymorphic ventricular tachycardia in adults without structural heart disease. Am J Cardiol 101(8):1142–1146

78. Pappas LK et al (2006) Exercise-induced second-degree atrioventricular block. Int J Cardiol 111(3):461–463

79. Beckerman J et al (2005) Exercise-induced ventricular arrhythmias and cardiovascular death. Ann Noninvasive Electrocardiol 10(1):47–52

80. Morshedi-Meibodi A et al (2004) Clinical correlates and prognostic significance of exercise-induced ventricular premature beats in the community: the Framingham Heart Study. Circulation 109(20):2417–2422

81. Bunch TJ et al (2004) The prognostic significance of exercise-induced atrial arrhythmias. J Am Coll Cardiol 43(7):1236–1240

82. Partington S et al (2003) Prevalence and prognostic value of exercise-induced ventricular arrhythmias. Am Heart J 145(1):139–146

83. Sharma AD et al (1987) Sensitivity and specificity of invasive and noninvasive testing for risk of sudden death in Wolff-Parkinson-White syndrome. J Am Coll Cardiol 10(2):373–381

84. Gibbons RJ et al (1997) ACC/AHA guidelines for exercise testing: executive summary. A report of the American College of Cardiology/American Heart Association Task Force on Practice Guidelines (committee on exercise testing). Circulation 96(1):345–354

85. Podrid PJ, Graboys TB (1984) Exercise stress testing in the management of cardiac rhythm disorders. Med Clin North Am 68(5):1139–1152

86. Graboys TB et al (1982) Long-term survival of patients with malignant ventricular arrhythmia treated with antiarrhythmic drugs. Am J Cardiol 50(3):437–443

87. Falk RH (1989) Flecainide-induced ventricular tachycardia and fibrillation in patients treated for atrial fibrillation. Ann Intern Med 111(2):107–111

88. Bricker JT et al (1985) Exercise testing in children with Wolff-Parkinson-White syndrome. Am J Cardiol 55(8):1001–1004

89. Farrell TG et al (1991) Risk stratification for arrhythmic events in postinfarction patients based on heart rate variability, ambulatory electrocardiographic variables and the signal-averaged electrocardiogram. J Am Coll Cardiol 18(3):687–697

90. Stevenson WG, Ridker PM (1996) Should survivors of myocardial infarction with low ejection fraction be routinely referred to arrhythmia specialists? JAMA 276(6):481–485

91. Gardner PI et al (1985) Electrophysiologic and anatomic basis for fractionated electrograms recorded from healed myocardial infarcts. Circulation 72(3):596–611

92. Richards DA et al (1984) Electrophysiologic substrate for ventricular tachycardia: correlation of properties in vivo and in vitro. Circulation 69(2):369–381

93. Steinberg JS, Berbari EJ (1996) The signal-averaged electrocardiogram: update on clinical applications. J Cardiovasc Electrophysiol 7(10):972–988

94. Korhonen P et al (2006) QRS duration in high-resolution methods and standard ECG in risk assessment after first and recurrent myocardial infarctions. Pacing Clin Electrophysiol 29(8):830–836

95. Folino AF et al (2006) Long-term follow-up of the signal-averaged ECG in arrhythmogenic right ventricular cardiomyopathy: correlation with arrhythmic events and echocardiographic findings. Europace 8(6):423–429

96. Bauce B et al (2010) Differences and similarities between arrhythmogenic right ventricular cardiomyopathy and athlete's heart adaptions. Br J Sports Med 44(2):148–154

97. Denes P et al (1983) Quantitative analysis of the high-frequency components of the terminal portion of the body surface QRS in normal subjects and in patients with ventricular tachycardia. Circulation 67(5):1129–1138

98. Simson MB (1981) Use of signals in the terminal QRS complex to identify patients with ventricular tachycardia after myocardial infarction. Circulation 64(2):235–242

99. Breithardt G et al (1983) Prognostic significance of late ventricular potentials after acute myocardial infarction. Eur Heart J 4(7):487–495

100. Goldberger JJ et al (1994) Assessment of effects of autonomic stimulation and blockade on the signal-averaged electrocardiogram. Circulation 89(4):1656–1664

101. Gomes JA et al (2001) Prediction of long-term outcomes by signal-averaged electrocardiography in patients with unsustained ventricular tachycardia, coronary artery disease, and left ventricular dysfunction. Circulation 104(4):436–441

102. Gottlieb S et al (1995) Improvement in the prognosis of patients with acute myocardial infarction in the 1990s compared with the prethrombolytic era: an analysis by age subgroups. Am J Geriatr Cardiol 4(6):17–31

103. Pedretti R et al (1992) Influence of thrombolysis on signal-averaged electrocardiogram and late arrhythmic events after acute myocardial infarction. Am J Cardiol 69(9):866–872

104. Denes P et al (1994) Prognostic significance of signal-averaged electrocardiogram after thrombolytic therapy and/or angioplasty during acute myocardial infarction (CAST substudy). Cardiac Arrhythmia Suppression Trial (CAST) SAECG substudy investigators. Am J Cardiol 74(3):216–220

105. Steinberg JS et al (1994) Effects of thrombolytic therapy administered 6 to 24 hours after myocardial infarction on the signal-averaged ECG. Results of a multicenter randomized trial. LATE ancillary study investigators. Late Assessment of Thrombolytic Efficacy. Circulation 90(2):746–752

106. Bauer A et al (2005) Reduced prognostic power of ventricular late potentials in post-infarction patients of the reperfusion era. Eur Heart J 26(8):755–761

107. Hartikainen JE et al (1996) Distinction between arrhythmic and nonarrhythmic death after acute myocardial infarction based on heart rate variability, signal-averaged electrocardiogram, ventricular arrhythmias and left ventricular ejection fraction. J Am Coll Cardiol 28(2):296–304

108. Kuchar DL, Rosenbaum DS (1989) Noninvasive recording of late potentials: current state of the art. Pacing Clin Electrophysiol 12(9):1538–1551

109. Middlekauff HR et al (1990) Comparison of frequency of late potentials in idiopathic dilated cardiomyopathy and ischemic cardiomyopathy with advanced congestive heart failure and their usefulness in predicting sudden death. Am J Cardiol 66(15):1113–1117

110. Poll DS et al (1985) Abnormal signal-averaged electrocardiograms in patients with nonischemic congestive cardiomyopathy: relationship to sustained ventricular tachyarrhythmias. Circulation 72(6):1308–1313

111. Keeling PJ et al (1993) Usefulness of signal-averaged electrocardiogram in idiopathic dilated cardiomyopathy for identifying patients with ventricular arrhythmias. Am J Cardiol 72(1):78–84

112. Mancini DM, Wong KL, Simson MB (1993) Prognostic value of an abnormal signal-averaged electrocardiogram in patients with nonischemic congestive cardiomyopathy. Circulation 87(4):1083–1092

113. Fauchier L et al (2000) Long-term prognostic value of time domain analysis of signal-averaged electrocardiography in idiopathic dilated cardiomyopathy. Am J Cardiol 85(5):618–623

114. Silverman ME et al (1995) Prognostic value of the signal-averaged electrocardiogram and a prolonged QRS in ischemic and nonischemic cardiomyopathy. Am J Cardiol 75(7):460–464

115. Turrini P et al (1999) Late potentials and ventricular arrhythmias in arrhythmogenic right ventricular cardiomyopathy. Am J Cardiol 83(8):1214–1219

116. Blomstrom-Lundqvist C et al (1988) Quantitative analysis of the signal-averaged QRS in patients with arrhythmogenic right ventricular dysplasia. Eur Heart J 9(3):301–312

117. Epstein AE et al (2008) ACC/AHA/HRS 2008 guidelines for device-based therapy of cardiac rhythm abnormalities: a report of the American College of Cardiology/American Heart Association Task Force on Practice Guidelines (writing committee to revise the ACC/AHA/NASPE 2002 guideline update for implantation of cardiac pacemakers and antiarrhythmia devices) developed in collaboration with the American Association for Thoracic Surgery and Society of Thoracic Surgeons. J Am Coll Cardiol 51(21):e1–e62

118. Haghjoo M, Arya A, Sadr-Ameli MA (2006) Microvolt T-wave alternans: a review of techniques, interpretation, utility, clinical studies, and future perspectives. Int J Cardiol 109(3):293–306

119. Narayan SM (2008) T-wave alternans testing for ventricular arrhythmias. Prog Cardiovasc Dis 51(2):118–127

120. Adam DR et al (1984) Fluctuations in T-wave morphology and susceptibility to ventricular fibrillation. J Electrocardiol 17(3):209–218

121. Selvaraj RJ et al (2007) Endocardial and epicardial repolarization alternans in human cardiomyopathy: evidence for spatiotemporal heterogeneity and correlation with body surface T-wave alternans. J Am Coll Cardiol 49(3):338–346

122. Narayan SM (2007) T-wave alternans and human ventricular arrhythmias: what is the link? J Am Coll Cardiol 49(3):347–349

123. Chinushi M et al (1998) Electrophysiological basis of arrhythmogenicity of QT/T alternans in the long-QT syndrome: tridimensional analysis of the kinetics of cardiac repolarization. Circ Res 83(6):614–628

124. Koller ML et al (2005) Altered dynamics of action potential restitution and alternans in humans with structural heart disease. Circulation 112(11):1542–1548

125. Bloomfield DM, Hohnloser SH, Cohen RJ (2002) Interpretation and classification of microvolt T wave alternans tests. J Cardiovasc Electrophysiol 13(5):502–512

126. Smith JM et al (1988) Electrical alternans and cardiac electrical instability. Circulation 77(1):110–121

127. Richter S, Duray G, Hohnloser SH (2005) How to analyze T-wave alternans. Heart Rhythm 2(11):1268–1271

128. Bloomfield DM et al (2006) Microvolt T-wave alternans and the risk of death or sustained ventricular arrhythmias in patients with left ventricular dysfunction. J Am Coll Cardiol 47(2):456–463

129. Chow T et al (2006) Prognostic utility of microvolt T-wave alternans in risk stratification of patients with ischemic cardiomyopathy. J Am Coll Cardiol 47(9):1820–1827

130. Chow T et al (2007) Microvolt T-wave alternans identifies patients with ischemic cardiomyopathy who benefit from implantable cardioverter-defibrillator therapy. J Am Coll Cardiol 49(1):50–58

131. Costantini O et al (2009) The ABCD (Alternans Before Cardioverter Defibrillator) trial: strategies using T-wave alternans to improve efficiency of sudden cardiac death prevention. J Am Coll Cardiol 53(6):471–479

132. Gold MR et al (2000) A comparison of T-wave alternans, signal averaged electrocardiography and programmed ventricular stimulation for arrhythmia risk stratification. J Am Coll Cardiol 36(7):2247–2253

133. Rashba EJ et al (2004) Enhanced detection of arrhythmia vulnerability using T wave alternans, left ventricular ejection fraction, and programmed ventricular stimulation: a prospective study in subjects with chronic ischemic heart disease. J Cardiovasc Electrophysiol 15(2):170–176

134. Shalaby AA et al (2007) Microvolt T-wave alternans during atrial and ventricular pacing. Pacing Clin Electrophysiol 30(Suppl 1):S178–S182

135. Chow T et al (2008) Does microvolt T-wave alternans testing predict ventricular tachyarrhythmias in patients with ischemic cardiomyopathy and prophylactic defibrillators? The MASTER (Microvolt T wave alternans testing for risk stratification of post-myocardial infarction patients) trial. J Am Coll Cardiol 52(20):1607–1615

136. Salerno-Uriarte JA et al (2007) Prognostic value of T-wave alternans in patients with heart failure due to nonischemic cardiomyopathy: results of the ALPHA study. J Am Coll Cardiol 50(19):1896–1904

137. Gold MR et al (2008) Role of microvolt T-wave alternans in assessment of arrhythmia vulnerability among patients with heart failure and systolic dysfunction: primary results from the T-wave alternans Sudden Cardiac Death in Heart Failure Trial substudy. Circulation 118(20):2022–2028

138. Grimm W et al (2003) Noninvasive arrhythmia risk stratification in idiopathic dilated cardiomyopathy: results of the Marburg cardiomyopathy study. Circulation 108(23):2883–2891

139. Stein PK et al (1994) Heart rate variability: a measure of cardiac autonomic tone. Am Heart J 127(5):1376–1381

140. Heart rate variability (1996) Standards of measurement, physiological interpretation, and clinical use. Task force of the European society of cardiology and the North American Society of Pacing and Electrophysiology. Eur Heart J 17(3):354–381

141. Odemuyiwa O et al (1991) Comparison of the predictive characteristics of heart rate variability index and left ventricular ejection fraction for all-cause mortality, arrhythmic events and sudden death after acute myocardial infarction. Am J Cardiol 68(5):434–439

142. Ortak J et al (2005) Changes in heart rate, heart rate variability, and heart rate turbulence during evolving reperfused myocardial infarction. Pacing Clin Electrophysiol 28(Suppl 1):S227–S232

143. Chiou CW, Zipes DP (1998) Selective vagal denervation of the atria eliminates heart rate variability and baroreflex sensitivity while preserving ventricular innervation. Circulation 98(4):360–368

144. La Rovere MT, Pinna GD, Raczak G (2008) Baroreflex sensitivity: measurement and clinical implications. Ann Noninvasive Electrocardiol 13(2):191–207

145. Adamson PB, Vanoli E (2001) Early autonomic and repolarization abnormalities contribute to lethal arrhythmias in chronic ischemic heart failure: characteristics of a novel heart failure model in dogs with postmyocardial infarction left ventricular dysfunction. J Am Coll Cardiol 37(6):1741–1748

146. Schwartz PJ, La Rovere MT, Vanoli E (1992) Autonomic nervous system and sudden cardiac death. Experimental basis and clinical observations for post-myocardial infarction risk stratification. Circulation 85(1 Suppl):I77–I91

147. Stein PK, Deedwania P (2009) Usefulness of abnormal heart rate turbulence to predict cardiovascular mortality in high-risk patients with acute myocardial infarction and left ventricular dysfunction (from the EPHESUS study). Am J Cardiol 103(11):1495–1499

148. Exner DV et al (2007) Noninvasive risk assessment early after a myocardial infarctions, the REFINE study. J Am Coll Cardiol 50(24):2275–2284

149. Moore RK et al (2006) Heart rate turbulence and death due to cardiac decompensation in patients with chronic heart failure. Eur J Heart Fail 8(6):585–590

150. Balcioglu S et al (2007) Heart rate variability and heart rate turbulence in patients with type 2 diabetes mellitus with versus without cardiac autonomic neuropathy. Am J Cardiol 100(5):890–893

151. Yang A et al (2005) Influence of obstructive sleep apnea on heart rate turbulence. Basic Res Cardiol 100(5):439–445

152. Winfree AT (1983) Sudden cardia death: a problem in topology. Sci Am 248(5):144–149, 152–157, 160–161

153. Baumert M et al (2004) Forecasting of life threatening arrhythmias using the compression entropy of heart rate. Methods Inf Med 43(2):202–206

154. Baumert M et al (2002) Heart rate and blood pressure interaction in normotensive and chronic hypertensive pregnancy. Biomed Tech (Berl) 47(Suppl 1 Pt 2):554–556

155. Recommended guidelines for in-hospital cardiac monitoring of adults for detection of arrhythmia (1991) Emergency Cardiac Care Committee members. J Am Coll Cardiol 18(6):1431–143

6

Electrophysiology Study: Indications and Interpretations

Karen E. Thomas and Peter J. Zimetbaum

CONTENTS

Abstract

The electrophysiology study is central to the field of cardiac electrophysiology. This chapter begins by describing maneuvers performed in a basic electrophysiology study. Indications for an electrophysiology study are then discussed. They include (1) evaluation of syncope, (2) diagnosis of an arrhythmia, (3) evaluation of patients with Wolff–Parkinson–White, and (4) risk stratification of sudden cardiac death. The role of EP studies in non-ischemic cardiomyopathies is also addressed.

From: *Contemporary Cardiology: Management of Cardiac Arrhythmias*
Edited by: Gan-Xin Yan, Peter R. Kowey, DOI 10.1007/978-1-60761-161-5_6
© Springer Science+Business Media, LLC 2011

Key Words: Arrhythmogenic right ventricular cardiomyopathy; AV node function; AV Wenckebach; bradyarrhythmias; corrected sinus node recovery time; electrophysiology study; His bundle; His Purkinje function; HV interval; hypertrophic cardiomyopathy; inducible ventricular tachycardia; intracardiac intervals; Multicenter Automatic Defibrillator Implantation Trial (MADIT); Multicenter Unsustained Tachycardia Trial (MUSTT); non-ischemic cardiomyopathy; sinus node function; sinus node recovery time; sinoatrial conduction time; supraventricular arrhythmias; syncope; ventricular arrhythmias; ventricular stimulation; Wolff-Parkinson-White ECG pattern; Wolff-Parkinson-White syndrome.

INTRODUCTION

Central to the field of cardiac electrophysiology and cardiac arrhythmia management is the electrophysiology study (EPS). In broad terms, a diagnostic electrophysiology study is an invasive, catheter-based procedure which makes intracardiac recordings of baseline cardiac intervals in sinus rhythm, as well as intracardiac recordings during supraventricular and ventricular arrhythmias. Additionally, fixed cycle length pacing and extrastimulus testing can be performed to evaluate a patient's native conduction system and to help induce and determine the nature of an arrhythmia. Finally, an electrophysiology study can be therapeutic and potentially curative when radiofrequency ablation is performed.

Indications and interpretations of an electrophysiology study is the subject of the current chapter. Major indications for an EPS include (1) the evaluation of syncope, (2) definitive diagnosis of subjective palpitations or of a documented cardiac arrhythmia, (3) evaluation of patients with Wolff-Parkinson-White, and (4) risk stratification of sudden cardiac death. Interpretations of the electrophysiology study will be included in the relevant indication for the EPS. Specific details regarding the role of the electrophysiology study in the evaluation and treatment of supraventricular and ventricular arrhythmias will not be discussed in this chapter, but will be the topic of subsequent chapters.

THE BASIC ELECTROPHYSIOLOGY STUDY

A basic electrophysiology study is performed in a dedicated electrophysiology lab where, with fluoroscopic guidance, catheters are placed in the cardiac chambers. In our lab, the right and left femoral veins are the most common access sites. From the femoral veins, catheters are passed via the inferior vena cava into the right atrium and right ventricle. If required, a transseptal puncture performed from the right atrium can be used to access the left atrium. In our lab, we prefer to use the femoral artery to access the left ventricle via the retrograde aortic approach. Alternatively, a transseptal approach can be employed. It is also possible to use the antecubital, brachial, or subclavian veins for catheter placement in the right heart, particularly the coronary sinus.

Four catheters are generally used for a complete diagnostic electrophysiology study. One catheter is placed in the high posterolateral wall of the right atrium, designated high right atrium (HRA). Catheter placement is near the junction of the right atrium and superior vena cava in the region of the sinus node. A second catheter is placed in the coronary sinus (CS). The CS catheter allows for indirect left atrial recording and stimulation. Direct catheter placement in the left atrium, via transseptal puncture, is not usually required for a diagnostic EPS. A third catheter is placed in the right ventricle (RV) and is most often positioned in the right ventricular apex, but can be positioned anywhere along the intraventricular septum as well as the right ventricular outflow tract. A fourth catheter is placed across the tricuspid annulus in the region of the His bundle electrogram. Ideally the most proximal His bundle potential is recorded. Often, the proximal His bundle electrogram is present when the atrial and ventricular potentials are of approximately equal size *(1)*. Notably, a His bundle electrogram can be recorded from the left side of the heart when the catheter is placed in the noncoronary cusp of the aortic valve. See Figs. 1 and 2 for RAO and LAO views of diagnostic catheter position.

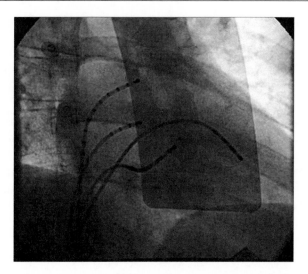

Fig. 1. Right anterior oblique (RAO) projection of diagnostic catheter position.

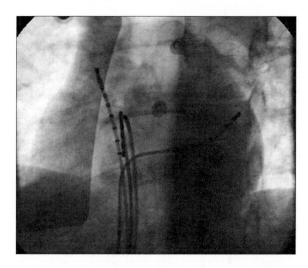

Fig. 2. Left anterior oblique (LAO) projection of diagnostic catheter position.

BASIC INTRACARDIAC INTERVALS

An electrophysiology study begins with measurements of the basic intracardiac intervals. The atrio-His (AH) interval represents conduction time from the low right atrium through the (atrio-ventricular) AV node to the His bundle. Conduction through the AV node constitutes the majority of the AH interval and as such the AH interval largely represents AV nodal function. The AH interval is measured from the atrial electrogram seen on the His bundle recording to the onset of the His deflection. It is important to note that a patient's autonomic state can dramatically affect conduction through the AV node and therefore the AH interval. Thus, the absolute value of an AH interval should not represent a definite assessment of AV nodal function. Instead the response of the AH interval to pacing maneuvers or drugs provides the most meaningful information about the functional state of the AV node (1).

A normal AH interval is 60–125 msec. Causes of AH prolongation include heightened vagal tone, ischemia (during inferior myocardial infarction), infectious processes such as Lyme disease, and fibrocalcific degeneration. Causes of AH shortening include heightened sympathetic tone or rarely an atrio-His bypass tract *(2)*.

The His-ventricular (HV) interval is the time from the earliest recorded His potential to the *earliest* recorded ventricular deflection measured on either the His tracing or on the surface QRS. It is important to emphasize that earliest ventricular deflection may not be on the His-bundle catheter, but rather on the surface ECG.

A normal HV interval is 35–55 msec. Unlike the AH interval, the HV interval is not significantly affected by autonomic tone. Causes of HV prolongation include aortic and mitral annular calcification, infiltrative processes, surgery, or anti-arrhythmic medications. Conduction over an accessory pathway can cause shortening of the HV interval. Occasionally, HV measurements are falsely shortened. This can occur when premature ventricular contractions cause retrograde activation of the His or when a right bundle potential is mistaken for a His bundle potential. See Fig. 3 for basic intracardiac recordings and AH and HV interval measurements.

Basic intracardiac intervals

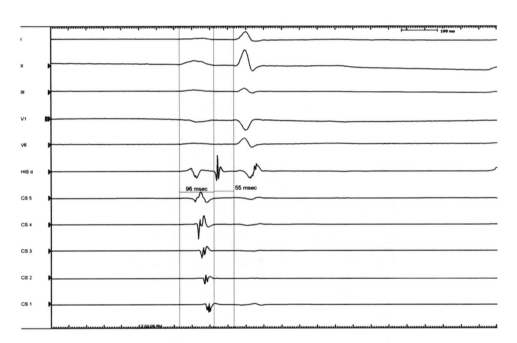

Fig. 3. Basic intracardiac intervals are shown on this intracardiac tracing in sinus rhythm. AH interval measures 96 msec. HV interval measures 55 msec.

In addition to recording baseline cardiac intervals, the basic electrophysiology study includes performing several pacing maneuvers. Fixed cycle length pacing and pacing with the introduction of premature stimuli are typically performed to assess a patient's conduction system and to induce arrhythmias. Fixed cycle length pacing is performed by introducing electrical stimuli (S1) at a fixed cycle length (i.e., 600, 500 msec). This pacing technique is used to assess the functional properties of the sinus node, the AV node, and His-Purkinje system and is discussed below. Pacing with the introduction of premature stimuli is performed by pacing at a fixed cycle length for a predefined number of beats followed by the introduction of premature stimuli. Typically, eight beats (S1) at a cycle length of 600 msec are followed by a premature stimuli (S2) at 400 msec. The interval of the premature stimuli (S2) is then shortened by 10–20 msec increments until the extrastimuli fails to capture the myocardium.

The introduction of multiple stimuli (S2, S3, S4) may be used to induce reentrant arrhythmias. In general, premature stimuli are not introduced at a coupling interval shorter than 180 msec to prevent the induction of atrial or ventricular fibrillation.

Complications of the EP study include pain and minor bleeding at the access sites, usually the femoral veins. Rarely, significant hemorrhage, groin or retroperitoneal hematoma formation, pseudoanerysm or fistula formation can occur. Phlebitis or thromboembolism may occur although these are relatively rare in a diagnostic EPS. Catheter placement and manipulation can cause vascular damage and extremely rarely lead to perforation of the atrium or ventricle causing tamponade. More often, the regrettable complications of an electrophysiology study including tamponade, heart attack, and stroke occur during radiofrequency ablation, particularly in the left atrium or ventricle. Despite these potential complications, the electrophysiology study, particularly a diagnostic electrophysiology study, is considered a relatively safe procedure which is performed worldwide on a daily basis.

INDICATIONS FOR ELECTROPHYSIOLOGY STUDY

As mentioned, major indications for a diagnostic electrophysiology study include the evaluation of syncope, diagnosis of subjective palpitations or a documented arrhythmia, evaluation of patients with Wolff-Parkinson-White, and risk stratification of sudden cardiac death.

INDICATIONS FOR AN ELECTROPHYSIOLOGY STUDY FOR THE EVALUATION OF SYNCOPE

Syncope is the sudden and transient loss of consciousness accompanied by a loss of postural tone. There are many etiologies of true syncope including bradyarrhythmias and tachyarrhythmias. For many patients, the etiology of syncope can be determined by history and physical examination alone. This is often the case with vasovagal syncope. Additional evaluation, including ECG, telemetry monitoring, and ECHO, can definitively determine the etiology of syncope in some patients (i.e., patients with conversion pauses caught on telemetry).

For some patients who continue to have unexplained syncope after initial evaluation, an electrophysiology study is warranted. The current ACC/AHA recommendation regarding patients with unexplained syncope in whom an electrophysiology study is warranted is: "EP testing can be useful in patients with syncope when bradyarrhythmias or tachyarrhythmias are suspected and in whom noninvasive diagnostic are not conclusive" (3). Findings on ECG such as sinus bradycardia, prolonged AV conduction, and bundle branch block have been shown to predict bradyarrhythmic findings on EPS with 79% sensitivity. Findings of organic heart disease on ECHO or non-sustained ventricular tachycardia (NSVT) on Holter monitor have been demonstrated to predict ventricular tachyarrhythmias on EPS with 100% sensitivity (4). Thus, patients with electrocardiographic evidence of conduction disease or ventricular ectopy and those patients with structural heart disease deserve an electrophysiology study for unexplained syncope. The ACC/AHA makes a specific recommendation to perform an electrophysiology study in patients with unexplained syncope and impaired left ventricular function (3). This recommendation is likely due to the concern for the higher rate of ventricular arrhythmias in this group of patients.

Our general practice is consistent with the published ACC/AHA guidelines that patients with clinical characteristics suggestive of possible bradyarrhythmic or tachyarrhythmic causes of syncope undergo EPS. This includes patients with ECG and ECHO findings as mentioned above, as well as patients who have syncope and associated palpitations. Additionally, we believe that in patients with "concerning" syncope (i.e., syncope that was unheralded, syncope that resulted in significant trauma, or syncope in patients with high-risk jobs (e.g., pilot, firefighter)), an electrophysiology study may be warranted.

That said, we realize that published studies have shown that an electrophysiology study is relatively low yield in patients with normal ECG and normal ECHO *(4)*.

INTERPRETATIONS OF AN ELECTROPHYSIOLOGY STUDY FOR SYNCOPE

The goal of an electrophysiology study in patients with syncope should be to determine sinus node function, AV node function, and His-Purkinje function to evaluate for potential bradyarrhythmias. Subsequently, atrial and then ventricular stimulation should be performed to evaluate for supraventricular or ventricular arrhythmias that lead to hypotension and could potentially cause syncope.

BRADYARRHYTHMIAS

Sinus Node Function

In the electrophysiology lab, the study of bradyarrhythmias begins with the evaluation of sinus node function. Direct measurement of the sinus node electrogram is possible in a research setting, but is not routinely performed in the clinical EP lab. Instead, the response of the sinus node to sustained fixed cycle length atrial pacing and atrial premature depolarizations is used as an indirect measure of sinus node function.

Fixed cycle length atrial pacing causes overdrive suppression of the sinus node. The degree of overdrive suppression is a measure of sinus node function and is called the sinus node recovery time (SNRT). In the electrophysiology lab, sinus node recovery times are obtained by measuring the response to fixed cycle length pacing from the HRA catheter. Stimulation is begun at a cycle length just below the sinus node cycle length, is continued at a stable rate for 60 sec, and is then terminated. The interval from the last paced beat to the first sinus beat is the sinus node recovery time. The sinus node recovery time should be calculated at multiple fixed pacing cycle lengths. Generally, SNRT is performed at 100 msec increments from pacing rates just under the sinus rate to 200 msec. A patient's sinus node recovery time is considered the longest pause between the last paced atrial depolarization to the first sinus return cycle. Although there is some variation, in general, SNRT <1.5 sec is considered normal.

The corrected sinus node recovery time (CSRT) is a second way to evaluate the automaticity of the sinus node. The corrected sinus node recovery time was developed because evaluation of SNRT in patients with resting bradycardia can be inaccurate. The CSRT = SNRT – sinus cycle length. Normal CSRT are considered <550 msec.

Findings of abnormal SNRT or CSRT are clinically meaningful. Two studies performed by Gang and Engel nearly 30 ago revealed that prolonged pauses after the cessation of atrial pacing correlate with conversion pauses after atrial arrhythmias in patients with tachy-brady syndromes *(5, 6)*. Therefore, particularly in patients with atrial fibrillation or other supraventricular arrhythmias, findings of markedly abnormal SNRT or CSRT implicate a conversion pause as the cause of syncope.

Sinoatrial conduction time (SACT) is a third measure of sinus node function. Specifically, the SACT measures the time it takes for a sinus impulse to exit the sinus node and conduct to the surrounding atrial tissue. SACT is assessed by introducing premature atrial stimulation into sinus rhythm. Elevated SACT suggest a problem with sinus node conduction, whereas prolonged SNRT and CSRT suggest a problem with sinus node automaticity. In general, evaluations of sinus node automaticity are considered the more useful evaluations of sinus node conduction *(1)*.

Finally, the response to carotid sinus pressure can be evaluated in the clinic setting, but should be included in an EP study for the evaluation of syncope as well. A sinus pause >3 sec is thought be significant, particularly if it reproduces the patient's symptoms.

AV Node Function

AV nodal function is evaluated by determining the AV nodal Wenckebach cycle length. AV Wenckebach (AVWB) is determined by pacing at progressively rapid fixed cycle lengths. AVWB is reached when there is atrial capture without capture of the His bundle or ventricle. AV Wenckebach cycle length >500 msec is considered abnormal. AV nodal conduction is markedly affected by a patient's autonomic state as well as medications; interpretations of AV nodal Wenckebach measurements should be considered in this light.

Although an electrophysiology study can detect abnormalities in sinus node and AV nodal function, the EP study is relatively poor at detecting *transient* conduction disturbances that cause syncope. In a study by Fujimura, 21 patients with documented sinus pauses ($n = 8$) or AV block ($n = 13$) causing syncope underwent an electrophysiology study prior to pacer implantation. Of the eight patients with sinus pauses, three had abnormalities on EP study – one had a prolonged sinus node recovery time and two had carotid hypersensitivity. Of the 13 patients with documented AV or infranodal block, only two had findings on EP study consistent with AV conduction disease. In this study the sensitivity of the EP study to detect transient sinus node dysfunction was 37.5% and the sensitivity to detect transient AV nodal dysfunction was 15.4% *(7)*. This study, along with others, highlights the fact that transient conduction disturbances which cause syncope may not be detected on EP study. In other words, there is a relatively high false negative rate for EPS when considering transient bradyarrhythmias causing syncope. Thus, in patients with syncope, normal conduction on an electrophysiology study does not exclude a transient bradyarrhythmia as the cause of syncope.

When patients with syncope do have markedly abnormal findings of sinus or AV nodal function on electrophysiology study, a permanent pacer is recommended.

His-Purkinje Function

The final evaluation for potential bradyarrhythmias in patients with unexplained syncope involves evaluation of the infranodal conduction system or His-Purkinje system. The HV interval, as described above, normally measures 35–55 msec. Prolonged HV intervals are almost always associated with an abnormal QRS complex because impairment of infra-Hisian conduction is not homogenous *(1)*.

In patients with bundle branch block, measurement of the HV interval predicts progression to complete heart block. In a study by Scheinman, 313 patients with chronic bundle branch block underwent EP study and measurement of the HV interval. Patients were divided into groups according to measured HV intervals. Group I had normal HV intervals <55 msec. Group II had HV intervals 55–69 msec. Group III had HV intervals >70 msec. In 3-year follow-up, Groups I, II, and III had progression to high-degree heart block 4, 2, and 12% of the time. Of patients with markedly prolonged HV intervals (>100 msec), 24% developed high-degree block during follow-up *(8)*. This study demonstrated that patients with bundle branch block and prolonged HV intervals are at relatively high risk for developing high-grade block. Thus, transient high-grade block must be considered as the etiology of syncope in patients with bundle branch block and prolonged HV intervals on EPS.

Currently, the ACC/AHA guidelines state that permanent pacemaker implantation is reasonable for patients with a markedly prolonged HV interval (greater than or equal to 100 msec) *(3)*. This recommendation is based largely on the study by Scheinman. The ACC/AHA recommendation for pacer implantation applies to patients with syncope as well as asymptomatic patients who are incidentally found to have prolonged HV intervals on EPS.

In addition to HV interval measurement, fixed cycle length pacing can be performed to evaluate His-Purkinje function. Block in or below the His-Purkinje system at cycle lengths >400 msec is abnormal and an indication for implantation of a permanent pacemaker. At times block in the AV node impairs the ability to evaluate the His-Purkinje system. In these instances, atropine can be administered to improve conduction through the AV node to allow assessment of infranodal conduction.

Numerous studies have been performed to evaluate the ability of the electrophysiology study to identify the etiology of syncope. Although these studies vary somewhat in their inclusion criteria and method of EPS, in general, the results are similar. In patients with unexplained syncope, findings at EP study suggestive of bradyarrhythmias as the cause of syncope occur approximately 15% of the time *(9–11)*. Thus, the electrophysiology study is relatively low yield in identifying undiagnosed bradyarrhythmias as the cause of syncope although abnormalities on ECG may increase the sensitivity of an EPS slightly.

TACHYARRHYTHMIAS

Tachyarrhythmias, both supraventricular and ventricular, can be diagnosed during electrophysiology study and may be the etiology of syncope. As previously mentioned, patients with organic heart disease or non-sustained ventricular tachycardia and syncope have a higher rate of ventricular tachycardia on EPS *(4)*. Numerous studies have shown that, in general, in patients with undiagnosed syncope and *structurally normal hearts* who undergo EP study, approximately 10% are diagnosed with supraventricular arrhythmias and 15% are diagnosed with ventricular tachycardia *(9, 10, 12, 13)*.

SUPRAVENTRICULAR ARRHYTHMIAS

For patients with supraventricular arrhythmias, these arrhythmias can usually be induced on EPS. Whether or not a supraventricular arrhythmia identified at EP study is the cause of a patient's syncope can be difficult to determine. Including invasive arterial monitoring as part of the electrophysiology study can sometime be of help as it allows rapid demonstration of the hemodynamic consequences of an arrhythmia. In our experience, syncope with supraventricular tachycardia is relatively rare. When syncope does occur, it tends to occur at the onset of the SVT and is likely due to baroreceptor reflexes *(2)*.

Atrial fibrillation may be induced during an electrophysiology study. Easily inducible atrial fibrillation at electrophysiology study may suggest undiagnosed atrial fibrillation in a patient. Syncope in patients with paroxysmal atrial fibrillation is not usually due to the arrhythmia itself, but rather due to pauses at the time of conversion from atrial fibrillation to sinus rhythm.

VENTRICULAR ARRHYTHMIAS

The final portion of an electrophysiology study conducted for the evaluation of syncope is ventricular stimulation. Ventricular stimulation with single, double, or triple extrastimuli should be performed at two locations in the right ventricle, usually RV apex and RV outflow tract. (Please see the section on the role of the EPS in risk stratification for sudden cardiac death for detailed description of ventricular stimulation.)

The ability to induce ventricular tachycardia by ventricular stimulation is highly dependent on a patient's underlying myocardial substrate. In patients with ischemic heart disease and structurally abnormal hearts, stable monomorphic tachycardia can be induced in approximately 30% of patients *(14)*. These patients should be identified as high risk for ventricular tachycardia prior to EP study based on abnormal findings on ECG and echocardiography. Identifying patients by electrophysiology study with ischemic heart disease and abnormal left ventricular systolic function who are at risk for sudden cardiac death will be discussed in detail later in this chapter.

In patients without structural heart disease, induction of ventricular tachycardia at electrophysiology study occurs at a rate of 10–15% *(13, 15)*. Aggressive stimulation protocols may be more likely to induce ventricular tachycardia, but these may be false-positive results. In general, ventricular stimulation in patients with unexplained syncope is highest when restricted to up to stimulation from two sights *(2)*.

INDICATIONS FOR AN ELECTROPHYSIOLOGY STUDY TO DIAGNOSE AN ARRHYTHMIA

Evaluation of subjective palpitations or documented arrhythmia is a second indication for an electrophysiology study. Supraventricular and ventricular arrhythmias are often experienced by the patient as palpitations or heart racing, potentially with associated with shortness of breath, chest pressure, dizziness, or syncope.

All patients with a history of palpitations should undergo history, physical examination, and ECG. Occasionally, a baseline sinus rhythm ECG can suggest the cause of palpitations, as for example in patients with Wolff-Parkinson-White syndrome. If there is no documentation of the patient's arrhythmia, a 2-week event monitor should be ordered to document a patient's palpitations. In many instances, sinus tachycardia will be documented. At other times, a symptomatic arrhythmia will be documented. At times these arrhythmias can be diagnosed on the event monitor, as in cases of atrial fibrillation or atrial flutter. Other times, a narrow complex arrhythmia may be documented on the monitor, but the nature of the arrhythmia cannot be determined. In fact, in many instances, even when a 12 lead ECG is obtained of a supraventricular tachycardia, a definitive diagnosis cannot be made. In these instances of undifferentiated SVT, an electrophysiology study is warranted to definitively diagnose (and potential cure via radiofrequency ablation) the patient's arrhythmia. While an EP study can be performed for diagnosis and treatment purposes of a supraventricular arrhythmia, it is not required. For non-life threatening supraventricular arrhythmias, empiric medical management with a beta-blocker or calcium channel blocker is a reasonable initial approach. In our practice, decisions regarding performing an EP study are largely influenced by patient preference.

In some instances, patients who present with palpitations have a documented wide complex tachycardia (WCT). Like for narrow complex arrhythmias, at times it is difficult to determine the true etiology of the WCT. For patients with undifferentiated WCT, an electrophysiology study is indicated.

At times patients describe subjective palpitations, but no arrhythmia can be documented. In some instances, particularly if patients have concerning associated symptoms, like syncope, an EP study is warranted to determine if there is any arrhythmia present and the nature of the arrhythmia.

ACC/AHA have not published widely applicable recommendations regarding indications for EP study in patients with symptomatic palpitations or in patients with documented undifferentiated narrow or wide complex arrhythmias. In patients with coronary heart disease and wide-QRS complex tachycardias, the ACC/AHA states that "EP testing is useful for diagnostic evaluation" *(3)*. The North American Society of Pacing and Electrophysiology (now Heart Rhythm Society) published guidelines in 2002 regarding recommendations for catheter ablation of specific tachycardias, but no mention is made regarding indications for a diagnostic EP study to diagnose these arrhythmias. Thus, in the absence of published guidelines, our general approach is outlined above.

THE ROLE OF THE ELECTROPHYSIOLOGY STUDY IN PATIENTS WITH WOLFF-PARKINSON-WHITE

Patients with manifest AV accessory pathways, characterized by short PR interval and delta wave on the surface ECG, have Wolff-Parkinson-White (WPW) ECG. The accessory AV bypass tract in these patients predisposes them to AV reentrant tachycardias. Patients with manifest preexcitation on surface ECG and documented supraventricular tachycardia have WPW syndrome. In general, patients with WPW syndrome should undergo electrophysiology study for curative ablation of the AV accessory pathway. It is important to note that atrial fibrillation occurs in 10–30% of patients with WPW syndrome and can be life-threatening when atrial fibrillation conducts rapidly to the ventricle over the bypass tract causing ventricular fibrillation *(16, 17)*. This concern contributes, in part, to the rationale to study and ablation patients with symptomatic WPW.

For asymptomatic patients with WPW ECG, the role of the electrophysiology study is controversial. Indeed, a recent "Controversies in Cardiovascular Medicine" was published in *Circulation* to address the question: "Should catheter ablation be performed in asymptomatic patients with Wolff-Parkinson-White Syndrome?" *(18, 19)*.

Proponents of performing an EPS in asymptomatic patients with WPW argue that some patients have ventricular fibrillation as their first "symptomatic" episode of WPW and that an EPS can identify some features of asymptomatic patients who are considered "high risk" *(20–22)*. Timmermans et al., and others, have demonstrated that short anterograde refractory period of the accessory pathway and RR intervals <200 msec during atrial fibrillation on an EP study correlate with increased risk of sudden death. Moreover, in the past several years Pappone et al. have published data which demonstrated that: (1) asymptomatic patients with WPW with inducible arrhythmias on EPS were more likely to develop symptomatic SVT in the future, (2) patients with inducible arrhythmias at EPS who undergo ablation were less likely to develop arrhythmias, and (3) patients who do not undergo ablation continued to have arrhythmias, including asymptomatic atrial fibrillation, which in some cases lead to ventricular fibrillation and death *(19, 23, 24)*.

Opponents of performing an EPS in asymptomatic patients with WPW argue that Pappone's arguments are flawed. In his portion of "Controversies in Cardiovascular Medicine" Wellens submits that: (1) the electrophysiological properties of the AV node and accessory pathway change over time, (2) inducibility on EP study is not stable over time, and (3) Pappone reported a much higher incidence of serious arrhythmias in his studies than previously published reports. Moreover, Wellens points out that EP studies are not without risks and that non-invasive methods can help risk stratify asymptomatic patients with WPW *(18)*.

The ACC/AHA/ESC take a neutral stand on the EP study in asymptomatic patients with WPW. The 2003 guidelines for the management of patients with supraventricular arrhythmias states, "The role of electrophysiological testing and catheter ablation in asymptomatic patients with pre-excitation is controversial." "Patients with asymptomatic pre-excitation should be encouraged to seek medical expertise whenever arrhythmia related symptoms occur. The potential value of electrophysiological testing in identifying high-risk patients who may benefit from catheter ablation must be balanced against the approximately 2% risk of a major complication associated with catheter ablation" *(25)*. Our practice is similar to that recommended by the ACC/AHA. Most patients with asymptomatic WPW undergo non-invasive testing and are found to be "low risk". There is a rare asymptomatic patient with WPW for whom we believe EP study and ablation is warranted.

THE ROLE OF THE EP STUDY IN RISK STRATIFICATION FOR SUDDEN CARDIAC DEATH

A final indication for an electrophysiology study is risk stratification for sudden cardiac death. It is well known that patients with coronary artery disease and depressed left ventricular systolic function are at increased risk for ventricular tachycardia and sudden cardiac death. However, only a minority of patients with ischemic cardiomyopathies will develop ventricular tachycardia. Thus, tools to stratify patients with structural heart disease according to their risk of sudden cardiac death have been developed.

The electrophysiology study and ventricular stimulation in particular have long been thought to predict future risk of sudden cardiac death. Decades ago numerous small studies demonstrated that inducible ventricular tachycardia in patients with ischemic heart disease predicted future arrhythmic events *(26–28)*. More recently, data from the Multicenter Unsustained Tachycardia Trial (MUSTT) and Multicenter Automatic Defibrillator Implantation Trial II (MADIT II) have demonstrated that an invasive EP study has a modest ability to predict future arrhythmic events. Reviewing data from these two contemporary studies is worthwhile as it helped shape the current ACC/AHA recommendations regarding the role of the EP study for risk stratification.

Multicenter Unsustained Tachycardia Trial

The Multicenter Unsustained Tachycardia Trial (MUSTT) trial, published in 1999, studied patients with coronary artery disease, left ventricular ejection fraction ≤40%, and asymptomatic unsustained ventricular tachycardia. A total of 2202 eligible patients underwent electrophysiology study prior to enrollment. Seven hundred and four patients were found to have inducible ventricular arrhythmias at EP study and were enrolled in the trial. 1397 patients had no sustained ventricular tachyarrhythmia at EP study and were followed in a registry.

Of the 704 trial patients, 351 were randomized to electrophysiology-guided antiarrhythmic therapy and 353 to no antiarrhythmic therapy. Of the 351 patients assigned to EP-guided therapy, 196 received an ICD, and 155 were treated with antiarrhythmic medication. The 1397 patients enrolled in the registry were not treated and were followed for outcomes.

Results of MUSTT revealed 2-year rate of cardiac arrest or death from arrhythmia in patients with no antiarrhythmic therapy was 18%; in patients with EP-guided therapy it was 12%. The 5-year event rate was 32% in those with no antiarrhythmic therapy, and 25% in those with EP-guided therapy *(29)*. These differences were statistically significant and the MUSTT investigators concluded that EP-guided therapy, and ICDs in particular, benefit patients at high risk for sudden cardiac death.

One year after the publication of MUSTT, the same investigators published an article comparing the outcomes of inducible patients in the trial who did not receive therapy to noninducible patients enrolled in the registry. In other words, patients with positive EP study and no therapy were compared to patients with negative EP study. This comparison allowed for accurate determination of the diagnostic accuracy of the EP study.

The major finding from this study was the 2-year rate of cardiac arrest and death due to an arrhythmia was 12% in non-inducible patients and 18% for inducible patients assigned to no antiarrhythmic therapy. The 5-year event rates were 24% and 32% respectively. In regards to spontaneous ventricular tachycardia, at 5 years 6% of patients who were non-inducible had VT, whereas 21% of patients who were inducible had VT *(30)*. Please see Table 1 for these results.

In summary, data from the MUSTT investigators revealed that inducibility on EP study accurately predicts increased risk of ventricular tachycardia, cardiac arrest, and death due to arrhythmia. Patients

Table 1
Results from Multicenter Unsustained Tachycardia Trial and MUSTT-EPS

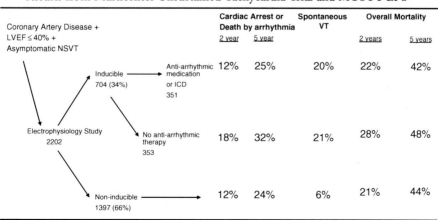

Coronary Artery Disease + LVEF ≤ 40% + Asymptomatic NSVT		Cardiac Arrest or Death by arrhythmia		Spontaneous VT	Overall Mortality	
		2 year	5 year		2 years	5 years
Inducible 704 (34%) → Anti-arrhythmic medication or ICD 351		12%	25%	20%	22%	42%
No anti-arrhythmic therapy 353		18%	32%	21%	28%	48%
Non-inducible 1397 (66%)		12%	24%	6%	21%	44%

Electrophysiology Study 2202

with a positive EP study had higher event rates than those patients who were non-inducible. However, these studies also revealed that the ability of the EP study to predict future events is limited. Differences in event rates between the two groups were statistically significant, but small. At 5 years the difference in rates of cardiac death and death due to an arrhythmia was only 12%. Thus, although an EP study can distinguish between patients who are at high and low risk, the differences between these two groups is small.

Multicenter Automatic Defibrillator Implantation Trial

The MADIT II trial is the second large contemporary trial which gives data regarding the predictive value of the electrophysiology study. The Multicenter Automatic Defibrillator Implantation Trial II (MADIT II) published in 2002 enrolled 1232 patients with prior myocardial infarction and left ventricular ejection fraction $\leq 30\%$. Patients were randomized in a 3:2 fashion to ICD (742 patients) or conventional medical therapy (490 patients). The primary outcome was death from any cause.

MADIT II did not require inducibility on EP study for enrollment in the trial, but in patients assigned to the ICD arm, an EP study was strongly encouraged at the time of ICD implantation. After publication of MADIT II, II investigators published a substudy of patients who underwent elective EP study at the time of ICD implantation. Of the 720 patients in the ICD arm, 593 underwent an EP study. Of those, 207(36%) met a "standard" definition of inducibility. Patients who were found to be inducible on EP study were subsequently compared to patients who were non-inducible on EP study. The primary endpoint of this substudy was the incidence of spontaneous VT or VF on ICD interrogation.

Results from the MADIT II substudy revealed the rates of ventricular tachycardia and ventricular fibrillation (VF) in patients who were inducible (by the standard definition) were similar to rates of patients who were non-inducible. At 2 years, the incidence of ICD therapy for VT or VF was 29.4% in inducible patients and 25.5% in non-inducible patients *(14)*. This suggests that the EP study cannot differentiate among patients who will receive appropriate shocks.

MADIT II investigators then employed a "narrow" definition of inducibility, namely induction of sustained monomorphic ventricular tachycardia, and evaluated arrhythmic outcomes. In this setting, the prognostic ability of the EP study was dramatically improved. Patients in whom sustained monomorphic VT was induced on EP study were significantly more likely to develop both VT (hazard ratio 1.89) and VT or VF (hazard ratio 1.56) than patients who were not inducible *(14)*. Thus, when sustained monomorphic ventricular tachycardia is induced, it accurately predicts future ventricular tachycardia.

In conclusion, among patients with chronic coronary artery disease and reduced left ventricular systolic function electrophysiology studies can identify patients who are at high risk for sudden cardiac death. Data collected as part of MUSTT and MADIT II trials revealed that patients with coronary artery disease and reduced left ventricular ejection fraction who are inducible on EP testing are at increased risk of spontaneous stable ventricular tachycardia, cardiac arrest, and death by arrhythmia. Although, this increased risk may be relatively small when compared to patients who are non-inducible. With this available data, the ACC/AHA/ESC guidelines state: "EP testing is reasonable for risk stratification in patients with remote MI, NSVT, and LVEF equal to or less than 40%" *(3)*. This is a Class IIa recommendation.

THE ROLE OF THE ELECTROPHYSIOLOGY STUDY IN NON-ISCHEMIC CARDIOMYOPATHIES

In addition to patients with ischemic cardiomyopathies, there are other subgroups of patients who are known to be at increased risk of sudden cardiac death due to ventricular arrhythmias. These subgroups include patients with non-ischemic dilated cardiomyopathy, hypertrophic cardiomyopathy, arrhythmogenic right ventricular cardiomyopathy, Brugada syndrome, and long QT syndrome. In general, the role of the EP study for risk stratification in these patients is less well characterized, although in some cases it may be of minor benefit.

In patients with non-ischemic dilated cardiomyopathy, studies have shown mixed results in regards to the ability of EP study to predict future arrhythmic events (31–33). Thus, the ACC/AHA do not recommend to undertake extrastimulus testing in this group of patients for the purposes of risk stratification. For patients with non-ischemic cardiomyopathies who have documented ventricular tachycardia, an EP study can be useful as bundle-branch reentry is relatively common in these patients. The ACC/AHA make a Class I recommendation in this regarding stating, "EP testing is useful to diagnose bundle-branch reentrant tachycardia and to guide ablation in patients with nonischemic dilated cardiomyopathy" (3). In patients with hypertrophic cardiomyopathy, the role of the electrophysiology study is controversial. In general, inducibility on EP study is not thought to have predictive power in this patient population. As such, the ACC/AHA make a Class IIb recommendation that "EP testing may be considered for risk assessment for SCD in patients with HCM"(3). As a general rule, we do not undertake extrastimulus testing in patients with hypertrophic cardiomyopathy.

In patients with arrhythmogenic right ventricular cardiomyopathy (ARVC), the ACC/AHA state: "EP testing might be useful for risk assessment of SCD in patients with ARVC." Historically, EP testing had been used not so much for risk stratification, but to guide ablation in patients with ventricular tachycardia. Recent studies have shown that voltage mapping of the right ventricle shows promise in helping to diagnose this type of cardiomyopathy (34).

In patients with Brugada syndrome and long QT syndrome, the ACC/AHA does not make a recommendation regarding EP testing, as its role is debated at this time.

PERFORMANCE AND INTERPRETATION OF EP STUDY PERFORMED FOR RISK STRATIFICATION

The electrophysiology study performed to stratify patients according to their risk for sudden death follows a relatively standard protocol. In general, programmed stimulation is performed with a fixed cycle length pacing (S1) of eight beats immediately followed by single, double, and triple ventricular extrastimuli (S2, S3, S4) (35, 36). The standard protocol includes at least two different cycle lengths (typically 600 and 400 msec) as well as stimulation in sinus rhythm.

The optimal number of extrastimuli that should be used during ventricular stimulation is debatable. In general, the greater the number of extrastimuli used, the higher the sensitivity, but lower the specificity of the resulting arrhythmia. We believe the use of up to three extrastimuli is optimal. Stimulation should be performed in two different sites, typically the right ventricular apex and right ventricular outflow tract. The protocol described by Josephson by which single ventricular extra stimuli (VES) are delivered at all sites and all cycle lengths before double VES, and double VES before triple VES is recommended (1). This format is less likely to result in ventricular fibrillation at one site which would require ending stimulation for the safety of the patient, when another site could produce monomorphic ventricular tachycardia.

Additional maneuvers can be employed to induce ventricular tachycardia. These include: (1) pacing from alternative sites (left ventricle or atrium), (2) infusing medication (isoproterenol or a type I agent like procainamide), (3) increasing the current used, and (4) using long-short sequences. However, these are not standard when performing ventricular stimulation for the purposes of risk stratification.

When a standard electrophysiology study is performed and no ventricular arrhythmias are induced, it is considered a negative EPS and the patient non-inducible. However, an electrophysiology study in which a ventricular arrhythmia is induced is not necessarily considered positive. The nature and duration of the ventricular arrhythmia need to be considered, as does the stimuli which induced it.

While the induction of some arrhythmias suggests a patient is at high risk for future spontaneous ventricular arrhythmias, the induction of other arrhythmias is non-specific and may be of no clinical import.

The strictest definition of a positive EPS is one in which monomorphic ventricular tachycardia is reproducibly induced and is sustained (>15 sec) or is hemodynamically unstable requiring cardioversion. This is the definition we employ in our lab. A broader definition of a positive EP study includes patients who develop sustained monomorphic VT, or polymorphic VT or ventricular fibrillation with one or two extrastimuli. Responses that are not interpreted as a positive EPS include nonsustained monomorphic or polymorphic ventricular tachycardia, bundle branch reentry ventricular tachycardia, repetitive polymorphic response, or polymorphic ventricular tachycardia or ventricular fibrillation induced with three extrastimuli.

It is important to note that sustained monomorphic ventricular tachycardia, especially in patients with coronary artery disease, can be reproducibly initiated on electrophysiology studies over time *(37, 38)*. If VT can be induced today, it will be induced one year from now. This finding supports the idea that in patients with chronic ischemic heart disease the myocardial scar that forms the substrate of ventricular arrhythmias is fixed and stable over time.

In accordance with the evidence and the ACC/AHA/ESC guidelines, it is our general practice to perform programmed ventricular stimulation on patients with coronary artery disease and LVEF 31–40% to evaluate for inducibility. Patients in whom sustained monomorphic or polymorphic ventricular tachycardia, or ventricular fibrillation, are induced subsequently undergo ICD implantation. Although we realized that non-inducible patients are still at moderately high risk for ventricular arrhythmias, we do not implant ICDs in these patients.

CONCLUSION

In conclusion, there are numerous indications for a diagnostic electrophysiology study. As described, these include determining the etiology of unexplained syncope, making a definitive diagnosis of subjective palpitations or documented narrow or wide complex tachycardia, evaluate patients with Wolff-Parkinson-White syndrome, and stratifying a patient's risk of sudden cardiac death, particularly patients with coronary artery disease and depressed left ventricular function.

As mentioned, the EP study is limited in its ability to determine a bradyarrhythmic or tachyarrhythmic etiology of syncope. Moreover, the EP study is limited in its ability to broadly distinguish between patients who are at high and low risk of sudden cardiac death. However, the EP study is excellent, indeed the gold standard, for determining the nature of a narrow complex or wide complex tachycardia. Much of electrophysiology is based on the ability of the EP study to make these diagnoses. These days, once a diagnostic EP study has made a definitive diagnosis of a particular arrhythmia, the EP study can be therapeutic with the application of radiofrequency ablation. It is for this reason that the EP study will remain at the heart of the field of electrophysiology.

REFERENCES

1. Josephson ME (2002) Clinical cardiac electrophysiology: techniques and interpretations. Lippincott Williams & Wilkins, Philadelphia
2. Zimetbaum PJ, Josephson ME (2009) Practical clinical electrophysiology. Lippincott, Williams & Wilkins, Philadelphia
3. Zipes DP, Camm AJ, Borggrefe M, Buxton AE, Chaitman B, Fromer M et al (2006) ACC/AHA/ESC 2006 guidelines for management of patients with ventricular arrhythmias and the prevention of sudden cardiac death: a report of the American college of cardiology/American heart association task force and the European society of cardiology committee for practice guidelines (writing committee to develop guidelines for management of patients with ventricular arrhythmias and the prevention of sudden cardiac death). J Am Coll Cardiol 48(5):e247–e346

4. Bachinsky WB, Linzer M, Weld L, Estes NA III (1992) Usefulness of clinical characteristics in predicting the outcome of electrophysiologic studies in unexplained syncope. Am J Cardiol 69(12):1044–1049

5. Engel TR, Luck JC, Leddy CL, Gonzalez AD (1979) Diagnostic implications of atrial vulnerability. Pacing Clin Electrophysiol 2(2):208–214

6. Gang ES, Reiffel JA, Livelli FD Jr, Bigger JT Jr (1983) Sinus node recovery times following the spontaneous termination of supraventricular tachycardia and following atrial overdrive pacing: a comparison. Am Heart J 105(2):210–215

7. Fujimura O, Yee R, Klein GJ, Sharma AD, Boahene KA (1989) The diagnostic sensitivity of electrophysiologic testing in patients with syncope caused by transient bradycardia. N Engl J Med 321(25):1703–1707

8. Scheinman MM, Peters RW, Suave MJ, Desai J, Abbott JA, Cogan J et al (1982) Value of the H-Q interval in patients with bundle branch block and the role of prophylactic permanent pacing. Am J Cardiol 50(6):1316–1322

9. Brembilla-Perrot B, Beurrier D, de la Chaise AT, Suty-Selton C, Jacquemin L, Thiel B et al (1996) Significance and prevalence of inducible atrial tachyarrhythmias in patients undergoing electrophysiologic study for presyncope or syncope. Int J Cardiol 53(1):61–69

10. Doherty JU, Pembrook-Rogers D, Grogan EW, Falcone RA, Buxton AE, Marchlinski FE et al (1985) Electrophysiologic evaluation and follow-up characteristics of patients with recurrent unexplained syncope and presyncope. Am J Cardiol 55(6):703–708

11. Hess DS, Morady F, Scheinman MM (1982) Electrophysiologic testing in the evaluation of patients with syncope of undetermined origin. Am J Cardiol 50(6):1309–1315

12. Denes P, Uretz E, Ezri MD, Borbola J (1988) Clinical predictors of electrophysiologic findings in patients with syncope of unknown origin. Arch Intern Med 148(9):1922–1928

13. Morady F, Scheinman MM (1983) The role and limitations of electrophysiologic testing in patients with unexplained syncope. Int J Cardiol 4(2):229–234

14. Daubert JP, Zareba W, Hall WJ, Schuger C, Corsello A, Leon AR et al (2006) Predictive value of ventricular arrhythmia inducibility for subsequent ventricular tachycardia or ventricular fibrillation in multicenter automatic defibrillator implantation trial (MADIT) II patients. J Am Coll Cardiol 47(1):98–107

15. Denniss AR, Ross DL, Richards DA, Uther JB (1992) Electrophysiologic studies in patients with unexplained syncope. Int J Cardiol 35(2):211–217

16. Campbell RW, Smith RA, Gallagher JJ, Pritchett EL, Wallace AG (1977) Atrial fibrillation in the preexcitation syndrome. Am J Cardiol 40(4):514–520

17. Wellens HJ, Durrer D (1974) Wolff-Parkinson-White syndrome and atrial fibrillation. Relation between refractory period of accessory pathway and ventricular rate during atrial fibrillation. Am J Cardiol 34(7):777–782

18. Wellens HJ (2005) Should catheter ablation be performed in asymptomatic patients with Wolff-Parkinson-White syndrome? When to perform catheter ablation in asymptomatic patients with a Wolff-Parkinson-White electrocardiogram. Circulation 112(14):2201–2207

19. Pappone C, Manguso F, Santinelli R, Vicedomini G, Sala S, Paglino G et al (2004) Radiofrequency ablation in children with asymptomatic Wolff-Parkinson-White syndrome. N Engl J Med 351(12):1197–1205

20. Klein GJ, Bashore TM, Sellers TD, Pritchett EL, Smith WM, Gallagher JJ (1979) Ventricular fibrillation in the Wolff-Parkinson-White syndrome. N Engl J Med 301(20):1080–1085

21. Montoya PT, Brugada P, Smeets J, Talajic M, Della BP, Lezaun R et al (1991) Ventricular fibrillation in the Wolff-Parkinson-White syndrome. Eur Heart J 12(2):144–150

22. Timmermans C, Smeets JL, Rodriguez LM, Vrouchos G, van den DA, Wellens HJ (1995) Aborted sudden death in the Wolff-Parkinson-White syndrome. Am J Cardiol 76(7):492–494

23. Pappone C, Santinelli V, Rosanio S, Vicedomini G, Nardi S, Pappone A et al (2003) Usefulness of invasive electrophysiologic testing to stratify the risk of arrhythmic events in asymptomatic patients with Wolff-Parkinson-White pattern: results from a large prospective long-term follow-up study. J Am Coll Cardiol 41(2):239–244

24. Pappone C, Santinelli V, Manguso F, Augello G, Santinelli O, Vicedomini G et al (2003) A randomized study of prophylactic catheter ablation in asymptomatic patients with the Wolff-Parkinson-White syndrome. N Engl J Med 349(19):1803–1811

25. Blomstrom-Lundqvist C, Scheinman MM, Aliot EM, Alpert JS, Calkins H, Camm AJ et al (2003) ACC/AHA/ESC guidelines for the management of patients with supraventricular arrhythmias–executive summary: a report of the American college of cardiology/American heart association task force on practice guidelines and the European society of cardiology committee for practice guidelines (writing committee to develop guidelines for the management of patients with supraventricular arrhythmias). Circulation 108(15):1871–1909

26. Richards DA, Byth K, Ross DL, Uther JB (1991) What is the best predictor of spontaneous ventricular tachycardia and sudden death after myocardial infarction? Circulation 83(3):756–763

27. Wilber DJ, Olshansky B, Moran JF, Scanlon PJ (1990) Electrophysiological testing and nonsustained ventricular tachycardia. Use and limitations in patients with coronary artery disease and impaired ventricular function. Circulation 82(2):350–358

28. Schmitt C, Barthel P, Ndrepepa G, Schreieck J, Plewan A, Schomig A et al (2001) Value of programmed ventricular stimulation for prophylactic internal cardioverter-defibrillator implantation in postinfarction patients preselected by noninvasive risk stratifiers. J Am Coll Cardiol 37(7):1901–1907

29. Buxton AE, Hafley GE, Lehmann MH, Gold M, O'Toole M, Tang A et al (1999) Prediction of sustained ventricular tachycardia inducible by programmed stimulation in patients with coronary artery disease. Utility of clinical variables. Circulation 99(14):1843–1850

30. Buxton AE, Lee KL, DiCarlo L, Gold MR, Greer GS, Prystowsky EN et al (2000) Electrophysiologic testing to identify patients with coronary artery disease who are at risk for sudden death. Multicenter unsustained tachycardia trial investigators. N Engl J Med 342(26):1937–1945

31. Turitto G, Ahuja RK, Caref EB, el Sherif N (1994) Risk stratification for arrhythmic events in patients with nonischemic dilated cardiomyopathy and nonsustained ventricular tachycardia: role of programmed ventricular stimulation and the signal-averaged electrocardiogram. J Am Coll Cardiol 24(6):1523–1528

32. Milner PG, Dimarco JP, Lerman BB (1988) Electrophysiological evaluation of sustained ventricular tachyarrhythmias in idiopathic dilated cardiomyopathy. Pacing Clin Electrophysiol 11(5):562–568

33. Brembilla-Perrot B, Donetti J, de la Chaise AT, Sadoul N, Aliot E, Juilliere Y (1991) Diagnostic value of ventricular stimulation in patients with idiopathic dilated cardiomyopathy. Am Heart J 121(4 Pt 1):1124–1131

34. Avella A, d'Amati G, Pappalardo A, Re F, Silenzi PF, Laurenzi F et al (2008) Diagnostic value of endomyocardial biopsy guided by electroanatomic voltage mapping in arrhythmogenic right ventricular cardiomyopathy/dysplasia. J Cardiovasc Electrophysiol 19(11):1127–1134

35. Waldo AL, Akhtar M, Brugada P, Henthorn RW, Scheinman MM, Ward DE et al (1985) The minimally appropriate electrophysiologic study for the initial assessment of patients with documented sustained monomorphic ventricular tachycardia. J Am Coll Cardiol 6(5):1174–1177

36. Vandepol CJ, Farshidi A, Spielman SR, Greenspan AM, Horowitz LN, Josephson ME (1980) Incidence and clinical significance of induced ventricular tachycardia. Am J Cardiol 45(4):725–731

37. Josephson ME, Almendral JM, Buxton AE, Marchlinski FE (1987) Mechanisms of ventricular tachycardia. Circulation 75(4 Pt 2):III41–III47

38. Roy D, Marchand E, Theroux P, Waters DD, Pelletier GB, Cartier R et al (1986) Long-term reproducibility and significance of provokable ventricular arrhythmias after myocardial infarction. J Am Coll Cardiol 8(1):32–39

IV   SPECIFIC ARRHYTHMIAS

7 Supraventricular Arrhythmias

Khalid Almuti, Babak Bozorgnia, and Steven A. Rothman

CONTENTS

INTRODUCTION
NONINVASIVE DIAGNOSIS OF SVT
MECHANISMS OF SVT
NON-INVASIVE AND PHARMACOLOGIC THERAPIES FOR SVT
PHARMACOTHERAPY
ELECTROPHYSIOLOGIC TESTING AND TACHYCARDIA ABLATION
CATHETER ABLATION OF AVNRT
ATRIAL TACHYCARDIA
SUMMARY
REFERENCES

Abstract

Paroxysmal supraventricular tachycardia is a common arrhythmia with multiple etiologies, including atrio-ventricular nodal reentrant tachycardia, atrio-ventricular reentrant tachycardia, and atrial tachycardia. Treatment of these arrhythmias depends greatly upon the proper diagnosis as well as an understanding of the arrhythmia's mechanism. A preliminary diagnosis can be often be inferred from the patient's history along with noninvasive testing and can help guide initial management strategies. Pharmacologic therapy, however, is often limited by side effects, compliance, and marginal efficacy. More definitive treatment of the arrhythmia requires an invasive electrophysiology study to confirm the diagnosis followed by catheter ablation of the arrhythmogenic substrate. The success rate for catheter ablation can approach 95% depending on the mechanism of the arrhythmia and is the treatment of choice for patients with severe symptoms.

Key Words: Activation mapping; adenosine; afterdepolarizations; amiodarone; antidromic atrioventricular reentrant tachycardia; atrial extrastimuli; atrial tachycardia; atrio-ventricular nodal reentrant tachycardia; atrio-ventricular reentrant tachycardia; automaticity; beta-blockers; digoxin, diltiazem; dofetilide; entrainment; flecainide; ibutilide; isoproterenol; macroreentry; metoprolol; microreentry; orthodromic atrio-ventricular reentrant tachycardia; pace mapping; para-Hisian pacing; pharmacotherapy; proarrhythmia; procainamide; propafeone; propranolol; radiofrequency catheter ablation; sotalol; supraventricular tachycardia; triggered activity; ventricular extrastimuli; verapamil; Wolff–Parkinson–White syndrome.

From: *Contemporary Cardiology: Management of Cardiac Arrhythmias*
Edited by: Gan-Xin Yan, Peter R. Kowey, DOI 10.1007/978-1-60761-161-5_7
© Springer Science+Business Media, LLC 2011

INTRODUCTION

The term "supraventricular tachycardia" (SVT) technically refers to arrhythmias originating above the AV node. This includes rhythms as disparate as sinus tachycardia and atrial fibrillation (AF), but in practice, the term "supraventricular tachycardia" is mostly used to refer to a finite number of abnormal rhythms that are paroxysmal in nature and include atrio-ventricular nodal reentrant tachycardia (AVNRT), atrio-ventricular reentrant tachycardia (AVRT), atrial tachycardia (AT), and, less commonly, junctional ectopic tachycardia and sino-atrial reentrant tachycardia. The prevalence of these paroxysmal SVT's is 2.25 per 1000 persons with a female preponderance especially before age 65 years *(1)*. In this chapter, the most common paroxysmal supraventricular arrhythmias (AVNRT, AVRT, and AT) will be discussed. AF and atrial flutter will be covered in more detail in separate chapters.

NONINVASIVE DIAGNOSIS OF SVT

History

In the absence of an electrocardiographic documentation of an SVT, history can be extremely helpful in differentiating SVT from other cardiac arrhythmias. If an SVT is documented on an ECG (or a cardiac monitor) then a detailed history can predict the mechanism of the SVT in a high percentage of patients *(2)*. Useful information includes descriptions of the onset and termination of the episode, instigating and terminating factors, symptoms during the episode, and age at the onset of symptoms *(3)*.

Reentrant SVTs such as AVNRT and AVRT are usually abrupt in onset and offset while automatic atrial arrhythmias, including sinus tachycardia, will usually initiate and subside gradually. Symptoms may include palpitations, dizziness, shortness of breath, and chest tightness. Some patients may experience diaphoresis, numbness in the extremities, and flushing. If asked, the patient will usually be able to tap out a rapid but regular demonstration of the episode. Many patients may also feel pulsations in the neck representing contraction of the atria against a closed AV valve. This phenomenon is more common in AVNRT *(2)*. More severe symptoms, such as syncope, are less frequent, but can occur in up to 20% of patients *(4)*.

Aside from the description of SVT episodes, history should also include any underlying cardiac diseases such as congenital heart disease or prior heart surgery. A history of heart surgery with resulting scar tissue may represent an arrhythmogenic substrate and makes a diagnosis of AT or atrial flutter more likely *(5)*. A history of prior catheter-based ablation therapy is also important to obtain for the same reason. The age and gender of the patient may, in some cases, help narrow the differential diagnosis of the SVT. For example, AVNRT tends to have a female preponderance with a bimodal age distribution *(2)*.

ECG Features

Several features on the cardiac electrocardiogram can be useful in determining the mechanism of SVT. Most important of these is the P wave location (Fig. 1). If discernable P waves are visible, then determining the length of the RP interval can be used to categorize the tachycardia as either a short- or a long-RP tachycardia. If the interval from the start of the P wave to the preceding QRS complex is shorter than the interval from the same P wave to the subsequent QRS complex, then the tachycardia is described as a short-RP tachycardia. The converse is true for a long-RP tachycardia *(6)*.

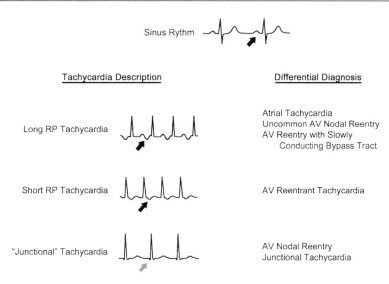

Fig. 1. Differential diagnosis of supraventricular tachycardia by P wave location. Representative rhythm strips are shown with the *black arrows* showing P wave location for sinus rhythm, long-RP tachycardia, and short-RP tachycardia. The *gray arrow* shows the location of the P wave, masked by the QRS, in a "junctional" tachycardia.

Short-RP tachycardias include most orthodromic AVRTs while long-RP tachycardias can represent atrial tachycardia, orthodromic AVRT with a slowly conducting bypass tract and atypical (fast–slow) AVNRT. If P waves are not visible, then the atrial activity may be occurring simultaneously with ventricular activation. Consequently, these P waves manifest as pseudo R' deflections in lead V1 or pseudo S waves in the inferior leads *(7)*. Such findings are highly specific for typical (slow–fast) AVNRT *(8)*. The presence of AV dissociation, or more P waves than QRS complexes, during tachycardia is useful because it rules out AVRT as the cause of the SVT since both the atria and the ventricles are critical limbs of the AVRT macroreentrant circuit; a 1:1 ratio of atrial and ventricular activity is required for all varieties of AVRT. While a P:QRS ratio >1 greatly favors AT, it does not completely exclude AVNRT since 2:1 block can occur in the lower AV nodal common pathway or His–Purkinje system *(9)*.

The initiation of the tachycardia, if captured on ECG or on a telemetry/cardiac monitor, can also be very helpful in determining the etiology of the arrhythmia *(6)*. A premature atrial contraction (PAC) that conducts with a prolonged PR interval and abruptly initiates an SVT is very suggestive of AVNRT, while an SVT that has a warm-up and/or a cooling-down period suggests an automatic atrial tachycardia. Initiation of SVT following a premature ventricular contraction (PVC) is suggestive of either orthodromic AVRT or uncommonly AVNRT. The presence of pre-excitation on sinus beats makes AVRT a very likely etiology.

When visible during SVT, the P wave morphology can be variable for both AT and orthodromic AVRT. With orthodromic AVRT, the morphology depends on the atrial insertion site of the bypass tract. Similarly, the P wave morphology is determined by the site of the arrhythmogenic focus in patient with AT. The morphology of the P wave can greatly aid in determining the approximate location of the bypass tract or the arrhythmogenic focus within the atria and in guiding ablation attempts. Examination of leads V1, aVL, and I can determine whether the focus is right or left atrial in origin while the morphology in the inferior leads can determine whether the focus is in the lower or higher portions of the atria. In patients with AVNRT and visible P waves, the morphology is negative in the inferior leads as activation of the right atrium occurs in a retrograde fashion beginning in the low posterior portion of the RA.

MECHANISMS OF SVT

Reentry

Reentry is the most common mechanism of narrow QRS complex tachycardia *(10)*. It requires two distinct pathways with different electrophysiologic properties that are linked proximally and distally, forming an anatomic or functional circuit *(5, 11)*. Reentry occurs when an impulse initially excites and conducts through the first pathway (or area of cardiac tissue), while failing to conduct through the second part of the circuit because it is refractory and therefore not excitable. Via the distal connection of the circuit, the impulse then enters the previously refractory tissue of the second pathway exciting it in a retrograde direction. The impulse must conduct sufficiently slowly within one limb of the circuit to allow the previously refractory tissue to recover excitability. If the impulse conducted in a retrograde manner in the second pathway reaches the proximal portion of the circuit when the first pathway is again excitable, then the impulse is able to reenter the first pathway resulting in a "circus movement" or reentrant arrhythmia.

The reentrant circuit may become repetitively activated, producing a sustained reentrant tachycardia. The type of arrhythmia that ensues is determined by the characteristics and location of the reentrant circuit. Reentry may use a large macroreentrant circuit (as in atrial flutter and AVRT) or small microreentrant circuits (as in some atrial tachycardias and AVNRT). Anatomic structures (e.g., the crista terminalis and eustachian ridge in the case of typical atrial flutter) or areas of fibrosis and scar may form the boundaries of the reentrant circuit *(12)*. Alternatively, the circuit may result from functional electrophysiologic properties of normal or diseased tissue that creates the milieu for reentry *(13)*.

Automaticity and Triggered Activity

A less common mechanism of narrow QRS complex tachycardia is automaticity. Automaticity is caused by enhanced diastolic phase 4 depolarization and when the firing rate exceeds the sinus rate, the abnormal rhythm will occur. Tissues capable of causing a narrow complex tachycardia due to automaticity may be found in the atria, AV junction, vena cava, and pulmonary veins. These rhythms can be either incessant or episodic.

Triggered activity is another arrhythmogenic mechanism due to abnormal impulse initiation *(14)*. This type of tachycardia results from interruptions of the repolarization process called an afterdepolarizations. When an afterdepolarization reaches a threshold, an action potential is triggered. Afterdepolarizations are characterized as either "early," occurring during repolarization, or "delayed" which occur at the end of repolarization or immediately after completion of repolarization *(15)*. Atrial tachycardias associated with digoxin toxicity or theophylline are examples of a triggered arrhythmia *(16)*.

Management of SVT

The management of SVT is based on the clinical presentation of the arrhythmia and the patient's preferences. While electrophysiologic testing may be used to assess the risk of life-threatening arrhythmias in patients with asymptomatic WPW *(17)*, treatment is typically not indicated for patients who have pre-excitation on their ECG without a clinical syndrome. Individuals with high-risk occupations (e.g., airplane pilots) and asymptomatic WPW, however, may require more aggressive management including "prophylactic" catheter-based ablation. Patients with mild, infrequent symptoms may benefit from intermittent pharmacologic therapy (e.g., "pill-in-pocket" approach), while patients with frequent symptomatic episodes are candidates for chronic therapy or catheter-based ablation. Patients with infrequent, but poorly tolerated arrhythmias also require a more definitive approach. An individual's lifestyle and personal preferences along with overall health and the presence of significant comorbidities should be considered when making long-term management decisions *(10)*.

NON-INVASIVE AND PHARMACOLOGIC THERAPIES FOR SVT

The development of catheter-based ablation technology for the treatment of SVT, providing high arrhythmia cure rates, has greatly diminished the role of pharmacologic therapy for SVT. Currently, the main role of pharmacotherapy is in the acute termination of an arrhythmia or for control of the ventricular response rate during SVT episodes. The chronic use of pharmacologic agents to suppress SVT is usually reserved for patients who are not candidates for catheter-based ablation procedures or patients who prefer a pharmacologic option.

PHARMACOTHERAPY

Acute Termination

In general, SVT is considered to be a non life-threatening condition with a good long-term prognosis. Nevertheless, certain episodes of SVT can present with hemodynamic compromise and/or significant symptoms. An acute intervention may be necessary to restore hemodynamic stability or to palliate severe symptoms. Pharmacotherapy, vagal maneuvers, and electrical cardioversion are options that can be used to achieve these goals.

Maneuvers that increase vagal tone, such as carotid sinus massage and the Valsalva maneuver, alter the refractoriness and conduction properties of the AV node and can terminate the SVT if the AV node is an integral part of the SVT circuit (e.g., AVNRT or AVRT) *(18)*. Alternatively, they can slow down the rate of the ventricular response to the SVT (i.e., in AT) and help differentiate the mechanism of the tachycardia *(6)*. If these measures are ineffective, then pharmacological intervention should be considered. Intravenous *verapamil* and adenosine are the drugs of choice for reentrant arrhythmias *(10, 19, 20)*. They exert their activity principally at the level of the AV node. Similar to vagal maneuvers, these agents may either terminate or slow down the tachycardia.

Adenosine's ultra-short duration of action makes it a preferred agent before resorting to emergent DC cardioversion in patients with a tenuous hemodynamic state. Caution has to be exercised when using adenosine due to a potential proarrhythmic effect stemming from a transient increase in atrial vulnerability to AF *(21–23)*. In patients with an AT, adenosine may result in transient AV block, helping determine the diagnosis. Occasionally, adenosine may terminate an AT, especially if the arrhythmia is due to a triggered or automatic mechanism *(24)*.

Intravenous verapamil is also effective for the acute termination of AVRT, but has a later onset of action and longer effect. It should not be used in patients with profound hypotension or those with severely depressed ventricular systolic function *(5)*. It should also be avoided in patients with pre-excited atrial fibrillation due to its potential to accelerate the ventricular response rate *(25, 26)*. Like adenosine, calcium channel blockers can occasionally terminate AT but the most common outcome is slowing down the ventricular response rate, making the tachycardia more hemodynamically stable without terminating it *(19, 27)*. Intravenous diltiazem and beta-blockers (*propranolol* and *metoprolol*) are also effective in the acute treatment of SVT.

Intravenous *procainamide* is a class IA agent that depresses conduction and prolongs refractoriness in atrial and ventricular myocardium, in accessory pathways, and in the His–Purkinje system *(28, 29)*. It may also cause slight shortening of the AV nodal refractory period but often has no discernable effect on AV nodal refractoriness *(13)*. Procainamide is most effective in terminating reentrant atrial tachycardia and AVRT; it is less effective in terminating AVNRT. In patients presenting with a wide QRS complex tachycardia of unknown etiology, procainamide is considered one of the safest and most effective drugs to administer *(30)*. Its electrophysiologic effects may result in the termination of both ventricular tachycardia and antidromic AVRT. Ibutilide can also be used in the acute management of patients with pre-excited atrial fibrillation *(10, 31)*.

Maintenance Pharmacotherapy

The goals of long-term maintenance therapy for SVT are to suppress future episodes and to control the rate of the ventricular response if episodes do recur. The selection of a pharmacologic agent is based on certain patient characteristics and on the unique electrophysiologic properties of the arrhythmia. Patient characteristics include existing comorbidities, baseline cardiac function, severity of symptoms during SVT, and drug sensitivities. Pharmacologic agents that are well tolerated with low organ toxicity are preferred.

Agents with AV nodal-specific activity (beta-blockers, calcium channel blockers, and to a lesser extent *digoxin*) are often used as first-line therapy and are most useful in suppressing reentrant arrhythmias that use the AV node for at least one limb of the tachycardia, especially AVNRT. Overall, these agents may improve symptoms in up to 60–80% of patients *(5)*, but are sometimes inadequate as monotherapy because of their inability to directly slow conduction and alter the refractoriness of an accessory pathway or to significantly reduce the frequency of arrhythmia-triggering ectopy *(32–34)*.

Class IC antiarrhythmic agents (i.e., flecainide and propafenone) prolong both antegrade and retrograde refractoriness in the accessory pathway *(35)* making them useful in the chronic treatment of AVRT and other paroxysmal SVTs *(36–40)*. An important contraindication to the use of these agents is the presence of known coronary disease or structural heart disease as the risk of proarrhythmic effects in those settings is considerable *(41)*. Other antiarrhythmic agents that are effective in the treatment of paroxysmal SVT include sotalol *(42, 43)*, dofetilide *(44, 45)*, and amiodarone *(46–48)*. These are best considered as second-line agents, however, due to their side effect profiles and increased risk of proarrhythmia.

Chronic drug therapy usually requires continuous dosing at regular intervals for an indefinite period of time. However, there are patients with infrequent and well-tolerated episodes of SVT that cause mild symptoms. Such patients may benefit from regimens of intermittent oral drugs or "pill-in-the-pocket" therapy *(49)* that terminate SVT episodes. Drugs that can be used in this manner include shorter acting beta-blockers, calcium channel blocker, and class IC AAD such as propafenone and flecainide *(50–53)*.

ELECTROPHYSIOLOGIC TESTING AND TACHYCARDIA ABLATION

The invasive electrophysiology procedure in patients with SVT has two purposes: determination of the mechanism of the arrhythmia and catheter ablation of the anatomic substrate causing the tachycardia. To evaluate the patient's clinical arrhythmia, the tachycardia must first be initiated in the electrophysiology laboratory. Reentrant arrhythmias can be initiated with a variety of pacing maneuvers, although intravenous isoproterenol, a beta agonist, may be needed to enhance conduction of the AV node *(54)*. Triggered arrhythmias usually require the addition of isoproterenol along with programmed stimulation for initiation while automatic arrhythmias are generally not inducible with programmed stimulation, but can be facilitated with isoproterenol *(55)*. In addition to its utility in initiating the clinical tachycardia, programmed stimulation can also be used to define the arrhythmogenic substrate.

Atrial extrastimuli (AES) are atrial premature depolarizations delivered at sequentially shorter coupling intervals (usually 10 msec decrements) after the last beat of a fixed cycle length drivetrain or during the spontaneous rhythm. Atrial extrastimuli are used to assess the refractory periods of supraventricular tissues and also to facilitate the induction of SVT. Measurement of the AH interval associated with each decremental AES will usually demonstrate a slight increase in the AH interval due to the decremental conduction properties of the AV node. Plotting of the AH interval as a function of the AES coupling interval results in an AV nodal conduction curve. Dual AV nodal physiology is demonstrated by a discontinuity in this curve *(56)* as well as by an abrupt increase in the AH interval (usually >50 msec) in response to a 10 msec decrement in the coupling interval of the AES (Fig. 2). AES can

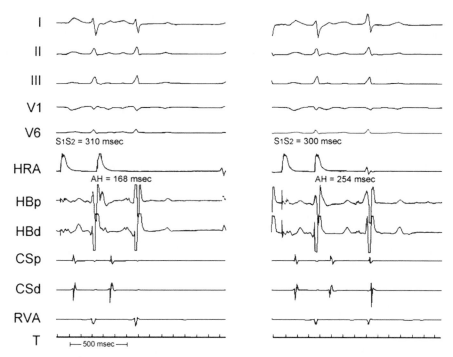

Fig. 2. Dual AV nodal pathways. AV nodal conduction is measured (AH interval) in response to decremental atrial depolarizations delivered after an eight-beat pacing drive. The *left hand panel* shows an AH interval of 168 msec in response to a coupling interval of 310 msec. The *right hand panel* shows an abrupt increase in the AH interval to 254 msec in response to a 10 msec decrease in the coupling interval (300 msec). This abrupt increase is consistent with dual AV nodal pathways as the fast pathway is now refractory and conduction occurs over the slow pathway. An AV nodal echo beat also occurs as retrograde conduction is now present through the fast pathway. (Surface leads I, II, III, V1, and V6 are shown with intracardiac electrograms: HRA = high right atrium, HB = His bundle, CS = coronary sinus, RVA = right ventricular apex; p = proximal, d = distal, s = stimuli, T = time).

also be used to determine the refractory period of an accessory pathway's antegrade conduction, which could have prognostic implications should the patient develop AF with rapid conduction *(57)*.

Ventricular extrastimuli (VES) are ventricular premature beats that are also delivered at sequentially shorter coupling intervals after a fixed cycle length drivetrain or other spontaneous rhythm. The atrial activation sequence with normal retrograde AV nodal activation typically shows earliest atrial activity in the septal region near the His bundle recording site, although occasionally may be earliest in the posterior septum and proximal coronary sinus recordings. Accessory pathways located on the left free wall of the mitral annulus will have early atrial activity in the distal CS recordings while right free wall pathways will have early atrial activation in the lateral RA catheter. Measurement of the VA interval will allow assessment of the retrograde refractory periods of the AV node or accessory pathways. Retrograde dual AV nodal pathways may be manifested by an abrupt increase in the VA conduction time through the AV node (>50 msec) in response to a 10 msec decrement in the coupling interval.

Careful assessment of the atrial activation sequence during VES is very important. When more than one retrograde pathway is present (i.e., AV node and accessory pathway), fusion of atrial activation may result in early atrial activation at multiple sites. As the refractory period of one pathway is approached with decremental VES, a change in the atrial activation sequence may signifying a shift in retrograde conduction through only one of the pathways, confirming the presence of an accessory pathway. Multiple shifts in the retrograde atrial activation sequence can be seen in cases where more than one accessory pathway is present. Retrograde dual AV nodal pathways, however, may also cause a shift in atrial activation. Earliest activation may shift more posteriorly and inferiorly as AV nodal conduction changes from the fast to slow pathway *(58)*.

Para-Hisian pacing can also be performed to evaluate retrograde atrial activation and is used to differentiate anteroseptal accessory pathways from normal retrograde AV nodal conduction *(59)*. In the presence of an accessory pathway, pacing the His bundle without capturing local ventricular tissue will require atrial activation to occur via an impulse that must first conduct over the His–Purkinje system to the ventricle and then through the ventricular myocardium back to the accessory pathway. If local ventricular tissue is captured, however, then conduction occurs over a small area of ventricular tissue and directly then to the AP. This results in a shortening of the His (or pacing stimulus) to atrial interval (Fig. 3). Capture of local ventricular tissue without His bundle capture would also result in the shorter HA interval. Since AV nodal conduction requires conduction from the His bundle to the atrium via the AV node only, there would be no change with or without local ventricular capture. But if local ventricular capture occurs without His bundle stimulation, then the HA interval would lengthen (Fig. 4).

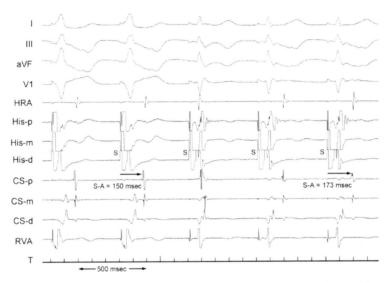

Fig. 3. Para-Hisian pacing in the presence of an accessory pathway. Pacing is performed from the anteroseptum with the first 2 complexes resulting in capture of both the His bundle and local ventricular tissue. Subsequent pacing stimuli show capture of only the His bundle with a narrowing of the QRS (i.e., pure His bundle capture). Local ventricular capture allows conduction back to the atrium to occur directly over the accessory pathway, resulting in a shorter stimulus to atrial electrogram (S–A) interval of 150 msec (surface leads I, III, aVF, and V1 are shown with intracardiac electrograms: HRA = high right atrium, His = His bundle, CS = coronary sinus, RVA = right ventricular apex; p = proximal, m = mid, d = distal, s = stimuli, T = time).

Induction of SVT

The induction of reentrant SVT with extrastimuli requires block in one pathway while the second pathway conducts with sufficient delay to allow recovery and retrograde conduction in the first *(15)*. In AV nodal reentry, the antegrade effective refractory period (ERP) of the fast AV nodal pathway is usually longer than the ERP of the slow pathway such that common type AVNRT can be induced with AES. The retrograde ERP of the fast AV nodal pathway, however, tends to be shorter than the slow

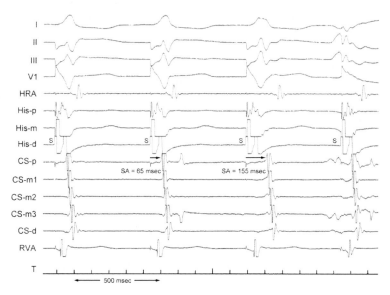

Fig. 4. Para-Hisian pacing in the absence of an accessory pathway. Pacing is performed from the anteroseptum with the second complex showing capture of both the His bundle and local ventricular tissue and the third complex showing capture of only local ventricular tissue (wider QRS duration). The stimulus to atrial electrogram (SA) interval is lengthened when His bundle capture is lost since ventriculoatrial conduction is AV nodal dependent (surface leads I, II, III, and V1 are shown with intracardiac electrograms: HRA = high right atrium, His = His bundle, CS = coronary sinus, RVA = right ventricular apex; p = proximal, m = mid, d = distal, s = stimuli, T = time).

pathway and typical AVNRT is usually not induced with VES. When the retrograde slow pathway ERP is shorter than the fast pathway ERP, however, uncommon AVNRT can be induced with VES *(60)*. Rapid atrial pacing near the AV nodal Wenckebach cycle length (CL) can also be used to induce common AVNRT.

In patients with Wolff–Parkinson–White syndrome, if the antegrade accessory pathway ERP is longer than the AV nodal pathway ERP, and there is sufficient prolongation of AV nodal conduction, then AVRT can be induced with AES. For patients with concealed accessory pathways, only sufficient prolongation in AV nodal conduction is usually necessary to induce AVRT as antegrade block is already present in the accessory pathway. More commonly, AVRT can be induced with ventricular extrastimuli as the retrograde refractory period of the accessory pathway is usually shorter than that of the AV node. Delivering VES at shorter drive cycle lengths can be helpful as AV nodal refractoriness will increase while most bypass tract refractory periods will decrease.

Atrial tachycardias can be either reentrant, triggered or automatic and each mechanism typically requires a different mode of induction *(55)*. For microreentrant atrial tachycardia, multiple extrastimuli are commonly needed to achieve block in one limb of the circuit and cause significant prolongation of conduction in the other to allow reentry. Rapid (burst) atrial pacing is commonly used to induce triggered arrhythmias, especially during the infusion of an intravenous catecholamine, such as isoproterenol. Automatic AT is usually not initiated with either AES or burst pacing, but may be enhanced by isoproterenol.

Electrophysiologic Diagnostic Techniques

Once SVT is initiated, careful assessment of the ventricular and atrial timing, along with programmed stimulation and rapid pacing, can be used to differentiate the mechanism of the SVT. If spontaneous AV block is observed, then AVRT is definitively ruled out and atrial tachycardia is the most likely diagnosis. Rarely, AVNRT can have a 2:1 AV ratio due to block in the lower common AV nodal pathway or His bundle *(9)*. For tachycardias with a VA time of <60 msec, measured from the onset of ventricular activation to the earliest atrial activation, a diagnosis of AVNRT is most likely *(61)*. In AVRT, conduction from the ventricle to the atrium, via the bypass tract, would be expected to take longer than 60 msec. Atrial tachycardia with a prolonged PR interval, such that the P wave falls on the preceding QRS, would be an exception to this.

Other observations can also be helpful in diagnosing the SVT mechanism. Bundle branch block that results in an increase in the tachycardia CL or a >20 msec increase in the VA interval is consistent with AVRT utilizing an ipsilateral accessory pathway *(62)* (Fig. 5). This is due to the extra time required to traverse a circuit with conduction proceeding down the opposite bundle branch and then across the septum. If spontaneous termination is observed, then it should be noted if the last beat ends with ventricular activation (VA block) or atrial activation (AV block). If the tachycardia reproducibly terminates with atrial activation, then an atrial tachycardia would be very unlikely since both block in the atrial circuit and AV nodal block would have to occur simultaneously.

The effect caused by ventricular stimulation during His bundle refractoriness can also be very useful in differentiating the tachycardia mechanism *(63)*. Ventricular extrastimuli are delivered either simul-

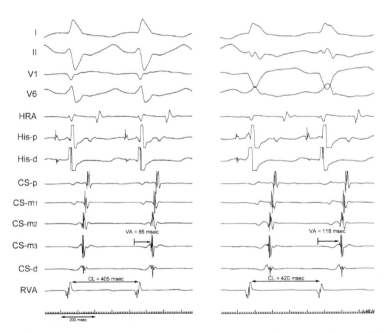

Fig. 5. Orthodromic SVT with bundle branch block. The panel on the left shows surface and intracardiac recordings of orthodromic SVT utilizing a left lateral accessory pathway. The VA interval from earliest ventricular activation to earliest atrial activation is 86 msec. The panel on the right shows the same orthodromic SVT with left bundle aberration. Because conduction must now proceed via the right bundle branch and then across the septum to the left ventricle, there is an increase in the VA interval to 118 msec and an increase in the orthodromic SVT cycle length to 420 msec (surface leads I, II, V1, and V6 are shown with intracardiac electrograms: HRA = high right atrium, His = His bundle, CS = coronary sinus, RVA = right ventricular apex; p = proximal, m = mid, d = distal).

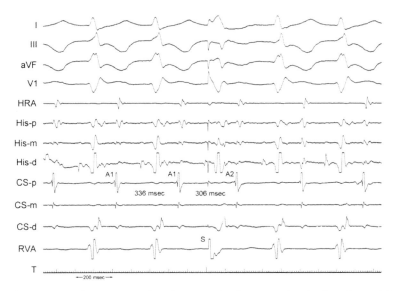

Fig. 6. His bundle refractory ventricular extrastimuli. A ventricular extrastimulus is delivered during orthodromic SVT when the His bundle is refractory due to antegrade activation, prohibiting retrograde conduction over the His bundle and AV node. The subsequent atrial activation is advanced by 30 msec demonstrating the presence of an accessory pathway over which retrograde conduction can occur (surface leads I, III, aVF, and V1 are shown with intracardiac electrograms: HRA = high right atrium, His = His bundle, CS = coronary sinus, RVA = right ventricular apex; p = proximal, m = mid, d = distal, s = stimulus, T = time).

taneously or up to 55 msec before the expected His bundle activation, such that retrograde conduction through the AV node is prevented. Any effect on the subsequent atrial activation or cycle length would therefore require a separate retrograde pathway. Several responses can be observed as follows:

(1) Atrial activation is advanced (Fig. 6):

- AP is present if the atrial activation sequence remains unchanged and the tachycardia resets
- A bystander AP is present if the atrial activation sequence is changed

(2) Atrial activation is prolonged (Fig. 7):

- An AP with decremental conduction is present and participating in the circuit

(3) Tachycardia breaks without atrial activation:

- AP is present and participating in the circuit

(4) Atria activation is not advanced while ventricular activation advances 30 msec without modification of tachycardia CL:

- Excludes the presence of a bypass tract

Overdrive ventricular pacing is another diagnostic maneuver and is performed by pacing from the ventricle at a cycle length faster than the tachycardia CL by 10–20 msec *(64)*. The SVT is entrained if 1:1 VA conduction is maintained. If the SVT resumes at the end of ventricular pacing, then the pattern of continuation can be helpful in differentiating AVNRT and AVRT (VAVA pattern) from AT (VAAV pattern). The post-pacing interval (or return cycle length) can also be measured. A PPI minus

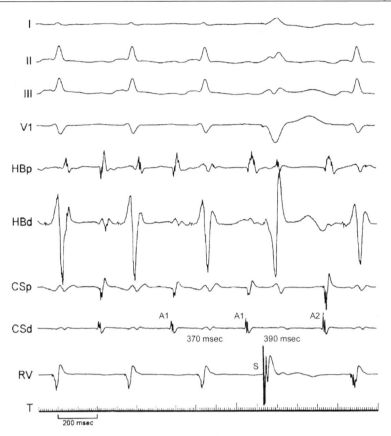

Fig. 7. His bundle refractory ventricular extrastimuli in the presence of slowly conducting accessory pathway. A ventricular extrastimulus is delivered during His bundle refractoriness, resulting in a delay in the subsequent atrial activation (A2) by 20 msec due to conduction over a decrementally conducting accessory pathway (surface leads I, II, III, and V1 are shown with intracardiac electrograms: HB = His bundle, CS = coronary sinus, RVA = right ventricular apex; p = proximal, d = distal, s = stimulus, T = time).

the tachycardia CL of >115 msec supports a diagnosis of AVNRT *(65)*. If the tachycardia terminates, then a termination pattern of VAVA would support AVNRT or AVRT. In contrast, a termination pattern of VAAV would support a diagnosis of AT.

Differentiation of AVNRT from AVRT can often be done by measuring the HA interval during SVT and comparing it to the HA interval with ventricular pacing at the tachycardia CL. In typical AVNRT, the SVT circuit involves reentry between antegrade conduction down the slow AV nodal pathway and retrograde through the fast pathway. Usually, the conducted impulse enters the fast pathway in a retrograde manner while continuing antegrade conduction through a lower "common pathway" of tissue before activating the His bundle. Measuring the HA interval may therefore result in a false shortening of the HA interval when compared with ventricular pacing, which must conduct through both the "common lower pathway" and fast pathway in series (Fig. 8).

For AVRT, the HA interval measured during SVT requires conduction through the His–Purkinje system, ventricular tissue, and finally the AP. In contrast, ventricular pacing will result in conduction from the passing point through ventricular tissue to the AP, while simultaneously conducting through the His–Purkinje system to the His bundle. Therefore, the HA interval measured during ventricular pacing will be shorter than that during SVT, opposite to that seen during AVNRT (Fig. 9).

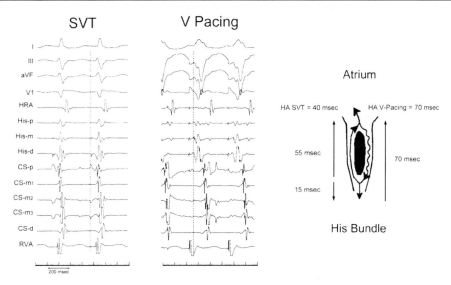

Fig. 8. Differential HA interval with ventricular pacing during AV nodal reentrant SVT. During AV nodal reentry, early retrograde conduction over the fast pathway occurs simultaneously with conduction over a common lower pathway. This may result in a false shortening of the His bundle to atrial electrogram (HA) interval when compared to ventricular pacing, which requires conduction over both the lower common AV nodal tissue and the retrograde fast pathway (surface leads I, III, and V1 are shown with intracardiac electrograms: HB = His bundle, CS = coronary sinus, RVA = right ventricular apex; p = proximal, m= mid, d = distal).

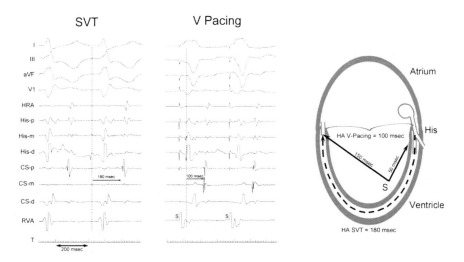

Fig. 9. Differential HA interval with ventricular pacing during AV reentrant SVT. During AV reentry, the reentrant circuit from the His bundle to atria involves conduction through the lower His–Purkinje system and then over ventricular myocardium to the accessory pathway. During ventricular pacing, conduction will occur simultaneously retrograde through the His–Purkinje system to the His bundle and over the ventricular myocardium to the accessory pathway. This results in a shorter HA interval during ventricular pacing when compared to the HA interval during SVT (surface leads I, III, aVF, and V1 are shown with intracardiac electrograms: HRA = right atrium, His = His bundle, CS = coronary sinus, RVA = right ventricular apex; p = proximal, m= mid, d = distal, s= stimuli, T = time).

CATHETER ABLATION OF AVNRT

The approach to the catheter ablation of AVNRT is based upon the concept of dual, or multiple, AV nodal pathways. These pathways are thought of as being anatomically continuous and possessing different electrophysiologic properties making them functionally separate and distinct *(66–68)*. In the typical and most common form of AVNRT, the dual pathways have the following characteristics: (1) A "fast" pathway with rapid conduction and relatively long refractory period and (2) a "slow" pathway with relatively slower conduction, but possessing a shorter refractory period.

During normal sinus rhythm, a sinus beat conducts down both the fast and slow pathways, but the rapid conduction of the fast pathway allows the impulse to reach the His bundle region first. The impulse traveling down the slow pathway will usually be unable to activate the His bundle region since it is still refractory, nor can it conduct retrograde up the fast pathway since that pathway is also still refractory. This scenario results in a single impulse reaching the ventricle and the PR interval is usually normal in length.

Atrial premature beats, however, may encounter the fast AV nodal pathway while it is still refractory and preferentially conduct down the slow pathway (now excitable due to its shorter refractory period). This is manifested on the surface ECG by a long PR interval. In addition, the long conduction time down the "slow" pathway will allow recovery of the fast pathway and the impulse can then conduct retrograde to the atrium and initiate a reentrant tachycardia that conducts back down the slow pathway. The resulting rhythm is typical AVNRT and accounts for approximately 90% of all cases of AVNRT. Atypical forms of AVNRT account for the other 10% of cases and involve either the reverse circuit, with antegrade conduction down the fast pathway and retrograde conduction up a slow pathway (fast-slow tachycardia) or a circuit in which both the antegrade and retrograde limbs are relatively "slow" pathways with distinct electrophysiologic properties (slow–slow AVNRT).

AV Node Modification Using Radiofrequency Energy

The target in catheter ablation of AVNRT is to modify or eliminate the SP of the AV node while carefully preserving FP conduction. The SP is usually found in the mid to posterior low septal region (Koch's triangle) *(68)*. The exact target site is usually determined by the anatomic position on fluoroscopic views and by the morphology of the intracardiac electrogram *(69)*. Ablation of the slow pathway preserves fast pathway function with a normal PR interval after the ablation and has a lower risk of complete heart block than fast pathway modification *(70)*.

Using fluoroscopic guidance, the ablation electrode is typically positioned near the tricuspid valve annulus at the level of the coronary sinus ostium and along its anterior lip. A good ablation site records a small fractionated or multicomponent atrial potential with an atrial amplitude that is 10–15% of the local ventricular amplitude *(71, 72)* (Fig. 10). Approximately 90% of successful slow pathway ablation sites are found between the coronary sinus ostium and the tricuspid valve. The occurrence of transient junctional rhythm during RF energy application is indicative of a potentially effective site for ablation *(73)*. Fast junctional rhythms with CLs <350 msec, however, may predict a higher risk of conduction block and energy application should be terminated during such lesions *(74)*. Successful ablation is confirmed by the inability to reinduce the tachycardia and either elimination of the slow pathway or modification of the slow pathway with prolongation of the refractory period *(75)*. In patients with atypical forms of AVNRT, ablation can be performed in a similar manner or by targeting the site of earliest retrograde atrial activity during the atypical AVNRT *(76)*.

ABLATION SUCCESS RATE

In experienced hands, the posterior approach described above successfully eliminates arrhythmia recurrence in over 95% of patients *(71, 77–80)*. Evidence of dual pathway physiology can persist in one-third to one-half of cases since it is not necessary to eliminate all slow pathway conduction to

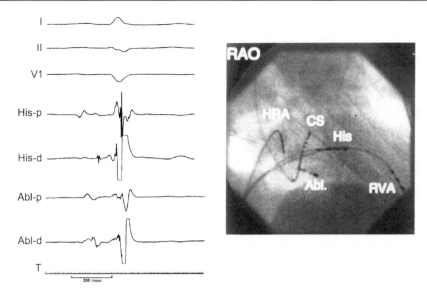

Fig. 10. Catheter position for radiofrequency modification of the AV nodal slow pathway. Fluoroscopic imaging in an RAO projection is shown of the ablation catheter position on the posterior septum. The intracardiac electrogram recording at this position is shown on the *left-hand side* (surface leads I, II, and V1 are shown with intracardiac electrograms: His = His bundle, Abl = ablation catheter; p = proximal, d = distal, T = time. Position of the high right atrial (HRA), coronary sinus (CS), His bundle (His), right ventricular apical (RVA), and ablation (Abl) catheters are shown on the fluoroscopic image).

achieve clinical success (i.e., elimination of arrhythmia recurrence). If the slow pathway is damaged but not completely abolished, a "jump" and single atrial echoes may still be present *(77, 75, 81)*. Persistence of double echo beats is not acceptable as an endpoint since the substrate for AVNRT is still intact.

ATRIAL TACHYCARDIA

Focal atrial tachycardia represents a rapid, usually narrow QRS rhythm emanating from an atrial source other than the sinus node and then spreading centrifugally to activate the rest of the atria *(30)*. The arrhythmogenic focus may originate in either the right or the left atrium, with the region of the crista terminalis and the pulmonary vein ostias being frequent locations. Up to 80% of focal AT arises from the right atrium *(82, 83)*. Overall, AT is less common than AVNRT and AVRT, accounting for only 5–15% of all adult SVT's seen in clinical practice, and is frequently associated with structurally abnormal hearts *(55, 84)*.

Atrial tachycardias can be caused by one of three mechanisms: (1) enhanced or abnormal automaticity, (2) triggered activity, or (3) reentry *(55)*. Focal AT is usually associated with a tachycardia cycle length (CL) of ≥250 ms (heart rate <240 bpm) *(30)*. While the surface ECG is not helpful in determining the exact tachycardia mechanism, the P wave morphology can be used to determine the approximate site of the arrhythmogenic focus. In contrast to macroreentrant atrial flutter, the surface ECG in a focal AT usually demonstrates isoelectric baselines between P waves. When due to an automatic mechanism, the focal AT may be associated with an onset characterized by a progressively faster rate (warm-up) and termination with progressive slowing of the rate (cool-down). The tachycardia cycle length can vary over time. In contrast, microreentrant and triggered focal ATs are characterized by acute onset and termination.

Diagnosis and Ablation

Finding the target area for ablation can be challenging given the large number of potential locations and the need to be precise in delivering RF ablation lesions to abolish the tachycardia. Determining the mechanism of the tachycardia is helpful when ablating the tachycardia as different mechanisms have different local electrogram characteristics and responses to pacing maneuvers. Surface ECG P wave morphology examination can suggest possible starting areas for mapping *(83)*. Further localization can be performed using a combination of activation mapping, pace mapping, and entrainment.

ACTIVATION MAPPING

Activation mapping aims at identifying the earliest site of activation in the atria. The site would be at the center of the centrifugal activation waves that activate atrial tissue. A mapping and ablation catheter is inserted into the right or left atrium and endocardial mapping is performed either visually or with the aid of three-dimensional electroanatomical mapping systems.

If surface ECG P waves are discernable, then the clearest P wave is chosen as a reference point for comparison reasons. Otherwise, a relatively stable intracardiac atrial electrogram signal is used for that purpose (i.e., a signal on a coronary sinus catheter). An activation map of one or both atria is then constructed by comparing the timing of the local signal at the distal tip of the mapping catheter to the chosen reference point. The goal is to find the local signal with the earliest timing compared to the reference. For focal ATs of an autonomic or triggered mechanism, local atrial activation may precede the onset of the P wave by up to 20–60 msec *(85, 86)*. For microreentrant mechanisms, mid-diastolic activity may be present at the successful ablation site.

Three-dimensional electroanatomic mapping systems can aid in visualizing the tachycardia focus. The location with the earliest and latest activation timing compared to the reference are designated by different colors with a variety of other colors in between. If the tachycardia is truly focal in nature, the result is a color map with progressively larger color rings spreading out from the arrhythmogenic focus (Fig. 11). For tachycardias that are difficult to sustain, a 3D multi-electrode balloon mapping catheter can acquire an activation map with hundreds of points from few tachycardia beats *(87)*.

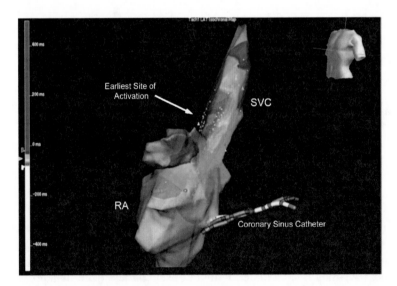

Fig. 11. Three-dimensional mapping of a focal atrial tachycardia. A three-dimensional image of the right atrium (RA) and superior vena cava (SVC) is shown and color coded to the local atrial activation time. Atrial activation propagates from a focal site of origin at the SVC–RA junction.

PACE MAPPING

For atrial tachycardias that are difficult to induce during the electrophysiology study, pace mapping is a technique that may aid in locating an arrhythmogenic focus in a small area of potential targets for ablation. Pace mapping requires ECG documentation of the tachycardia P wave morphology along with the pattern of intracardiac chamber activation. The mapping catheter is moved to various positions within the suspected chamber and pacing is initiated at the lowest output needed for capture of the atria. The paced P wave morphology and pattern of chamber activation is then compared to the clinical tachycardia *(88)*. An area with a high level of concordance in surface and intracardiac electrogram signals is suggestive of proximity to the arrhythmogenic focus. Unlike ventricular arrhythmias where pace mapping utilizes the usually clear QRS signals, P wave morphology is much more difficult to discern. Often, the P wave is superimposed on the T wave preventing attempts at morphologic comparisons. Rapid pacing to create AV block and separate the P waves from adjoining T waves may be necessary at times.

ENTRAINMENT MAPPING

Entrainment mapping is used in cases of microreentrant tachycardia to assess whether areas of mid-diastolic activity are necessary in the reentrant circuit and therefore potentially successful sites for ablation. Using the mapping catheter during SVT, sites of early atrial activation and mid diastolic activity are located (Fig. 12). Pacing is then performed for a brief period at cycle lengths of 20–30 msec shorter than that of the tachycardia itself. If the tachycardia continues at the termination of pacing then the return cycle length (defined as the time from the last pacing impulse to the first

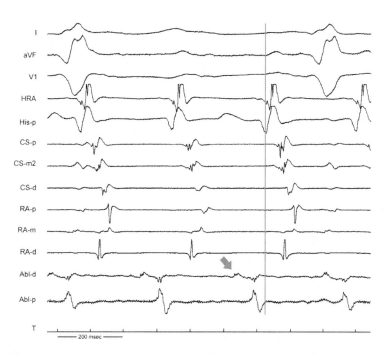

Fig. 12. Activation mapping of a focal atrial tachycardia. Local mid-diastolic, atrial activity is present on the distal ablation electrogram (Abl-d). The fractionated signal precedes the onset of the P wave by 95 msec *(arrow)* (surface leads I, aVF, and V1 are shown with intracardiac electrograms: HRA = right atrium, His = His bundle, CS = coronary sinus, RA = right atrial, Abl = ablation/mapping catheter; p = proximal, m= mid, d = distal, s= stimuli, T = time).

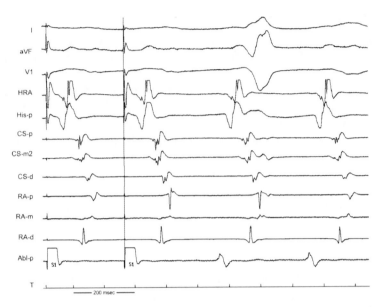

Fig. 13. Entrainment mapping of a focal atrial tachycardia with concealed fusion. Pacing is performed from the ablation catheter at the site of mid-diastolic atrial activity (see Fig. 12). Surface P wave morphology and the intracardiac atrial activation sequence are identical to that of the clinical atrial tachycardia (surface leads I, aVF, and V1 are shown with intracardiac electrograms: HRA = right atrium, His = His bundle, s= stimuli, T = time).

recorded local electrical impulse on the ablation catheter) is documented. If the return cycle length is equal or close to the tachycardia cycle length, the finding would be suggestive that the tip of the mapping catheter is within the reentrant circuit. Concealed fusion occurs with the paced P wave morphology and intracardiac activation pattern is identical to the clinical tachycardia and signifies a site with high success for termination of the tachycardia (Fig. 13) *(86)*.

Catheter Ablation

Once a focus for the AT is identified, then ablation can be targeted at that location. Depending on the location, radiofrequency (RF) energy (with or without cooling) or cryoablation can be used. In arrhythmias of an automatic or triggered mechanism, the initiation of RF energy causes heating of the local tissue, often leading to transient acceleration of the tachycardia with subsequent termination. In cases of a reentrant arrhythmia, slowing of the tachycardia may precede termination. In either case, if termination is not achieved within approximately 15 sec, despite adequate energy delivery, then ablation should be halted and re-evaluation of the site with further mapping performed. If AT terminates, then additional lesions may be delivered to the small area of tissue surrounding the target to assure destruction of the arrhythmogenic focus. Thereafter, attempts at re-induction of the tachycardia are necessary to confirm abolition of the tachycardia.

In recent years, ablation of focal AT has been associated with an overall success rate of greater than 80%. Tachycardias with right and left atrial origins have higher ablation success rates compared to AT's originating from septal foci *(80, 86, 89)*. Complications related to ablation of tachycardia are relatively uncommon, occurring in 1–2% of cases *(80, 89)*. These include vascular injury, cardiac perforation, and injury to surrounding intra- and extra-cardiac structures. Atrial tachycardias arising from the posterolateral aspect of the right atrium may result in damage to the phrenic nerve *(90)*. In these regions, high output pacing can be performed to assess for diaphragmatic capture, signifying the location of the phrenic nerve, and varying techniques or different energy sources for ablation can be used to avoid diaphragmatic paralysis (91).

Catheter Ablation of AVRT

The approach for catheter ablation of AVRT is more complicated than AVNRT. While the ablation site for AVNRT is fairly well defined and limited to the posterior septum, potential ablation sites for AVRT are as variable as the locations of the accessory pathways. Most pathways, however, are left lateral in location followed by paraseptal and right lateral tracts. In addition, up to 10% of patients with AVRT may have more than one bypass tract (92–94). Successful ablation in up to 94% of patients with accessory pathways has been reported in large series of patients with AVRT (92, 95).

Mapping of the accessory pathway location can be performed by determining the earliest antegrade ventricular activation during sinus rhythm if pre-excitation is present or by the earliest retrograde atrial activation during either orthodromic SVT or ventricular pacing. In the case of left-sided pathways, placement of the coronary sinus catheter should be performed such that the earliest retrograde atrial activation is "bracketed" by more proximal and distal electrode pairs. For right-sided pathways, placement of a circular catheter around the tricspid annulus can be helpful in localizing the bypass tract. The retrograde atrial activation of septal accessory pathways is best mapped during orthodromic AVRT or with fast enough ventricular pacing to avoid fusion with retrograde atrial activation via the AV node.

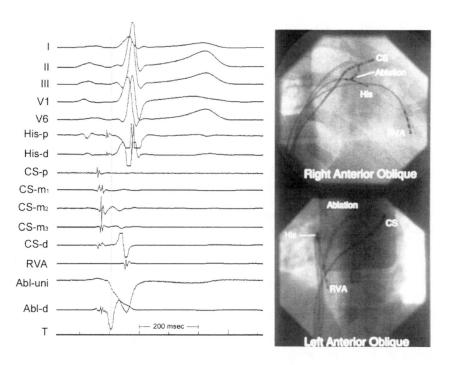

Fig. 14. Catheter ablation of an accessory pathway. Right and left anterior oblique fluoroscopic images of the catheter positions for ablation of a left lateral accessory pathway are demonstrated on the *right-hand panel*. The intracardiac electrogram recordings at these sites are shown on the *left-hand panel* (surface leads I, II, III, V1, and V6 are shown with intracardiac electrograms: His = His bundle, CS = coronary sinus, RVA = right ventricular apex, Abl = ablation/mapping catheter; p = proximal, m= mid, d = distal, uni = unipolar. Position of the coronary sinus (CS), His bundle (His), right ventricular apical (RVA), and ablation catheters are shown on the fluoroscopic images).

Local electrogram characteristics will vary depending on the method of mapping. Mapping antegrade conduction of the acessory pathway will locate the ventricular insertion of the pathway and the local ventricular electrogram should precede the onset of the surface ECG delta wave by up to 20 msec (Fig. 14) *(96)*. Unipolar recordings are particularly helpful and will show a QS deflection, demonstrating that all ventricular activation is propagating from that point *(97)*. The local bipolar electrogram will show a continuous signal with a local atrio-ventricular interval of less than or equal to 40 msec *(98)*. A discrete accessory pathway potential, when present, also predicts a higher probability of success *(99)*.

In mapping the atrial insertion of an accessory pathway, the onset of earliest atrial activation is located during either orthodromic SVT or ventricular pacing. The bipolar electrogram will typically demonstrate continuous electrical activity *(100)* with a local ventriculoatrial interval of less than 60 msec and a surface QRS onset to local atrial electrogram time of 80 msec *(98, 101)*. Pacing at ventricular CLs that result in 2:1 block, or with ventricular premature depolarizations that block in the bypass tract, is sometimes needed to determine which part of the signal is atrial or ventricular in origin. The presence of possible accessory pathway potentials is seen in only 30% of successful ablation sites *(101)*.

SUMMARY

The paroxysmal supraventricular tachycardias are a diverse group of arrhythmias with the majority being due to either AV nodal reentry or atrio-ventricular reentry. While pharmacologic therapy is still used for suppression and treatment, especially for the atrial arrhythmias, efficacy and side effects have limited their application. Radiofrequency catheter ablation has become the treatment of choice for most symptomatic patients due to the procedure's high rate of success and infrequent complications. Catheter ablation, however, still requires a diligent approach in determining the diagnosis and mechanism of the arrhythmia during the invasive electrophysiology procedure.

REFERENCES

1. Orejarena LA, Vidaillet HJ, DeStefano F, Nordstrom DL, Vierkant RA, Smith PN, Hayes JJ (1998) Paroxysmal supraventricular tachycardia in the general population. J Am Coll Cardiol 31:150–157
2. Gonzalez-Torrecilla E, Almendral J, Arenal A, Atienza F, Atea LF, del Castillo S, Fernandez-Aviles F (2009) Combined evaluation of bedside clinical variables and the electrocardiogram for the differential diagnosis of paroxysmal atrioventricular reciprocating tachycardias in patients without pre-excitation. J Am Coll Cardiol 53:2353–2358
3. Zimetbaum P, Josephson ME (1998) Evaluation of patients with palpitations. N Engl J Med 338:1369–1373
4. Wood KA, Drew BJ, Scheinman MM (1997) Frequency of disabling symptoms in supraventricular tachycardia. Am J Cardiol 79:145–149
5. Ferguson JD, DiMarco JP (2003) Contemporary management of paroxysmal supraventricular tachycardia. Circulation 107:1096–1099
6. Wellens HJ (1996) The value of the ECG in the diagnosis of supraventricular tachycardias. Eur Heart J 17(Suppl C):10–20
7. Kumar UN, Rao RK, Scheinman MM (2006) The 12-lead electrocardiogram in supraventricular tachycardia. Cardiol Clin 24:427–37, ix
8. Kalbfleisch SJ, el-Atassi R, Calkins H, Langberg JJ, Morady F (1993) Differentiation of paroxysmal narrow QRS complex tachycardias using the 12-lead electrocardiogram. J Am Coll Cardiol 21:85–89
9. Man KC, Brinkman K, Bogun F, Knight B, Bahu M, Weiss R, Goyal R, Harvey M, Daoud EG, Strickberger SA, Morady F (1996) 2:1 atrioventricular block during atrioventricular node reentrant tachycardia. J Am Coll Cardiol 28:1770–1774
10. Blomstrom-Lundqvist C, Scheinman MM, Aliot EM, Alpert JS, Calkins H, Camm AJ, Campbell WB, Haines DE, Kuck KH, Lerman BB, Miller DD, Shaeffer CWJ, Stevenson WG, Tomaselli GF, Antman EM, Smith SCJ, Alpert JS, Faxon DP, Fuster V, Gibbons RJ, Gregoratos G, Hiratzka LF, Hunt SA, Jacobs AK, Russell ROJ, Priori SG, Blanc JJ, Budaj A, Burgos EF, Cowie M, Deckers JW, Garcia MA, Klein WW, Lekakis J, Lindahl B, Mazzotta G, Morais JC, Oto A, Smiseth O, Trappe HJ (2003) ACC/AHA/ESC guidelines for the management of patients with supraven-

tricular arrhythmias–executive summary: a report of the American college of cardiology/American heart association task force on practice guidelines and the European society of cardiology committee for practice guidelines (writing committee to develop guidelines for the management of patients with supraventricular arrhythmias). Circulation 108: 1871–1909

11. Ganz LI, Friedman PL (1995) Supraventricular tachycardia. N Engl J Med 332:162–173

12. Shah D, Jais P, Haissaguerre M (2002) Electrophysiological evaluation and ablation of atypical right atrial flutter. Card Electrophysiol Rev 6:365–370

13. Akhtar M, Jazayeri MR, Sra J, Blanck Z, Deshpande S, Dhala A (1993) Atrioventricular nodal reentry. Clinical, electrophysiological, and therapeutic considerations. Circulation 88:282–295

14. Cranefield PF (1977) Action potentials, afterpotentials, and arrhythmias. Circ Res 41:415–423

15. Wit AL, Rosen MR (1983) Pathophysiologic mechanisms of cardiac arrhythmias. Am Heart J 106: 798–811

16. Akhtar M, Tchou PJ, Jazayeri M (1988) Mechanisms of clinical tachycardias. Am J Cardiol 61:9A–19A; Marchlinski FE, Miller JM (1985) Atrial arrhythmias exacerbated by theophylline. Response to verapamil and evidence for triggered activity in man. Chest 88:931–934

17. Pappone C, Santinelli V, Rosanio S, Vicedomini G, Nardi S, Pappone A, Tortoriello V, Manguso F, Mazzone P, Gulletta S, Oreto G, Alfieri O (2003) Usefulness of invasive electrophysiologic testing to stratify the risk of arrhythmic events in asymptomatic patients with Wolff-Parkinson-White pattern: results from a large prospective long-term follow-up study. J Am Coll Cardiol 41:239–244

18. Waxman MB, Wald RW, Sharma AD, Huerta F, Cameron DA (1980) Vagal techniques for termination of paroxysmal supraventricular tachycardia. Am J Cardiol 46:655–664

19. Gonzalez R, Scheinman MM (1981) Treatment of supraventricular arrhythmias with intravenous and oral verapamil. Chest 80:465–470

20. DiMarco JP, Sellers TD, Berne RM, West GA, Belardinelli L (1983) Adenosine: electrophysiologic effects and therapeutic use for terminating paroxysmal supraventricular tachycardia. Circulation 68:1254–1263

21. Pelleg A, Pennock RS, Kutalek SP (2002) Proarrhythmic effects of adenosine: one decade of clinical data. Am J Ther 9:141–147

22. Kaltman JR, Tanel RE, Shah MJ, Vetter VL, Rhodes LA (2006) Induction of atrial fibrillation after the routine use of adenosine. Pediatr Emerg Care 22:113–115

23. Strickberger SA, Man KC, Daoud EG, Goyal R, Brinkman K, Knight BP, Weiss R, Bahu M, Morady F (1997) Adenosine-induced atrial arrhythmia: a prospective analysis. Ann Intern Med 127:417–422

24. Iwai S, Markowitz SM, Stein KM, Mittal S, Slotwiner DJ, Das MK, Cohen JD, Hao SC, Lerman BB (2002) Response to adenosine differentiates focal from macroreentrant atrial tachycardia: validation using three-dimensional electroanatomic mapping. Circulation 106:2793–2799

25. Gulamhusein S, Ko P, Carruthers SG, Klein GJ (1982) Acceleration of the ventricular response during atrial fibrillation in the Wolff-Parkinson-White syndrome after verapamil. Circulation 65:348–354

26. Jacob AS, Nielsen DH, Gianelly RE (1985) Fatal ventricular fibrillation following verapamil in Wolff-Parkinson-White syndrome with atrial fibrillation. Ann Emerg Med 14:159–160

27. Markowitz SM, Stein KM, Mittal S, Slotwiner DJ, Lerman BB (1999) Differential effects of adenosine on focal and macroreentrant atrial tachycardia. J Cardiovasc Electrophysiol 10:489–502

28. Wellens HJ, Durrer D (1974) Effect of procaine amide, quinidine, and ajmaline in the Wolff-Parkinson-White syndrome. Circulation 50:114–120

29. Windle J, Prystowsky EN, Miles WM, Heger JJ (1987) Pharmacokinetic and electrophysiologic interactions of amiodarone and procainamide. Clin Pharmacol Ther 41:603–610

30. Saoudi N, Cosio F, Waldo A, Chen SA, Iesaka Y, Lesh M, Saksena S, Salerno J, Schoels W (2001) Classification of atrial flutter and regular atrial tachycardia according to electrophysiologic mechanism and anatomic bases: a statement from a joint expert group from the Working Group of Arrhythmias of the European society of cardiology and the North American society of pacing and electrophysiology. J Cardiovasc Electrophysiol 12:852–866

31. Glatter KA, Dorostkar PC, Yang Y, Lee RJ, Van Hare GF, Keung E, Modin G, Scheinman MM (2001) Electrophysiological effects of ibutilide in patients with accessory pathways. Circulation 104:1933–1939

32. Akhtar M, Tchou P, Jazayeri M (1989) Use of calcium channel entry blockers in the treatment of cardiac arrhythmias. Circulation 80:IV31–IV39

33. Gmeiner R, Ng CK (1982) Metoprolol in the treatment and prophylaxis of paroxysmal reentrant supraventricular tachycardia. J Cardiovasc Pharmacol 4:5–13

34. Lindsay BD, Saksena S, Rothbart ST, Herman S, Barr MJ (1987) Long-term efficacy and safety of beta-adrenergic receptor antagonists for supraventricular tachycardia. Am J Cardiol 60:63D–67D

35. Hellestrand KJ, Nathan AW, Bexton RS, Spurrell RA, Camm AJ (1983) Cardiac electrophysiologic effects of flecainide acetate for paroxysmal reentrant junctional tachycardias. Am J Cardiol 51:770–776

36. Dorian P, Naccarelli GV, Coumel P, Hohnloser SH, Maser MJ (1996) A randomized comparison of flecainide versus verapamil in paroxysmal supraventricular tachycardia. The Flecainide multicenter investigators group. Am J Cardiol 77:89A–95A

37. Ward DE, Jones S, Shinebourne EA (1986) Use of flecainide acetate for refractory junctional tachycardias in children with the Wolff-Parkinson-White syndrome. Am J Cardiol 57:787–790

38. Musto B, D'Onofrio A, Cavallaro C, Musto A (1988) Electrophysiological effects and clinical efficacy of propafenone in children with recurrent paroxysmal supraventricular tachycardia. Circulation 78:863–869

39. Musto B, D'Onofrio A, Cavallaro C, Musto A, Greco R (1988) Electrophysiologic effects and clinical efficacy of flecainide in children with recurrent paroxysmal supraventricular tachycardia. Am J Cardiol 62:229–233

40. Kim SS, Lal R, Ruffy R (1986) Treatment of paroxysmal reentrant supraventricular tachycardia with flecainide acetate. Am J Cardiol 58:80–85

41. Echt DS, Liebson PR, Mitchell LB, Peters RW, Obias-Manno D, Barker AH, Arensberg D, Baker A, Friedman L, Greene HL et al (1991) Mortality and morbidity in patients receiving encainide, flecainide, or placebo. The Cardiac arrhythmia suppression trial.N Engl J Med 324:781–788

42. Mitchell LB, Wyse DG, Duff HJ (1987) Electropharmacology of sotalol in patients with Wolff-Parkinson-White syndrome. Circulation 76:810–818

43. Kunze KP, Schluter M, Kuck KH (1987) Sotalol in patients with Wolff-Parkinson-White syndrome. Circulation 75:1050–1057

44. Tendera M, Wnuk-Wojnar AM, Kulakowski P, Malolepszy J, Kozlowski JW, Krzeminska-Pakula M, Szechinski J, Droszcz W, Kawecka-Jaszcz K, Swiatecka G, Ruzyllo W, Graff O (2001) Efficacy and safety of dofetilide in the prevention of symptomatic episodes of paroxysmal supraventricular tachycardia: a 6-month double-blind comparison with propafenone and placebo. Am Heart J 142:93–98

45. Kobayashi Y, Atarashi H, Ino T, Kuruma A, Nomura A, Saitoh H, Hayakawa H (1997) Clinical and electrophysiologic effects of dofetilide in patients with supraventricular tachyarrhythmias. J Cardiovasc Pharmacol 30:367–373

46. Rosenbaum MB, Chiale PA, Ryba D, Elizari MV (1974) Control of tachyarrhythmias associated with Wolff-Parkinson-White syndrome by amiodarone hydrochloride. Am J Cardiol 34:215–223

47. Wellens HJ, Lie KI, Bar FW, Wesdorp JC, Dohmen HJ, Duren DR, Durrer D (1976) Effect of amiodarone in the Wolff-Parkinson-White syndrome. Am J Cardiol 38:189–194

48. Feld GK, Nademanee K, Weiss J, Stevenson W, Singh BN (1984) Electrophysiologic basis for the suppression by amiodarone of orthodromic supraventricular tachycardias complicating pre-excitation syndromes. J Am Coll Cardiol 3:1298–1307

49. Alboni P, Tomasi C, Menozzi C, Bottoni N, Paparella N, Fuca G, Brignole M, Cappato R (2001) Efficacy and safety of out-of-hospital self-administered single-dose oral drug treatment in the management of infrequent, well-tolerated paroxysmal supraventricular tachycardia. J Am Coll Cardiol 37:548–553

50. Rae AP (1998) Placebo-controlled evaluations of propafenone for atrial tachyarrhythmias. Am J Cardiol 82:59 N–65 N

51. Musto B, Cavallaro C, Musto A, D'Onofrio A, Belli A, De Vincentis L (1992) Flecainide single oral dose for management of paroxysmal supraventricular tachycardia in children and young adults. Am Heart J 124: 110–115

52. Rose JS, Bhandari A, Rahimtoola SH, Wu D (1986) Effective termination of reentrant supraventricular tachycardia by single dose oral combination therapy with pindolol and verapamil. Am Heart J 112:759–765

53. Yeh SJ, Lin FC, Chou YY, Hung JS, Wu D (1985) Termination of paroxysmal supraventricular tachycardia with a single oral dose of diltiazem and propranolol. Circulation 71:104–109

54. Cossu SF, Rothman SA, Chmielewski IL, Hsia HH, Vogel RL, Miller JM, Buxton AE (1997) The effects of isoproterenol on the cardiac conduction system: site-specific dose dependence. J Cardiovasc Electrophysiol 8: 847–853

55. Chen SA, Chiang CE, Yang CJ, Cheng CC, Wu TJ, Wang SP, Chiang BN, Chang MS (1994) Sustained atrial tachycardia in adult patients. Electrophysiological characteristics, pharmacological response, possible mechanisms, and effects of radiofrequency ablation. Circulation 90:1262–1278

56. Wu D, Denes P, Dhingra R, Wyndham C, Rosen KM (1975) Determinants of fast- and slow-pathway conduction in patients with dual atrioventricular nodal pathways. Circ Res 36:782–790

57. Patruno N, Critelli G, Pulignano G, Urbani P, Villanti P, Reale A (1989) [Asymptomatic pre-excitation. Identification of potential risk using transesophageal pacing]. Cardiologia 34:777–781

58. Sung RJ, Waxman HL, Saksena S, Juma Z (1981) Sequence of retrograde atrial activation in patients with dual atrioventricular nodal pathways. Circulation 64:1059–1067

59. Hirao K, Otomo K, Wang X, Beckman KJ, McClelland JH, Widman L, Gonzalez MD, Arruda M, Nakagawa H, Lazzara R, Jackman WM (1996) Para-Hisian pacing. A new method for differentiating retrograde conduction over an accessory AV pathway from conduction over the AV node. Circulation 94:1027–1035

60. Strasberg B, Swiryn S, Bauernfeind R, Palileo E, Scagliotti D, Duffy CE, Rosen KM (1981) Retrograde dual atrioventricular nodal pathways. Am J Cardiol 48:639–646

61. Benditt DG, Pritchett EL, Smith WM, Gallagher JJ (1979) Ventriculoatrial intervals: diagnostic use in paroxysmal supraventricular tachycardia. Ann Intern Med 91:161–166
62. Coumel P, Attuel P (1974) Reciprocating tachycardia in overt and latent preexcitation. Influence of functional bundle branch block on the rate of the tachycardia. Eur J Cardiol 1:423–436
63. Sellers TDJ, Gallagher JJ, Cope GD, Tonkin AM, Wallace AG (1976) Retrograde atrial preexcitation following premature ventricular beats during reciprocating tachycardia in the Wolff-Parkinson-White syndrome. Eur J Cardiol 4: 283–294
64. Knight BP, Ebinger M, Oral H, Kim MH, Sticherling C, Pelosi F, Michaud GF, Strickberger SA, Morady F (2000) Diagnostic value of tachycardia features and pacing maneuvers during paroxysmal supraventricular tachycardia. J Am Coll Cardiol 36:574–582
65. Michaud GF, Tada H, Chough S, Baker R, Wasmer K, Sticherling C, Oral H, Pelosi FJ, Knight BP, Strickberger SA, Morady F (2001) Differentiation of atypical atrioventricular node re-entrant tachycardia from orthodromic reciprocating tachycardia using a septal accessory pathway by the response to ventricular pacing. J Am Coll Cardiol 38: 1163–1167
66. McGuire MA, Lau KC, Johnson DC, Richards DA, Uther JB, Ross DL (1991) Patients with two types of atrioventricular junctional (AV nodal) reentrant tachycardia. Evidence that a common pathway of nodal tissue is not present above the reentrant circuit. Circulation 83:1232–1246
67. Janse MJ, Anderson RH, McGuire MA, Ho SY (1993) "AV nodal" reentry: part I: "AV nodal" reentry revisited. J Cardiovasc Electrophysiol 4:561–572
68. McGuire MA, Bourke JP, Robotin MC, Johnson DC, Meldrum-Hanna W, Nunn GR, Uther JB, Ross DL (1993) High resolution mapping of Koch's triangle using sixty electrodes in humans with atrioventricular junctional (AV nodal) reentrant tachycardia. Circulation 88:2315–2328
69. Kalbfleisch SJ, Strickberger SA, Williamson B, Vorperian VR, Man C, Hummel JD, Langberg JJ, Morady F (1994) Randomized comparison of anatomic and electrogram mapping approaches to ablation of the slow pathway of atrioventricular node reentrant tachycardia. J Am Coll Cardiol 23:716–723
70. Lee MA, Morady F, Kadish A, Schamp DJ, Chin MC, Scheinman MM, Griffin JC, Lesh MD, Pederson D, Goldberger J et al (1991) Catheter modification of the atrioventricular junction with radiofrequency energy for control of atrioventricular nodal reentry tachycardia. Circulation 83:827–835
71. Jackman WM, Beckman KJ, McClelland JH, Wang X, Friday KJ, Roman CA, Moulton KP, Twidale N, Hazlitt HA, Prior MI et al (1992) Treatment of supraventricular tachycardia due to atrioventricular nodal reentry, by radiofrequency catheter ablation of slow-pathway conduction. N Engl J Med 327:313–318
72. Yamabe H, Okumura K, Tsuchiya T, Tabuchi T, Iwasa A, Yasue H (1998) Slow potential-guided radiofrequency catheter ablation in atrioventricular nodal reentrant tachycardia: characteristics of the potential associated with successful ablation. Pacing Clin Electrophysiol 21:2631–2640
73. Jentzer JH, Goyal R, Williamson BD, Man KC, Niebauer M, Daoud E, Strickberger SA, Hummel JD, Morady F (1994) Analysis of junctional ectopy during radiofrequency ablation of the slow pathway in patients with atrioventricular nodal reentrant tachycardia. Circulation 90:2820–2826
74. Lipscomb KJ, Zaidi AM, Fitzpatrick AP, Lefroy D (2001) Slow pathway modification for atrioventricular node re-entrant tachycardia: fast junctional tachycardia predicts adverse prognosis. Heart 85:44–47
75. Lindsay BD, Chung MK, Gamache MC, Luke RA, Schechtman KB, Osborn JL, Cain ME (1993) Therapeutic end points for the treatment of atrioventricular node reentrant tachycardia by catheter-guided radiofrequency current. J Am Coll Cardiol 22:733–740
76. Strickberger SA, Kalbfleisch SJ, Williamson B, Man KC, Vorperian V, Hummel JD, Langberg JJ, Morady F (1993) Radiofrequency catheter ablation of atypical atrioventricular nodal reentrant tachycardia. J Cardiovasc Electrophysiol 4:526–532
77. Clague JR, Dagres N, Kottkamp H, Breithardt G, Borggrefe M (2001) Targeting the slow pathway for atrioventricular nodal reentrant tachycardia: initial results and long-term follow-up in 379 consecutive patients. Eur Heart J 22: 82–88
78. Haissaguerre M, Gaita F, Fischer B, Commenges D, Montserrat P, d'Ivernois C, Lemetayer P, Warin JF (1992) Elimination of atrioventricular nodal reentrant tachycardia using discrete slow potentials to guide application of radiofrequency energy. Circulation 85:2162–2175
79. Calkins H, Yong P, Miller JM, Olshansky B, Carlson M, Saul JP, Huang SK, Liem LB, Klein LS, Moser SA, Bloch DA, Gillette P, Prystowsky E (1999) Catheter ablation of accessory pathways, atrioventricular nodal reentrant tachycardia, and the atrioventricular junction: final results of a prospective, multicenter clinical trial. The Atakr multicenter investigators group. Circulation 99:262–270
80. Scheinman MM, Huang S (2000) The 1998 NASPE prospective catheter ablation registry. Pacing Clin Electrophysiol 23:1020–1028

81. Hummel JD, Strickberger SA, Williamson BD, Man KC, Daoud E, Niebauer M, Bakr O, Morady F (1995) Effect of residual slow pathway function on the time course of recurrences of atrioventricular nodal reentrant tachycardia after radiofrequency ablation of the slow pathway. Am J Cardiol 75:628–630

82. Kistler PM, Roberts-Thomson KC, Haqqani HM, Fynn SP, Singarayar S, Vohra JK, Morton JB, Sparks PB, Kalman JM (2006) P-wave morphology in focal atrial tachycardia: development of an algorithm to predict the anatomic site of origin. J Am Coll Cardiol 48:1010–1017

83. Tang CW, Scheinman MM, Van Hare GF, Epstein LM, Fitzpatrick AP, Lee RJ, Lesh MD (1995) Use of P wave configuration during atrial tachycardia to predict site of origin. J Am Coll Cardiol 26:1315–1324

84. Porter MJ, Morton JB, Denman R, Lin AC, Tierney S, Santucci PA, Cai JJ, Madsen N, Wilber DJ (2004) Influence of age and gender on the mechanism of supraventricular tachycardia. Heart Rhythm 1:393–396

85. Walsh EP, Saul JP, Hulse JE, Rhodes LA, Hordof AJ, Mayer JE, Lock JE (1992) Transcatheter ablation of ectopic atrial tachycardia in young patients using radiofrequency current. Circulation 86:1138–1146

86. Lesh MD, Van Hare GF, Epstein LM, Fitzpatrick AP, Scheinman MM, Lee RJ, Kwasman MA, Grogin HR, Griffin JC (1994) Radiofrequency catheter ablation of atrial arrhythmias. Results and mechanisms. Circulation 89: 1074–1089

87. Schmitt C, Zrenner B, Schneider M, Karch M, Ndrepepa G, Deisenhofer I, Weyerbrock S, Schreieck J, Schomig A (1999) Clinical experience with a novel multielectrode basket catheter in right atrial tachycardias. Circulation 99: 2414–2422

88. Tracy CM, Swartz JF, Fletcher RD, Hoops HG, Solomon AJ, Karasik PE, Mukherjee D (1993) Radiofrequency catheter ablation of ectopic atrial tachycardia using paced activation sequence mapping. J Am Coll Cardiol 21:910–917

89. O'Hara GE, Philippon F, Champagne J, Blier L, Molin F, Cote JM, Nault I, Sarrazin JF, Gilbert M (2007) Catheter ablation for cardiac arrhythmias: a 14-year experience with 5330 consecutive patients at the Quebec heart institute, Laval Hospital. Can J Cardiol 23(Suppl B):67B–70B

90. Swallow EB, Dayer MJ, Oldfield WL, Moxham J, Polkey MI (2006) Right hemi-diaphragm paralysis following cardiac radiofrequency ablation. Respir Med 100:1657–1659

91. Lee JC, Steven D, Roberts-Thomson KC, Raymond JM, Stevenson WG, Tedrow UB (2009) Atrial tachycardias adjacent to the phrenic nerve: recognition, potential problems, and solutions. Heart Rhythm 6:1186–1191; Bastani H, Insulander P, Schwieler J, Tabrizi F, Braunschweig F, Kenneback G, Drca N, Sadigh B, Jensen-Urstad M (2009) Safety and efficacy of cryoablation of atrial tachycardia with high risk of ablation-related injuries. Europace 11:625–629

92. Calkins H, Langberg J, Sousa J, el-Atassi R, Leon A, Kou W, Kalbfleisch S, Morady F (1992) Radiofrequency catheter ablation of accessory atrioventricular connections in 250 patients. Abbreviated therapeutic approach to Wolff-Parkinson-White syndrome. Circulation 85:1337–1346

93. Lesh MD, Van Hare GF, Schamp DJ, Chien W, Lee MA, Griffin JC, Langberg JJ, Cohen TJ, Lurie KG, Scheinman MM (1992) Curative percutaneous catheter ablation using radiofrequency energy for accessory pathways in all locations: results in 100 consecutive patients. J Am Coll Cardiol 19:1303–1309

94. Weng KP, Wolff GS, Young ML (2003) Multiple accessory pathways in pediatric patients with Wolff-Parkinson-White syndrome. Am J Cardiol 91:1178–1183

95. Chen YJ, Chen SA, Tai CT, Chiang CE, Lee SH, Chiou CW, Ueng KC, Wen ZC, Yu WC, Huang JL, Feng AN, Chang MS (1997) Long-term results of radiofrequency catheter ablation in patients with Wolff-Parkinson-White syndrome. Zhonghua Yi Xue Za Zhi (Taipei) 59:78–87

96. Lin JL, Schie JT, Tseng CD, Chen WJ, Cheng TF, Tsou SS, Chen JJ, Tseng YZ, Lien WP (1995) Value of local electrogram characteristics predicting successful catheter ablation of left-versus right-sided accessory atrioventricular pathways by radiofrequency current. Cardiology 86:135–142

97. Grimm W, Miller J, Josephson ME (1994) Successful and unsuccessful sites of radiofrequency catheter ablation of accessory atrioventricular connections. Am Heart J 128:77–87

98. Silka MJ, Kron J, Halperin BD, Griffith K, Crandall B, Oliver RP, Walance CG, McAnulty JH (1992) Analysis of local electrogram characteristics correlated with successful radiofrequency catheter ablation of accessory atrioventricular pathways. Pacing Clin Electrophysiol 15:1000–1007

99. Calkins H, Kim YN, Schmaltz S, Sousa J, el-Atassi R, Leon A, Kadish A, Langberg JJ, Morady F (1992) Electrogram criteria for identification of appropriate target sites for radiofrequency catheter ablation of accessory atrioventricular connections. Circulation 85:565–573

100. Haissaguerre M, Fischer B, Warin JF, Dartigues JF, Lemetayer P, Egloff P (1992) Electrogram patterns predictive of successful radiofrequency catheter ablation of accessory pathways. Pacing Clin Electrophysiol 15:2138–2145

101. Swartz JF, Tracy CM, Fletcher RD (1993) Radiofrequency endocardial catheter ablation of accessory atrioventricular pathway atrial insertion sites. Circulation 87:487–499

8 Pharmacologic Management of Atrial Fibrillation and Flutter

Deepak Saluja, Kathleen Hickey, and James A. Reiffel

CONTENTS

Abstract

Atrial fibrillation is the most commonly encountered arrhythmia requiring therapy and is associated with significant morbidity, a reduced quality of life, an increased risk for mortality, a significant likelihood of hospitalization, an increased risk for stroke and systemic embolism, and significant costs. Both rate control and rhythm control have been shown to improve quality of life. Neither as a strategy has been proven to reduce mortality versus the other; however, in some series the attainment and maintenance of sinus rhythm has had superior outcomes if risks from therapy are not encountered (especially those of amiodarone). In patients with markers of an increased risk for stroke, anticoagulation with warfarin is essential. In all patients, rate control is also necessary so as to reduce both symptoms and the risk for a tachycardia-induced cardiomyopathy. The choice of rhythm control strategy must be individualized based on patient characteristics. This chapter will review the considerations necessary for choosing appropriate pharmacologic therapies as well as the therapeutic agents themselves.

Key Words: Atrial fibrillation; Atrial flutter; Antiarrhythmic drugs; Rate control; Rhythm control; Anticoagulation.

INTRODUCTION

Atrial fibrillation (AF) is the most commonly encountered sustained arrhythmia in clinical practice, affecting an estimated 2.3–5.1 million people in the United States, with the prevalence expected to triple by 2050 as the population ages *(1)*. AF is associated with physical symptoms, a shortened life expectancy, and reduced quality of life (QoL).

From: *Contemporary Cardiology: Management of Cardiac Arrhythmias*
Edited by: Gan-Xin Yan, Peter R. Kowey, DOI 10.1007/978-1-60761-161-5_8
© Springer Science+Business Media, LLC 2011

The impact AF can have on a patient's health may take several forms. AF can cause palpitations, angina, dyspnea, lightheadedness, chronic fatigue, and/or impaired exercise tolerance. Even in the absence of such symptoms, AF may lead to several potentially significant associated conditions, including tachycardia-induced cardiomyopathy and thromboembolism.

Quality of life is adversely affected by the presence of AF in most populations, either due to the presence of symptoms, side effects of medications, or due to lifestyle disruptions associated with anticoagulation (2). All-cause mortality in patients with AF is 1.5–1.9 fold higher than those without AF, regardless of the presence of symptoms (3). This may be due to the effects of AF itself, toxicities associated with treatment, or comorbidities such as hypertension, heart failure, and valvular disease more commonly seen in AF patients.

While antiarrhythmic drug (AAD) therapy can mitigate both symptoms and decreased QoL by maintaining sinus rhythm (SR), clinical trials have thus far failed to conclusively demonstrate that the pursuit of SR with currently available AADs decreases mortality (4–7). Further analysis of these trials has suggested the absence of AF may be associated with decreased mortality in those who can achieve it without significant proarrhythmia or toxicity (8). Although this may become achievable with the development of newer agents such as dronedarone, which was recently shown in the ATHENA trial to be associated with a reduction in a combined endpoint of cardiovascular hospitalization and death in a high-risk AF population (9), given the currently available data, the main focus of drug treatment of AF at present remains improving symptoms and QoL in a way that minimizes the side effects and risks from therapy. While rate control and anticoagulation to reduce the risk of thromboembolism remain vital components in achieving this goal, it must be emphasized that many patients will not have adequate relief of symptoms until a normal rhythm is established, even after controlling the ventricular rate. Rhythm control, therefore, remains an important and commonly employed (10) part of the physician's armamentarium in treating AF in selected cases.

PATTERNS OF AF

Characterizing the pattern of AF is critical in selecting the appropriate rate or rhythm control treatment strategy for an individual patient (Table 1). Treatment algorithms in the 2006 ACC/AHA/ESC Guidelines for the Treatment of Patients with Atrial Fibrillation are based on this division (11). While several systems have been proposed to classify AF based on various characteristics, the system that is most practical for clinical use divides AF into groups based on duration of AF episodes and therapeutic history.

Table 1
Classification of Patterns of AF

Patterns of AF
Paroxysmal Episodes of AF last less than 1 week Terminates spontaneously, without electrical or pharmacological cardioversion
Persistent Episodes of AF last longer than 1 week *or* Electrical or pharmacologic cardioversion is used to terminate AF
Permanent A strategy of rhythm control has been abandoned or never tried *and* AF is continually present

AF is termed *paroxysmal* when it terminates without drug or electrical cardioversion therapy and recurs within 1 week; *persistent* when self-terminating episodes last longer than 1 week or when therapy is delivered to terminate the rhythm; and *permanent* when a strategy of rhythm control has been either abandoned or never tried and the patient remains in AF indefinitely. The paroxysmal and persistent categories are not mutually exclusive, as both may be seen in a particular individual at different times. The classification of a patient who presents with AF for the first time presents a special situation, since the history and clinical decision making required for classification under this system has not yet been established. In this case, some time may be necessary to assess the patient's likelihood for spontaneous termination, recurrence, and response to any treatments delivered. In all categories, it is assumed that the duration of any episode of AF is > 30 sec, and that AF is not due to reversible causes (hyperthyroidism, pneumonia, pericarditis, etc.) *(11)*.

Paroxysmal AF

By definition, paroxysmal AF is self-terminating and limited in duration. The choice of therapy is therefore dependent on the presence and severity of symptoms during episodes of AF. Asymptomatic patients whose rates are controlled off of medications may not require AAD therapy. Patients with rapid ventricular responses require rate control, which may be sufficient to control symptoms in certain cases. Rhythm monitoring devices such as 24-h Holter monitors can be valuable tools to ensure that rates are reasonable not only at rest but also during daily activities. Rhythm control strategies are most often reserved for those patients who have intolerable symptoms during AF not alleviated by rate controlling medications.

Persistent AF

Patients with persistent AF have either self-terminating episodes of AF that last longer than 1 week or episodes in which therapy is delivered for rhythm conversion. Patients in this category occasionally have more significant degrees of abnormalities in left ventricular ejection fraction, left atrial size, and left atrial contractile function than paroxysmal patients; abnormalities that may be reversible with the restoration of sinus rhythm *(12)*. For those patients who have disabling symptoms that are not alleviated by rate control, a rhythm control strategy is indicated. Electrical or pharmalcologic cardioversion may be used to terminate events. For patients with infrequent events, as-needed cardioversion without further antiarrhythmic therapy may suffice. Pharmacologic cardioversion can be achieved with either a single dose of an AAD at the onset of episodes (the so-called "pill-in-the-pocket" approach) *(13)*, or daily dosing of an AAD over a limited period of time. Alternatively, for patients in whom intermittent therapy is inadequate or inconvenient, longer term daily maintenance antiarrhythmic drug (AAD) therapy may be used. For those patients who fail AAD therapy or for those who are intolerant of or unwilling to take them, catheter ablation therapy is an efficacious method of rhythm control in the paroxysmal and persistent AF populations whose availability is increasing *(14)*. As with PAF, anticoagulation of patients at "high risk" for thromboembolism with warfarin is employed. It should be continued even if sinus rhythm is restored.

Permanent AF

By definition, a patient with permanent AF is one in whom a rhythm control strategy has been abandoned. Pharmacologic therapy in these patients therefore consists of rate control and, in "high-risk" patients, anticoagulation. As recent advances in catheter ablation techniques expand the population of patients in whom maintenance of sinus rhythm can be achieved to include certain patients with long-term AF *(15)* as well as left ventricular dysfunction *(16)*, it may become necessary to reconsider the possibility of achieving sinus rhythm in the patient with permanent AF. In many of these patients, adequate rhythm control may require adjunctive AAD therapy in addition to ablation.

GOALS OF TREATMENT

Rate Control vs. Rhythm Control

The goal in the treatment of pharmacological treatment of AF is, as in any other disease, to improve the quality and, if possible, the quantity of life while minimizing any potential toxic effects of therapy. Other therapeutic goals specific to the treatment of AF include preventing or reversing structural changes caused by the persistence of AF and the prevention of thromboembolism.

In general, the approach to AF therapy has been divided into two possible strategies: (1) controlling the ventricular rate during AF episodes (rate control) and (2) preventing AF from recurring (rhythm control). Although this division is useful conceptually, it is somewhat artificial in clinical practice, since a strategy of rhythm control does not assure that achievement and maintenance of SR occur, and a strategy of rate control in PAF patients does not define the overall burden of AF. Nevertheless, treatment decisions are based on such factors as the severity and type of symptoms, the presence of other comorbidities such as atherosclerotic disease and ventricular hypertrophy, the functionality of the AV node, the toxicities of the treatments under consideration, and the preferences of the patient. In recent years, several trials have been done in order to establish an evidence basis to guide decision making *(4–7, 17, 18)*. Below is a discussion of the relative efficacy of these two treatment strategies in achieving selected endpoints.

Mortality

As noted above, AF is associated with a significant increase in all-cause mortality compared to patients with SR *(3)*. It was reasonably expected, therefore, that if this association was causal, the maintenance of SR should lead to reduced mortality. Maintaining SR would then become an endpoint in its own right, without consideration to the presence or severity of symptoms. Several trials have been completed in recent years addressing this hypothesis *(4–7, 17, 18)*.

The largest such trial completed to date is the AFFIRM trial, a study of 4060 patients aged 65 or older with AF and other risk factors for stroke or death randomized to either a rate control or rhythm control strategy. In the rate control arm, patients were treated with a combination of β (beta)-blockers, calcium channel blockers, and digoxin. Patients in the rhythm control arm were treated generally with Class III AADs (largely amiodarone). Overall mortality (the primary endpoint) was not statistically different between the two groups. There was, in fact, a trend toward increased mortality in the rhythm control arm *(7)*.

Other, smaller, trials have found similar results. The RACE trial compared rate and rhythm control strategies in 522 patients with persistent AF and mild-to-moderate heart failure. The rates of achievement of a combined endpoint that included mortality, heart failure hospitalization, pacemaker implantation, hemorrhage, thrombotic complications, and severe adverse events were no different between the two groups *(6)*. AF-CHF, the first trial to compare rhythm and rate control strategies in heart failure patients, found no difference in total mortality, with a higher rate of hospitalizations in the rhythm control group *(17)*. Other smaller randomized trials of treatment strategies in AF including STAF *(4)*, HOT-CAFÉ *(5)*, and PIAF *(18)* similarly found no differences in mortality between groups (although none were adequately powered to do so). These findings are also in keeping with the results obtained from subanalyses of AAD therapy in other populations, including DIAMOND-AF *(19)* and CHF-STAT *(20)*. A metaanalysis of available rate vs. rhythm control therapy trials came to the same conclusion and further found that a rhythm control strategy was associated with higher health-care utilization and costs *(21)*.

Several features of these trials bear noting. First, they were designed to compare different *treatment strategies*, as opposed to different *rhythms*. This distinction is necessary because many patients with AF in whom rate control is pursued may continue to have periods of SR, while those seeking rhythm control may be in AF a significant proportion of time despite AAD or ablative therapy. Second, there was a high overall degree of crossover between groups (14.9% from the rate control group and 37.5% in the rhythm control group at 5 years in the AFFIRM trial), such that in intention-to-treat analyses, a fair number of patients were analyzed as belonging to a treatment assignment that they did not remain in during the study *(7)*.

Although an orthodox analysis of the randomized data described consistently fails to demonstrate a survival advantage for a strategy of rhythm control, there are data that suggest that when sinus rhythm can be maintained and the toxicities of AAD therapy avoided, patients do significantly better than when left in AF. An on-treatment reanalysis of the AFFIRM data that classified patients into subgroups based on which treatment they actually received, as opposed to which treatment they were randomized to, found that the presence of SR was associated with a lower risk of mortality, and AAD therapy was associated with increased mortality after adjustment for the presence of SR *(8)*. This suggests that beneficial effects of SR may have been cancelled out by a harmful effect of the drugs used to achieve it (again, largely amiodarone, which was associated with an increase in non-cardiovascular mortality). Other data from the DIAMOND-AF *(19)* and the CHF-STAT *(20)* found a similar positive survival benefit for the presence of SR, although similar analyses in some other drug trials have not duplicated these results *(4–6, 18)*.

An additional point to consider is that patients enrolled in the above-mentioned rate vs. rhythm control trials had to be willing to be randomized to either strategy. Patients who were already rate controlled and still symptomatic were highly unlikely to enroll in such trials; hence, such trials should not be taken to indicate that rate control is a reasonable strategy for all AF patients. Similarly, these trials enrolled patients at increased risk for thromboembolism or death. Hence, their results should not be generalized to a lower risk population for whom AAD therapy may be less problematic.

Taken together, the above data suggest that an a priori strategy of rhythm control with currently available AADs should not be undertaken with the expectation of a survival advantage. It is important to emphasize, however, that given the lack of clear increased mortality with rhythm control agents, these data do not suggest that a strategy of rhythm control be withheld from specific patients who have intolerable symptoms in AF in the presence of a controlled rate. It is possible that newer AADs with more favorable safety profiles will deliver the benefits of SR without the toxicities of current therapies, as was suggested by the ATHENA data *(9)*.

Quality of Life and Exercise Tolerance

It is known that AF can adversely effect patients' QoL, exercise tolerance, and functional status in ways unrelated to objective measures of its severity *(22)*, and treatment of AF can improve these endpoints compared to leaving AF untreated *(7, 18)*.

In randomized trials, treatment with a strategy of rhythm control has not conclusively been found to deliver QoL improvements superior to those attained by a strategy of rate control *(23–25)*. Most studies have found, however, that those patients that are able to achieve SR do appear to have improvements in QoL that exceed those in who remain in AF *(24, 26)*. An important exception is the AFFIRM trial, in which QoL was comparable whether patients were in sinus rhythm or in AF *(25)*. One explanation for this discrepancy may be the relatively low number of highly symptomatic patients enrolled in the older AFFIRM population.

Rhythm control may be superior to rate control in improving exercise tolerance. In several trials, exercise capacity improved more in patients treated with rhythm control strategies than with a rate control strategy *(5, 18, 26, 27)*.

Ventricular and Atrial Structure and Function

AF is associated with changes in the electrical, contractile, and structural functions of the heart. In the atria, structural changes are thought to play a role in the persistence of AF *(28)* and may explain why SR is more difficult to maintain after cardioversion in patients with a longer duration of preceding AF *(29)*.

Maintenance of SR has been associated with benefits in chamber remodeling in patients with and without clinical heart failure at baseline in some trials *(12, 30, 31)*. In the RACE, SR was associated with improvements in LV function and reduction in atrial sizes in patients with mild-to-moderate heart failure. Similar improvements were not seen in patients whom the ventricular rate was controlled, although it did prevent deterioration in LV function *(30)*. In a small study of patients with AF and heart failure that underwent catheter ablation, patients who achieved SR had reductions in LA and LV sizes and increases in ejection fraction, while those that remained in AF showed none of these changes *(31)*. Similar changes were noted in a larger study of patients undergoing catheter ablation who had relatively preserved baseline LV function *(12)*. Changes in electrophysiological parameters are also seen with the achievement of SR. Patients who maintain SR 1 week after cardioversion have increased atrial refractory periods and decreased sinus node recovery times and P-wave durations compared to immediately after cardioversion *(32)*.

Prevention of Thromboembolism

AF can be associated with a substantially increased rate of thromboembolic events that is reduced with the use of oral anticoagulants *(33, 34)*. Warfarin therapy, however, can be inconvenient *(2)*, carries its own risks, and does not completely eliminate thromboembolism *(35)*. In years past, a strategy of rhythm control was often used with the anticipated goal of discontinuing oral anticoagulant therapy. Data from both the RACE and AFFIRM trials showed that the rates of thromboembolism were higher in rhythm control patients than in rate control patients, illustrating that SR by itself does not eliminate embolic risk in patients with risk markers associated with their prior AF *(6, 7)*. Among the rhythm control patients with thromboembolism, most had stopped taking warfarin. Important to note is that most of these patients were in SR at the time of their event.

Several observations may explain the above findings. First, restoring electrical normality to a fibrillating atrium does not immediately restore mechanical normality *(36)*, and the persistence of atrial dysfunction may result in a continued risk of stroke after SR is restored. Second, recurrences of AF can be asymptomatic and may go unnoticed unless rhythm monitoring is continuous *(37)*. Third, AF may either cause or be a marker of biochemical alterations at the endothelial and intraatrial level that may increase stroke risk independent of mechanical considerations and that may persist after SR has been restored *(38)*. That is, AF and clot propensity may both be downstream effects of atrial dysfunction and that AF itself may not be the (sole) causative factor of increased thromboembolic risk.

The above suggests that stroke risk persists in "high-risk" patients with AF even after SR has been restored. As a general rule, patients in AF with indications for anticoagulation (see below) should be continued on it even after rhythm conversion. Pursuing rhythm control in an AF patient with stroke risk factors has not yet been shown to reduce their risk of stroke and should not be undertaken for this purpose alone.

SPECIFIC DRUGS FOR MAINTENANCE OF OR CONVERSION TO SINUS RHYTHM

Antiarrhythmic drugs are commonly divided into classes based on the Vaughan-Williams classification system, which divides drugs based on their major mechanism of action (Table 2). This section will review the role of these drugs in the conversion to and maintenance of sinus rhythm in AF.

Table 2
The Vaughan-Williams Antiarrhythmic Drug Classification

Vaughan-Williams classification					
Na+ channel			β-receptor[1]	K+ channel	Ca+ channel
Ia	Ib	Ic	II	III	IV
Procainamide	Lidocaine	Propafenone	Metoprolol	Amiodarone	Diltiazem
Quinidine	Mexilitine	Flecainide	Propranolol	Sotalol	Verapamil
Disopyrimide			Esmolol		
			Cavedilol[2]		

[1] Among other β-receptor antagonists

[2] Carvedilol also exhibits α-receptor blocking properties

Class Ia

Class Ia agents include quinidine, disopyrimide, and procainamide. They are sodium channel blocking agents that prolong the action potential in a use dependent fashion, although drugs in this class also have other important ion channel and autonomic effects, such as Ik_r inhibition in the case of all three of these agents, I_{to} inhibition in the case of quinidine, and vagolytic effects in the case of disopyrimide and less so, quinidine. They have been used for the acute conversion of AF as well as maintenance of SR after conversion. The potassium channel inhibitory effects may be associated with Torsades de Pointes type (TdP) proarrhythmia. This risk may be highest with quinidine.

QUINIDINE

Quinidine is among the first used and best studied of the AADs in AF. Oral quinidine has found to increase the odds of SR maintenance over placebo by about twofold in a recent systematic review of 44 antiarrhythmic trials *(39)*. It can also be used for the conversion of AF to SR. The PAFAC trial showed that the combination of quinidine plus verapamil maintained sinus rhythm after electrical cardioversion in 65% of treated patients *(40)*. This efficacy was equally to sotalol and better than placebo. In this trial, verapamil appeared to have substantially reduced the risk of TdP from quinidine. Overall, however, results have been more variable, success rates varying from 20 to 80% in different reports *(41, 42)*. Its use has always been limited by its substantial side effect profile, which includes diarrhea and upper GI intolerance in up to a quarter of patients. More concerning, however, are several reports linking the use of quinidine with an increase in overall mortality *(43, 44)*. If used for AF, quinidine must be initiated in-hospital.

PROCAINAMIDE

Procainamide has an efficacy for the conversion of AF that is approximately equal to that of quinidine *(45)*. Negative inotropic effects, QT prolongation, and hypotension complicate intravenous administration for this purpose. In one series, intravenous procainamide converted 52% of treated patients, although serious side effects occurred in 10%, including hypotension, bradycardia, and heart block *(45)*. While these concerns limit its use in most circumstances, it continues to be a drug option in the pharmacological conversion of AF in patients with WPW, where administration of conventional rate controlling agents is limited by concerns over AV nodal suppression and acceleration of ventricular response through enhanced accessory conduction.

Its long-term use for the maintenance of SR is limited by a side effect profile that includes rash, GI intolerance, neutropenia, and the development of a lupus-like syndrome in up to 30% of long-term users. Oral procainamide is now very difficult to obtain in the United States as a result of significant market decline over the past decade.

DISOPYRIMIDE

There are limited amount of data regarding the use of disopyrimide for the treatment of AF. One trial reported efficacy vs. placebo in the maintenance of SR after electrical cardioversion *(46)*. Substantial negative inotropic and vagolytic effects can limit its use in most patients. Its vagolytic actions may be of some benefit in patients with vagally mediated AF, such as those patients with lone AF that develops nocturnally.

Due to the side effects outlined above, concerns over mortality, and the availability of other classes of drugs, current guidelines no longer consider Class Ia drugs as playing a role drug treatment of AF in the majority of patients *(11)*.

Class Ib

Drugs of this class include lidocaine, mexiletine, and phenytoin. They have little effect on atrial myocardium and do not play a role in treating AF.

Class Ic

Class Ic agents include flecainide, propafenone, encainide, and moricizine. These class Ic agents potently block sodium channels in a use-dependent manner, have slow association/dissociation characteristics, and have little effect on action potential duration. Flecainide and propafenone have been used for the acute conversion of AF as well as maintenance of SR. Moricizine is no longer available in the United States.

PROPAFENONE AND FLECAINIDE

The largest studies of propafenone for maintenance of SR were the RAFT and ERAFT studies. RAFT (done in the US and Canada) and ERAFT (done in Europe) were two trials with similar designs that studied the efficacy of twice-daily sustained-release propafenone in patients with PAF. Together these trials studied over 1100 patients with PAF and randomized them to 325 mg twice a day, 425 mg twice a day, or placebo. In RAFT, a 225 mg twice-daily arm was studied as well. There was a dose-responsive increase in the time to recurrent symptomatic AF over placebo in all propafenone arms *(47, 48)*. This is consistent with other trials, which have reported similar efficacy *(49)*. The absolute efficacy rates for the same doses were greater in the RAFT than in the ERAFT trial; a result of a population in ERAFT that had a longer history of AF, a history of more frequent AF events, and more prior therapy resistance.

Flecainide has been found to prolong time to first AF relapse and time between symptomatic episodes in patients with PAF. In one placebo-controlled study, patients treated with flecainide had on average 27 days between symptomatic attacks vs. 6 days for placebo patients *(50)*. The efficacy of flecainide is probably similar to that of propafenone; one study comparing the drugs head to head in 200 patients found the chances of safe and effective treatment to be 77% for flecainide-treated and 75% for propafenone-treated patients *(51)*.

Immediate release propafenone, given as 600 mg orally, has been studied for the acute conversion of AF (initially in the observed setting), where it has been found to achieve SR in 62% of patients 8 h after administration (about double that of placebo) *(52)*. Other trials have conversion rates at 8 h of ~70–80% with both single doses of immediate release propafenone (600 mg) or single doses of flecainide (300 mg). Intravenous administration is equally efficacious, but not commercially available in the US *(53)*.

Recently the safety and efficacy of single out-of-hospital doses of AADs for the conversion of AF have been established. Alboni et al. studied this "pill-in-the-pocket" approach by giving either weight-based doses of flecainide (200 or 300 mg) or propafenone (450 or 600 mg) to patients with PAF and recurrent AF in whom pharmacologic conversion was initially achieved in the hospital. Both drugs were effective in terminating palpitations within 6 h in 94% of episodes and markedly reduced the number of hospitalizations vs. before the trial began *(13)*. When used, the first administration of these agents is usually given under observation and in successful respondents, subsequent events may be treated at home. This is especially true of patients with unknown sinus and AV node function. In patients without concomitant sinus node disease, conduction disease, or associated structural heart disease, however, initial administration as an outpatient may be employed. We have done so in over 150 patients during the past 5 years without difficulty. In patients with known dysfunction, caution should be used when administering Ic drugs in any setting.

Propafenone and flecainide are generally considered safe drugs for the chronic suppression of AF in patients with no or minimal heart disease. Perhaps the most serious cardiac side effect of these drugs is the risk of conversion to atrial flutter, which can occasionally conduct 1:1. To prevent this potentially dangerous situation, many physicians administer these drugs with nodal blocking agents. Non-cardiac side effects of flecainide include dizziness and visual changes. The most common side effects of propafenone are taste disturbance and GI intolerance. While generally well tolerated, some trials have reported excessive rates of discontinuation due to these effects *(54)*. In RAFT and ERAFT, discontinuation rates in excess of placebo were only seen with the highest dose, and serious adverse events did not exceed placebo event rates with any dose *(47, 55)*.

The use of Ic agents is limited to patients without coronary disease and with structurally normal ventricles. This major limitation is in large part due to the results of the CAST trial. CAST studied the effects of flecainide, encainide, and moricizine on mortality in patients with premature ventricular depolarizations after myocardial infarction. The trial was stopped early after it was shown that patients in the encainide and flecainide arms had a higher rate of total mortality (3.0%) as well as fatal and nonfatal arrhythmic events (4.5%) and than patients in the placebo arm (1.6 and 1.7%, respectively) *(56)*. Similar results were later reported in the moricizine arm *(57)*.

As a result of the above findings, patients with risk factors for coronary disease must undergo stress testing for inducible ischemia before the administration of a Class Ic agent, and these agents must be discontinued in those patients with clinical ischemic events. Likewise, Class Ic agents should not be administered to patients with other ventricular pathophysiological states in which cell-to-cell conduction may be impaired, such as by fibrosis, infiltration, or inflammation, or in the presence of significant ventricular hypertrophy.

Class II

Class II agents block β (beta)1 and β (beta)2-adrenergic receptors in the heart and vasculature with varying proportional affinity, and are conventionally known as β (beta)-blockers. Some agents have effects on α (alpha)-adrenergic receptors as well.

While β (beta)-blockade is generally prescribed for control of the ventricular rate in AF, some basic and clinical data suggest that it may have direct effects in preventing AF occurrence. Data from experiments using isolated human right atrial cardiomyoctes show that chronic treatment with β (beta)-blockers decreases I_{to} current density and phase 1 of the action potential, which prolongs action potential duration and the atrial refractory period (58). Clinical data support this association. Observational data have suggested a link between β (beta)-blockers use and a decreased incidence of AF (59), and randomized data studying the role of β (beta)-blockers after cardioversion suggest an effect in maintaining sinus rhythm. One placebo-controlled trial of extended release metoprolol showed a decrease in the rate of relapse after cardioversion for persistent AF from 59.9% in the placebo arm to 48.7% (60). Atenolol and bisoprolol have also been studied in similar circumstances and have been found to be equally effective as sotalol in decreasing AF recurrence after cardioversion without the risk of life-threatening Torsades (61, 62).

Randomized and metaanalysis data (63) suggest that β (beta)-blockade appears to have particular efficacy in preventing AF after cardiac surgery. The administration of metoprolol after cardiac surgery decreases the incidence of AF occurrence modestly (39% vs. 31% in the placebo arm in one trial) (64). This efficacy of metoprolol is increased substantially by the use of a strategy 48-h titrated-dose intravenous metoprolol infusion (65). Carvedilol may be particularly effective in post-cardiac surgery AF prevention, having been shown to superior to both placebo (66) and metoprolol for this purpose. In one randomized active treatment comparison, the incidence of post-heart surgery AF was reduced from 36% in the metoprolol arm to 16% in the carvedilol arm (67).

Less evidence is available regarding the ability of β (beta)-blockers to achieve conversion to SR without electrical cardioversion. Although in one small trial, 50% of the patients given intravenous esmolol converted to SR compared with 12% of patients given verapamil (68), no placebo-controlled data are available, and the administration of β (beta)-blockers for this purpose alone is not recommended (11).

Class III

The most commonly used Class III agents in AF are amiodarone, sotalol, dofetilide, and ibutilide. They all have in common their ability to block K$^+$ current during repolarization, which has the effect of prolonging the APD and the surface QT interval, although they differ in their route of administration, pharmacology, and full spectrum of antiarrhythmic effects. Ibutilide is only available intravenously for rapid cardioversion. Dofetilide is only available orally. Sotalol is only available orally in the United States, but is available both orally and for IV administration in parts of Europe, where it is used for both cardioversion (IV) and sinus rhythm maintenance (orally).

The major limitation to the use of Class III antiarrhythmics is the risk of TdP, a specific type of polymorphic ventricular tachycardia characterized by a rotating axis and QRS amplitude. The basis of the increased risk of TdP with Class III agents is potassium channel inhibition, which prolongs repolarization and with it, early afterdepolarizations, and phase 2 reentry. Although TdP most commonly terminates spontaneously, sustained episodes yielding syncope as well as degeneration to ventricular fibrillation can occur. Although all Class III agents have this effect on the QT, some Class III agents (dofetilide, ibutilide, sotalol) appear to have a greater propensity to cause TdP than others (amiodarone, azimilide) (69). These differences may be a result of degree of ion channel specificity or of differences in the degree of use dependence (70). Patient factors appear to be important as well. For example, women have a longer QT interval than men at baseline and are twice as likely to develop TdP with all Class III agents. Risk increases in the setting of hypokalemia, hypomagnesemia, and bradycardia (71). It also increases in the presence of ventricular hypertrophy and impaired metabolism/elimination of the causative drugs. Vigilance in monitoring the QT interval, electrolyte status, renal function is required to mitigate proarrhythmic risk. The time of greatest risk in AF patients given these drugs is at the time of conversion when post-conversion pauses or bradycardia may occur.

An important issue in the assessment of proarrhythmic risk is the difficulty in accurately measuring the QT interval in AF. Commonly used corrections do not account for variability in the RR interval and are inaccurate at the extremes of heart rate often seen in AF. Recently, a new QT correction formula has been derived for use in AF that appears to be more accurate than conventional corrections *(72)*.

AMIODARONE

Amiodarone is a complicated antiarrhythmic that, while classified as Class III, displays characteristics of all antiarrhythmic drug classes. It has a very large volume of distribution due to extensive accumulation in various locations and therefore must be "loaded" before steady-state dosages can be prescribed. It has an extensive side effect profile, including optic nerve, pulmonary, neurologic, skin, thyroid, and liver toxicity that necessitates long-term follow-up and screening of liver function, thyroid, eye, and pulmonary status on a scheduled basis, regardless of the absence of symptoms for those chronically exposed. Additionally, amiodarone may increase defibrillation thresholds in patients with implantable defibrillators. Amiodarone is burdened with innumerable drug interactions. No drug should be co-administered with amiodarone without first checking on the interaction potential and required dosing adjustment. Despite this formidable description, data from several randomized trials indicate that amiodarone is the most effective antiarrhythmic currently available for rhythm control in treatment of AF *(73–77)*.

The CTAF trial studied 403 patients with persistent and paroxysmal AF with least one episode in the preceding 6 months to open-label amiodarone or another AAD. The other AAD was either propafenone or sotalol (in randomized modest doses), given sequentially in an order that was determined in a second randomization. After initial cardioversion, 65% of amiodarone-treated patients were free from recurrent AF (defined as symptomatic AF lasting at least 10 min) compared with 37% of the propafenone or sotalol treated patients. Among those with AF relapse, amiodarone was associated with a longer time to first recurrence than propafenone and sotalol (>498 compared with 98 days). There was a trend toward increased discontinuation of study medication due to side effects in the amiodarone arm (18% vs. 11%) *(73)*. Some, but not all, additional comparisons of amiodarone to propafenone *(76)* and sotalol *(77)* in patients with paroxysmal AF are consistent with the above findings.

Amiodarone has also been studied in patients with persistent AF. In the SAFE-T trial, 665 patients were randomized to amiodarone, sotalol, or placebo in a blinded fashion. At 1 year, SR was maintained in 52% of amiodarone, 32% of sotalol, and 13% of placebo-treated patients. The median time of recurrence of AF was 487, 74, and 6 days, respectively. In subgroup analysis, patients with ischemic disease, median time to recurrence was not significantly different between amiodarone and sotalol. Restoration and maintenance of SR were associated with improvements in QoL and exercise capacity *(74)*.

The results described above are supported by data obtained from the AFFIRM trial, where amiodarone was associated with a greater frequency of cardioversion-free SR maintenance than either sotalol or Class I agents *(75)*, as well as by results of a systematic metaanalysis of 44 trials, which found that amiodarone was the most effective drug for the treatment of AF (odds ratios of 0.19, 0.31, and 0.43 for the maintenance of SR compared to placebo, Class I drugs, and sotalol, respectively) *(39)*. Amiodarone's efficacy may be lowered somewhat by a side effect profile that may be higher than with other AADs. One trial found that when taking both tolerability and efficacy into account, propafenone was favored over amiodarone in maintaining SR *(76)*.

Intravenous amiodarone is also effective in converting AF to SR, although its particular pharmacokinetics require a substantial dosing period (usually >24 h) and total dose (usually 1–2 gm) before adequate tissue levels accumulate, reducing its immediate-term efficacy. Slowing of ventricular rate, however, may occur with as little as 300–400 mg of IV amiodarone. For the acute conversion of recent-onset AF, one metaanalysis concluded that oral amiodarone was minimally more effective than placebo for conversion at 6–8 but significantly so at 24 h, *(78)* while another found an odds ratio of

4.33 for conversion to SR after 48 h but 1.4 before *(79)*. In AF of more chronic duration, amiodarone was found to be equally as efficacious as sotalol in the SAFE-T trial after 28 days of treatment (27% vs. 24% respectively) *(74)* and equal to propafenone in another study (47% vs. 41% respectively) *(80)*. Although efficacy was equal in this latter study, all conversions on amiodarone occurred after 7 days of therapy.

Amiodarone is also effective at increasing the efficacy of electrical cardioversion of patients with chronic AF who do not achieve spontaneous cardioversion on drug. Amiodarone pretreatment renders electrical cardioversion in chronic AF more effective than placebo or diltiazem pretreatment (68–88% efficacy) *(81, 82)*. It also decreases the frequency (37% amiodarone vs. 80% placebo) and duration (8.8 months amiodarone vs. 2.7 months placebo) of relapses after cardioversion *(81)*.

SOTALOL

Sotalol is a medication with both Class II (β (beta)-blocking) and Class III (K^+-channel blocking) effects. It is administered as a racemic mixture of L- and D-sotalol, and has efficacy for both ventricular and atrial arrhythmias. Although both isomers contribute to sotalol's Class III properties by blocking the rapid component of the delayed rectifier current (Ik_r) and thereby prolonging repolarization, the L-isomer is responsible for virtually all of sotalol's β (beta)-blocking properties. As opposed to amiodarone, sotalol may decrease defibrillation thresholds in patients with implantable defibrillators *(83)*.

Oral sotalol has generally been found to be ineffective for the conversion of AF to SR *(84–86)* and is not recommended for this purpose *(11)*. It has, however, been found to be effective for the maintenance of SR *(87, 88)*. In a double-blind placebo-controlled multicenter trial comparing 80, 120, and 160 mg twice-daily sotalol regimens with placebo in 253 patients with AF who were in SR at the time of enrollment, time to recurrence of AF was significantly longer in the groups taking the higher two dosages of sotalol (229 and 175 days) than placebo (27 days) *(87)*. Similar results were found in another trial that included patients with paroxysmal supraventricular tachycardias in addition to AF *(88)*. No deaths or episodes of TdP were reported in either trial, which followed strict exclusion and dosing protocols.

Direct comparisons of sotalol with amiodarone have generally found sotalol to be the inferior agent for the maintenance of SR *(73–75)*. As mentioned above, both the CTAF and SAFE-T trials found greater efficacy for amiodarone than sotalol in freedom from recurrence of AF *(73, 74)*. Analysis of the AFFIRM data as well as systematic metaanalysis reached the same conclusion *(39, 75)*. A possible exception may be in patients with ischemic disease. In the SAFE-T trial, the median time to AF recurrence among ischemic patients was equal between the amiodarone and sotalol groups *(74)*.

Although less efficacious than amiodarone, sotalol has generally been found to have an efficacy equal to Class Ic agents. A 100 patient randomized trial of propafenone and sotalol in patients who failed previous treatment with Ia agents found no difference between the drugs, with ~40% of patients in each group maintaining SR *(89)*. This is consistent with data from the CTAF trial, where an equal percentage of patients (37%) in the propafenone and sotalol arms were free of AF at 1 year *(73)*. One of sotalol's biggest advantages over Class Ic agents is that its β (beta)-blocking properties make it more effective in controlling the ventricular rate during periods of AF breakthrough. In fact, β (beta)-blockers are often administered with Ic agents to mitigate the risk of rapid conduction after conversion of AF to atrial flutter. The β (beta)-blocking effects of sotalol begin at doses as low as 80 mg/d and plateau at doses between 240 and 320 mg/d while, in the presence of normal renal function, its Class III effects only begin at doses of 160 mg/d and increase linearly with dose thereafter. Because of the risk of TdP, sotalol should not be used only as a rate control agent.

The most important concerns regarding sotalol, which is not organ toxic, are bradycardia, which is dose dependent, and proarrhythmic TdP. The risk of TdP is 2–4% for all indications, although it is highest in those treated for sustained VT and VF and lower in those treated for AF *(90)*. TdP pointes is more common at higher doses of sotalol (>320 mg/day), in the presence of decreased renal function (the drug is renally excreted), and female gender *(71, 91)*. Sotalol may be given to patients with heart failure, but caution should be used in patients with congestive symptoms. In the heart failure population, sotalol is associated with an increased risk of TdP *(91)* but a decrease in the incidence of shocks in those with an implantable defibrillator *(92)*. Due to concerns about increased risk of TdP in hypertrophic hearts, the current guidelines do not recommend the use of sotalol in patients with more than minimal hypertrophy *(11)*.

Dofetilide

Dofetilide is a highly specific blocker of the rapid component of the delayed rectifier potassium current (Ik_r). Its effects on the action potential are similar to that of other Class III agents; namely, prolongation of phases 2 and 3 and therefore the surface QT interval. Its main drawback is the potential for proarrhythmic TdP (see below), which is influenced by dose, QT interval, and renal function. Dofetilide also has numerous drug interactions, including some with verapamil and diltiazem that must be noted. For these reasons, it is only available for prescription by individuals who have completed specialized training administered by the manufacturer. In its clinical AF trials, TdP was often not self-terminating.

Dofetilide can be used for the conversion of AF to SR. Intravenous dofetilide, which is not available in the United States, converted 31% of patients with either AF or atrial flutter into SR compared to 0% with placebo, although efficacy was significantly greater in patients with atrial flutter (54%) than those with AF (15%) *(93)*. Other trials using oral dofetilide have found comparable conversion rates from AF as well as atrial flutter *(19, 94, 95)*, but the availability of ibutilide, an available and established intravenous Ik_r blocker, coupled with the need for in-hospital initiation of dofetilide makes its use for this purpose unusual.

Oral dofetilide has been studied in several randomized trials and shown to be efficacious in the maintenance of SR. The SAFIRE-D trial evaluated three doses of dofetilide in patients with AF and atrial flutter. Among 250 patients who converted to SR, all doses of dofetilide achieved higher rates of SR maintenance at 1 year (up to 58% for 500 mcg BID dofetilide) than placebo. Adverse events included TdP in 0.8% (two patients) and one sudden cardiac death, thought to be arrhythmic *(95)*. The SAFIRE data are consistent with the findings of the EMERALD trial, in which 671 patients with AF were randomized to dofetilide (in one of three dosages), sotalol, or placebo. Dofetilide was more effective than either sotalol or placebo. The findings of the EMERALD trial may be limited, however, in that the dosage of sotalol used (80 mg) was comparatively low for the treatment of AF, and that the trial was only presented in abstract form.

The DIAMOND trial was a study of the effect of dofetilide compared to placebo on mortality in patients with heart failure with or without ischemic heart disease. Overall survival was not different between the two groups. Among those patients with AF or atrial flutter, cardioversion occurred in 59% compared with 34% with placebo and was maintained at 1 year in 79 and 42% of patients, respectively. Restoration of SR was associated with decreased mortality, and dofetilide treatment overall was associated with a decreased rate of hospitalizations. Torsades occurred in four patients (1.6%) with no fatalities *(19)*.

Overall, dofetilide is an effective drug for the conversion of AF or maintenance of SR. Although dofetilide probably has a neutral effect on mortality in patients with heart failure *(96)*, it does have a measurable, if low, risk of TdP, which may not be self-terminating. It must therefore be initiated in a monitored setting, with careful dose adjustments for changes in creatinine clearance (it is renally excreted) and QTc. Since direct comparisons to other AADs with more established efficacy and safety profiles are lacking, it is not considered first line in the current guidelines *(11)*.

IBUTILIDE

Ibutilide, like dofetilide, is a blocker of Ik_r, although it also delays inactivation of the slow inward sodium currents that occur during early repolarization to some degree (likely more so in ventricular than in atrial tissue). In addition to prolonging the QT interval, ibutilide may cause some mild slowing of the sinus rate *(97, 98)*. Ibutilide is only available as intravenous infusion and is therefore only used for acute arrhythmia termination.

Two separate trials of ibutilide in patients with AF or atrial flutter of relatively recent onset using two 10-min 1 mg infusions separated by 10 min showed acute conversion rates of 35–47% *(99, 100)*. Conversion was more common in patients with atrial flutter (63%) than in those with AF (31%), in those with a shorter duration of arrhythmia, and in those with a normal left atrial size *(99)*. Conversion rates of acute AF and atrial flutter after cardiac surgery have been even higher. Concomitant administration of 4 g of intravenous magnesium with ibutilide enhanced the efficacy of conversion and attenuate increases in QT interval in one trial *(101)*. Alternatively, $MgSO_4$ may be administered upon conversion to SR or upon the development of ventricular ectopy to reduce the subsequent risk of TdP.

The rate of TdP with ibutilide has been 1.7% (sustained) to 8.3% (overall) in large trials *(99, 100, 102)* and is more common in woman *(103)*. Like sotalol, ibutilide exhibits reverse use dependence. Prolongation of the QT is therefore exaggerated at slower heart rates, which may explain an increased propensity toward Torsades during bradycardia.

Class IV

Non-dihydropyridine calcium channel antagonists block L-type calcium current in cardiomyocytes and AV nodal tissue. Like β (beta)-blockers, they are generally used for the control of ventricular rate in AF. Several studies have investigated potential inherent antiarrhythmic effects of calcium channel blockade. Some studies have suggested that treatment with verapamil can abrogate atrial electrical remodeling seen in acute AF *(104–106)*, suggesting it may have particular benefits when used for rate control in these patients. Some studies, however, have suggested possible proarrhythmic effects of acute calcium blocker administration *(107)*. Although some data have suggested a modest effect in preventing atrial arrhythmias after thoracic surgery compared to placebo *(108)*, data for its use in maintaining SR after cardioversion have been disappointing *(109)*.

Overall, the data supporting a role for calcium channel blockers in AF outside of rate control are weak, and they are not recommended for this purpose *(11)*.

Newer Agents

Several new agents are under development for the treatment of AF. Some have novel mechanisms of action, and others have safety profiles that are improved over existing agents of the same class. A full review of newer agents is beyond the scope of this chapter. Several agents that are in particularly advanced stages of development or well studied are described below.

DRONEDARONE

Dronedarone is a non-iodinated benzfuran derivative of amiodarone that shows promise in exhibiting many of amiodarone's beneficial antiarrhythmic effects without thyroid or pulmonary toxicities seen in trials to date. At the time of writing, it was awaiting FDA approval for use. Approval came in July 2009.

In similarly designed phase III trials (ADONIS and EURIDIS) of dronedarone in patients with paroxysmal or persistent AF that had been cardioverted, dronedarone was associated with a significant increase in time to recurrence compared with placebo (158 vs. 59 days in ADONIS and 96 vs. 41 days in EURIDIS) and a decrease in the ventricular rate during recurrent episodes *(110)*. Enthusiasm for dronedarone waned after the results of the ANDROMEDA trial, which evaluated the effect of dronedarone on mortality on patients with Class IV heart failure in which a trend toward increased mortality with dronedarone therapy was noted *(111)*. However, in a retrospective analysis, mortality was increased only in those patients in whom angiotensin converting enzyme (ACE) inhibitors and angiotensin receptor blockers (ARBs) had been discontinued.

Insufficiently appreciated at the time, dronedarone decreases renal tubular secretion of creatinine, increasing serum creatinine levels without actually effecting filtration rate, creating the false impression of renal dysfunction. Inappropriate withdrawal of the ACE inhibitors and ARBs, stalwarts of heart failure therapy, rather than a direct effect of dronedarone, may have been an important contributor to the ANDROMEDA results. Subsequent to ANDROMEDA, the results of the ATHENA trial, which evaluated the safety of dronedarone on mortality and rhythm control in 2628 high-risk patients with AF were reported. Without any excessive discontinuation of ACE inhibitors in this trial, which studied patients with similar characteristics to those in AFFIRM, there was a 24% decrease in the combination of all-cause mortality and cardiovascular hospitalization (the trial's primary endpoint) *(9)*. Reductions in arrhythmic death, acute coronary syndrome, and other clinically important endpoints, including AF, also occurred. In the U.S. dronedarone was approved to decrease cardiovascular hospitalization in non permanent AF patients with characteristics similar to ATHENA trial enrollees, who do not have Class IV heart failure or recent decompensation.

VERNAKALANT

Vernakalant is an atrial-specific AAD that blocks the ultra-rapid K^+ current (Ik_{ur}), the transient outward current (I_{to}), and has a mild effect on Na^+ channels. Trials of intravenous vernakalant in medical patients have found it to have an efficacy for the acute conversion of relatively recent-onset AF of 38% compared with 3% of placebo-treated patients. Vernakalant was not efficacious in converting atrial flutter, and there were no reported instances of TdP *(112)*. Intravenous vernakalant was submitted to the FDA for an indication of AF conversion. An additional trial to increase the size of the overall population studied has been requested prior to approval. Oral vernakalant is in an earlier stage of development.

AZIMILIDE

Azimilide is a Class III medication that, similar to amiodarone, has a long half-life and blocks Ik_r, Ik_s, sodium, and calcium currents without use dependence. Trials evaluating azimilide in AF have been mixed. Initial trials showed increased arrhythmia-free survival in patients with a history of AF or atrial flutter *(113)* with a neutral effect in overall mortality and a low incidence of TdP in a large population with ischemic heart disease *(114)*. More recently, however, larger multicenter trials have failed to show significant efficacy in AF rhythm control in the dose used and some increased risk of both TdP and neutropenia *(55, 113, 115)*. Based on this data, the manufacturer of azimilide is no longer seeking FDA approval for use in AF.

Non-antiarrhythmic Drugs

Many drugs that do not directly affect the action potential and are not conventionally classified as antiarrhythmics have been studied for their ability to treat AF. These agents include statins, fish oil, and ACE-I/ARBs. A full review of these medications is beyond the scope of this chapter, but the interested reader is referred to recent reviews *(116, 117)*.

SPECIFIC DRUGS FOR THE CONTROL OF VENTRICULAR RATE IN AF

The main determinant of the ventricular response to AF in patients without an accessory AV nodal connection is the functional refractory period of the AV node, which is in turn determined by intrinsic factors and the balance of sympathetic and parasympathetic tone. Drugs used to slow the ventricular response in AF act either by increasing directly altering AV nodal refractory properties or by changing autonomic characteristics. Multiple drugs are available for this function, including β (beta)-blockers, non-dihydropyridine calcium channel antagonists, digoxin, and, much less commonly, clonidine. Other medications usually reserved for control of the atrial rhythm, including amiodarone, sotalol, and to a lesser extent, propafenone, also have rate-slowing effects in AF but are seldom used for this purpose alone, although dronedarone may find a role for this purpose in part of its clinical profile, and it has been approved for such in Europe.

Drugs for rate control can be combined, especially in patients with normal ventricular function. Negative inotropy is a concern in patients with systolic failure, while combination therapy may increase the risk of bradycardia, especially in those patients with paroxysmal AF. Permanent pacing may be indicated for paroxysmal patients in whom the ventricular rate in AF cannot be controlled without periods of symptomatic bradycardia in SR or for permanent AF patients who have large rate swings in the arrhythmia with rapid rates requiring AV nodal suppression but slow rates necessitating pacer implantation.

Class I

Class I agents are not used for the control of ventricular rate in AF. Propafenone has weak β (beta)-blocking properties (~1/40th the potency of propranolol on a milligram for milligram basis) that is too small to provide any clinically meaningful ventricular rate control. Other Cass I agents, such as procainamide and disopyrimide, have vagolytic effects and have the potential to increase AV nodal conduction.

Class II

By inhibiting adrenergic input into the AV node, β (beta)-blockers act to increase AV nodal refractoriness, thereby prolonging the functional refractory period of the AV node. They are especially effective under circumstances of increased sympathetic tone, such as post-operatively. Although used mainly for this purpose, they may also have antiarrhythmic effects in certain circumstances, as noted above.

For the acute control of rapid AF, intravenous formulations of β (beta)-blockers such as metoprolol, atenolol, and propranolol can effectively control ventricular rate. Esmolol, a short-acting selective β (beta)1-antagonist, can be particularly useful as a continuous infusion in difficult-to-control cases.

For long-term management, oral β (beta)-blockers such as metoprolol, atenolol, nadolol, bisoprolol, carvedilol, or propranolol (among others) may be given. A systematic review of the use of β (beta)-blockers for rate control found that compared to placebo, β (beta)-blockers are effective for the control of ventricular rate in AF both at rest and during exercise, usually without deleterious effects on exercise tolerance. Among those β (beta)-blockers studied, nadolol and atenolol were the most efficacious *(118)*. In the AFFIRM trial, β (beta)-blockers were the most effective class of drugs for rate control, achieving target heart rates in 70% of patients vs. 54% for calcium channel blockers *(119)*.

Newer agents such as carvedilol, a non-selective agent with β (beta)- and α (alpha)-adrenergic blocking activity, are also effective in controlling ventricular rate in AF. In the heart failure population, in whom β (beta)-blocker administration is indicated for its beneficial effects on overall survival *(120)*, carvedilol has been shown to decrease the ventricular rate both at rest and during exercise *(121)*. The efficacy of β (beta)-blockade in this population is of substantial clinical utility, as the administration of diltiazem has been associated with increased mortality events in patients with baseline reductions in ejection fraction *(122)*. In patients with the brady–tachy syndrome, pindolol is the beta-blocker of choice as its intrinsic sympathomimetic actions prevent worsening of sinus bradyarrhythmias in about 85% of such patients while its beta-blocking effects are useful in control of the ventricular rate in AF *(123)*.

Class III

Both amiodarone and sotalol can slow the ventricular rate in AF, although their toxicities and availability of alternative rate control agents limit their use for this purpose alone. Sotalol has effective β (beta)-blocking properties at higher doses and has an advantage over other antiarrhythmics in that breakthrough AF occurs at a slower rate. In one study, sotalol was more effective in controlling ventricular rate during exercise than metoprolol *(83)*.

Amiodarone also has rate-slowing effects for in patients that do not achieve conversion. It may have a limited role in rate control in critically ill patients with rapid AF in whom intravenous administration of conventional agents may precipitate or exacerbate hypotension, and in whom electrical cardioversion in contraindicated or not desirable. In one study, intravenous amiodarone decreased the mean heart rate in critically ill patients with rapid AF by 37 beats per minute and increased mean blood pressure, while intravenous esmolol, diltiazem, and digoxin had no effect on the heart rate and reduced mean blood pressure overall *(124)*. Dronedarone, in addition to its effects on preventing AF, is useful for slowing the ventricular rate, as was shown in the ERATO trial *(125)*. Rates at rest on Holter monitoring and rates during exercise testing were both improved with this agent (averaging about 10–15 bpm).

Class IV

Calcium channel blockers slow the ventricular response in AF by decreasing L-type calcium current in the AV node, which reduces the height of the action potential, prolongs its duration, and increases the AV nodal functional refractory period.

Both of the most common non-dihydropyridine calcium channel blockers currently in use, diltiazem and verapamil, are effective medications for rate control in AF. They are subject to the same cautions noted above as β (beta)-blockers with regards to bradycardia and decreased inotropy in specific populations *(122)*. Chronic treatment of patients with systolic function may be a particular issue, as noted above, although calcium channel blockers may be particularly helpful in patients with bronchospastic disease which β (beta)-blockers may aggravate.

Diltiazem and verapamil appear to be equally effective in decreasing ventricular response in AF both at rest and with exercise, and may provide more benefits in QoL and exercise tolerance than β (beta)-blockers *(126, 127)*. A systematic review of calcium channel blockers for control of ventricular rate in AF found similar results *(118)*. Intravenous formulations may be useful for the acute control of ventricular rate, although infusions are generally required, and hypotension may be a limiting side effect *(128)*.

Digoxin

Digoxin is a cardiac glycoside derived from the foxglove plant. Its main effects are to increase parasympathetic tone, decreasing the functional refractory period of the AV node. It also increases inotropy by inhibiting the Na^+/K^+ ATPase pump, which indirectly increases myocyte Ca^{2+} availability. It is renally cleared, and doses must therefore be adjusted in renal failure.

Digoxin has no role in the conversion of AF, having been shown in randomized trials to be ineffective for this purpose *(129, 130)*. Digoxin is, however, extensively used for the control of the ventricular rate in AF. However, because of its mechanism of action, it is most efficacious under conditions in which modulation of parasympathetic tone is most relevant. For example, in a systematic review, the majority of trials of rate controlling agents in AF that involved digoxin found that while it was effective in slowing resting heart rate, it did not control the ventricular response under exercise conditions *(118)*. Although some data have suggested that digoxin can be as effective as other agents at rate control in AF *(119)*, most active patients will not achieve adequate control with digoxin monotherapy and must be managed with at least one additional agent. It is therefore most appropriate to use for rate control in sedentary patients and in those with systolic heart failure. Digitalis may increase vagal-induced AF.

DRUG SELECTION IN SPECIFIC POPULATIONS

In all cases, a thorough history and physical exam including basic laboratory tests and evaluation of cardiac function should be performed in every AF patient in order to identify possible reversible causes and precipitants of AF, such as valvular disease, metabolic abnormalities, and thyroid function. The effects of lesser recognized factors, such as caffeine, stress, alcohol, and obesity on the initiation of AF should not be underestimated. One recent study demonstrated acute stress, high coffee consumption, and body mass index over 30 as independent risk factors for the development of AF, and acute ingestion of excessive amounts of alcohol is known to precipitate AF in otherwise healthy individuals. These issues should be addressed in all patients with AF.

When the decision to initiate antiarrhythmic therapy has been made, drug selection in a particular patient is based on the balance of efficacy and safety of the various available agents in particular patient populations. The relevant patient characteristics include left ventricular systolic function, ventricular mass, presence of coronary disease, previous infarction, and renal function (Table 3). Current recommendations are outlined in the 2006 ACC/AHA/ESC AF practice guidelines and summarized in Table 4 *(11)*.

Table 3
Important Clinical Characteristics in Choosing AADs for AF

Important clinical characteristics in choosing AADs
LV function Congestive symptoms preclude sotalol use Arrhythmic risk precludes Class Ic use Amiodarone considered first line Dofetilide may be considered as second line
LV mass Significant LVH precludes Class Ic, sotalol, or dofetilide use Amiodarone considered first line
Coronary artery disease Class Ic agents contraindicated in those with previous infarction Class Ic generally withheld in those with CAD but without infarction Sotalol considered first line Amiodarone considered second line due to toxicities
Impaired renal function Toxic metabolites may accumulate with procainamide use Proarrhythmic risk precludes sotalol use Dofetilide contraindicated with severe renal dysfunction Caution advised with Class Ic use
Prolonged baseline QT interval Increased proarrhythmic risk with procainamide, sotalol, dofetilide, ibutilide

Table 4
Trials of Anticoagulation for the Prevention of Stroke in Nonvalvular AF

sTrial	Summary	References
	Stroke prevention trials in AF	
EAFT	Wafarin vs placebo (secondary prevention)	*(139)*
BAATAF	Low-intensity warfarin vs. placebo (or ASA)	*(148)*
SPAF I	Warfarin vs. ASA vs. placebo	*(149)*
AFASAK	Warfarin vs. ASA	*(150)*
CAFA	Warfarin vs. placebo	*(151)*
VA Study	Low-intensity wafarin vs. placebo	*(152)*

Minimal Disease

For patients with structurally normal ventricles and normal renal function, first-line drugs include propafenone and flecainide as well as sotalol. These agents are both safe and efficacious in this population and can spare patients the toxicities of long-term amiodarone use. All three are essentially devoid of organ toxicity. The Class Ic AADs are also essentially devoid of ventricular proarrhythmic risk in this population and the TdP risk of sotalol in this circumstance should be less than 1–2% if administered properly. Dronedarone is also reasonable in this patient group.

Although the use of Ia agents for AF rhythm control is discouraged, and they no longer appear in the latest practice guidelines, the vagolytic properties of disopyrimide may be of benefit for those cases in which vagal tone is known to be a substantial AF precipitant.

Coronary Disease

For patients with coronary disease who require drug therapy beyond β (beta)-blockade, amiodarone *(131, 132)*, sotalol *(133)*, and azimilide *(114)* have neutral effects on mortality in the general post-infarct population. As noted earlier, however, azimilide is not available clinically. Sotalol is considered first-line therapy given its β (beta)-blocking capacity, although dofetilide plus a rate control agent may also be used. Amiodarone, although effective, is reserved for second-line therapy given its toxicities.

For patients with coronary disease and previous infarction, Class Ic agents are contraindicated given an increased mortality when used in this population *(56)*. These agents are also generally withheld in patients with coronary disease who have not yet had infarction given concern over the potential for proarrhythmia in even reversible ischemia. Their use in patients without coronary disease but with substantial risk factors is up to the discretion of the physician but requires vigilance in screening for the development of coronary lesions. In CAD patients without severe heart failure dronedarone is another alternative.

Heart Failure

Patients with left ventricular systolic dysfunction and congestive failure are generally treated with ACE inhibitors/ARB and β (beta)-blocker for their beneficial effects on overall survival. These medications, by improving overall hemodynamics and possibly independently, may lower the AF burden in this population. In two large trials of carvedilol in patients with congestive failure *(134, 135)* patients treated with carvedilol had lower rates of AF and atrial flutter than those treated with placebo.

For patients who require additional drug therapy, the risk of proarrhythmia precludes the use of Ic agents and congestive symptoms would preclude sotalol. Amiodarone is the preferred agent in this population, given its established safety and efficacy *(136)*. Dofetilide may also be considered as it has been shown to have efficacy in the heart failure population with a neutral effect on overall mortality. If heart failure is severe, dronedarone is contraindicated.

LVH

Substantial left ventricular hypertrophy is a risk factor for thromboembolism in AF *(33)*, is a risk factor for coronary disease and demand ischemia, and is thought to increase the risk of TdP *(137, 138)*. What constitutes "substantial" is not well established, but in practice a cutoff wall thickness of 14 mm is commonly used. Because of these concerns, current guidelines advise against the routine use of Class Ic agents, sotalol, or dofetilide in the presence of substantial LVH. Class Ia agents should also be avoided when LVH is present for the same reason. Amiodarone, which carries a lower risk of TdP, is the first and only medication recommended by the guidelines when substantial LVH is present. Those patients with conditions that have a predisposition toward LVH, such as hypertension, but who have minimal or no hypertrophy on imaging, are treated in the algorithm as if they have no cardiac disease. Ongoing management of their underlying condition, however, is essential.

ANTICOAGULATION

Stroke is one of the most feared complications of AF, occurring in 5% of AF patients per year overall, and 14% of those who have already had a stroke *(139)*. Clinical characteristics that increase the risk of stroke include female sex, diabetes, hypertension, clinical heart failure, prior stroke, and possibly coronary disease *(140–142)*. In one study, the relative risk of stroke was 1.4 for patients with congestive failure, 1.6 for hypertension, 1.7 for diabetes, and 2.5 for prior stroke. Age is also an important risk factor, with a continuous relative risk of 1.4 per decade of life *(143)*. In patients over 75, AF accounts for half of all strokes, and AF is the most common cause of disabling strokes among elderly women *(144, 145)*. Patients under age 60 with none of the above risk factors (so-called lone AF) have an extremely low incidence of stroke over the long term (1.3% in 15 years) *(146)*.

Although there is some evidence that time spent in AF is related to clot formation *(147)*, it appears that overall, patients with paroxysmal AF have about the same overall stroke risk as those with persistent AF *(148, 149)*. Similarly, as noted above, patients treated with a strategy of rhythm control have a continued risk of stroke that is at least equal to those treated with rate control. Current practice, therefore, is to continue preventative stroke therapy in indicated AF patients, even if they have periods of SR whether with or without antiarrhythmic therapy or ablation.

The mainstay of stroke prevention in AF for those at highest risk is oral anticoagulation with warfarin. Several risk stratification tools have been created identify high-risk patients based on clinical characteristics. The most commonly used and best validated is the $CHADS_2$ score (Table 5), which was studied in a population of 1733 patients aged 65–95 with nonrheumatic AF. For each one-point increase in the $CHADS_2$ score, the risk of stroke without treatment increases by 1.5-fold *(33)*.

Six large clinical trials done published between 1989 and 1999 have largely provided the body of knowledge that has determined the current approach taken to reduce strokes in patients with AF (Table 6) *(141, 150–154)*. Together, these trials showed a 62% decrease in stroke for adjusted-dose warfarin monotherapy; significantly better than aspirin (ASA) or placebo. The benefit of warfarin is present in all age groups, risk profiles, and in those both with and without prior stroke *(141, 143, 155)*. The generally recommended INR range is 2–3. Stroke rates rise steeply at values below 2, while higher levels of anticoagulation increase rates of major bleeding without equal benefit in stroke prevention *(156, 157)*. The rate of increase in bleeding with INRs above 3.0 is more gradual than the steep increase in risk for embolism at INRs below 2.0.

Table 5
The CHADS$_2$ Risk Score and Associated Stroke Risk (33)

CHADS$_2$ score	
Clinical risk	Score
Congestive heart failure	1
Hypertension	1
Age $\geq$ 75	1
Diabetes mellitus	1
Stroke or TIA history	2

CHADS$_2$ score		
Score	Stroke rate per 100 patient-years	95% CI
0	1.9	1.2–3.0
1	2.8	2.0–3.8
2	4.0	3.1–5.1
3	5.9	4.6–7.3
4	8.5	6.3–11.1
5	12.5	8.2–17.5
6	18.2	10.5–27.4

Table 6
The Selection of AADs in Specific Populations

Approach to AAD selection for AF rhythm control		
Characteristic	First line	Second line
No or minimal disease	Flecainide Propafenone Sotalol	Amiodarone Dofetilide
Hypertension with LVH	Amiodarone	–
Coronary disease	Sotalol Dofetilide	Amiodarone
Heart failure	Amiodarone Dofetilide	–

The effect of ASA on stroke risk is more modest than that of warfarin and has not been seen in every trial. In one metaanalysis, ASA therapy was associated with a 20% reduction in stroke events overall, although it seems to be less effective in those at highest risk (139). Part of the utility of ASA may be in its superior prevention of non-cardioembolic stroke in patients with atherosclerotic risk factors (158). ASA appears to be most useful in patients judged to be at lower risk of stroke. One pooled analysis found that in patients aged 65–75 without other stroke risk factors, the baseline stroke rate (4.3%/year) was decreased to nearly the same degree by ASA therapy (1.4%/year) as with warfarin (1.1%/year) and concluded that ASA treatment seemed adequate in low-risk populations (155). There are no data regarding the effects of different ASA dosing regimens, although only 325 mg daily showed efficacy in the ASA–warfarin trials. Adding low-dose warfarin therapy to ASA is inferior to adjusted-dose warfarin monotherapy in stroke prevention, as shown in the SPAF III trail, and is not recommended (159). ASA therapy in combination with clopidogrel is inferior to warfarin (160) but superior to ASA therapy alone, although with a small increase in bleeding endpoints (161).

The greatest hazard of anticoagulant or antiplatelet therapy is the risk of bleeding, particularly intracranial hemorrhage. Hemorrhage risk is higher with warfarin therapy than with ASA *(162)* and is highest in those given combined therapy *(163)*. Particular care must be taken in elderly patients, in whom stroke prevention therapy is effective, although is associated with a higher risk of bleeding than in younger patients *(150, 164)*. Current guidelines have suggested that a lower INR range might be a reasonable compromise between toxicity and efficacy for patients above age 75 at high risk for bleeding *(11)*.

In practice, warfarin therapy with an INR of 2–3 is given to patients with a CHADS$_2$ score of 2 or greater who have paroxysmal or persistent AF and do not have contraindications to anticoagulation therapy. Patients with CHADS$_2$ scores of 0 that are below age 60 are at extremely low risk of stroke and can probably be followed without ASA or warfarin. Patients with a CHADS$_2$ score of 0 that are above age 60 or those with a CHADS$_2$ score of 1 are often treated with warfarin or ASA, the choice being dependent on factors such as the assessment of bleeding risk, the availability of timely monitoring, and patient preference.

In the near future, easier to use and possibly more effective alternatives to warfarin are likely to appear. Many direct thrombin inhibots and factor Xa inhibitors are under study, with one, dabigatran, currently under consideration by the FDA.

ATRIAL FLUTTER

Atrial flutter can be defined generally by surface EKG as a non-sinus atrial arrhythmia with an atrial rate between 200 and 400 bpm *(165)*. Defined mechanistically, "atrial flutter" as will be discussed here refers to a reentrant circuit rotating around the tricuspid valve. Also known as "typical" flutter, this rhythm most commonly travels in a counterclockwise manner and produces characteristic negative sawtooth flutter waves in the inferior leads on EKG.

Both atrial flutter and AF may occur in the same patient. Most often, periods of AF initiate flutter by forming functional components of the flutter circuit *(166)*, although atrial flutter may exist in the absence of AF. A large population cohort study showed that among patients hospitalized with an episode of atrial flutter, nearly 50% were hospitalized with AF in the ensuing 5 years *(167)*.

Atrial flutter can cause a similar spectrum of symptoms as AF, including thromboembolism. In some patients, because of the rapid organized manner of impulses reaching the AV node, the ventricular response to atrial flutter is more rapid and more difficult to control in AF than during AF. Conduction that occurs in a 1:1 manner may be poorly tolerated and result in syncope. The goals of treatment in atrial flutter are therefore similar to those in AF. That is, the alleviation of symptoms, prevention of thromboembolism, and the minimization of treatment toxicities.

One of the main differences in treatment of AF and atrial flutter is that since atrial flutter is caused by a defined circuit that can be easily accessed through the venous system, catheter ablation can be accomplished in with little morbidity and with an approximately 90% cure rate *(168)*. As a result, ablation is considered much earlier in the course of treatment than in AF. When ablation is not pursued or desired, AAD treatment may be used for the pharmacologic conversion, as an adjunct to electrical cardioversion, and for the long-term maintenance of SR. Although Class Ia agents *(45, 54)* have been shown to be effective for cardioverting atrial flutter, the best evidence is for Class III drugs, particularly dofetilide and ibutilide. Intravenous administration of ibutilide has a 63% efficacy rate for the conversion of atrial flutter to SR compared to 31% for AF *(99)*, while oral treatment with dofetilide is significantly more likely to maintain SR when given for atrial flutter than for AF *(95)*. Studies of AADs in atrial flutter have generally included AF patients, so efficacy in this population alone has not been well established for most drugs. As with AF, clinical characteristics must be taken into account to choose an AAD that maximizes safety.

Anticoagulation for the prevention of systemic embolization is an important component of atrial flutter therapy, as it is with AF. The risk of stroke may be slightly lower for patients solely with atrial flutter than with AF, but it remains elevated compared to normal controls, and the frequent coexistence of the two rhythms makes this distinction unnecessary in many patients *(167, 169)*. Patients with atrial flutter are therefore treated with the same anticoagulation strategy as those with AF described above. That is, adjusted-dose warfarin therapy for those patients with clinical risk factors for stroke.

REFERENCES

1. Miyasaka Y, Barnes ME, Gersh BJ et al (2006) Secular trends in incidence of atrial fibrillation in Olmsted County, Minnesota, 1980 to 2000, and implications on the projections for future prevalence. Circulation 114(2):119–125
2. Luderitz B, Jung W (2000) Quality of life in patients with atrial fibrillation. Arch Intern Med 160(12):1749–1757
3. Benjamin EJ, Wolf PA, D'Agostino RB et al (1998) Impact of atrial fibrillation on the risk of death: the Framingham heart study. Circulation 98(10):946–592
4. Carlsson J, Miketic S, Windeler J et al (2003) Randomized trial of rate-control versus rhythm-control in persistent atrial fibrillation: the strategies of treatment of atrial fibrillation (STAF) study. J Am Coll Cardiol 41(10):1690–1696
5. Opolski G, Torbicki A, Kosior DA et al (2004) Rate control vs rhythm control in patients with nonvalvular persistent atrial fibrillation: the results of the polish how to treat chronic atrial fibrillation (HOT CAFE) Study. Chest 126(2): 476–486
6. Van Gelder IC, Hagens VE, Bosker HA et al (2002) A comparison of rate control and rhythm control in patients with recurrent persistent atrial fibrillation. N Engl J Med 347(23):1834–1840
7. Wyse DG, Waldo AL, DiMarco JP et al (2002) A comparison of rate control and rhythm control in patients with atrial fibrillation. N Engl J Med 347(23):1825–1833
8. Corley SD, Epstein AE, DiMarco JP et al (2004) Relationships between sinus rhythm, treatment, and survival in the atrial fibrillation follow-up investigation of rhythm management (AFFIRM) study. Circulation 109(12):1509–1513
9. Hohnloser SH, Crijns HJ, van Eickels M et al (2009) Effect of dronedarone on cardiovascular events in atrial fibrillation. N Engl J Med 360(7):668–678
10. Reiffel J (2009) Current assignment of rate vs rhythm control for atrial fibrillation by US cardiologists: the AFFECTS registry. Heart Rhythm 6(5):S104–S105
11. Fuster V, Ryden LE, Cannom DS et al (2006) ACC/AHA/ESC 2006 Guidelines for the management of patients with atrial fibrillation: a report of the American college of cardiology/American heart association task force on practice guidelines and the European society of cardiology committee for practice guidelines (writing committee to revise the 2001 guidelines for the management of patients with atrial fibrillation): developed in collaboration with the European heart rhythm association and the heart rhythm society. Circulation 114(7):e257–e354
12. Reant P, Lafitte S, Jais P et al (2005) Reverse remodeling of the left cardiac chambers after catheter ablation after 1 year in a series of patients with isolated atrial fibrillation. Circulation 112(19):2896–2903
13. Alboni P, Botto GL, Baldi N et al (2004) Outpatient treatment of recent-onset atrial fibrillation with the "pill-in-the-pocket" approach. N Engl J Med 351(23):2384–2391
14. O'Neill MD, Jais P, Hocini M et al (2007) Catheter ablation for atrial fibrillation. Circulation 116(13):1515–1523
15. Oral H, Pappone C, Chugh A et al (2006) Circumferential pulmonary-vein ablation for chronic atrial fibrillation. N Engl J Med 354(9):934–941
16. Hsu LF, Jais P, Sanders P et al (2004) Catheter ablation for atrial fibrillation in congestive heart failure. N Engl J Med 351(23):2373–2383
17. Roy D, Talajic M, Nattel S et al (2008) Rhythm control versus rate control for atrial fibrillation and heart failure. N Engl J Med 358(25):2667–2677
18. Hohnloser SH, Kuck KH, Lilienthal J (2000) Rhythm or rate control in atrial fibrillation – pharmacological intervention in atrial fibrillation (PIAF): a randomised trial. Lancet 356(9244):1789–1794
19. Pedersen OD, Bagger H, Keller N et al (2001) Efficacy of dofetilide in the treatment of atrial fibrillation-flutter in patients with reduced left ventricular function: a Danish investigations of arrhythmia and mortality on dofetilide (diamond) substudy. Circulation 104(3):292–296
20. Deedwania PC, Singh BN, Ellenbogen K et al (1998) Spontaneous conversion and maintenance of sinus rhythm by amiodarone in patients with heart failure and atrial fibrillation: observations from the veterans affairs congestive heart failure survival trial of antiarrhythmic therapy (CHF-STAT). The department of veterans affairs CHF-STAT investigators. Circulation 98(23):2574–2579
21. Vidaillet H, Greenlee RT (2005) Rate control versus rhythm control. Curr Opin Cardiol 20(1): 15–20
22. Dorian P, Jung W, Newman D et al (2000) The impairment of health-related quality of life in patients with intermittent atrial fibrillation: implications for the assessment of investigational therapy. J Am Coll Cardiol 36(4):1303–1309

23. Gronefeld GC, Lilienthal J, Kuck KH et al (2003) Impact of rate versus rhythm control on quality of life in patients with persistent atrial fibrillation. Results from a prospective randomized study. Eur Heart J 24(15): 1430–1436

24. Hagens VE, Ranchor AV, Van Sonderen E et al (2004) Effect of rate or rhythm control on quality of life in persistent atrial fibrillation. Results from the rate control versus electrical cardioversion (RACE) study. J Am Coll Cardiol 43(2):241–247

25. Jenkins LS, Brodsky M, Schron E et al (2005) Quality of life in atrial fibrillation: the atrial fibrillation follow-up investigation of rhythm management (AFFIRM) study. Am Heart J 149(1):112–120

26. Singh SN, Tang XC, Singh BN et al (2006) Quality of life and exercise performance in patients in sinus rhythm versus persistent atrial fibrillation: a veterans affairs cooperative studies program substudy. J Am Coll Cardiol 48(4): 721–730

27. Chung MK, Shemanski L, Sherman DG et al (2005) Functional status in rate- versus rhythm-control strategies for atrial fibrillation: results of the atrial fibrillation follow-up investigation of rhythm management (AFFIRM) functional status substudy. J Am Coll Cardiol 46(10):1891–1899

28. Lin CS, Pan CH (2008) Regulatory mechanisms of atrial fibrotic remodeling in atrial fibrillation. Cell Mol Life Sci 65(10):1489–1508

29. Dittrich HC, Erickson JS, Schneiderman T et al (1989) Echocardiographic and clinical predictors for outcome of elective cardioversion of atrial fibrillation. Am J Cardiol 63(3):193–197

30. Hagens VE, Crijns HJ, Van Veldhuisen DJ et al (2005) Rate control versus rhythm control for patients with persistent atrial fibrillation with mild to moderate heart failure: results from the RAte control versus electrical cardioversion (RACE) study. Am Heart J 149(6):1106–1111

31. Efremidis M, Sideris A, Xydonas S et al (2008) Ablation of atrial fibrillation in patients with heart failure: reversal of atrial and ventricular remodelling. Hellenic J Cardiol 49(1):19–25

32. Raitt MH, Kusumoto W, Giraud G et al (2004) Reversal of electrical remodeling after cardioversion of persistent atrial fibrillation. J Cardiovasc Electrophysiol 15(5):507–512

33. Gage BF, Waterman AD, Shannon W et al (2001) Validation of clinical classification schemes for predicting stroke: results from the national registry of atrial fibrillation. JAMA 285(22):2864–2870

34. Stroke Prevention in Atrial Fibrillation Investigators (1994) Warfarin versus aspirin for prevention of thromboembolism in atrial fibrillation: stroke prevention in atrial fibrillation II study. Lancet 343(8899):687–691

35. Hart RG, Halperin JL (1999) Atrial fibrillation and thromboembolism: a decade of progress in stroke prevention. Ann Intern Med 131(9):688–695

36. Manning WJ, Silverman DI, Katz SE et al (1994) Impaired left atrial mechanical function after cardioversion: relation to the duration of atrial fibrillation. J Am Coll Cardiol 23(7):1535–1540

37. Page RL, Wilkinson WE, Clair WK et al (1994) Asymptomatic arrhythmias in patients with symptomatic paroxysmal atrial fibrillation and paroxysmal supraventricular tachycardia. Circulation 89(1):224–227

38. Cai H, Li Z, Goette A et al (2002) Downregulation of endocardial nitric oxide synthase expression and nitric oxide production in atrial fibrillation: potential mechanisms for atrial thrombosis and stroke. Circulation 106(22): 2854–2858

39. Lafuente-Lafuente C, Mouly S, Longas-Tejero MA et al (2006) Antiarrhythmic drugs for maintaining sinus rhythm after cardioversion of atrial fibrillation: a systematic review of randomized controlled trials. Arch Intern Med 166(7):719–728

40. Fetsch T, Bauer P, Engberding R et al (2004) Prevention of atrial fibrillation after cardioversion: results of the PAFAC trial. Eur Heart J 25(16):1385–1394

41. Volgman AS, Carberry PA, Stambler B et al (1998) Conversion efficacy and safety of intravenous ibutilide compared with intravenous procainamide in patients with atrial flutter or fibrillation. J Am Coll Cardiol 31(6):1414–1419

42. Kirpizidis C, Stavrati A, Geleris P et al (2001) Safety and effectiveness of oral quinidine in cardioversion of persistent atrial fibrillation. J Cardiol 38(6):351–354

43. Flaker GC, Blackshear JL, McBride R et al (1992) Antiarrhythmic drug therapy and cardiac mortality in atrial fibrillation. The stroke prevention in atrial fibrillation investigators. J Am Coll Cardiol 20(3):527–532

44. Lafuente-Lafuente C, Mouly S, Longas-Tejero MA et al (2007) Antiarrhythmics for maintaining sinus rhythm after cardioversion of atrial fibrillation. Cochrane Database Syst Rev (4):CD005049

45. Stiell IG, Clement CM, Symington C et al (2007) Emergency department use of intravenous procainamide for patients with acute atrial fibrillation or flutter. Acad Emerg Med 14(12):1158–1164

46. Karlson BW, Torstensson I, Abjorn C et al (1988) Disopyramide in the maintenance of sinus rhythm after electroconversion of atrial fibrillation. A placebo-controlled one-year follow-up study. Eur Heart J 9(3):284–290

47. Meinertz T, Lip GY, Lombardi F et al (2002) Efficacy and safety of propafenone sustained release in the prophylaxis of symptomatic paroxysmal atrial fibrillation (The European rythmol/rytmonorm atrial fibrillation trial *(ERAFT)* study). Am J Cardiol 90(12):1300–1306

48. Pritchett EL, Page RL, Carlson M et al (2003) Efficacy and safety of sustained-release propafenone (propafenone SR) for patients with atrial fibrillation. Am J Cardiol 92(8):941–946

49. Stroobandt R, Stiels B, Hoebrechts R (1997) Propafenone for conversion and prophylaxis of atrial fibrillation. Propafenone atrial fibrillation trial investigators. Am J Cardiol 79(4):418–423

50. Anderson JL, Gilbert EM, Alpert BL et al (1989) Prevention of symptomatic recurrences of paroxysmal atrial fibrillation in patients initially tolerating antiarrhythmic therapy. A multicenter, double-blind, crossover study of flecainide and placebo with transtelephonic monitoring. Flecainide supraventricular tachycardia study group. Circulation 80(6): 1557–1570

51. Chimienti M, Cullen MT Jr, Casadei G (1996) Safety of long-term flecainide and propafenone in the management of patients with symptomatic paroxysmal atrial fibrillation: report from the flecainide and propafenone Italian study investigators. Am J Cardiol 77(3):60A–75A

52. Capucci A, Boriani G, Rubino I et al (1994) A controlled study on oral propafenone versus digoxin plus quinidine in converting recent onset atrial fibrillation to sinus rhythm. Int J Cardiol 43(3):305–313

53. Boriani G, Capucci A, Lenzi T et al (1995) Propafenone for conversion of recent-onset atrial fibrillation. A controlled comparison between oral loading dose and intravenous administration. Chest 108(2):355–358

54. Aliot E, Denjoy I (1996) Comparison of the safety and efficacy of flecainide versus propafenone in hospital outpatients with symptomatic paroxysmal atrial fibrillation/flutter. The flecainide AF French study group. Am J Cardiol 77(3):66A–71A

55. Pritchett EL, Kowey P, Connolly S et al (2006) Antiarrhythmic efficacy of azimilide in patients with atrial fibrillation. Maintenance of sinus rhythm after conversion to sinus rhythm. Am Heart J 151(5):1043–1049

56. Ruskin JN (1989) The cardiac arrhythmia suppression trial (CAST). N Engl J Med 321(6):386–388

57. The Cardiac Arrhythmia Suppression Trial II Investigators (1992) Effect of the antiarrhythmic agent moricizine on survival after myocardial infarction. N Engl J Med 327(4):227–233

58. Workman AJ, Kane KA, Russell JA et al (2003) Chronic beta-adrenoceptor blockade and human atrial cell electrophysiology: evidence of pharmacological remodelling. Cardiovasc Res 58(3):518–525

59. Psaty BM, Manolio TA, Kuller LH et al (1997) Incidence of and risk factors for atrial fibrillation in older adults. Circulation 96(7):2455–2461

60. Kuhlkamp V, Schirdewan A, Stangl K et al (2000) Use of metoprolol CR/XL to maintain sinus rhythm after conversion from persistent atrial fibrillation: a randomized, double-blind, placebo-controlled study. J Am Coll Cardiol 36(1): 139–146

61. Steeds RP, Birchall AS, Smith M et al (1999) An open label, randomised, crossover study comparing sotalol and atenolol in the treatment of symptomatic paroxysmal atrial fibrillation. Heart 82(2):170–175

62. Plewan A, Lehmann G, Ndrepepa G et al (2001) Maintenance of sinus rhythm after electrical cardioversion of persistent atrial fibrillation; sotalol vs bisoprolol. Eur Heart J 22(16):1504–1510

63. Crystal E, Connolly SJ, Sleik K et al (2002) Interventions on prevention of postoperative atrial fibrillation in patients undergoing heart surgery: a meta-analysis. Circulation 106(1):75–80

64. Connolly SJ, Cybulsky I, Lamy A et al (2003) Double-blind, placebo-controlled, randomized trial of prophylactic metoprolol for reduction of hospital length of stay after heart surgery: the beta-blocker length of stay (BLOS) study. Am Heart J145(2):226–232

65. Halonen J, Hakala T, Auvinen T et al (2006) Intravenous administration of metoprolol is more effective than oral administration in the prevention of atrial fibrillation after cardiac surgery. Circulation 114(1 Suppl):I1–I4

66. Tsuboi J, Kawazoe K, Izumoto H et al (2008) Postoperative treatment with carvedilol, a beta-adrenergic blocker, prevents paroxysmal atrial fibrillation after coronary artery bypass grafting. Circ J 72(4):588–591

67. Acikel S, Bozbas H, Gultekin B et al (2008) Comparison of the efficacy of metoprolol and carvedilol for preventing atrial fibrillation after coronary bypass surgery. Int J Cardiol 126(1):108–113

68. Platia EV, Michelson EL, Porterfield JK et al (1989) Esmolol versus verapamil in the acute treatment of atrial fibrillation or atrial flutter. Am J Cardiol 63(13):925–929

69. Wolbrette DL (2003) Risk of proarrhythmia with class III antiarrhythmic agents: sex-based differences and other issues. Am J Cardiol 91(6A):39D–44D

70. Shantsila E, Watson T, Lip GY (2007) Drug-induced QT-interval prolongation and proarrhythmic risk in the treatment of atrial arrhythmias. Europace 9(Suppl 4):iv37–iv44

71. Gowda RM, Khan IA, Wilbur SL et al (2004) Torsade de pointes: the clinical considerations. Int J Cardiol 96(1):1–6

72. Saluja D, Guyotte J, Reiffel J (2008) An improved QT correction method for use in atrial fibrillation and a comparison with the assessment of QT in sinus rhythm. J Atrial Fib 1(1):1–11

73. Roy D, Talajic M, Dorian P et al (2000) Amiodarone to prevent recurrence of atrial fibrillation. Canadian trial of atrial fibrillation investigators. N Engl J Med 342(13):913–920

74. Singh BN, Singh SN, Reda DJ et al (2005) Amiodarone versus sotalol for atrial fibrillation. N Engl J Med 352(18):1861–1872

75. Maintenance of sinus rhythm in patients with atrial fibrillation: an AFFIRM substudy of the first antiarrhythmic drug (2003). J Am Coll Cardiol 42(1):20–29

76. Kochiadakis GE, Igoumenidis NE, Hamilos MI et al (2004) Long-term maintenance of normal sinus rhythm in patients with current symptomatic atrial fibrillation: amiodarone vs propafenone, both in low doses. Chest 125(2):377–383

77. Kochiadakis GE, Igoumenidis NE, Marketou ME et al (2000) Low dose amiodarone and sotalol in the treatment of recurrent, symptomatic atrial fibrillation: a comparative, placebo controlled study. Heart 84(3):251–257

78. Chevalier P, Durand-Dubief A, Burri H et al (2003) Amiodarone versus placebo and class Ic drugs for cardioversion of recent-onset atrial fibrillation: a meta-analysis. J Am Coll Cardiol 41 (2):255–262

79. Letelier LM, Udol K, Ena J et al (2003) Effectiveness of amiodarone for conversion of atrial fibrillation to sinus rhythm: a meta-analysis. Arch Intern Med 4163(7):777–785

80. Kochiadakis GE, Igoumenidis NE, Parthenakis FI et al (1999) Amiodarone versus propafenone for conversion of chronic atrial fibrillation: results of a randomized, controlled study. J Am Coll Cardiol 33(4):966–971

81. Galperin J, Elizari MV, Chiale PA et al (2001) Efficacy of amiodarone for the termination of chronic atrial fibrillation and maintenance of normal sinus rhythm: a prospective, multicenter, randomized, controlled, double blind trial. J Cardiovasc Pharmacol Ther 6(4):341–350

82. Capucci A, Villani GQ, Aschieri D et al (2000) Oral amiodarone increases the efficacy of direct-current cardioversion in restoration of sinus rhythm in patients with chronic atrial fibrillation. Eur Heart J 21(1):66–73

83. Anderson JL, Prystowsky EN (1999) Sotalol: an important new antiarrhythmic. Am Heart J 137(3):388–409

84. Hohnloser SH, van de Loo A, Baedeker F (1995) Efficacy and proarrhythmic hazards of pharmacologic cardioversion of atrial fibrillation: prospective comparison of sotalol versus quinidine. J Am Coll Cardiol 26(4):852–858

85. Halinen MO, Huttunen M, Paakkinen S et al (1995) Comparison of sotalol with digoxin-quinidine for conversion of acute atrial fibrillation to sinus rhythm (the sotalol-digoxin-quinidine trial). Am J Cardiol 76(7):495–498

86. Singh S, Saini RK, DiMarco J et al (1991) Efficacy and safety of sotalol in digitalized patients with chronic atrial fibrillation. The sotalol study group. Am J Cardiol 68(11):1227–1230

87. Benditt DG, Williams JH, Jin J et al (1999) Maintenance of sinus rhythm with oral D,L-sotalol therapy in patients with symptomatic atrial fibrillation and/or atrial flutter. D,L-sotalol atrial fibrillation/flutter study group. Am J Cardiol 84(3): 270–277

88. Wanless RS, Anderson K, Joy M et al (1997) Multicenter comparative study of the efficacy and safety of sotalol in the prophylactic treatment of patients with paroxysmal supraventricular tachyarrhythmias. Am Heart J 133(4):441–446

89. Reimold SC, Cantillon CO, Friedman PL et al (1993) Propafenone versus sotalol for suppression of recurrent symptomatic atrial fibrillation. Am J Cardiol 71(7):558–563

90. MacNeil DJ, Davies RO, Deitchman D (1993) Clinical safety profile of sotalol in the treatment of arrhythmias. Am J Cardiol 72(4):44A–50A

91. Lehmann MH, Hardy S, Archibald D et al (1996) Sex difference in risk of torsade de pointes with D,L-sotalol. Circulation 94(10):2535–2541

92. Pacifico A, Hohnloser SH, Williams JH et al (1999) Prevention of implantable-defibrillator shocks by treatment with sotalol. D,L-sotalol implantable cardioverter-defibrillator study group. N Engl J Med 340(24):1855–1862

93. Falk RH, Pollak A, Singh SN et al (1997) Intravenous dofetilide, a class III antiarrhythmic agent, for the termination of sustained atrial fibrillation or flutter. Intravenous dofetilide investigators. J Am Coll Cardiol 29(2):385–390

94. Ferguson JJ (1999) Meeting highlights. Highlights of the 71st scientific sessions of the American heart association. Circulation 99(19):2486–2491

95. Singh S, Zoble RG, Yellen L et al (2000) Efficacy and safety of oral dofetilide in converting to and maintaining sinus rhythm in patients with chronic atrial fibrillation or atrial flutter: the symptomatic atrial fibrillation investigative research on dofetilide (SAFIRE-D) study. Circulation 102(19):2385–2390

96. Pritchett EL, Wilkinson WE (1999) Effect of dofetilide on survival in patients with supraventricular arrhythmias. Am Heart J 138(5 Pt 1):994–997

97. Lee KS (1992) Ibutilide, a new compound with potent class III antiarrhythmic activity, activates a slow inward Na+ current in guinea pig ventricular cells. J Pharmacol Exp Ther 262(1):99–108

98. Buchanan LV, Kabell G, Brunden MN et al (1993) Comparative assessment of ibutilide, D-sotalol, clofilium, E-4031, and UK-68,798 in a rabbit model of proarrhythmia. J Cardiovasc Pharmacol 22(4):540–549

99. Stambler BS, Wood MA, Ellenbogen KA et al (1996) Efficacy and safety of repeated intravenous doses of ibutilide for rapid conversion of atrial flutter or fibrillation. Ibutilide repeat dose study investigators. Circulation 94(7):1613–1621

100. Abi-Mansour P, Carberry PA, McCowan RJ et al (1998) Conversion efficacy and safety of repeated doses of ibutilide in patients with atrial flutter and atrial fibrillation. Study investigators. Am Heart J 136(4 Pt 1):632–642

101. Tercius AJ, Kluger J, Coleman CI et al (2007) Intravenous magnesium sulfate enhances the ability of intravenous ibutilide to successfully convert atrial fibrillation or flutter. Pacing Clin Electrophysiol 30(11):1331–1335

102. Ellenbogen KA, Stambler BS, Wood MA et al (1996) Efficacy of intravenous ibutilide for rapid termination of atrial fibrillation and atrial flutter: a dose-response study. J Am Coll Cardiol 28(1):130–136

103. Gowda RM, Khan IA, Punukollu G et al (2004) Female preponderance in ibutilide-induced torsade de pointes. Int J Cardiol 95(2–3):219–222

104. Tieleman RG, De Langen C, Van Gelder IC et al (1997) Verapamil reduces tachycardia-induced electrical remodeling of the atria. Circulation 95(7):1945–1953

105. Daoud EG, Knight BP, Weiss R et al (1997) Effect of verapamil and procainamide on atrial fibrillation-induced electrical remodeling in humans. Circulation 96(5):1542–1550

106. Moriguchi M, Niwano S, Yoshizawa N et al (2003) Verapamil suppresses the inhomogeneity of electrical remodeling in a canine long-term rapid atrial stimulation model. Pacing Clin Electrophysiol 26(11):2072–2082

107. Shenasa M, Kus T, Fromer M et al (1988) Effect of intravenous and oral calcium antagonists (diltiazem and verapamil) on sustenance of atrial fibrillation. Am J Cardiol 62(7):403–407

108. Amar D, Roistacher N, Rusch VW et al (2000) Effects of diltiazem prophylaxis on the incidence and clinical outcome of atrial arrhythmias after thoracic surgery. J Thorac Cardiovasc Surg 120(4):790–798

109. Villani GQ, Piepoli MF, Terracciano C et al (2000) Effects of diltiazem pretreatment on direct-current cardioversion in patients with persistent atrial fibrillation: a single-blind, randomized, controlled study. Am Heart J 140(3):e12

110. Singh BN, Connolly SJ, Crijns HJ et al (2007) Dronedarone for maintenance of sinus rhythm in atrial fibrillation or flutter. N Engl J Med 357(10):987–999

111. Kober L, Torp-Pedersen C, McMurray JJ et al (2008) Increased mortality after dronedarone therapy for severe heart failure. N Engl J Med 358(25):2678–2687

112. Roy D, Pratt CM, Torp-Pedersen C et al (2008) Vernakalant hydrochloride for rapid conversion of atrial fibrillation: a phase 3, randomized, placebo-controlled trial. Circulation 117(12):1518–1525

113. Pritchett EL, Page RL, Connolly SJ et al (2000) Antiarrhythmic effects of azimilide in atrial fibrillation: efficacy and dose-response. Azimilide supraventricular arrhythmia program 3 (SVA-3) investigators. J Am Coll Cardiol 36(3):794–802

114. Camm AJ, Pratt CM, Schwartz PJ et al (2004) Mortality in patients after a recent myocardial infarction: a randomized, placebo-controlled trial of azimilide using heart rate variability for risk stratification. Circulation 109(8):990–996

115. Kerr CR, Connolly SJ, Kowey P et al (2006) Efficacy of azimilide for the maintenance of sinus rhythm in patients with paroxysmal atrial fibrillation in the presence and absence of structural heart disease. Am J Cardiol 98(2):215–218

116. Morrow JP, Reiffel JA (2009) Drug therapy for atrial fibrillation: what will its role be in the era of increasing use of catheter ablation? Pacing Clin Electrophysiol 32(1):108–118

117. Morrow JP, Cannon CP, Reiffel JA (2007) New antiarrhythmic drugs for establishing sinus rhythm in atrial fibrillation: what are our therapies likely to be by 2010 and beyond? Am Heart J 154(5):824–829

118. Segal JB, McNamara RL, Miller MR et al (2000) The evidence regarding the drugs used for ventricular rate control. J Fam Pract 49(1):47–59

119. Olshansky B, Rosenfeld LE, Warner AL et al (2004) The atrial fibrillation follow-up investigation of rhythm management (AFFIRM) study: approaches to control rate in atrial fibrillation. J Am Coll Cardiol 43(7):1201–1208

120. Packer M, Bristow MR, Cohn JN et al (1996) The effect of carvedilol on morbidity and mortality in patients with chronic heart failure. US carvedilol heart failure study group. N Engl J Med 334(21):1349–1355

121. Agarwal AK, Venugopalan P (2001) Beneficial effect of carvedilol on heart rate response to exercise in digitalised patients with heart failure in atrial fibrillation due to idiopathic dilated cardiomyopathy. Eur J Heart Fail 3(4):437–440

122. Goldstein RE, Boccuzzi SJ, Cruess D et al (1991) Diltiazem increases late-onset congestive heart failure in postinfarction patients with early reduction in ejection fraction. The adverse experience committee; and the multicenter diltiazem postinfarction research group. Circulation 83(1):52–60

123. Reiffel JA (1992) Improved rate control in atrial fibrillation. Am Heart J 123(4 Pt 1):1094–1098

124. Clemo HF, Wood MA, Gilligan DM et al (1998) Intravenous amiodarone for acute heart rate control in the critically ill patient with atrial tachyarrhythmias. Am J Cardiol 81(5):594–598

125. Davy JM, Herold M, Hoglund C et al (2008) Dronedarone for the control of ventricular rate in permanent atrial fibrillation: the efficacy and safety of dRonedArone for the control of ventricular rate during atrial fibrillation (ERATO) study. Am Heart J 156(3):527 e1–e9

126. Tamariz LJ, Bass EB (2004) Pharmacological rate control of atrial fibrillation. Cardiol Clin 22(1):35–45

127. Lundstrom T, Ryden L (1990) Ventricular rate control and exercise performance in chronic atrial fibrillation: effects of diltiazem and verapamil. J Am Coll Cardiol 16(1):86–90

128. Delle Karth G, Geppert A, Neunteufl T et al (2001) Amiodarone versus diltiazem for rate control in critically ill patients with atrial tachyarrhythmias. Crit Care Med 29(6):1149–1153

129. Jordaens L, Trouerbach J, Calle P et al (1997) Conversion of atrial fibrillation to sinus rhythm and rate control by digoxin in comparison to placebo. Eur Heart J 18(4):643–648

130. Falk RH, Knowlton AA, Bernard SA et al (1987) Digoxin for converting recent-onset atrial fibrillation to sinus rhythm. A randomized, double-blinded trial. Ann Intern Med 106(4):503–506

131. Julian DG, Camm AJ, Frangin G et al (1997) Randomised trial of effect of amiodarone on mortality in patients with left-ventricular dysfunction after recent myocardial infarction: EMIAT. European myocardial infarct amiodarone trial investigators. Lancet 349(9053):667–674

132. Cairns JA, Connolly SJ, Roberts R et al (1997) Randomised trial of outcome after myocardial infarction in patients with frequent or repetitive ventricular premature depolarisations: CAMIAT. Canadian amiodarone myocardial infarction arrhythmia trial investigators. Lancet 349(9053):675–682

133. Julian DG, Prescott RJ, Jackson FS et al (1982) Controlled trial of sotalol for one year after myocardial infarction. Lancet 1(8282):1142–1147

134. Packer M, Coats AJ, Fowler MB et al (2001) Effect of carvedilol on survival in severe chronic heart failure. N Engl J Med 344(22):1651–1658

135. Dargie HJ (2001) Effect of carvedilol on outcome after myocardial infarction in patients with left-ventricular dysfunction: the CAPRICORN randomised trial. Lancet 357(9266):1385–1390

136. Massie BM, Fisher SG, Radford M et al (1996) Effect of amiodarone on clinical status and left ventricular function in patients with congestive heart failure. CHF-STAT investigators. Circulation 93(12):2128–2134

137. Ben-David J, Zipes DP, Ayers GM et al (1992) Canine left ventricular hypertrophy predisposes to ventricular tachycardia induction by phase 2 early afterdepolarizations after administration of BAY K 8644. J Am Coll Cardiol 20(7): 1576–1584

138. Prystowsky EN (2000) Management of atrial fibrillation: therapeutic options and clinical decisions. Am J Cardiol 85(10A):3D–11D

139. Hart RG, Benavente O, McBride R et al (1999) Antithrombotic therapy to prevent stroke in patients with atrial fibrillation: a meta-analysis. Ann Intern Med 131(7):492–501

140. Hart RG, Pearce LA, McBride R et al (1999) Factors associated with ischemic stroke during aspirin therapy in atrial fibrillation: analysis of 2012 participants in the SPAF I-III clinical trials. The stroke prevention in atrial fibrillation (SPAF) investigators. Stroke 30(6):1223–1229

141. EAFT (1993) Secondary prevention in non-rheumatic atrial fibrillation after transient ischaemic attack or minor stroke. EAFT (European atrial fibrillation trial) study group. Lancet 342(8882):1255–1262

142. Fang MC, Singer DE, Chang Y et al (2005) Gender differences in the risk of ischemic stroke and peripheral embolism in atrial fibrillation: the Anticoagulation and Risk factors In Atrial fibrillation (ATRIA) study. Circulation 112(12): 1687–1691

143. Risk factors for stroke and efficacy of antithrombotic therapy in atrial fibrillation (1994) Analysis of pooled data from five randomized controlled trials. Arch Intern Med 154(13):1449–1457

144. Moulton AW, Singer DE, Haas JS (1991) Risk factors for stroke in patients with nonrheumatic atrial fibrillation: a case-control study. Am J Med 91(2):156–161

145. Boysen G, Nyboe J, Appleyard M et al (1988) Stroke incidence and risk factors for stroke in Copenhagen, Denmark. Stroke 19(11):1345–1353

146. Kopecky SL, Gersh BJ, McGoon MD et al (1987) The natural history of lone atrial fibrillation. A population-based study over three decades. N Engl J Med 317(11):669–674

147. Capucci A, Santini M, Padeletti L et al (2005) Monitored atrial fibrillation duration predicts arterial embolic events in patients suffering from bradycardia and atrial fibrillation implanted with antitachycardia pacemakers. J Am Coll Cardiol 46(10):1913–1920

148. Hart RG, Pearce LA, Rothbart RM et al (2000) Stroke with intermittent atrial fibrillation: incidence and predictors during aspirin therapy. Stroke prevention in atrial fibrillation investigators. J Am Coll Cardiol 35(1):183–187

149. Hohnloser SH, Pajitnev D, Pogue J et al (2007) Incidence of stroke in paroxysmal versus sustained atrial fibrillation in patients taking oral anticoagulation or combined antiplatelet therapy: an ACTIVE W Substudy. J Am Coll Cardiol 50(22):2156–2161

150. The effect of low-dose warfarin on the risk of stroke in patients with nonrheumatic atrial fibrillation (1990) The Boston area anticoagulation trial for atrial fibrillation investigators. N Engl J Med 323(22):1505–1511

151. Stroke Prevention in Atrial Fibrillation Study (1991) Final results. Circulation 84(2):527–539

152. Petersen P, Boysen G, Godtfredsen J et al (1989) Placebo-controlled, randomised trial of warfarin and aspirin for prevention of thromboembolic complications in chronic atrial fibrillation. The Copenhagen AFASAK study. Lancet 1(8631):175–179

153. Connolly SJ, Laupacis A, Gent M et al (1991) Canadian atrial fibrillation anticoagulation (CAFA) study. J Am Coll Cardiol 18(2):349–355

154. Ezekowitz MD, Bridgers SL, James KE et al (1992) Warfarin in the prevention of stroke associated with nonrheumatic atrial fibrillation. Veterans affairs stroke prevention in nonrheumatic atrial fibrillation investigators. N Engl J Med 327(20):1406–1412

155. Ezekowitz MD, Levine JA (1999) Preventing stroke in patients with atrial fibrillation. JAMA 281(19): 1830–1835

156. Hylek EM, Skates SJ, Sheehan MA et al (1996) An analysis of the lowest effective intensity of prophylactic anticoagulation for patients with nonrheumatic atrial fibrillation. N Engl J Med 335(8):540–546

157. Optimal oral anticoagulant therapy in patients with nonrheumatic atrial fibrillation and recent cerebral ischemia (1995) The European atrial fibrillation trial study group. N Engl J Med 333(1):5–10

158. The efficacy of aspirin in patients with atrial fibrillation (1997) Analysis of pooled data from 3 randomized trials. The atrial fibrillation investigators. Arch Intern Med 157(11):1237–1240

159. Stroke Prevention in Atrial Fibrillation III randomised clinical trial (1996) Adjusted-dose warfarin versus low-intensity, fixed-dose warfarin plus aspirin for high-risk patients with atrial fibrillation. Lancet 348(9028):633–638

160. Connolly S, Pogue J, Hart R et al (2006) Clopidogrel plus aspirin versus oral anticoagulation for atrial fibrillation in the Atrial fibrillation Clopidogrel Trial with Irbesartan for prevention of Vascular Events (ACTIVE W): a randomised controlled trial. Lancet 367(9526):1903–1912

161. Connolly SJ, Pogue J, Hart RG et al (2009) Effect of clopidogrel added to aspirin in patients with atrial fibrillation. N Engl J Med 360(20):2066–2078

162. van Walraven C, Hart RG, Singer DE et al (2002) Oral anticoagulants vs aspirin in nonvalvular atrial fibrillation: an individual patient meta-analysis. JAMA 288(19):2441–2448

163. Hart RG, Benavente O, Pearce LA (1999) Increased risk of intracranial hemorrhage when aspirin is combined with warfarin: a meta-analysis and hypothesis. Cerebrovasc Dis 9(4):215–217

164. Shireman TI, Howard PA, Kresowik TF et al (2004) Combined anticoagulant-antiplatelet use and major bleeding events in elderly atrial fibrillation patients. Stroke 35(10):2362–2367

165. Surawicz B, Knilans T (2001) Atrial flutter and atrial fibrillation. In: Chou's electrocardiography in clinical practice, 5th edn. Saunders, Philadelphia, PA, p 345

166. Waldo AL (2003) Inter-relationships between atrial flutter and atrial fibrillation. Pacing Clin Electrophysiol 26(7 Pt 2):1583–1596

167. Biblo LA, Yuan Z, Quan KJ et al (2001) Risk of stroke in patients with atrial flutter. Am J Cardiol 87(3):346–349, A9

168. Andrew P, Montenero AS (2007) Atrial flutter: a focus on treatment options for a common supraventricular tachyarrhythmia. J Cardiovasc Med (Hagerstown) 8(8):558–567

169. Ghali WA, Wasil BI, Brant R et al (2005) Atrial flutter and the risk of thromboembolism: a systematic review and meta-analysis. Am J Med 118(2):101–107

9 Catheter Ablation of Atrial Flutter and Atrial Fibrillation

Joseph E. Marine and Hugh Calkins

CONTENTS

Abstract

Atrial flutter and atrial fibrillation are two of the most common arrhythmias seen in clinical practice and the most common indications for referral for catheter ablation. While they are historically grouped together, research over the past 20 years has shown that atrial flutter and atrial fibrillation are distinct arrhythmias with different electrophysiological mechanisms. This review will consider the development of and current approach to catheter ablation of atrial flutter and atrial fibrillation.

Key Words: Atrial fibrillation; atrial flutter; atrioventricular (AV) conduction; entrainment; cavotricuspid isthmus; reentry; catheter ablation; anticoagulation; meta-analysis; complications; pericardial tamponade; stroke; fluoroscopy; cardioversion; guidelines; counterclockwise atrial flutter; clockwise atrial flutter; programmed stimulation; electroanatomical mapping; perimitral flutter; phrenic nerve injury; transseptal puncture; antiarrhythmic drug; multiple wavelet hypothesis; atrial fibrosis; rate control; rhythm control; AFFIRM trial; AV junction ablation; Maze-III procedure; linear ablation; pulmonary veins; focal triggers; pulmonary vein stenosis; pulmonary vein isolation; circumferential ablation; mitral isthmus; proarrhythmia; vagal denervation; ganglionated plexi; complex fractionated atrial electrogram (CFAE); stepwise approach (to AF ablation); amiodarone; paroxysmal atrial fibrillation; persistent atrial fibrillation; esophagus; atrial-esophageal fistula; randomized trial; quality of life; worldwide survey; HRS expert consensus statement; cryoablation; remote navigation.

INTRODUCTION

Atrial flutter and atrial fibrillation are two of the most common arrhythmias seen in clinical practice and the most common indications for referral for catheter ablation. While they are historically grouped together, research over the past 20 years has shown that atrial flutter and atrial fibrillation are distinct arrhythmias with different electrophysiological mechanisms. While they share common risk factors, cause similar symptoms, and often coexist in the same patients, ablation strategies for the two arrhythmias differ and depend critically upon an understanding of their distinct natural histories and

From: *Contemporary Cardiology: Management of Cardiac Arrhythmias*
Edited by: Gan-Xin Yan, Peter R. Kowey, DOI 10.1007/978-1-60761-161-5_9
© Springer Science+Business Media, LLC 2011

mechanisms. This review will therefore largely consider catheter ablation for atrial flutter and atrial fibrillation separately, although we will point out several important points of overlap between them.

ATRIAL FLUTTER

Historical Background

Since its first electrocardiographic description, atrial flutter has been recognized as a common atrial tachyarrhythmia causing palpitations, fatigue, congestive heart failure, and thromboembolism. By ECG criteria, atrial flutter is distinguished from atrial fibrillation by the presence of regular, organized atrial activity, usually at a rate of 240–320 beats per minute (bpm) with 2:1 conduction to the ventricles. In patients with relatively slower atrial rates of 200–250 bpm and short atrioventricular (AV) nodal refractory periods, 1:1 AV conduction may be seen. Other patients may have 3:1, 4:1, or variable AV conduction. In most cases, the atrial activation is seen on the ECG as a "sawtooth" waveform in the inferior leads (II, III, and aVF) with positive P-waves in lead V1 and negative P-waves in lead V6.

Since its first description in 1913 through the 1960s, electrophysiologists debated whether the mechanism of the arrhythmia is focal or reentrant. However, since the 1970s, evidence mounted favoring reentry as the fundamental mechanism. Waldo et al. demonstrated that most cases of atrial flutter after cardiac surgery can be entrained and terminated with atrial pacing *(1)*. Josephson and others demonstrated that the arrhythmia could be reproducibly and specifically induced with programmed atrial stimulation in patients who demonstrated the arrhythmia clinically *(2)*.

By 1990, several investigators had demonstrated by multipolar catheter recordings in patients with atrial flutter that right atrial activation showed a stereotypical reentrant pattern with the wave of depolarization spreading up the interatrial septum, over the top of the right atrium, down the lateral wall, through the floor of the right atrium, and then up the interatrial septum again in a counterclockwise pattern when the right atrium is viewed in a left anterior oblique position *(3)*. The left atrium is activated passively and is not required for the maintenance of the arrhythmia. Other investigators using intracardiac ultrasound and pacing entrainment mapping demonstrated that the tricuspid valve annulus forms the anterior border of the reentrant circuit while the Eustachian ridge and crista terminalis form the posterior border of the reentrant circuit *(4, 5)*.

Typical Atrial Flutter Pathway: Contemporary Model

In normal sinus rhythm, atrial depolarization begins in the sinus node, at the anterolateral junction of the superior vena cava and the right atrium. From there, depolarization spreads simultaneously down the anterolateral wall, posterior wall, and interatrial septum until reaching the AV node. The atrium is then electrically silent until another wave of depolarization is initiated from the pacemaker in the sinus node. In typical atrial flutter, there is no physiologic pacemaker regulating the atrial rate. Rather, a continuous reentrant wave of depolarization drives atrial activity, spreading down the anterolateral wall, through the relatively narrow cavotricuspid isthmus, up the interatrial septum, over the roof of the RA, and then down the anterolateral wall again. The left atrium is activated passively from right to left. The rate of the flutter is determined by the length of the circuit (which is longer in dilated right atria) and conduction velocity of the atrial myocardium (which may be affected by intrinsic disease, autonomic tone, electrolyte status, and antiarrhythmic drugs). Of central importance is the observation that the continuity of the circuit depends on conduction through the relatively narrow cavotricuspid isthmus region. The work of numerous investigators in the late 1980s and 1990s showed that disrupting conduction in the isthmus region both terminates typical atrial flutter acutely and renders it noninducible.

Catheter Ablation of Atrial Flutter: Evolution of Technique

Ablation of atrial flutter was first reported by Guiraudon and Klein in 1986 using open-heart surgical techniques *(6)*. The arrhythmia was mapped intraoperatively and ablated surgically near the ostium of the coronary sinus in the right atrium. Within a few years, several groups reported replicating the technique using transvenous radiofrequency (RF) catheter ablation in the right atrium in the region between the tricuspid valve and inferior vena cava, known as the cavotricuspid isthmus *(7, 8)*. The initial technique, using 4-mm-tipped catheters, involved ablation in the cavotricuspid isthmus until the arrhythmia terminated, followed by demonstration that it could no longer be induced with programmed atrial stimulation.

By the mid-1990s, the limitations of the initial RF catheter ablation techniques for atrial flutter became apparent, with reports of short-term recurrence rates of 20–30%. In 1996, several investigators reported improved electrophysiological endpoints, the most important of which is demonstration of electrical block across the ablated region of the cavotricuspid isthmus *(9)*. Another important advance of the later 1990s was introduction of larger-tipped RF ablation catheters (8–10 mm) and irrigated-tipped catheters, both of which allow for more rapid and reliable creation of the larger ablation lesions needed to achieve this electrical conduction block *(10, 11)*. Together, these advances improved the acute success rate to 90–95% and reduced recurrence rates of atrial flutter to 3–5%.

Atrial Flutter Ablation: A Contemporary Technique

The patient is brought to the EP laboratory after overnight fast. As with electrical cardioversion, patients with persistent atrial flutter are therapeutically anticoagulated for at least 3 weeks before the procedure; alternatively, pre-procedural transesophageal echocardiography may be performed to exclude intracardiac thrombus. We generally prefer to continue therapeutic anticoagulation with warfarin during the peri-procedural period, rather than holding warfarin prior to the procedure and bridging with low molecular weight heparin and/or unfractionated heparin. Moderate intravenous sedation with midazolam and fentanyl can be used as needed for patient anxiety and discomfort. Using local anesthesia, sheaths are placed in the right and/or left femoral veins and quadripolar pacing catheters are positioned in the right ventricular apex and His bundle region under fluoroscopic guidance. A long steerable catheter with 10 electrode bipoles spaced every 1 cm (20-pole catheter) is positioned with the tip, and first 3–4 bipoles in the coronary sinus and the remaining poles in the cavotricuspid isthmus and anterolateral right atrium (Fig. 1). Alternatively, separate multipolar catheters can be used for the

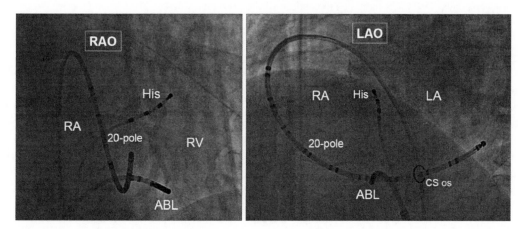

Fig. 1. Right anterior oblique (RAO – A) and left anterior oblique (LAO – B) fluoroscopic views of catheter placement for ablation of typical atrial flutter. RA indicates right atrium; RV, right ventricle; ABL, ablation catheter positioned in the cavotricuspid isthmus; LA, left atrium; CS, coronary sinus.

coronary sinus and anterolateral right atrium. A radiofrequency ablation catheter with 8–10 mm tip or 4 mm irrigated tip is positioned in the cavotricuspid isthmus.

If the patient is in sinus rhythm, attempts are made to induce atrial flutter using programmed atrial stimulation. The arrhythmia is then mapped to determine the right atrial activation pattern and to prove that the cavotricuspid isthmus is an obligate part of the reentrant circuit. The ablation catheter is then positioned in the cavotricuspid isthmus and advanced so that the tip lies on the tricuspid valve annulus (Fig. 2). RF energy is then applied, which causes resistive heating and necrosis of the myocardium lying in immediate contact with the tip. Every 30–60 sec, the tip is pulled back several millimeters toward the inferior vena cava until a complete line has been created connecting the tricuspid valve annulus with the inferior vena cava. Ablation is continued until atrial flutter terminates to sinus rhythm.

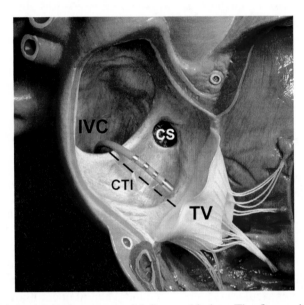

Fig. 2. Anatomy of the right atrium relevant to atrial flutter ablation. The figure shows right anterior oblique view of a heart model of the right atrium and right ventricle with the anterolateral walls removed. The ablation catheter is positioned on the annulus of the tricuspid valve (TV) in the cavotricuspid isthmus (CTI), the starting point for ablation. Dashed line shows the path along which the catheter is withdrawn to create a line of block to the inferior vena cava (IVC). CS indicates the ostium of the coronary sinus.

After termination, pacing on each side of the ablation line is performed to prove that no electrical conduction across the line is possible. If bidirectional conduction block is not present, the isthmus region is probed with the ablation catheter to find gaps of viable myocardium, which allow conduction. Once bidirectional block is present and stable over a brief observation period, an atrial pacing protocol is repeated to confirm noninducibility of the clinical arrhythmia and to look for other arrhythmias. Catheters and sheaths are then removed. Typical total procedure times are 2–3 h from start of sheath insertion, with fluoroscopy times of 10–20 min and RF ablation time of 10–20 min. Patients who do not require immediate intravenous anticoagulation can often be discharged after a 4-h observation period, with the remainder leaving after an overnight stay. Patients who arrive for the ablation procedure in atrial flutter are effectively being cardioverted to sinus rhythm, and therefore require continuous therapeutic anticoagulation for at least 4 weeks afterward.

Atrial Flutter Ablation: Results

In a recently published meta-analysis, Perez et al. examined 158 studies reporting results of atrial flutter ablation involving a total of 10,719 patients with a mean of 14.3 ± 0.3 months of follow-up *(12)*.

Adjusting for potential reporting bias, the overall acute success rate was 91.1% with an adjusted recurrence rate of atrial flutter of 10.9%. To reflect contemporary practice, the authors also examined the 49 studies (3098 patients) in which 8–10 mm or irrigated-tipped RF ablation catheters were used with a procedural endpoint of bidirectional cavotricuspid isthmus block. In this contemporary subgroup, the adjusted acute success rate was improved to 93.6% with a recurrence rate of atrial flutter of 6.7%.

Two randomized controlled trials of catheter ablation for atrial flutter have been reported, both showing marked superiority of the procedure compared with medical therapy. Natale et al. randomized 61 patients with at least two episodes of atrial flutter to either undergo RF catheter ablation or to receive sequential trials of antiarrhythmic drug therapy *(13)*. During a mean follow-up period of 21 ± 11 months, atrial flutter recurred in 93% of the medically treated group vs. only 6% of the group treated with catheter ablation. Quality of life was shown to be significantly improved in the catheter ablation group.

Da Costa et al. randomized 104 patients after a single episode of symptomatic atrial flutter to treatment with either RF catheter ablation or medical therapy with amiodarone *(14)*. After a mean follow-up of 13 ± 6 months, 30% of amiodarone-treated patients experienced recurrence of atrial flutter vs. only 4% of the ablation-treated group. Moreover, there were no complications of catheter ablation during the trial while 10% of the medically treated group experienced complications of amiodarone treatment, including sinus node dysfunction (4%) and thyroid abnormalities (6%). The high recurrence rates of atrial flutter with medical treatment in these trials is also supported by a study of Babaev et al., who followed 53 patients after initial hospital presentation with the first onset of atrial flutter *(15)*. All patients were cardioverted and medically treated, 36% with antiarrhythmic drugs. After a mean follow-up of 22 ± 12 months, 92% of patients experienced recurrence of atrial flutter, with a 42% recurrence rate in the first month alone.

An important limitation to catheter ablation of atrial flutter that has been noted in numerous studies is a high incidence of atrial fibrillation in follow-up, likely due to common atrial substrate and risk factors shared by the two arrhythmias. A prior history of atrial fibrillation is the most potent predictor of atrial fibrillation after successful atrial flutter ablation. In the Perez meta-analysis, the overall adjusted occurrence of atrial fibrillation after atrial flutter ablation was 33.6%. The adjusted incidence of post-ablation atrial fibrillation was 52.7% among patients with a prior history of atrial fibrillation, vs. 23.1% among those with no history of atrial fibrillation. The meta-analysis also showed that incidence of atrial fibrillation after atrial flutter ablation increases with duration of follow-up. Other investigators have shown that risk of post-procedural atrial fibrillation is also increased by coexisting heart failure and left ventricular dysfunction. In an analysis of 110 patients after atrial flutter ablation, Paydak et al. found that 74% of patients with both pre-procedural atrial fibrillation and left ventricular dysfunction experienced atrial fibrillation in follow-up, vs. only 10% of patients with no history of atrial fibrillation and normal left ventricular function *(16)*.

Atrial Flutter Ablation: Risks

Catheter ablation of atrial flutter has a long track record of safety, and significant complications of the procedure are uncommon. As with most cardiac endovascular procedures, femoral hematoma is the most common complication, but rarely requires intervention. Deep venous thrombosis and infection of the vascular access occur with similarly low frequency as in standard cardiac catheterization. Atrial pacing protocols may induce atrial fibrillation, which may require electrical or chemical cardioversion; ventricular arrhythmias are rarely seen.

Pericardial tamponade due to perforation and hemopericardium has been reported in about 0.5% of cases in large series of catheter ablations for SVT *(17)*. These series report procedure-related mortality of 0.1–0.3%, which also includes complications related to ablation on the left side of the heart. To our knowledge, no case of death caused by atrial flutter ablation has been reported to date.

RF ablation can potentially injure cardiac structures adjacent to the area being ablated, such as the tricuspid valve, AV node, and right coronary artery. The risk is minimized, however, with appropriate training and experience, as well as with careful monitoring of electrograms and fluoroscopic images during ablation. Rare cases of AV block requiring pacemaker placement have been reported when the medial or septal cavotricuspid isthmus region is targeted. As with electrical or chemical cardioversion, stroke is a potential complication of ablation in a patient with persistent atrial flutter, which can be minimized with appropriate anticoagulation and/or screening with transesophageal echocardiography.

In a recent meta-analysis of atrial flutter ablation, complication rates in 93 studies which included 6293 patients were summarized (12). The overall complication rate was 2.6%. Of the 77 specific complications reported in these studies, significant vascular injury occurred in 26 patients (0.4%), complete AV block in 12 (0.2%), pericardial effusion in 8 (0.1%), stroke in 3 (0.05%), and myocardial infarction due to right coronary injury in 1 (0.02%).

Atrial Flutter Ablation: Evidence-Based Guidelines

Because of the high degree of efficacy and safety, catheter ablation for atrial flutter has become the first-line therapy for treatment of symptomatic arrhythmia, and is clearly superior to antiarrhythmic drug therapy. In the 2003 American Heart Association (AHA) – American College of Cardiology (ACC) – European Society of Cardiology (ESC) Guidelines for Management of Patients with Supraventricular Arrhythmias, catheter ablation carries a class I recommendation for the treatment of atrial flutter that is recurrent or poorly tolerated (18). For a first occurrence of well-tolerated atrial flutter, catheter ablation has a class IIa recommendation. In contrast, almost all antiarrhythmic drugs for recurrent atrial flutter carry a class IIb recommendation, based on Level C (limited) evidence of efficacy.

Atrial Flutter: Atypical Forms

The preceding discussion has generally referred to the common or typical form of atrial flutter which has classical appearance on 12-lead ECG and requires conduction through the cavotricuspid isthmus for its maintenance. This typical form comprises approximately 90% of atrial flutters seen in clinical practice. The remaining 10% form a spectrum of arrhythmias, which may involve the right or left atrium and utilize a variety of reentrant pathways (Table 1).

Table 1
Types of Atypical Atrial Flutter

Right atrial origin
Cavotricuspid isthmus-dependent
    1. Clockwise typical atrial flutter
    2. Type Ic atrial flutter
    3. Lower loop reentry
Non-isthmus dependent
    1. Incisional reentry (post-cardiac surgery)
    2. Upper loop reentry

Left atrial origin
  Perimitral flutter
  Incisional reentry (post-cardiac surgery)
  Post-ablation for atrial fibrillation

One of the more common variants is so-called "clockwise" typical atrial flutter. This arrhythmia utilizes the same reentrant pathway in the right atrium as typical counterclockwise atrial flutter, but in the opposite direction. This variant can be induced with programmed stimulation in most patients with typical atrial flutter, but for unknown reasons is far less common clinically (19). The ablation technique, success rates, and risks of catheter ablation are same similar to typical atrial flutter.

Another variant of typical atrial flutter is that seen after antiarrhythmic drug treatment of atrial fibrillation, or so-called "type Ic" atrial flutter (20). This arrhythmia has been described mainly after treatment with type Ic sodium channel-blocking antiarrhythmic drugs (flecainide and propafenone) as well as with amiodarone. Almost all cases utilize the same reentrant right atrial circuit as with typical atrial flutter, and the ablation technique used is the same. Rates of acute success of catheter ablation as well as recurrence rates of atrial flutter are felt to be similar to those for typical atrial flutter ablation. Importantly, successful ablation of atrial flutter in this group does not obviate the need for continuation of antiarrhythmic drug therapy to suppress atrial fibrillation. However, recurrences of atrial fibrillation are often seen in this group, even with the continuation of antiarrhythmic drug therapy.

Most other forms of atrial flutter do not utilize the cavotricuspid isthmus and therefore will be unaffected by the standard ablation technique for typical atrial flutter. In these so-called "atypical" forms of atrial flutter, a large variety of electrocardiographic patterns have been described, and there is no ECG pattern that has been found to be characteristic of any type of reentrant circuit. In these atypical forms, the reentrant circuit travels around one or more fixed anatomical or functional barriers. In these cases, one or more barriers is often created as a result of atrial fibrosis from surgical incision, pericardiotomy, placement of surgical patches for treatment of congenital heart disease, or prior catheter or surgical ablation of atrial fibrillation (21). Atypical atrial flutter is occasionally seen in patients who have never undergone cardiac procedures; such patients are usually found to have developed spontaneous atrial fibrosis as a component of a cardiomyopathy.

Atypical Atrial Flutter: Ablation Technique

The technique for mapping and ablation of atypical flutters is different from that for typical atrial flutter. After placement of standard electrophysiological catheters, atrial pacing maneuvers are performed to identify whether the right atrium or left atrium is the site of origin of the arrhythmia. Once this is determined, that atrium undergoes electroanatomical mapping. In this procedure, the cardiac chamber of interest (in this case, the right or left atrium) is mapped in a point-by-point fashion using one of several specialized computer systems that can integrate electrical and spatial information. After approximately 50–100 points are gathered over a 15–30 min period, a three-dimensional shell of the mapped atrium is created with activation and voltage encoded in color format. If created accurately and in sufficient detail, the activation pathway of the atypical flutter is usually apparent. An ablation strategy is then devised, which usually involves ablation of a critical narrow portion of the circuit by connecting two or more electrical barriers.

One of the most common forms of atypical flutter occurs after right atriotomy, and usually consists of a reentrant circuit which revolves around a lateral right atrial scar. In such cases, the atrial flutter is usually easily ablated by connecting the lateral right atrial scar to the ostium of the inferior vena cava with a 1–2 cm ablation line (Fig. 3). Less commonly, right atrial flutter circuits may form around posterior or septal scars or patches. Ablation of such atrial flutters usually involves connecting the scar to the ostium of the inferior vena cava or the tricuspid valve annulus. The most difficult forms of right atrial flutter usually result from complex congenital heart disease and associated corrective operations. Nakagawa et al. described a series of such cases, some of which had 6–8 distinct flutter circuits (22). With lengthy procedures involving extremely detailed electroanatomical mapping and ablation lines connecting a number of scars and other barriers, they were able to render approximately 70% of patients free of atrial arrhythmias.

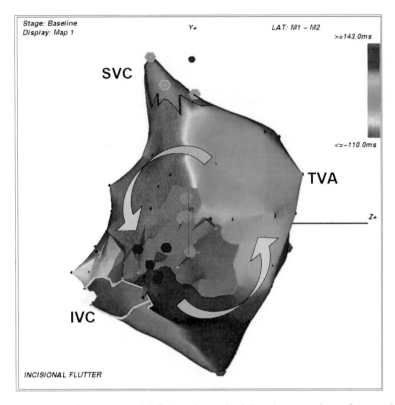

Fig. 3. Electroanatomical map of atypical atrial flutter due to incisional reentry late after surgical repair of atrial septal defect. Figure shows a right lateral view of electroanatomical map of right atrium during atypical atrial flutter in a 44-year-old woman who underwent surgical repair of atrial septal defect 20 years previously. Area of scar, probably representing a surgical incision, is shown in gray. The large *red dots* represent RF ablation lesions. Direction of depolarization during atrial flutter is indicated by *arrows*. SVC indicates superior vena cava; TVA, tricuspid valve annulus, IVC, inferior vena cava.

With the rise in utilization of ablation therapy for atrial fibrillation, this has become the most common cause for the development of atypical atrial flutter arising in the left atrium *(23)*. The most common form of left atrial flutter, so-called "perimitral flutter," utilizes a circuit which travels around the mitral valve annulus. Ablation of this form of atypical atrial flutter generally involves creating a line of ablation lesions, which connects the mitral valve annulus to one of the left-sided pulmonary veins (Fig. 4). Creating a full transmural ablation line in this region may be very challenging, and may require ablation within the coronary sinus to achieve complete conduction block. Other forms of left atrial flutter may utilize one or more pulmonary veins as a central barrier. Ablation in these cases may involve connecting the ostia of the right and left superior pulmonary veins and/or connecting the ostium of one or more pulmonary veins to the mitral valve annulus. As with atypical right atrial flutters, many different pathways are possible, and successful ablation usually requires careful electroanatomical mapping of the reentrant circuit and its associated barriers in order to formulate a successful ablation strategy *(24)*.

In addition to macro-reentrant forms of atypical atrial flutter following ablation of atrial fibrillation, it is also common to observe atypical atrial flutter with a presumed micro-reentrant mechanism due to a gap in an ablation line. These micro-reentrant forms of atypical atrial flutter can be recognized by their centrifugal spread of activation as well as a more discrete P-wave morphology with a clear isoelectric interval on the 12-lead ECG *(25)*.

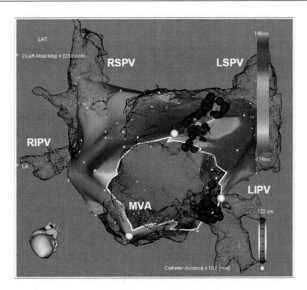

Fig. 4. Two approaches to ablation of peri-mitral left atrial flutter occurring after AF ablation. Left anterior oblique view of an electroanatomical map of the left atrium is shown. The *lower line* of *red dots* indicate ablation lesions connecting the mitral valve annulus (MVA) to the ostium of the left inferior pulmonary vein (LIPV), which is the standard approach. The *upper line* indicates alternative approach connecting the MVA to the left superior pulmonary vein (LSPV). RSPV indicates right superior pulmonary vein; RIPV, right inferior pulmonary vein.

Atypical Atrial Flutter: Results, Risks, and Guidelines

Compared with ablation of typical right atrial flutter, there is much less published data on the results of catheter ablation of atypical atrial flutter. Most data have been reported in the form of case series, usually with fewer than 25 patients and less than 1 year of follow-up. In general, success rates of 70–80% have been reported, considerably less than what has been achieved with catheter ablation of typical atrial flutter. Recurrence rates have not been well described in the literature, but are likely higher than the 5–10% reported for typical atrial flutter owing to the more complex nature of the atrial substrate that gives rise to these arrhythmias.

Complication rates cannot be precisely determined from the limited literature on this subject, but are probably similar to those for ablation of typical atrial flutter described above when only right atrial ablation is performed. One potential additional complication that may result from ablation of atypical right atrial flutter is right phrenic nerve injury resulting in temporary or permanent right hemi-diaphragmatic paralysis. This complication usually arises from ablation along the posterolateral right atrium and/or lateral ostium of the superior vena cava, and may be reduced testing with high-output pacing looking for diaphragmatic stimulation at each high-risk site prior to delivering RF ablation. In addition, the risk of AV block may be higher when ablating atypical atrial flutter in the septal region, and AV conduction must be carefully monitored whenever delivering RF lesions near the interatrial septum. Ablation of atypical left atrial flutter likely carries a higher complication rate than that of right atrial flutters owing to the need for transseptal puncture and catheterization as well as delivery of RF lesions in the left atrium. Some of these potential risks will be covered in the later sections on ablation of atrial fibrillation.

Because of the more complex nature of atypical atrial flutters and the broad diversity of atrial substrates and cardiac and noncardiac comorbidities, including history of atrial fibrillation, patient selection for catheter ablation of atypical atrial flutter must be individualized, and uniform treatment recommendations cannot be make. In contrast to typical atrial flutter, a trial of antiarrhythmic drug therapy may be warranted, and a rate control strategy may be effective in the occasional patient with minimal or no symptoms. Reflecting this clinical heterogeneity, the 2003 ACC/AHA/ESC Guidelines for Treatment of Supraventricular Arrhythmias accord ablation of atypical atrial flutter a class IIa recommendation *(18)*.

Summary: Catheter Ablation of Atrial Flutter

RF catheter ablation of typical, cavotricuspid isthmus-dependent atrial flutter is a safe and highly effective curative treatment for this troublesome atrial arrhythmia and is recommended as first-line therapy for most symptomatic patients. Atypical atrial flutter is a heterogeneous clinical problem and requires individualized clinical decision-making. Successful ablation of atypical atrial flutter usually requires careful electroanatomical mapping with ablation of all induced sustained atrial flutter circuits. Development of atrial fibrillation after successful ablation of atrial flutter remains a significant clinical problem.

ATRIAL FIBRILLATION

Clinical Background

Atrial fibrillation (AF) is the most common sustained arrhythmia, with an estimated prevalence of at least 2 million in the United States, a number which is likely to rise due to the aging of the population *(26)*. Prevalence increases with age in a nearly exponential fashion, with estimated prevalence of 10% in people over the age of 80 years, and the estimated lifetime risk for developing AF for a 40-year-old is about 25% *(27)*. Patients with AF may be asymptomatic or suffer from a variety of symptoms, including palpitations, dyspnea, chest discomfort, fatigue, malaise, and loss of exercise tolerance. In some cases, tachycardia-induced cardiomyopathy may result from uncontrolled ventricular rate. It is an important cause of stroke, with estimated attributable risk of 20–25%. Quality of life is reduced in most patients, and epidemiologic studies have linked AF to increased risk of mortality.

For most of the past 50 years, the dominant model of AF mechanism has been the multiple wavelet hypothesis of Moe and Allessie *(28)*. According to this model, six to eight randomly moving reentrant wavelets are required to maintain AF. The wavelets do not follow any fixed pathways, but do observe fixed anatomical boundaries and may collide with one another, extinguish, and reform, resulting in an apparently chaotic pattern of atrial activation. In recent years, increasing attention has focused on electrophysiologic triggers of AF, particularly focal arrhythmias arising from the pulmonary veins. Contemporary research has also established that, in contrast to other supraventricular arrhythmias, AF is often a progressive disease which becomes increasingly self-sustaining and resistant to treatment over time due to electrical and anatomical remodeling, resulting in atrial fibrosis and enlargement.

Management of AF begins with medical control of ventricular rate and anticoagulation if stroke risk factors are present. A trial of cardioversion is appropriate for most patients who first present with sustained AF, although it is recognized that some older patients with minimal or no symptoms may be managed successfully in permanent AF. Longer-term treatment is guided by the patient's age, symptoms, comorbidities, and personal preferences. Disease management has been affected by the AFFIRM and RACE trials, which showed no reduction in stroke risk or overall mortality in patients with AF who were treated with antiarrhythmic drugs to maintain sinus rhythm over a simpler rate control and anticoagulation strategy *(29, 30)*. Subgroup analysis of the AFFIRM trial, however, did show improved outcomes in the subset of patients who successfully maintained sinus rhythm, suggesting that there may be significant benefit to maintaining sinus rhythm, which is offset by adverse effects and relative inefficacy of antiarrhythmic drugs *(31)*.

Patients enrolled in the AFFIRM and RACE trials had either asymptomatic or minimally symptomatic AF, thereby making them appropriate candidates for either rate or rhythm control strategy. It is therefore inappropriate to conclude that rate and rhythm control are equivalent treatment strategies for patients with symptomatic AF. Since publication of the AFFIRM trial in 2002, the safety and efficacy of catheter ablation of AF has improved significantly, and it is continuing to improve further. In addition, committing a patient to a rate control strategy will likely to render the atrium more resistant to AF ablation several years later due to progressive atrial remodeling. We are therefore reluctant to commit younger patients (<70 years) to a rate control strategy without attempting an initial rhythm control approach. On the other hand, we quickly move to a rate control strategy for very elderly AF patients who are either asymptomatic or minimally symptomatic.

For those patients with recurrent AF who do not have acceptable symptom control with rate control medications, rhythm control generally begins with a choice of antiarrhythmic drug therapy. Randomized trials have shown that antiarrhythmic drugs maintain sinus rhythm in 30–60% of patients over a 1–2 year follow-up period (32, 33). Success rates of antiarrhythmic drugs depend upon cardiac comorbidities, left atrial size and fibrosis, and duration of AF. Selection of antiarrhythmic drug therapy depends upon patients' comorbidities, other medications, renal function, and personal preferences. A useful algorithm can be found in the 2006 ACC/AHA/ESC Guidelines for the management of patients with atrial fibrillation (26).

For patients with symptomatic AF who cannot tolerate or achieve acceptable symptom control with either a rate control strategy or with antiarrhythmic drug therapy, catheter ablation has evolved from an investigational procedure to one that is now performed on thousands of patients annually in many medical centers throughout the world. The growing acceptance of this procedure has been brought about by a growing number of reports showing safety and efficacy of catheter ablation of AF targeting the pulmonary veins and posterior left atrium. The remainder of this section will review the development of catheter ablation procedures, highlighting current techniques, outcomes, complications, and remaining questions.

Catheter Ablation of AF: Historical Background

The era of catheter ablation therapy for cardiac arrhythmias began in 1982 with reports of direct current ablation of the AV junction for control of ventricular rate in patients with intractable supraventricular tachyarrhythmias, including AF (34). While rarely performed now for other supraventricular arrhythmias, catheter ablation of the AV junction with permanent pacemaker implantation remains a useful treatment for selected AF patients with refractory symptoms due to uncontrolled ventricular response despite medical therapy, particularly in elderly patients (35). In recent years, biventricular pacemakers have been increasingly used in patients undergoing AV junction ablation who have preexisting heart failure symptoms due to left ventricular dysfunction and/or mitral regurgitation, due to the well-established risk for right ventricular apical pacing to exacerbate these problems (36). In the early 1990s, several groups reported success in modifying AV node conduction with partial catheter ablation with acceptable ventricular rate control, but without complete AV block or need for pacemaker implantation. These early results proved not to be durable, with a majority of patients either regressing to rapid ventricular response or progressing to high-degree AV block and pacemaker-dependency, and AV node modification is now rarely performed for AF.

Concurrently with the development of catheter ablation techniques described above, Cox and colleagues developed a series of surgical techniques for the disruption of AF, first in a canine model and then in series of patients (37). The most advanced version of the operation, the Maze-III procedure, was based upon the multiple wavelet hypothesis, in which maintenance of the arrhythmia requires maintenance of a critical number of circulating wavelets of reentry, each of which requires a critical mass of atrial tissue to sustain it. In the Maze-III operation, after induction of cardiopulmonary bypass, a series of transmural incisions are made in the left and right atria, with preservation of the sinus node and an uninterrupted corridor of atrial tissue to allow conduction to the AV node. In addition, the right and left atrial appendages are removed, which may further reduce stroke risk. The end result of the procedure is that the atria are divided into electrically isolated subsections such that maintenance of AF is prevented regardless of the mode of initiation. In the course of their research, these investigators found that the left atrial lesion set was largely sufficient to prevent AF, while right atrial lesions were required to prevent development of atrial flutter. Interestingly, isolation of the pulmonary veins and posterior left atrium was a feature common to all successful iterations of the procedure.

With the Maze-III approach, Cox and colleagues have reported maintenance of sinus rhythm in 95% of patients at long-term follow-up with stroke rates of 0.1%/year *(38)*. Fifteen percent of patients required permanent pacemakers, and 7% lost left atrial transport function. Several other surgical series in other centers have reported success rates nearly as high, above 85%. Widespread application of the Maze-III operation as a stand-alone treatment for AF has been limited by the complexity of the procedure and the morbidity and risk associated with sternotomy/thoracotomy and cardiopulmonary bypass, as well as by limited adoption among cardiothoracic surgeons. However, long-term results of the Maze-III operation still stand as the gold standard for what can be achieved with catheter and surgical ablation techniques.

Catheter Ablation of AF – Linear Approach

The success of the Maze-III procedure in the early 1990s led some interventional cardiac electrophysiologists to attempt to reproduce the procedure with RF catheter lesions using a transvenous approach. In 1994, Schwartz and colleagues reported reproducing the Maze-III lesion set in a small series of patients using specially designed sheaths and standard RF ablation catheters *(39)*. Efficacy was modest, complication rates were high, and procedure and fluoroscopy times exceedingly long, and further attempts to reproduce the full Maze-III lesion set were abandoned. However, this report demonstrated a proof-of-concept that led others to try to improve the catheter-based approach.

In 1996, Haissaguerre and colleagues reported the outcomes of linear catheter ablation in 45 patients undergoing right and/or left atrial ablation for paroxysmal AF *(40)*. They found that right atrial ablation (with two or more procedures in 19 patients) led to rhythm control in 15 patients (33%), 9 of whom required antiarrhythmic drugs. Ten patients in whom right atrial ablation was unsuccessful then underwent left atrial ablation via transseptal approach, leading to rhythm control in six patients (60%). Further refinement of linear catheter ablation technique by this group was reported in 1999, in a series of 44 patients (91% with paroxysmal AF) who underwent RF catheter ablation to create specific lesions sets in the right (2 lines) and left (3–4 lines) atria *(41)*. A mean of 2.7 +/– 1.3 procedures were required to complete the lesions and to ablate post-procedure atrial flutters, which occurred in 70% patients and were generally observed to be caused by incomplete lines of block. Interestingly, 29 patients (66%) were observed to have areas of focal electrical discharge initiating AF and underwent attempted ablation of these foci, 97% of which were located in the pulmonary veins.

Of the 44 patients in this study, maintenance of sinus rhythm was achieved without antiarrhythmic drugs in 25 (57%) and 27% had improved rhythm control on antiarrhythmic drugs. The investigators noted significant complications in nine patients (20%). In retrospect, it is likely that ablation of initiating pulmonary vein foci significantly improved their results compared with a pure linear approach. Multicenter trials of linear ablation of AF using novel multipolar ablation catheters were attempted, but were terminated prematurely due to high complication rates and poor efficacy. On the basis of these observations, and the rapid advances in ablation of AF targeting initiating focal triggers, the catheter-based linear ablation approach for AF has been largely abandoned.

Catheter Ablation of AF: Focal Approach

One important observation which came from the early work of Haissaguerre and colleagues in linear ablation of AF was the fact that some patients with paroxysmal AF appear to have a focal source of electrical activity triggering some or all paroxysms of AF. They published findings of a series of 45 patients in a landmark publication in 1998 *(42)*. Patients had a mean age of 54 +/– 11 years and had frequent (often daily) paroxysms of drug-refractory AF for a mean of 6 +/– 6 years. Most patients (69%) had structurally normal hearts. Patients also had at least 700 isolated premature atrial ectopic beats on a 24-h Holter. All patients underwent intracardiac mapping to localize the source of the premature atrial ectopic beats; 69 ectopic foci were found and targeted for ablation. Remarkably, 65 foci (94%) originated within pulmonary veins, most within 2–4 cm of the ostium. AF was initiated with a burst of rapid firing from the foci and was abolished with RF ablation at the site of origin. After a follow-up period of 8 +/– 6 months, 28 patients (62%) were free of AF off antiarrhythmic drugs, a substantial effect given the frequency and long duration of symptoms preceding the procedure. These findings were soon replicated by other groups.

The electrophysiologic basis of these focal sources appeared to be sleeves of left atrial muscle investing the pulmonary veins, an anatomic observation that had been made decades ago. One or more veins develop abnormal, paroxysmal, rapid automaticity, triggering AF as a result *(43)*. Despite extensive research, the pathophysiology of this process remains poorly understood. Further research established that non-pulmonary vein foci were an important source of AF in some patients, although percentages vary among different groups from 5 to 20% *(44)*. Sources identified included several thoracic veins: the vein/ligament of Marshall (a remnant of the fetal left superior vena cava on the posterior left atrial wall), the coronary sinus, and the superior vena cava. Other reported sources include the left atrial posterior wall and various right atrial sites. Rare cases of AF triggered by ectopic foci in the inferior vena cava and in a persistent left superior vena cava have been described.

With increasing use of focal ablation of pulmonary vein triggers, the problem of pulmonary vein stenosis quickly became recognized due to its serious sequelae, including hemoptysis, pulmonary edema, and pulmonary hypertension. Another problem with the focal approach to pulmonary vein ablation was the recognition that after successful ablation, recurrence rates were high and remapping usually showed new foci in the ablated vein or in other veins rather than recurrence of the original focus. Paroxysmal AF appears to be a field effect, rendering patients susceptible to recurrences from multiple pulmonary vein foci. A final major limitation of this approach is that it requires direct observation of atrial premature beats triggering AF during the ablation procedure, limiting it to patients with frequent spontaneous or inducible atrial ectopy.

Catheter Ablation of AF: Segmental Ostial Approach

Recognition of these major limitations of focal ablation led to techniques to electrically isolate the entire pulmonary vein. Because the pulmonary vein musculature conducts to left atrial musculature by discrete connections, investigators targeted those connections using multipolar catheters shaped into rings or baskets *(45, 46)*. After placement of a diagnostic electrophysiology catheter in the coronary sinus, two long sheaths are placed across the interatrial septum with a double transseptal technique. After defining pulmonary vein anatomy with contrast venography, a circular mapping catheter is placed at the ostium of the targeted pulmonary vein. Ablation is performed with a separate roving catheter through the second transseptal sheath at the site of earliest activation sequentially until pulmonary vein electrical activity disappears or becomes dissociated from left atrial activity. Using this strategy, between 20% and 60% of the pulmonary vein circumference is typically targeted for ablation. It was found that by ablating at or just outside the pulmonary vein ostium, the incidence of significant pulmonary vein stenosis could be reduced to less than 5%. Pulmonary vein isolation has the additional advantage of simultaneously treating all triggering foci within the vein, thereby obviating the need to elicit and map those foci individually.

Marchlinski et al. compared their experience with focal vs. segmental ostial isolation for treatment of AF in 107 patients and found freedom from AF at 1 year in 80% of patients treated with pulmonary vein isolation vs. 45% of patients treated with focal ablation *(47)*. For similar reasons, investigators were soon led to attempt to isolate as many pulmonary veins as possible at the initial ablation session. Comparative case series ultimately demonstrated that empiric four vein isolation led to superior outcomes over isolating fewer veins.

Using this approach, electrophysiology centers began reporting success rates of 60–80% for patients with paroxysmal AF with medium-term follow-up. Success rates for this approach are clearly better for patients with paroxysmal atrial fibrillation than for those with persistent atrial fibrillation. Recurrences generally result from reconnection of previously isolated veins or ectopy in pulmonary veins not targeted at the initial procedure. A minority of recurrences have been shown to be due to electrical triggers outside of the pulmonary veins.

Table 2 summarizes the outcomes of eight case series or trials that have reported on the safety and efficacy of segmental ostial ablation for the treatment of AF *(46, 48–54)*. Medium-term success was achieved in 196 of 280 patients with paroxysmal AF (70%) and 21 of 70 patients with persistent atrial fibrillation (30%). The overall major complication rate was 6.3%, including stroke (0.7%), pericardial tamponade (1.2%), and significant pulmonary vein stenosis (4.3%).

The technique of segmental ostial pulmonary vein isolation represented an important advance in catheter treatment of AF over the focal approach. Medium-term success for patients with paroxysmal AF is good, but results are generally worse for persistent AF. It remains the preferred approach to paroxysmal AF in some centers, although most have moved toward techniques to modify left atrial substrate.

Catheter Ablation of AF: Circumferential Approach

Concurrently with the development of the segmental approach to pulmonary vein isolation, Pappone and colleagues working in Milan developed the circumferential approach using electroanatomic mapping *(55, 56)*. After placement of one or more diagnostic electrophysiology catheters, a single transseptal puncture is performed and a long transseptal sheath is placed in the left atrium. Using an electroanatomic mapping system, an anatomic shell is constructed with the mapping/ablation catheter, including the pulmonary veins. RF ablation is then performed circumferentially around each vein, well outside the ostium, with the endpoint of ablation being the elimination or marked reduction (80–90%) in the amplitude of electrical signals within the encircling lesions. In cases where the inferior and superior veins were closely spaced or shared a common ostium, a single large circumferential RF lesion set would be performed. Despite lack of evidence showing pulmonary veins treated in this way were completely electrically isolated from the left atrium, this group began reporting results for paroxysmal AF, which were as good or better than those working with the ostial segmental approach. Furthermore, patients with persistent AF treated with the circumferential approach achieved results nearly as good as those with paroxysmal AF, and far better than reports of patients treated with segmental pulmonary vein isolation.

In 2001, Pappone and colleagues reported results of this approach in 251 consecutive patients with drug-refractory AF (paroxysmal in 179 and persistent in 72) *(57)*. Electroanatomic mapping immediately after ablation showed an estimated 23 +/– 9% of the entire left atrial surface area was transformed to a low-voltage or electrically silent state. After a mean follow-up period of 10.4 +/– 4.5 months, 85% of patients with paroxysmal AF and 68% of patients with persistent AF were free of symptomatic AF.

Results from other centers using the circumferential approach have not been as favorable. Table 3 summarizes the outcomes of six case series or trials which have reported on the safety and efficacy of

Table 2
Summary of Clinical Studies of Segmental Pulmonary Vein (PV) Ablation

Study	Year	Follow-up (months)	Success			Complications			
			Overall	Paroxysmal AF	Persistent or permanent AF	PV stenosis (>50%)	Stroke	Cardiac tamponade	Mitral valve injury
Haissaguerre (46)	2000	4±5	51/70 (73)	51/70 (73)	–	0	0	0	0
Oral (48)	2002	5±3	44/70 (63)	41/58 (71)	3/12 (25)	0	1 (1.4)	0	0
Deisenhofer (49)	2003	8±4	38/75 (51)	N/A	N/A	6 (8)	0	4 (5.3)	0
Marrouche (50)	2003	14±5	271/315 (86)	N/A	N/A	22 (7)	2 (0.6)	0	0
Arentz (51)	2003	12	34/55 (62)	26/37 (70)	8/18 (44)	1 (1.8)	0	1 (1.8)	0
Oral (52)	2003	6	27/40 (67)	27/40 (67)	–	0	0	0	0
Mansour (53)	2004	21±5	22/40 (55)	19/33 (58)	3/7 (43)	0	0	2 (5)	0
Vasamreddy (54)	2004	11±8	39/75 (52)	32/42 (76)	7/33 (21)	3 (4)	2 (2.6)	2 (2.6)	1 (1.3)
Overall	–	–	526/740 (71)	196/280 (70)	21/70 (30)	32 (4.3)	5 (0.7)	9 (1.2)	1 (0.1)

Values are given as n (%); Success was defined as free of atrial fibrillation (AF) recurrence without antiarrhythmic drugs.

circumferential ablation for treatment of AF *(52, 53, 57–60)*. Medium-term success was achieved in 290 of 393 patients with paroxysmal AF (74%) and 73 of 149 patients with persistent/permanent AF (49%). The overall major complication rate was 2.4%, including stroke (0.4%), pericardial tamponade (0.7%), and PV stenosis (0.4%).

Catheter Ablation of AF: Additional Approaches

The reported success of the circumferential approach raised several important questions and has led investigators to attempt modifications to the standard circumferential lesion set, resulting in additional, hybrid approaches to ablation of AF. The first question is whether complete electrical isolation of the pulmonary veins is necessary to achieve clinical success. Several investigators have addressed this question and come to differing conclusions. Cappato et al. studied 43 patients with serial electrophysiology studies and found a high rate (80%) of recurrent conduction from previously disconnected veins *(61)*. However, freedom from AF was no more likely in those with recurrent conduction than in those without. Forty percent of patients who had recurrence of pulmonary vein conduction were free of AF.

In contrast, Gerstenfeld et al. who studied 34 patients with recurrent AF after initial pulmonary vein isolation, and with careful pulmonary vein mapping, found that 86% of recurrent triggers came from pulmonary veins which had either not been targeted for initial ablation (32%) or developed recurrent conduction (54%) *(62)*. Ouyang et al. treated 41 patients with paroxysmal AF with a modified circumferential ablation approach. In each patient, a single large extra-ostial circumferential lesion set was placed around inferior and superior pulmonary veins on each side while a circular mapping catheter was present in each of the two ipsilateral veins *(59)*. Ablation was continued until complete electrical isolation was achieved in all four pulmonary veins. Ten patients had early recurrence and nine underwent a second procedure – all nine patients showed recurrent conduction from a previously isolated pulmonary vein and underwent re-isolation of that pulmonary vein.

It is now clear throughout the world that nearly all patients who have recurrent AF after an initial attempt at AF ablation and return for a repeat procedure will demonstrate electrical reconnection of at least one, and usually several, pulmonary veins. It is also clear that in many patients reconnection of pulmonary vein conduction occurs soon after initial isolation. We have previously examined the rate of early recurrence of pulmonary vein conduction 30 and 60 min after initial isolation *(63)*. Recovery of PV conduction was observed within the first 30 min in approximately one-third of veins and between 30 and 60 min in 17% of veins. Overall, results of these and other investigations suggest that complete and durable isolation of the pulmonary veins is important for long-term success of the procedure, particularly for patients with paroxysmal AF.

A second important question concerns the safety and efficacy of adding left atrial linear lesions to the basic circumferential pulmonary vein ablation lesion set. The two linear lesions most commonly added are a line connecting the right and left superior veins across the superior aspect of the left atrium (so-called "roof" line) and a line connecting the left inferior pulmonary vein to the mitral valve annulus (so-called "mitral isthmus" line). These lesions sets are designed to further modify electrical substrate to prevent AF as well as to prevent left atrial flutters, which might be formed by the large circumferential lines of block. Jais et al. have shown that achieving block with the mitral isthmus line in particular is technically challenging and sometimes requires ablation within the coronary sinus *(64)*. Whether these additional lines improve clinical success remains to be determined, with some studies suggesting that additional left atrial ablation lines may be unhelpful or proarrhythmic. Currently, many centers are adding these lesions in patients with persistent AF, in patients with inducible AF or left atrial flutter after the standard circumferential lesions are made, and in patients with recurrent AF after an initial procedure.

Table 3
Summary of Clinical Studies of Circumferential Pulmonary Vein (PV) Ablation

Study	Year	Follow-up (months)	Success			Complications			
			Overall	Paroxysmal AF	Persistent or permanent AF	PV stenosis (>50%)	Cardiac tamponade	Stroke	Left atrial flutter
Pappone (57)	2001	10±5	188/251 (75)	148/179 (83)	40/72 (56)	0	2 (0.8)	0	0
Oral (52)	2003	6	35/40 (88)	35/40 (88)	–	0	0	0	1 (2.5)
Mansour (53)	2004	11±3	25/40 (63)	21/32 (66)	4/8 (50)	0	1 (2.5)	1 (2.5)	0
Kottkamp (58)	2004	12	37/100 (37)	34/80 (43)	3/20 (15)	0	0	0	4 (5)
Ouyang (59)	2004	6±1	39/41(95)	39/41(95)	–	0	0	0	0
Vasamreddy (60)	2004	6±3	39/70 (56)	13/21 (62)	26/49 (53)	2 (2.8)	1 (1.4)	1 (1.4)	0
Overall	–	–	363/542 (67)	290/393 (74)	73/149 (49)	2 (0.4)	4 (0.7)	2 (0.4)	5 (0.9)

Values are given as *n* (%); Success was defined as free of atrial fibrillation (AF) recurrence without antiarrhythmic drugs.

A third major question is whether modification of autonomic innervation of the left atrium plays a significant role in procedural success. Pappone et al. studied 297 patients undergoing circumferential ablation for paroxysmal AF and found that 34% of them showed evidence of cardiac vagal denervation during the ablation procedure and in follow-up *(65)*. They found that ablation along the posterior left atrium in their standard lesion set sometimes produced a vagal reflex, resulting in sinus bradycardia and transient AV block. When ablation was continued at these sites, loss of the reflex occurred, suggesting vagal denervation, which was confirmed by indices of heart rate variability on follow-up Holter monitoring. A remarkable 99% of 100 patients who achieved complete vagal denervation were free of AF at 12 months, vs. 85% of the remaining patients.

More recently, Po et al. reported on the results of a specific ablation approach targeting the left atrial ganglionated plexi, which serve as integration centers of the cardiac autonomic nervous system *(66)*. After transseptal catheterization, they first localized the sites of ganglionated plexi (typically 4 per patient) using high-frequency pacing stimulation looking for a parasympathetic cardiac response (>50% increase in R–R interval). Interestingly, the ganglionated plexi were generally found to be located near the ostia of each of the pulmonary veins, and would therefore be typically encompassed in a standard wide-area circumferential ablation approach. After localization, RF ablation was performed at each site, until the parasympathetic response was eliminated. Twelve months after a single procedure, 80% of patients were free of symptomatic AF. While results of these two reports are interesting and encouraging, the role systematic modification of cardiac autonomic innervation is not yet well-established.

A fourth major question concerns the role of targeting complex fractionated atrial electrograms in the right and left atrium. Nademanee et al. studied 121 patients with drug-refractory paroxysmal (57 patients) and persistent/permanent (64 patients) atrial fibrillation and used a novel approach to mapping of the substrate and performing ablation *(67)*. During atrial fibrillation in all patients (spontaneous or induced), biatrial electroanatomical mapping was performed. Areas of complex, fractionated electrical (CFAE) potentials were noted and tagged. These sites were targeted for ablation, using a mean of 64 +/– 36 pulses. Sites were spread over nine areas of both atria and were not confined to the pulmonary veins, which were not specifically targeted for isolation. Using this approach, termination of AF occurred during ablation in 91% of patients. At 12-month follow-up, 70% of patients were free of AF off antiarrhythmic drugs; with a second procedure, success rate increased to 83%. Complication rate was comparable to other approaches.

This novel approach to ablation of AF has generated considerable interest in the subject of electrogram characteristics and the role in maintenance of atrial fibrillation. CFAE potentials have been shown to be reproducible and temporally stable in a given patient *(68)*. It remains unknown whether they represent sites of "rotors", which generate wavelets, sites of autonomic innervation from ganglionated plexi, or areas of atrial fibrosis. While Nademanee et al. have reported similarly favorable results in a larger series of patients with longer follow-up duration, these results have not been replicated at other centers *(69)*. Furthermore, addition of CFAE ablation to standard pulmonary vein isolation procedures has not yet been demonstrated to significantly improve outcome.

A final major question in the field is the role of more extensive catheter ablation of the atria to treat patients with longstanding persistent AF, defined as continuously present for at least 1 year. This form of AF is regarded as a more advanced stage of the disease, and is usually accompanied by left atrial enlargement and more extensive fibrosis. Results of standard pulmonary vein isolation procedures with these patients in most centers have been disappointing. Haissaguerre and colleagues in Bordeaux have reported on a more extensive ablative technique, which they term the "stepwise approach" *(70, 71)*. The technique involves initial pulmonary vein isolation followed by isolation of other thoracic veins, and then atrial tissue ablation targeting all regions with rapid or heterogeneous activation (termed "defragmentation"). A final step may include creation of sequential linear lesions on the left atrial roof, coronary sinus, mitral isthmus, and other left atrial regions, with a goal of achieving termination of arrhythmia during ablation. Prolongation of mean AF cycle length in the atrial appendages is frequently noted prior to termination or organization to atrial flutter.

In an initial series of 60 patients undergoing the procedure, a remarkable 87% achieved acute termination of arrhythmia. Most patients organized to one or more morphologies of atrial tachycardia or flutter, which then required further ablation, and most patients required multiple procedures to finish all the required ablation components and/or ablate resulting atrial tachycardias and flutters. After multiple procedures, 95% maintained sinus rhythm at mean 11 +/– 6 months of follow-up. These excellent results in patients who are often resistant to other techniques stand as a benchmark. This success rate, however, reflects multiple ablation procedures with concomitant use of antiarrhythmic drugs in some patients; single-procedure long-term success rate free of antiarrhythmic drug therapy for patients with longstanding persistent AF is less than 40%.

Catheter Ablation of AF: A Contemporary Approach

At Johns Hopkins Hospital, we offer catheter ablation to patients with symptomatic paroxysmal or persistent AF despite treatment with at least one antiarrhythmic drug. There are no specific age, left atrial size, or LV ejection fraction cutoffs for the procedure. In general, we find that patients under 75 years, those with left atrial size 5 cm or less, and those without severe heart failure or major comorbidities tolerate the procedure better and have better outcomes. Patients undergo pre-procedural CT or MRI scanning to define pulmonary vein anatomy and to import the left atrial image into the electroanatomic mapping system used during the ablation procedure. Pre-procedural transesophageal echocardiography is performed in most patients to exclude left atrial thrombus, including all patients with persistent AF and patients with CHADS$_2$ score of 2 or more *(72)*. Patients with stroke risk factors are treated with therapeutic warfarin for a month prior to the ablation and bridged with enoxaparin.

The ablation procedure may be performed with moderate sedation or general anesthesia, depending on patient comorbidities, anticipated procedure time, and patient/operator preference. A radio-opaque temperature probe is placed in the esophagus to monitor and minimize ablation near this critical structure. Right femoral venous access is obtained and a monitoring femoral arterial line is placed. A multipolar diagnostic catheter is placed in the coronary sinus. After intravenous heparin is given, two transseptal punctures are performed and long sheaths passed into the left atrium. Contrast pulmonary venography is performed and used to create a merged electroanatomical image to guide the ablation procedure. Using a 4-mm open-irrigated tip ablation catheter and 25–30 W power settings, wide-area circumferential ablation around the left and right pulmonary venous antra is performed, staying 0.5–1 cm outside the ostium of each vein (Fig. 5). If the anatomy allows, ablation is generally performed between the superior and inferior pulmonary veins, in the so-called "carina" region *(73)*.

After circumferential ablation is completed, a circular multipolar electrode mapping catheter is introduced into the second transseptal sheath and the ostium of each pulmonary vein is mapped looking for residual electrical potentials and evidence of electrical isolation (Fig. 6). Additional ablation lesions guided by the mapping catheter are delivered until the vein is electrically isolated with evidence of both entrance and exit block, or dissociation of pulmonary vein potentials (Fig. 7). This procedure is repeated for each pulmonary vein. Each vein is reexamined with the mapping catheter 30–60 min after the last RF lesion is given to ensure persistent electrical isolation is present. If not, additional RF lesions are delivered to reisolate the vein.

At the first ablation procedure, additional ablation lines and ablation of CFAE sites are generally not performed. In patients undergoing re-do procedures for persistent AF, CFAE mapping and ablation is performed. If AF persists, additional RF ablation lines, including left atrial roof line and mitral isthmus line, may be added. Atypical atrial flutters, if present, may be specifically mapped and ablated. In general, cavotricuspid isthmus ablation is not performed unless there is clinical evidence of typical atrial flutter. Likewise, superior vena cava isolation is generally not performed unless the patient shows evidence that it is a focal source of triggering ectopy.

Total procedure times of 3–5 h and RF ablation times of 30–60 min are typical. After ablation is completed, heparinization is reversed with protamine and sheaths are removed. Anticoagulation is resumed after several hours during overnight observation in the hospital. Patients are bridged with enoxaparin to therapeutic anticoagulation with warfarin, which is continued for at least 2–3 months. Patients are seen in the office after 3 months, and Holter and/or event monitoring is performed every 3 months for the first year and afterward if symptoms indicate. Long-term anticoagulation management is determined by the patient's rhythm status, CHADS$_2$ score, and individual risk tolerance.

Risks of Catheter Ablation for AF

As with any medical procedure, potential risks need to be considered and balanced against potential benefits and likelihood of success in deciding what to recommend for a particular patient. Some of the risks of catheter ablation of atrial fibrillation are listed in Table 4. In addition to risks common to all catheter-based cardiac procedures, several of these risks are unique to or increased with ablation of AF.

Pericardial tamponade is a complication common to all invasive cardiac procedures, but appears to be higher in ablation of AF, likely due to prolonged procedure duration, transseptal access, multiple ablation lesions, and need for prolonged high-dose heparinization during the procedure. The rate of pericardial tamponade was 107/8745 procedures (1.22%) in the Worldwide Survey on Ablation of Atrial Fibrillation *(74)*. Occasional cases may be fatal, especially if the condition is not recognized prior to hemodynamic collapse.

The risk of pulmonary vein stenosis is increased with ablation within the ostium of the pulmonary vein and with multiple high-energy lesions around the circumference of the ostium *(75)*. Rates of significant pulmonary vein stenosis as high as 10% were seen with early experience with focal ablation, and have been reduced to about 1% with circumferential ablation. No procedural technique has proven to be entirely free of this risk, and variation in incidence may depend on how stenosis is measured and defined and how vigorously it is sought after the procedure. Due to its low incidence in contem-

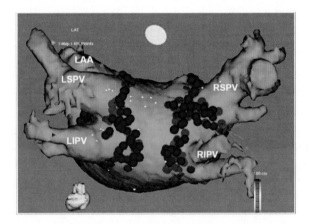

Fig. 5. Circumferential pulmonary vein ablation using electroanatomical mapping. The figure shows posteroanterior view of an electroanatomical map merged with computed tomographic scan of the left atrium. Each *red dot* represents approximately 5–10 sec of radiofrequency application performed during circumferential pulmonary vein isolation. LSPV indicates left superior pulmonary vein; LIPV, left inferior pulmonary vein; RSPV, right superior pulmonary vein; RIPV, right inferior pulmonary vein.

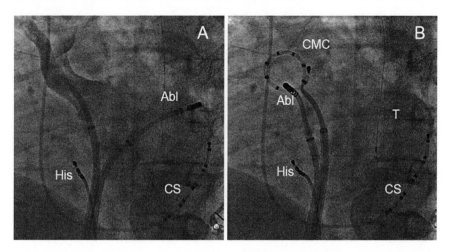

Fig. 6. Use of multielectrode circular mapping catheter to guide electrical isolation of the right superior pulmonary vein (RSPV). *Panel A* shows left anterior oblique fluoroscopy view of the left atrium during contrast injection of the right superior pulmonary vein. *Panel B* shows same view with circular mapping catheter (CMC) inserted just inside the ostium of the RSPV, with the ablation catheter (Abl) deployed near the venous ostium to complete electrical isolation of the vein. CS indicates the coronary sinus catheter; T, radio-opaque temperature probe; His, the His bundle catheter.

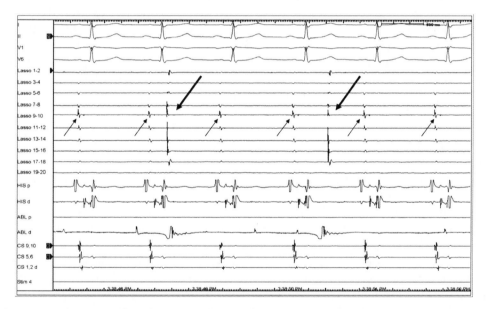

Fig. 7. Demonstration of electrical dissociation of the left superior pulmonary vein from the left atrium after catheter ablation. Figure shows electrogram recordings taken during pulmonary vein isolation. *Small arrows* point to far-field atrial potential on the circular mapping catheter (Lasso 1–20) during sinus rhythm. The *large arrows* point to slow, dissociated pulmonary vein potentials, indicating complete electrical isolation of the vein.

porary practice, we do not routinely screen for pulmonary vein stenosis, unless symptoms such as exertional dyspnea, chest pain, persistent cough, hemoptysis, or unexplained pneumonia occur. CT or MRI scanning with comparison to pre-procedural images is the most effective way to make the diagnosis. Treatment is challenging and may require angioplasty, stenting, or partial lung resection. In our

Table 4
Risks of Catheter Ablation of Atrial Fibrillation

Vascular injury
  Hematoma
  Pseudoaneurysm
  Arteriovenous fistula
Venous thromboembolus
Pericardial effusion/ tamponade
Stroke
Pulmonary vein stenosis
Phrenic nerve injury (R >> L)
Atrioesophageal fistula
Mitral valve injury
Coronary artery injury/myocardial infarction
Death

experience, pulmonary vein stenosis has become rare, and we have observed no symptomatic stenosis among the last 500 patients who have undergone AF ablation at our institution.

Stroke, although infrequent, continues to be an important issue. The Worldwide Survey on Ablation of Atrial Fibrillation found 20 strokes reported for 7154 left-sided ablation procedures, an event rate of 0.25%, including two deaths (74). The rate of transient ischemic attack was 0.66%. Potential sources of emboli include thrombi adherent to catheters and sheaths, endocardial disruption from the ablation lesions, thrombi or air passing through a patient foramen ovale or transseptal puncture site, and air introduced through transseptal sheaths. Careful attention to anticoagulation and sheath management should reduce risk, but the nature of the procedure with prolonged left-sided catheterization and extensive left atrial ablation in patients predisposed to stroke precludes eliminating it entirely. A history of prior stroke or transient ischemic attack and $CHADS_2$ score of 2 or more appear to be significant risk factors for this complication (76).

Permanent diaphragmatic paralysis was reported in 10/8745 cases (0.11%) in the Worldwide Registry and probably relates to ablation within the right superior pulmonary vein or superior vena cava and/or extensive linear ablation along the lateral right atrial wall. High-output pace-mapping at potential high-risk ablation sites may reduce, but does not entirely eliminate, risk. Diaphragmatic paralysis may resolve in 50–70% of cases, but may take up to a year for nerve regeneration to occur (77).

Left atrial-esophageal fistula is the most feared complication of AF ablation due to its high fatality rate, and is estimated to occur in approximately 0.1% of cases (78). Typically presenting days to weeks after otherwise uncomplicated procedures, premorbid symptoms may include dysphagia, fever, confusion, and hemetemesis. Stroke, sepsis syndrome, and sudden death are common sequelae. Diagnosis may be made with chest CT scanning, and endoscopy should be avoided if the diagnosis is suspected. When recognized, treatment includes total GI rest, avoidance of esophageal instrumentation, and either temporary esophageal stenting or surgical esophageal resection. Risk of this complication may be reduced by esophageal monitoring during the procedure using a radio-opaque temperature probe, and reduction of RF power settings during posterior left atrial ablation.

A recently reported multicenter survey of 162 centers found that 32 deaths occurred in 32,569 patients (0.1%) undergoing catheter ablation of AF (79). Causes of death included tamponade in 8 patients (25% of deaths), stroke in 5 (16%), atrioesophageal fistula in 5 (16%), and pneumonia in 2 (6%). A variety of miscellaneous causes accounted for each of the remaining deaths.

Results of AF Ablation: Randomized Trials and Multicenter Registries

To date, six randomized trials of AF ablation vs. medical therapy have been published in manuscript form, and they are summarized in Table 5 *(80–86)*. While varying in design, outcome measures, and ablation technique used, each one showed significantly improved outcome in the patients who received catheter ablation. Freedom from AF at 1 year ranged from 56 to 89% in the patients randomized to catheter ablation. Several of these studies also demonstrated improved quality of life and reduction in symptom burden in patients treated with ablation.

Khan et al. randomized 81 patients with drug-resistant paroxysmal or persistent AF associated with heart failure and left ventricular dysfunction (LVEF ≤ 40%) to undergo either pulmonary vein isolation or AV node ablation with biventricular pacing *(87)*. In the group undergoing pulmonary vein isolation, 71% were free of AF at 6 months without antiarrhythmic drug treatment. Patients randomized to pulmonary vein isolation showed improved quality of life scores, longer 6-min walk distance, and higher LVEF compared with the AV node ablation group.

The largest multicenter case series of AF ablation is the Worldwide Survey reported by Cappato et al. in 2005 *(74)*. Of the 777 centers contacted, 181 completed a standardized survey reporting outcomes of catheter ablation in 8745 patients between 1995 and 2002. Survey results showed widely varying procedure techniques and case volumes between centers, with a marked increase in procedure volume over time. Outcome of freedom of AF without use of antiarrhythmic drugs ranged from 30% at the lowest volume centers to 64% at the highest volume centers, with overall reported success rates of 52%. Including patients free of AF with continuation of antiarrhythmic drugs, overall success reported was 76%. The overall major complication rate was 6%.

A recent study reported the outcomes of two meta-analyses of the safety and efficacy of catheter ablation of AF and antiarrhythmic drug therapy *(88)*. The results of 63 AF ablation and 34 antiarrhythmic drug studies were included in these analyses. Patients enrolled in AF ablation studies tended to be younger (mean age 55 vs. 62 years), had longer duration of AF (6.0 vs. 3.1 years), and had failed a greater number of prior drug trials (2.6 vs. 1.7). The single procedure success rate of ablation off AAD therapy was 57% (95% CI 50–64%), the multiple procedure success rate off AAD was 71% (95% CI 65–77%), and the multiple procedure success rate on AAD or with unknown AAD usage was 77% (95% CI 73–81%). In comparison, the success rate for AAD therapy was 52% (95% CI 47–57%). A major complication of catheter ablation occurred in 4.9% of patients. Adverse events for AAD studies, while more common (30% vs. 5%), were less severe.

As of this writing, several large, multicenter randomized trials of catheter ablation for AF are being organized. The largest of these, the Catheter Ablation vs. Antiarrhythmic Drug Therapy for Atrial Fibrillation (CABANA) trial, plans to enroll several thousand patients to either catheter ablation or medical therapy for paroxysmal or persistent atrial fibrillation, with several years of follow-up and overall mortality as a primary outcome *(89)*. While results will not be expected until about 2015, this and other major trials should provide important information about patient selection, procedural technique, anticoagulation management, outcomes, and complications in AF patients.

HRS Consensus Document

The publication of the Expert Consensus Statement on Catheter and Surgical Ablation of Atrial Fibrillation in 2007 was a major milestone in the development of catheter ablation for AF and it provides a state-of-the-art review of the field *(90)*. The document reports the findings of a task force convened by the Heart Rhythm Society, which was charged with defining the indications, techniques, and outcomes of AF ablation procedures. It was written in partnership with the European Heart Rhythm Association and European Cardiac Arrhythmia Society, and was endorsed by the ACC and AHA. While there were few points of unanimity, broad consensus was reached on a number of important issues, and the doc-

Table 5
Randomized Trials of Catheter Ablation of Atrial Fibrillation vs. Medical Therapy

Study	N	Centers	AF type (paroxysmal/persistent)	Endpoint	Success ablation (%)	Success medical therapy (%)	p-value	Complications in ablation group
Krittayaphong (80)	30	1	Both	Freedom from AF at 1 year	79	40	0.018	1 stroke
Oral (81)	146	2	Persistent	Freedom from AF/AFl at 1 year without AAD or crossover to ablation	74	4	0.05*	None
Wazni (82)	70	3	Both	Freedom from AF at 1 year	87	37	<0.001	2 asymptomatic pulmonary vein stenoses
Stabile (83)	137	4	Both	Freedom from AF at 1 year	56	9	<0.001	1 tamponade, 1 stroke, 1 diaphragm paralysis
Jais (84)	112	7	Paroxysmal	Freedom from AF at 1 year	89	23	<0.0001	2 tamponades
Pappone (85)	198	1	Paroxysmal	Freedom from AF at 1 year off AAD	86	22	<0.001	1 TIA, 1 pericardial effusion

*p-value based on intention-to-treat analysis, AF indicates atrial fibrillation; TIA, transient ischemic attack

ument provides a framework for further development of the field. Among the most important findings of the Consensus Statement are:

1. Ablation is indicated for symptomatic AF refractory to at least one class I or III antiarrhythmic medication. Ablation may be appropriate as first-line therapy in rare clinical situations and in selected patients with heart failure and reduced LVEF. Presence of atrial thrombus is a contraindication.
2. Surgical ablation is indicated in symptomatic and selected asymptomatic AF patients undergoing cardiac surgery for other indications, and for patients who have failed one or more attempts at catheter ablation or cannot undergo catheter ablation due to contraindications.
3. Ablation strategies that target the pulmonary veins and or antral regions are the cornerstone for most AF ablation procedures. Complete electrical isolation should be the goal, and ablation within the ostia should be avoided.
4. If additional linear lesions are used, completeness should be demonstrated with mapping or pacing maneuvers. Cavotricuspid isthmus ablation should be performed only in patients with spontaneous or inducible typical atrial flutter.
5. Anticoagulation recommendations from the 2006 ACC/AHA/ESC Atrial Fibrillation Guidelines were endorsed. Pre-procedural transesophageal echocardiography is indicated for patients with persistent AF who are in AF at the time of the procedure. Enoxaparin or IV heparin bridging should be used and warfarin continued for at least 2 months afterward. Long-term warfarin treatment is recommended for patients with $CHADS_2$ scores of 2 or more regardless of cardiac rhythm.
6. Primary endpoint of AF ablation studies should be freedom from any atrial arrhythmia (AF, atrial flutter, or atrial tachycardia) lasting ≥ 30 sec off antiarrhythmic drug therapy after a single procedure. A blanking period of 3 months should be employed after ablation when reporting success, with a minimum follow-up of 12 months. Holter and continuous event monitoring should be performed at 3–6 month intervals and when indicated by symptoms.

Future Approaches to Catheter Ablation of Atrial Fibrillation

Further development of catheter technology for AF ablation can be anticipated as part of a continued effort to improve procedural success and long-term outcomes and to reduce complications rates. Techniques to deliver simplified circumferential ablation lesions using balloon-tipped catheters have been in development for several years. Cryoballoon technology, using cryoablation to achieve pulmonary vein isolation, is furthest in development. A study of 346 patients with paroxysmal ($n=293$) or persistent ($n=53$) AF has been reported, showing that 93% of pulmonary veins could be isolated with cryoballoon alone *(91)*. Maintenance of sinus rhythm was achieved in 74% of the paroxysmal patients and 42% of persistent patients. There were no cases of pulmonary vein stenosis or esophageal injury, but reversible right phrenic nerve injury occurred in 7.5% of patients with ablation in the right superior pulmonary vein. Other balloon technologies in development employ high-intensity focused ultrasound, laser energy, or radiofrequency energy. While attractive in principle, large-scale studies of safety and efficacy in comparison with standard catheter techniques will be needed.

Another important area of technological development is use of robotic and remote magnetic navigation capability. Use of the robotic remote navigation system (Hansen Medical, Mountain View, California) has been reported in a series of 71 patients undergoing catheter ablation of AF using two operators, one controlling the robotic sheath and ablation catheter from a computer console and the other manipulating the circular mapping catheter and other catheters at the bedside *(92)*. Pulmonary vein isolation was achieved with the system in 90% of patients. While 6-month success rate of 76% was comparable to standard catheter techniques, there was a higher than expected incidence of major complications, including five femoral vascular injuries, three cases of pericardial tamponade, and five cases of severe pulmonary vein stenosis. These complications were attributed in part to large size of the robotic sheath, more efficient energy delivery, and greater force applied at the tip of the catheter. Effective use of the remote magnetic navigation system (NIOBE II, Stereo-taxis, Inc., St. Louis, Missouri) has been reported by one very experienced center in a series of 40 patients, 38 of whom had successful pulmonary vein circumferential ablation with the system without any complications *(93)*. Overall, the remote magnetic navigation system appears safe, though questions remain about technical feasibility and the ability to deliver sufficient ablative energy to some regions of the heart. The system also has high initial capital equipment, structural, and maintenance costs.

Catheter Ablation of Atrial Fibrillation: Summary

In the 15 years since catheter ablation of AF was first reported, the procedure has undergone rapid evolution with corresponding improvement in procedural success and reduction in complications. When performed at experienced centers, catheter ablation is a safe and effective procedure for selected patients with symptomatic drug-refractory atrial fibrillation. More needs to be learned about the mechanism of AF in various patient populations and about how to apply this information to tailor the ablation procedure to individual patients. More uniform reporting of results and longer-term follow-up from multi-center studies are needed to confirm durability of the results reported to date. Because of the technical complexity of the procedure, and lower success rates and higher complication rates when compared with ablation of supraventricular tachycardia, catheter ablation of AF is best performed in experienced electrophysiology centers dedicated to carefully examining and reporting their results. Further advances in this very active field can be expected over the next 15 years.

REFERENCES

1. Waldo AL, MacLean WA, Karp RB, Kouchoukos NT, James TN (1977) Entrainment and interruption of atrial flutter with atrial pacing: studies in man following open heart surgery. Circulation 56:737–745
2. Watson RM, Josephson ME (1980) Atrial flutter. I. Electrophysiologic substrates and modes of initiation and termination. Am J Cardiol 45:732–741
3. Cosio FG, Goicolea A, López-Gil M et al (1990) Atrial endocardial mapping in the rare form of atrial flutter. Am J Cardiol 66:715–720
4. Olgin JE, Kalman JM, Fitzpatrick AP, Lesh MD (1995) Role of right atrial endocardial structures as barriers to conduction during human type I atrial flutter. Activation and entrainment mapping guided by intracardiac echocardiography. Circulation 92:1839–1848
5. Olgin JE, Kalman JM, Lesh MD (1996) Conduction barriers in human atrial flutter: correlation of electrophysiology and anatomy. J Cardiovasc Electrophysiol 7:1112–1126
6. Klein GJ, Guiraudon GM, Sharma AD, Milstein S (1986) Demonstration of macroreentry and feasibility of operative therapy in the common type of atrial flutter. Am J Cardiol 57:587–591
7. Saoudi N, Atallah G, Kirkorian G, Touboul P (1990) Catheter ablation of the atrial myocardium in human type I atrial flutter. Circulation 81:762–771
8. Feld GK, Fleck RP, Chen PS et al (1992) Radiofrequency catheter ablation for the treatment of human type I atrial flutter. Identification of a critical zone in the reentrant circuit by endocardial mapping techniques. Circulation 86: 1233–1240
9. Poty H, Saoudi N, Nair M, Anselme F, Letac B (1996) Further insights into the various types of isthmus block: application to ablation during sinus rhythm. Circulation 94:3204–3213
10. Jais P, Shah DC, Haissaguerre M, Hocini M, Garrigue S, Metayer PL, Clementy J (2000) Prospective randomized comparison of irrigated-tip versus conventional-tip catheters for ablation of common flutter. Circulation 101:772–776
11. Tsai CF, Tai CT, Yu WC et al (1999) Is 8-mm more effective than 4-mm tip electrode catheter for ablation of typical atrial flutter? Circulation 100:768–771
12. Perez FJ, Schubert CM, Parvez B et al (2009) Long-term outcomes after catheter ablation of cavo-tricuspid isthmus dependent atrial flutter: a meta-analysis. Circ Arrhythmia Electrophysiol published online Jun 23, 2009. doi:10.1161/CIRCEP.109.871665
13. Natale A, Newby K, Pisano E et al (2000) Prospective randomized comparison of antiarrhythmic therapy versus first-line radiofrequency ablation in patients with atrial flutter. J Am Coll Cardiol 35:898–904

14. Da Costa A, Thevienin J, Roche F et al (2006) Results from the Loire-Ardèche-Drôme-Isère-Puy-de-Dôme (LADIP) trial on atrial flutter, a multicentric prospective randomized study comparing amiodarone and radiofrequency ablation after the first episode of symptomatic atrial flutter. Circulation 114:1676–1681

15. Babaev A, Suma V, Tita C, Steinberg JS (2003) Recurrence rate of atrial flutter after initial presentation in patients on drug treatment. Am J Cardiol 92:1122–1124

16. Paydak H, Kall JG, Burke MC et al (1998) Atrial fibrillation after radiofrequency ablation of type I atrial flutter. Circulation 98:315–322

17. Calkins H, Yong P, Miller JM et al for the Atakr Multicenter Investigators Group (1999) Catheter ablation of accessory pathways, atrioventricular nodal reentrant tachycardia, and the atrioventricular junction: final results of a prospective, multicenter clinical trial. Circulation 99:262–270

18. Blomström-Lundqvist C, Scheinman MM, Aliot EM et al (2003) ACC/AHA/ESC guidelines for the management of patients with supraventricular arrhythmias–executive summary: a report of the American college of cardiology/American heart association task force on practice guidelines and the European society of cardiology committee for practice guidelines (writing committee to develop guidelines for the management of patients with supraventricular arrhythmias). Circulation 108: 1871–1909

19. Olgin JE, Kalman JM, Saxon LA, Lee RJ, Lesh MD (1997) Mechanism of initiation of atrial flutter in humans: site of unidirectional block and direction of rotation. J Am Coll Cardiol 29:376–384

20. Huang DT, Monahan KM, Zimetbaum P et al (1998) Hybrid pharmacologic and ablative therapy: a novel and effective approach for the management of atrial fibrillation. J Cardiovasc Electrophysiol 9:462–469

21. Saoudi N, Cosio F, Waldo A et al (2001) Classification of atrial flutter and regular atrial tachycardia according to electrophysiologic mechanism and anatomic bases: a statement from a joint expert group from the working group of arrhythmias of the European society of cardiology and the North American society of pacing and electrophysiology. J Cardiovasc Electrophysiol 12:852–866

22. Nakagawa H, Shah N, Matsudaira K et al (2001) Characterization of reentrant circuit in macroreentrant right atrial tachycardia after surgical repair of congenital heart disease: isolated channels between scars allow "focal" ablation. Circulation 103:699–709

23. Gerstenfeld EP, Marchlinski FE (2007) Mapping and ablation of left atrial tachycardias occurring after atrial fibrillation ablation. Heart Rhythm 4:S65–S72

24. Jaïs P, Shah DC, Haïssaguerre M et al (2000) Mapping and ablation of left atrial flutters. Circulation 101:2928–2934

25. Shah D, Sunthorn H, Burri H et al (2006) Narrow, slow-conducting isthmus dependent left atrial reentry developing after ablation for atrial fibrillation: ECG characterization and elimination by focal RF ablation. J Cardiovasc Electrophysiol 17:508–515

26. Fuster V, Ryden LE, Cannom DS et al (2006) ACC/AHA/ESC 2006 guidelines for the management of patients with atrial fibrillation: a report of the American college of cardiology/American heart association task force on practice guidelines and the European society of cardiology committee for practice guidelines (writing committee to revise the 2001 guidelines for the management of patients with atrial fibrillation). J Am Coll Cardiol 48:e149–246

27. Lloyd-Jones DM, Wang TJ, Leip EP et al (2004) Lifetime risk for development of atrial fibrillation: the Framingham heart study. Circulation 110:1042–1046

28. Moe GK, Abildskov JA (1959) Atrial fibrillation as a self-sustaining arrhythmia independent of focal discharge. Am Heart J 58:59–70

29. Wyse DG, Waldo AL, DiMarco JP et al (2002) Atrial fibrillation follow-up investigation of rhythm management (AFFIRM) investigators. A comparison of rate control and rhythm control in patients with atrial fibrillation. N Engl J Med 347:1825–1833

30. Van Gelder IC, Hagens VE, Bosker HA et al (2002) Rate control versus electrical cardioversion for persistent atrial fibrillation study group. A comparison of rate control and rhythm control in patients with recurrent persistent atrial fibrillation. N Engl J Med 347:1834–1840

31. Corley SD, Epstein AE, DiMarco JP et al (2004) AFFIRM Investigators. Relationships between sinus rhythm, treatment, and survival in the Atrial fibrillation follow-up investigation of rhythm management (AFFIRM) study. Circulation 109:1509–1513

32. Roy D, Talajic M, Dorian P et al (2000) Amiodarone to prevent recurrence of atrial fibrillation. Canadian trial of atrial fibrillation investigators. N Engl J Med 342:913–920

33. Singh BN, Singh SN, Reda DJ et al (2005) Sotalol amiodarone atrial fibrillation efficacy trial (SAFE-T) investigators. Amiodarone versus sotalol for atrial fibrillation. N Engl J Med 352:1861–1872

34. Scheinman MM, Morady F, Hess DS, Gonzalez R (1982) Catheter-induced ablation of the atrioventricular junction to control refractory supraventricular arrhythmias. JAMA 248:851–855

35. Kay GN, Ellenbogen KA, Giudici M et al (1998) The ablate and pace trial: a prospective study of catheter ablation of the AV conduction system and permanent pacemaker implantation for treatment of atrial fibrillation. APT investigators. J Interv Card Electrophysiol 2:121–135

36. Doshi RN, Daoud EG, Fellows C et al (2005) PAVE study group. Left ventricular-based cardiac stimulation post AV nodal ablation evaluation (the PAVE study). J Cardiovasc Electrophysiol 16:1160–1165

37. Cox JL, Schuessler RB, Lappas DG et al (1996) An 8 ½ year clinical experience with surgery for atrial fibrillation. Ann Surg 224:267–275

38. Prasad SM, Maniar HS, Camillo CJ et al (2003) The Cox maze III procedure for atrial fibrillation: long-term efficacy in patients undergoing lone versus concomitant procedures. J Thorac Cardiovasc Surg 126:1822–1828

39. Swartz JF, Pellersels G, Silvers J et al (1994) A catheter-based curative approach to atrial fibrillation in humans. Circulation 90:I–335

40. Haissaguerre M, Jais P, Shah DC et al (1996) Right and left atrial radiofrequency catheter therapy of paroxysmal atrial fibrillation. J Cardiovasc Electrophysiol 7:1132–1144

41. Jais P, Shah DC, Haissaguerre M et al (1999) Efficacy and safety of septal and left-atrial linear ablation for atrial fibrillation. Am J Cardiol 84:139R–146R

42. Haissaguerre M, Jais P, Shah DC et al (1998) Spontaneous initiation of atrial fibrillation by ectopic beats originating in the pulmonary veins. N Engl J Med 339:659–666

43. Chen SA, Hsieh MH, Tai CT et al (1999) Initiation of atrial fibrillation by ectopic beats originating from the pulmonary veins: electrophysiological characteristics, pharmacological responses, and effects of radiofrequency ablation. Circulation 100:1879–1886

44. Lin WS, Tai CT, Hsieh MH et al (2003) Catheter ablation of paroxysmal atrial fibrillation initiated by non-pulmonary vein ectopy. Circulation 107:3176–3178

45. Hocini M, Haissaguerre M, Shah D et al (2000) Multiple sources initiating atrial fibrillation from a single pulmonary vein identified by a circumferential catheter. Pacing Clin Electrophysiol 23:1828–1831

46. Haissaguerre M, Shah DC, Jais P et al (2000) Electrophysiological breakthroughs from the left atrium to the pulmonary veins. Circulation 102:2463–2465

47. Marchlinski FE, Callans D, Dixit S et al (2003) Efficacy and safety of targeted focal ablation versus PV isolation assisted by magnetic electroanatomic mapping. J Cardiovasc Electrophysiol 14:358–365

48. Oral H, Knight BP, Tada H et al (2002) Pulmonary vein isolation for paroxysmal and persistent atrial fibrillation. Circulation 105:1077–1081

49. Deisenhofer I, Schneider MA, Bohlen-Knauf M et al (2003) Circumferential mapping and electric isolation of pulmonary veins in patients with atrial fibrillation. Am J Cardiol 91:159–163

50. Marrouche NF, Martin DO, Wazni O et al (2003) Phased-array intracardiac echocardiography monitoring during pulmonary vein isolation in patients with atrial fibrillation: impact on outcome and complications. Circulation 107: 2710–2716

51. Arentz T, von Rosenthal J, Blum T et al (2003) Feasibility and safety of pulmonary vein isolation using a new mapping and navigation system in patients with refractory atrial fibrillation. Circulation 108:2484–2490

52. Oral H, Scharf C, Chugh A et al (2003) Catheter ablation for paroxysmal atrial fibrillation: segmental pulmonary vein ostial ablation versus left atrial ablation. Circulation 108:2355–2360

53. Mansour M, Ruskin J, Keane D (2004) Efficacy and safety of segmental ostial versus circumferential extra-ostial pulmonary vein isolation for atrial fibrillation. J Cardiovasc Electrophysiol 15:532–537

54. Vasamreddy CR, Lickfett L, Jayam VK et al (2004) Predictors of recurrence followingcatheter ablation of atrial fibrillation using an irrigated-tip ablation catheter. J Cardiovasc Electrophysiol 15:692–697

55. Pappone C, Rosanio S, Oreto G et al (2000) Circumferential radiofrequency ablation of pulmonary vein ostia: a new anatomic approach for curing atrial fibrillation. Circulation 102:2619–2628

56. Pappone C, Santinelli V (2004) The who, what, why, and how-to guide for circumferential pulmonary vein ablation. J Cardiovasc Electrophysiol 15:1226–1230

57. Pappone C, Oreto G, Rosanio S et al (2001) Atrial electroanatomic remodeling after circumferential radiofrequency pulmonary vein ablation: efficacy of an anatomic approach in a large cohort of patients with atrial fibrillation. Circulation 104:2539–2544

58. Kottkamp H, Tanner H, Kobza R et al (2004) Time courses and quantitative analysis of atrial fibrillation episode number and duration after circular plus linear left atrial lesions: trigger elimination or substrate modification: early or delayed cure? J Am Coll Cardiol 44:869–877

59. Ouyang F, Baensch D, Ernst S et al (2004) Complete isolation of the left atrium surrounding the pulmonary veins: new insights from the double-lasso technique in paroxysmal atrial fibrillation. Circulation 110:2090–2096

60. Vasamreddy CR, Dalal D, Eldadah Z et al (2005) Safety and efficacy of circumferential pulmonary vein catheter ablation of atrial fibrillation. Heart Rhythm 2:42–48

61. Cappato R, Negroni S, Pecora D et al (2003) Prospective assessment of late conduction recurrence across radiofrequency lesions producing electrical disconnection at the pulmonary vein ostium in patients with atrial fibrillation. Circulation 108:1599–1604

62. Gerstenfeld EP, Callans DJ, Dixit S et al (2003) Incidence and location of focal atrial fibrillation triggers in patients undergoing repeat pulmonary vein isolation: implications for ablation strategies. J Cardiovasc Electrophysiol 14: 685–690

63. Cheema A, Dong J, Dalal D et al (2007) Incidence and time course of early recovery of pulmonary vein conduction after catheter ablation of atrial fibrillation. J Cardiovasc Electrophysiol 18:387–391

64. Jaïs P, Hocini M, Hsu LF et al (2004) Technique and results of linear ablation at the mitral isthmus. Circulation 110:2996–3002

65. Pappone C, Santinelli V, Manguso F et al (2004) Pulmonary vein denervation enhances long-term benefit after circumferential ablation for paroxysmal atrial fibrillation. Circulation 109:327–334

66. Po SS, Nakagawa H, Jackman WM (2009) Localization of left atrial ganglionated plexi in patients with atrial fibrillation. J Cardiovasc Electrophysiol 20:1186–1189

67. Nademanee K, McKenzie J, Kosar E et al (2004) A new approach for catheter ablation of atrial fibrillation: mapping of the electrophysiologic substrate. J Am Coll Cardiol 43:2044–2053

68. Scherr D, Dalal D, Cheema A et al (2009) Long- and short-term temporal stability of complex fractionated atrial electrograms in human left atrium during atrial fibrillation. J Cardiovasc Electrophysiol 20:13–21

69. Nademanee K, Schwab MC, Kosar EM et al (2008) Clinical outcomes of catheter substrate ablation for high-risk patients with atrial fibrillation J Am Coll Cardiol 51:843–849

70. Haïssaguerre M, Hocini M, Sanders P et al (2005) Catheter ablation of long-lasting persistent atrial fibrillation: clinical outcome and mechanisms of subsequent arrhythmias. J Cardiovasc Electrophysiol 16:1138–1147

71. Haïssaguerre M, Sanders P, Hocini M (2005) Catheter ablation of long-lasting persistent atrial fibrillation: critical structures for termination. J Cardiovasc Electrophysiol 16:1125–1137

72. Scherr D, Dalal D, Chilukuri K et al (2009) Incidence and predictors of left atrial thrombus prior to catheter ablation of atrial fibrillation. J Cardiovasc Electrophysiol 20:379–384

73. Valles E, Fan R, Roux JF et al (2008) Localization of atrial fibrillation triggers in patients undergoing pulmonary vein isolation: importance of the carina region. J Am Coll Cardiol 52:1413–1420

74. Cappato R, Calkins H, Chen SA et al (2005) Worldwide survey on the methods, efficacy, and safety of catheter ablation for human atrial fibrillation. Circulation 111:1100–1105

75. Holmes DR Jr, Monahan KH, Packer D (2009) Pulmonary vein stenosis complicating ablation for atrial fibrillation: clinical spectrum and interventional considerations. JACC Cardiovasc Interv 2:267–276

76. Scherr D, Sharma K, Dalal D et al (2009) Incidence and predictors of periprocedural cerebrovascular accident in patients undergoing catheter ablation of atrial fibrillation. J Cardiovasc Electrophysiol. 2009 Jun 30. [Epub ahead of print]

77. Sacher F, Jais P, Stephenson K et al (2007) Phrenic nerve injury after catheter ablation of atrial fibrillation. Indian Pacing Electrophysiol J 7:1–6

78. Cummings JE, Schweikert RA, Saliba WI et al (2006) Brief communication: atrial-esophageal fistulas after radiofrequency ablation. Ann Intern Med 144:572–574

79. Cappato R, Calkins H, Chen SA et al (2009) Prevalence and causes of fatal outcome in catheter ablation of atrial fibrillation. J Am Coll Cardiol 53:1798–1803

80. Krittayaphong R, Raungrattanaamporn O, Bhuripanyo K et al (2003) A randomized clinical trial of the efficacy of radiofrequency catheter ablation and amiodarone in the treatment of symptomatic atrial fibrillation. J Med Assoc Thai 86(Suppl 1):S8–S16

81. Oral H, Pappone C, Chugh A et al (2006) Circumferential pulmonary-vein ablation for chronic atrial fibrillation. N Engl J Med 354:934–941

82. Wazni OM, Marrouche NF, Martin DO et al (2005) Radiofrequency ablation versus antiarrhythmic drugs as first-line treatment for symptomatic atrial fibrillation. J Am Med Assoc 293:2634–2640

83. Stabile G, Bertaglia E, Senatore G et al (2006) Catheter ablation treatment in patients with drug-refractory atrial fibrillation: a prospective, multi-centre, randomized, controlled study (Catheter ablation for the cure of atrial fibrillation study). Eur Heart J 27:216–221

84. Jaïs P, Cauchemez B, Macle L et al (2008) Catheter ablation versus antiarrhythmic drugs for atrial fibrillation: the A4 study. Circulation 118:2498–2505

85. Pappone C, Augello G, Sala S et al (2006) A randomized trial of circumferential pulmonary vein ablation versus antiarrhythmic drug therapy in paroxysmal atrial fibrillation: the APAF (ablation for paroxysmal atrial fibrillation) study. J Am Coll Cardiol 48:2340–2347

86. Nair GM, Nery PB, Diwakaramenon S et al (2009) A systematic review of randomized trials comparing radiofrequency ablation with antiarrhythmic medications in patients with atrial fibrillation. J Cardiovasc Electrophysiol 20:138–144

87. Khan MN, Jaïs P, Cummings J et al (2008) PABA-CHF Investigators. Pulmonary-vein isolation for atrial fibrillation in patients with heart failure. N Engl J Med 359:1778–1785

88. Calkins H, Reynolds MR, Spector P et al (2009) Treatment of atrial fibrillation with antiarrhythmic drugs or radiofrequency ablation: two systematic literature reviews and meta-analyses. Circ Arrhythmia Electrophysiol 2:349–361

89. Ablation Versus Anti-Arrhythmic (AA) Drug Therapy for AF - Pivotal Trial (CABANA). http://www.clinicaltrials.gov/ct2/show/NCT00911508?term=CABANA&rank=1. Accessed July 6, 2010

90. Calkins H, Brugada J, Packer DL et al (2007) HRS/EHRA/ECAS expert consensus statement on catheter and surgical ablation of atrial fibrillation: recommendations for personnel, policy, procedures and follow-up. Heart Rhythm 4: 816–861

91. Neumann T, Vogt J, Schumacher B et al (2008) Circumferential pulmonary vein isolation with the cryoballoon technique results from a prospective 3-center study. J Am Coll Cardiol 52:273–278

92. Wazni OM, Barrett C, Martin DO et al (2009) Experience with the Hansen Robotic system for atrial fibrillation ablation-lessons learned and techniques modified: Hansen in the real world. J Cardiovasc Electrophysiol 20:1193–1196

93. Pappone C, Vicedomini G, Manguso F et al (2006) Robotic magnetic navigation for atrial fibrillation ablation. J Am Coll Cardiol 47:1390–1400

10 Nonsustained Ventricular Tachycardia

Peem Lorvidhaya and Alfred E. Buxton

Contents

Abstract

Nonsustained ventricular tachycardia remains a common management problem in the medical community. Treatment is sometimes needed for the suppression of symptoms. More commonly, nonsustained ventricular tachycardia is asymptomatic and the clinician must determine the prognostic importance. The prognostic implications, the role of electrophysiologic study and other risk stratification strategies, and the potential role of pharmacologic and defibrillator intervention depend on the underlying cardiac substrate present in the individual patient. Currently available data regarding the entity are discussed in this chapter.

Key Words: Nonsustained ventricular tachycardia; ventricular tachycardia; ventricular fibrillation; implantable cardioverter-defibrillator; tachyarrhythmias; cardiac arrest; nonischemic dilated cardiomyopathy; hypertrophic cardiomyopathy; coronary artery disease; triggered activity; torsade de pointes; electrophysiologic study; sudden cardiac death; risk stratification; palpitations; syncope; catheter ablation.

INTRODUCTION

The patient with nonsustained ventricular tachycardia (NSVT) represents a common management problem for physicians. Most tachyarrhythmias come to our attention because of the symptoms they produce. In contrast, most NSVT does not cause symptoms. Rather, it derives its importance from the prognostic significance it carries in some patient populations. Thus, the discovery of NSVT requires the clinician to address the following questions: Is the patient symptomatic from the NSVT? What are the prognostic implications of NSVT in this patient? What interventions are warranted?

A variety of definitions have been used to signify the duration and rate of arrhythmia to qualify as NSVT. Currently, the most commonly used is three or more consecutive ventricular premature

From: *Contemporary Cardiology: Management of Cardiac Arrhythmias*
Edited by: Gan-Xin Yan, Peter R. Kowey, DOI 10.1007/978-1-60761-161-5_10
© Springer Science+Business Media, LLC 2011

depolarizations, up to a maximum duration of 30 sec before spontaneous termination. The most appropriate rate cutoff is greater than 100 beats per minute, based upon the observation that tachycardias having rates less than 100 beats per minute do not carry adverse prognostic significance, at least in persons with coronary artery disease *(1, 2)*.

NSVT is sometimes an important marker of increased risk for subsequent tachyarrhythmias capable of causing syncope, cardiac arrest, or sudden cardiac death. Of note, it is not entirely clear whether episodes of NSVT bear a cause-and-effect relationship with sustained tachyarrhythmias and sudden cardiac death, or if they are simply a surrogate marker of advanced cardiac dysfunction and electrical instability. However, it is clear that the prognostic significance of NSVT depends on the presence, type, and severity of the underlying heart disease. Therefore, in order to treat both the asymptomatic and the symptomatic patients with NSVT properly, the clinician must first have a thorough understanding of the underlying cardiac substrate in a particular patient. The prognosis hinges on whether this is a patient with a structurally normal heart, coronary artery disease with prior myocardial infarction, non-ischemic dilated cardiomyopathy, or hypertrophic cardiomyopathy. Knowing the anatomic substrate as well as the overall left ventricular systolic function determines the prognostic significance of the NSVT, the potential role of programmed electrical stimulation, and the appropriate management of the patient. In addition, the family history may be important for patients with NSVT attributable to ion channelopathies.

PREVALENCE OF NSVT

The prevalence of NSVT in individuals with no apparent cardiac disease is low (1–3%), without any significant difference between men and women *(3–13)*. The prevalence appears to increase with age (up to 11%) independent of the presence of structural heart disease *(8, 14, 15)*.

In patients with coronary artery disease, the prevalence of NSVT varies greatly depending on the disease stage. Patients who have documented chronic coronary artery disease by coronary angiography performed for ischemic symptoms demonstrate NSVT in approximately 5% *(9)*. NSVT has been shown to occur frequently (45%) in the acute phase (less than 48 h) of a myocardial infarction *(16, 17)*, but drops to around 7–16% 2–4 weeks after onset of the acute infarction in the prethrombolytic era *(1, 2, 18–22)*. One study reported NSVT in as many as 75% of patients following thrombolytic therapy *(23)*, which decreases to around 6.8% 2 weeks thereafter *(24)*. The incidence then remains fairly constant over the first year after infarction *(25)*.

The prevalence of NSVT is increased significantly in patients with other structural heart diseases as well, ranging from 20 to 28% in patients with hypertrophic cardiomyopathy *(26–32)*, 2–12% in patients with left ventricular hypertrophy *(33, 34)*, and up to 80% in patients with nonischemic dilated cardiomyopathy *(35–42)*.

PRESENTATIONS

Electrocardiographic

As is the case with sustained ventricular tachycardia, most episodes of NSVT are initiated with late-coupled VPDs *(2, 18, 25, 36, 43–45)* (see Fig. 1) with no clear correlation with the ambient sinus rate *(18, 25, 40, 45)*. The possibility that a nonsustained wide-complex tachycardia is supraventricular with aberrancy in nature also needs to be entertained.

The electrocardiographic morphology of NSVT may be uniform and constant, or polymorphic, varying constantly during individual episodes. There does not appear to be any relationship between the morphologic characteristics and the type of underlying heart disease, except for NSVT arising during

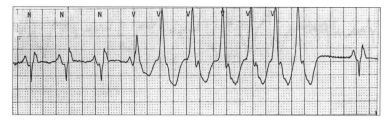

Fig. 1. Typical episode of NSVT in a patient with chronic coronary artery disease. The tachycardia appears to have a uniform morphology in this single monitor lead. The initial complex of the arrhythmia is a late-coupled ventricular premature beat.

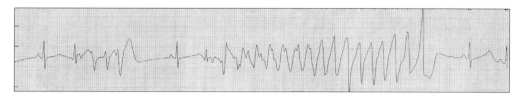

Fig. 2. Polymorphic ventricular tachycardia in the setting of long QT syndrome.

acute myocardial ischemia or in relation to long QT syndrome, which are generally polymorphic in nature (see Fig. 2).

Another group of patients without any apparent structural heart disease presents with a range of arrhythmias including isolated ventricular premature ventricular complexes, nonsustained tachycardia, and rarely, sustained ventricular tachycardia, all having the same morphology of either a left or right bundle branch block pattern with an inferior frontal plane axis *(46–49)* (see Figs. 3 and 4). Endocardial mapping most often localizes the origin of these to be from the right or left ventricular outflow tract, respectively, although tachycardias may arise from other sites *(47, 49)*.

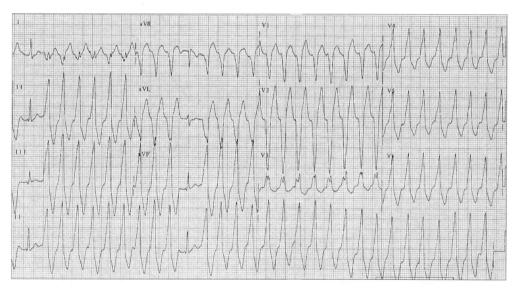

Fig. 3. 12-lead ECG typical of tachycardia originating in the right ventricular outflow tract in a patient without structural heart disease: left bundle branch pattern with an inferiorly-directed frontal plane QRS axis.

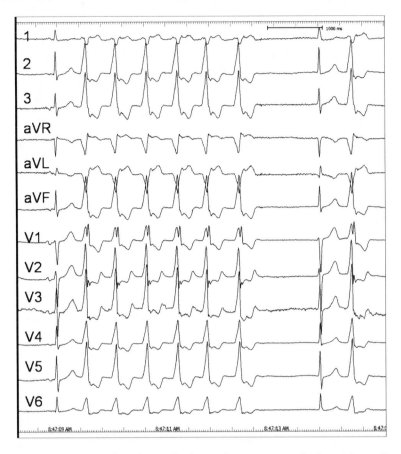

Fig. 4. 12-lead ECG of a left ventricular outflow tract ventricular tachycardia.

Symptoms and Clinical Manifestations

Symptoms related to NSVT are generally nonexistent to mild with palpitations being the most common. NSVT can also cause a pounding sensation in the neck, lightheadedness, or near syncope, potentially related to loss of AV synchrony. NSVT may cause syncope if the rate and duration are prolonged sufficiently to cause a marked decrease in cerebral blood flow. There is great variability as to when the symptoms are most prominent, although a quiet environment may make patients more aware of their episodes. The palpitations that the patient feels may provoke anxiety that many times initiates a vicious cycle of palpitations→anxiety →catecholamine surges→more episodes.

MECHANISMS

Triggered activity seems to be responsible for NSVT development in two principle clinical settings. Early afterdepolarizations arising in Purkinje cells or ventricular myocardium are responsible for the initiation of most episodes of polymorphic ventricular tachycardia (torsade de pointes) associated with congenital or acquired long QT syndrome *(50)*. If repetitive firing allows these afterdepolarizations to reach threshold potential, NSVT can be generated and perpetuate in a reentrant pattern *(51)*. The second setting in which triggered activity appears to be responsible for NSVT is in the syndrome of right ventricular outflow tract arrhythmias *(47)*. Increased intracellular calcium via cyclic AMP has been shown to mediate this type of triggered activity *(52)*.

Other settings in which experimental data suggest focal, non-reentrant mechanisms underlying NSVT are dilated nonischemic and ischemic cardiomyopathies. NSVT in a rabbit model of dilated cardiomyopathy appears to originate in the subendocardium *(53)* as in the canine model of ischemic cardiomyopathy *(54)*.

Reentry accounts for some NSVT in the setting of chronic coronary artery disease. It has been observed that subjects with NSVT and coronary artery disease have endocardial activation abnormalities that are a reflection of slow conduction, one of the prerequisites for reentry *(55)*. It is however important to realize that even in this setting that the mechanisms responsible for NSVT (noted above in experimental models) may differ from those responsible for inducible (and spontaneous) sustained ventricular tachycardia.

CLINICAL SCENARIOS

Structurally Normal Heart

The presence of NSVT in healthy individuals with a structurally normal heart does not correlate with an increased risk of sudden cardiac death *(9, 56)* although NSVT originating from the outflow tracts can be symptomatic and may require therapy to alleviate symptoms. Although rare cases of sudden death associated with these syndromes have been reported, we suspect most of these are related to unrecognized cardiomyopathy, especially right ventricular cardiomyopathy *(57)*.

Nonischemic Dilated Cardiomyopathy

In general, patients with dilated cardiomyopathy are at considerable risk of sudden death. Older studies reported 1-year mortality rates as high as 40–50% *(36, 58–60)*. However, total mortality with modern pharmacologic therapy is much lower, approximating 7% yearly *(61, 62)*. The prognostic significance of NSVT is variable, with little evidence that the occurrence of these arrhythmias is related specifically to an increased risk for sudden death, although they do correlate with increased overall cardiac mortality *(12, 35, 37, 39, 41, 42, 44, 58–60, 63)*. This lack of association may be due to the ubiquitous nature of NSVT in this population and the high overall mortality rates. However, the GESICA investigators found that the relative risk of sudden cardiac death was significantly increased (compared with nonsudden death) in patients with NSVT *(35)*. In contrast, the Veterans Administration trial (CHF–STAT) investigators did not find a specific increased risk for sudden cardiac death associated with NSVT *(39)*. A recent analysis suggests that the prognostic significance of NSVT in patients with dilated cardiomyopathy is dependent on EF. In this analysis, NSVT did not contribute prognostic information to patients with EF ≤35%. However, in patients with EF >35%, there was a threefold increased risk of arrhythmic events *(64)*.

Hypertrophic Cardiomyopathy

Hypertrophic cardiomyopathy is a genetically determined myocardial disease with a diverse natural history. A subset of patients with this disorder is at high risk for SCD *(26, 27)*. In addition to the important historical information (such as a history of syncope, cardiac arrest or a family history of unexpected sudden death in a young person), the presence of NSVT in patients with HCM appears to be a marker of increased risk of sudden death. In selected studies, the annual mortality rate among patients with hypertrophic cardiomyopathy and NSVT was 8–9% each year compared to 1% in patients without NSVT *(27, 28, 31)*. These studies were however done at tertiary referral institutions and these observations tended to include symptomatic patients or relatives of very symptomatic patients. Thus, the data may not be applicable to the majority of patients with this condition. A closer approximation of the risks in this population may be derived from a more recent community-based study where patients with NSVT had a sudden cardiac death incidence of 1.4% yearly compared to 0.6% in patients without NSVT over a 4.8 year follow-up period *(32)*. Thus, NSVT is a marker of increased risk for sudden cardiac death, but the magnitude of the risk assigned to this finding probably also depends on the presence of important clinical risk factors such as symptoms and a family history.

Coronary Artery Disease

Although patients with a myocardial infarction are at risk for reinfarction and related hemodynamic complications, sudden death accounts for 30–50% of deaths after an initial myocardial infarct. It appears that improvements in pharmacologic and mechanical coronary reperfusion strategies have lead to a decrease in the overall 1-year mortality rate after myocardial infarction. Importantly, at least one third of the deaths in the first year after myocardial infarction continue to be sudden and unexpected *(65)*.

The prognostic significance of NSVT with underlying coronary artery disease depends on the time the arrhythmia is discovered in the course of the disease. The occurrence of NSVT during the first 24–48 h of acute myocardial infarction was not thought previously to carry an increased risk for cardiac mortality or sudden death, either in-hospital or long-term *(17, 22, 66)*. However, one analysis demonstrated that the occurrence of NSVT may carry an adverse prognostic significance when it occurs 13 or more hours after the onset of infarction *(67)*.

The occurrence of NSVT in the first month after myocardial infarction more than doubles the risk of subsequent sudden death when compared to patients without NSVT. In the prethrombolytic era, frequent VPDs and NSVT were repeatedly shown to be independent risk factors for both overall cardiac death and sudden death *(2, 18, 68–70)*. NSVT detected 3 months to 1 year post-myocardial infarction is also associated with a significantly higher mortality rate *(71)*. It is important to note that although both the overall incidence of cardiac mortality and sudden death are higher in patients with NSVT, the proportion of sudden death compared to overall cardiac mortality is not increased in patients with frequent ectopy or NSVT *(2, 18, 20)*. This observation raises the question of the specificity of NSVT as a marker for subsequent arrhythmic events rather than a marker for overall poor cardiac function. Therefore, NSVT on the Holter monitor is an important observation, but alone it is not adequately specific in predicting tachyarrhythmic death to effectively guide antiarrhythmic or defibrillator therapy *(72, 73)*.

RISK STRATIFICATION OF PATIENTS WITH NSVT

Electrophysiologic Study

Sustained monomorphic ventricular tachycardia is seldom induced in asymptomatic patients with nonischemic dilated cardiomyopathy, and there is no correlation between inducibility of sustained ventricular tachycardia and subsequent arrhythmic events or total cardiac mortality *(74–78)*. In fact, sudden death occurred more frequently in patients without inducible ventricular tachycardia than in those with inducible arrhythmias. Thus, there appears to be no role for programmed electrical stimulation as a prognostic tool in this group of patients at present. However, a recent study from Germany suggests that ventricular fibrillation induced at EP study may have significant prognostic significance in patients with nonischemic dilated cardiomyopathy. In this study, patients who had survived spontaneous sustained VT or cardiac arrest underwent standard programmed stimulation prior to defibrillator implant. Patients in whom sustained polymorphic VT or VF were induced were significantly more likely to experience subsequent arrhythmias triggering the ICD. Interestingly, induced monomorphic VT did not predict arrhythmic event, consistent with earlier observations *(79)*. Whether similar results would occur in asymptomatic patients undergoing ICD implant for primary prevention of SCD is unclear.

The presence of inducible ventricular tachycardia in high-risk patients with hypertrophic cardiomyopathy indicates a poorer prognosis over a 28-month follow-up period *(80)*. In the subset of patients with NSVT on Holter monitoring, those who did not have induced sustained ventricular tachycardia had a 3% mortality compared to a 20% mortality in inducible patients. However, this study involved a highly selected population of patients, with the majority having survived episodes of cardiac arrest, syncope, or having a strong family history for sudden death. Thus it is not clear whether inducible ventricular tachycardia has independent prognostic utility in asymptomatic patients with a negative family history for sudden death. One other finding at electrophysiologic study has been suggested to have prognostic utility in this setting. Two groups of investigators have noted a correlation between the history of cardiac arrest and the development of fractionated electrograms in response to ventricular stimulation in this setting *(81, 82)*.

The results of programmed electrical stimulation in patients with coronary artery disease and NSVT are more encouraging. Programmed electrical stimulation appears capable of stratifying the risk for future sudden death in patients with a depressed ejection fraction and NSVT. Many earlier studies were limited in their ability to demonstrate the positive predictive value of inducible sustained ventricular tachycardia by virtue of small sample sizes and the lack of treatment control *(83–86)*. These earlier studies, although small, did suggest that patients with NSVT and EF >40% were at relatively low sudden death risk.

The Multicenter UnSustained Tachycardia Trial (MUSTT) enrolled 2202 patients with coronary artery disease, asymptomatic NSVT, and left ventricular ejection fraction ≤40%. Seven hundred and four patients with sustained tachyarrhythmias induced by programmed stimulation were randomized to either no antiarrhythmic therapy or EPS-guided therapy *(87)*. EPS-guided therapy included pharmacologic antiarrhythmic therapy and implantable defibrillators as indicated. Importantly, this trial included a broad group of patients studied and treated in both academic/tertiary care centers and private practice settings, suggesting that the findings are broadly applicable.

In MUSTT, inducible VT on EPS in untreated patients was associated with a 2-year risk of cardiac arrest or death from arrhythmia of 18%, which was statistically different from registry patients without inducible sustained VT (12%). The 2-year rate of overall mortality was also higher in the positive EPS group (28%) compared with the registry group (21%) *(88)*.

The risk of cardiac arrest or death from arrhythmia among patients who received treatment with defibrillators in the MUSTT study was significantly lower than those who did not receive defibrillator treatment (relative risk, 0.24; 95% confidence interval, 0.13–0.45; $p<0.001$) *(87)*. On the other hand, patients assigned to electrophysiology-guided therapy who were treated with only pharmacologic antiarrhythmic therapy had a similar rate of death and cardiac arrest to those in the control group who had not been treated with antiarrhythmic therapy. Thus, this study suggests that programmed stimulation not only carries prognostic significance, but can be used to guide the use of implantable defibrillators in patients with coronary disease and EF≤40%. Two other recent studies demonstrated similar results *(89, 90)*. Although not limited to patients with NSVT, many of the patients in these studies did have NSVT, and it seems likely results would be similar if only patients with NSVT were studied.

Signal-Averaged Electrocardiography

The signal-averaged electrocardiogram is a noninvasive test that identifies low-amplitude, high-frequency signals originating in myocardial regions in which slow conduction results in delayed activation. These signals have been correlated with the presence of inducible sustained ventricular tachycardia. Although a variety of techniques have been used, including analysis of signals in both the time and frequency domain, most data in this patient population have been derived using time domain signal processing techniques. The signal-averaged electrocardiographic variables that have been examined are the filtered QRS duration, the presence of late potentials (signals in the terminal 40 msec of the filtered QRS complex having a mean amplitude of less than 20–25 mV) and the duration of the low-amplitude signal in the terminal 40 msec of the filtered QRS complex.

Studies of heterogeneous patient populations with NSVT and/or complex ventricular ectopy show correlation of abnormal signal-averaged electrocardiograms with inducibility of sustained ventricular tachycardia with 92–100% sensitivity and 75–88% specificity *(91, 92)*. The negative predictive accuracy in predicting inducibility has been reported at 91% *(93, 94)*.

No study has directly examined the potential correlation between the signal-averaged electrocardiogram and sudden death in patients with NSVT and nonischemic dilated cardiomyopathy, although two groups have tried to examine the role of this test in patients with advanced congestive heart failure due to nonischemic dilated cardiomyopathy *(95, 96)*. Only one study found a fair correlation between abnormalities of the conventional time-domain signal-averaged electrocardiogram and subsequent sudden death *(95)*. The prognostic utility of the signal-averaged electrocardiogram in this population thus remains unclear.

Several earlier studies suggested that the signal-averaged electrocardiogram may identify patients with prior myocardial infarction likely to have ventricular tachycardia inducible by programmed stimulation *(70, 92–94, 97)*. Initial data from the MUSTT trial showed a poor correlation with the presence of inducible sustained ventricular tachycardia. However, preliminary analysis correlating abnormalities of the signal-averaged electrocardiogram with survival in the same trial suggest that this test may actually prove to be quite useful for risk stratification in this population *(98)*.

TREATMENT

There is a wide range of therapeutic options for patients with NSVT. The initial step is to establish whether there is any underlying structural heart disease and, if so, determine if the finding has a cause-and-effect relationship with NSVT. Once an underlying disease is identified, an appropriate risk stratification strategy needs to be carried out. The second major piece of information required is the determination of whether NSVT causes symptoms that require treatment. It is important to keep these two points separate in one's mind, because treatment aimed at relieving symptoms is quite different than treatment aimed at reducing risk of sudden death.

Structurally Normal Heart

In patients with grossly normal hearts, correlation of the symptoms and their arrhythmias is the initial step in deciding whether to initiate therapy. Repeated ECG monitoring may be needed to ascertain whether symptoms such as palpitations are indeed due to this arrhythmia since these patients appear to be at very low risk of sudden cardiac death. There is some accumulating evidence for occult pathology in apparently normal subjects who develop outflow tract tachycardias in this setting *(99–101)*. Patients with RVOT ventricular tachycardia might have subtle structural and functional abnormalities of the outflow tract as detected by magnetic resonance imaging *(99)* and the diagnosis of RVOT ventricular tachycardia needs to be differentiated from the diagnosis of arrhythmogenic right ventricular dysplasia *(102)*.

The first step is to explain the nature of the arrhythmia and its excellent overall prognosis. After such a discussion, the patient often feels relieved and reassurance alone is often adequate in the minimally symptomatic patient. Should a patient have significant symptoms and require pharmacologic intervention, beta-blocking agents are effective in up to 50% *(46–48, 103)*. Verapamil, propafenone, and amiodarone have also been used with varying degrees of success *(46–48)*. If a symptomatic patient with this type of arrhythmia does not respond to beta-blocker or calcium-blocker therapy, electrophysiology study and catheter ablation should be offered. In this setting, catheter ablation is successful in over 80% of cases with a low associated risk profile *(84, 104)*.

Structurally Abnormal Heart

In asymptomatic patients with structural heart disease, the potential indication for treatment is to reduce the risk of sudden death that has been associated with the presence of NSVT. In this case it is important to understand what is being treated. For prevention of sudden death, one does not necessarily need to suppress NSVT, as this in itself is not lethal. Rather, one is treating a presumed substrate for sustained tachyarrhythmias with which NSVT is associated.

Medical therapy remains the cornerstone of therapy for both ischemic and nonischemic cardiomyopathy. Specific beta-blockers, i.e., metoprolol succinate *(105)*, carvedilol *(106)*, and bisoprolol *(107)* have been shown to reduce mortality substantially. Nebivolol given to the elderly in heart failure reduced hospitalization but not mortality *(108)*. ACE inhibitors have also been shown to reduce mortality in these patients, with conflicting data whether they truly reduce the rate of sudden death or work more so through a decrease in worsening heart failure *(109–114)*. ARBs are largely equivalent in terms of mortality reduction from heart failure although there is some evidence that they may have less benefit in decreasing the rate of sudden cardiac death *(115)*. Major trials regarding aldosterone antagonists (aldactone *(116)* and eplerenone *(117)*) have shown significant decreases in sudden cardiac death compared with placebo (36 and 21%, respectively). Although not specifically studied in patients with CHF and NSVT, digoxin has been shown to have no mortality benefit, with a nonsignificant increase in arrhythmic death *(118)*.

THE ROLE OF ANTIARRHYTHMIC DRUGS

The prophylactic use of antiarrhythmic agents in patients with congestive heart failure has been discouraging. The Veterans Administration Heart Failure Trial (CHF-STAT) studied the effects of empiric therapy with amiodarone versus placebo in 666 patients (70% ischemic, 30% nonischemic cardiomyopathy) with nearly 80% of the study population having had NSVT on ambulatory monitoring *(119)*. The effect of amiodarone on survival in this study was neutral, even in patients with documented NSVT. One noteworthy aspect of these results is the fact that amiodarone did effectively suppress ventricular ectopy and although amiodarone had no beneficial effect on survival in the patients with coronary artery disease, there was a trend toward an improvement in survival with nonischemic cardiomyopathy patients. The GESICA trial *(120)*, which compared amiodarone with standard medical therapy, on the other hand, found significant reductions in overall mortality (28%), sudden cardiac death (27%), and death from heart failure (31%). This trial differed from the CHF-STAT study in that patients were not required to have arrhythmias to gain entry (although two-thirds of the patients did have NSVT) and congestive heart failure was attributed to coronary artery disease in only 39%.

Holter-guided pharmacologic therapy in an attempt to reduce the risk of sudden death in the setting of NSVT and coronary artery disease has been disappointing. The CAST (Cardiac Arrhythmia Suppression Trial) evaluated encainide, flecainide, and moricizine in survivors of recent myocardial infarction with frequent PVCs or NSVT *(72, 73)*. In order to be randomized, patients had to have demonstrated suppression of ventricular ectopy and NSVT with antiarrhythmic therapy. Although ventricular ectopy and NSVT were suppressed, the overall outcome was discouraging. Patients in this study in the treatment group receiving type IC antiarrhythmic therapy had a 4.5% incidence of sudden cardiac death compared to 1.2% in the placebo control group *(72)*. This finding suggests that suppression of NSVT or PVCs alone is not a meaningful endpoint and does not correlate with the overall effect on mortality. However, it is also possible that the observations of CAST relate to the toxicity of specific antiarrhythmic drugs; and if drugs could be identified that suppressed VPDs and

NSVT without the harmful effects of sodium channel blocking agents, mortality might be improved. Against this possibility are the results of trials with amiodarone.

Subsequently, the European Myocardial Infarction Amiodarone Trial (EMIAT) *(121)* enrolled patients with recent infarction and left ventricular ejection fraction ≤ 0.40 without screening for ventricular ectopy. The Canadian Myocardial Infarction Amiodarone Trial (CAMIAT) *(122)* on the other hand enrolled patients with recent infarction, frequent (≥ 10 VPDs/h) or NSVT, without regard for left ventricular ejection fraction. Patients were randomized to therapy with empiric amiodarone or conventional therapy alone. In each case, amiodarone had a neutral effect on total mortality, but did reduce the risk of sudden death. Thus, empiric therapy with amiodarone cannot be relied upon improving survival in high-risk patients with recent myocardial infarction. However, as there was no adverse effect on survival (as had been observed during earlier trials with Type I antiarrhythmic agents), it can be regarded as relatively safe to suppress other symptomatic arrhythmias, such as atrial fibrillation.

Several earlier nonrandomized, uncontrolled observational studies suggested that the response to antiarrhythmic therapy guided by programmed stimulation in patients with NSVT and coronary artery disease might be of significant value in improving survival *(83–86)*. The Multicenter UnSustained Tachycardia Trial (MUSTT) randomized 704 patients having inducible sustained ventricular tachycardia equally between two therapy arms *(87)*. The control group that received no antiarrhythmic treatment experienced a 32% arrhythmic death/arrest rate at 5 years. The active treatment group received antiarrhythmic therapy guided by electrophysiologic testing. The relative risk of arrhythmic events in the latter group was reduced by 27% (absolute risk reduction, 7%) in comparison to the group that received no antiarrhythmic therapy. A second significant finding of this study was the fact that pharmacologic antiarrhythmic therapy guided by electrophysiologic testing conferred no survival benefit. The improvement in survival associated with electrophysiologically guided therapy was due entirely to treatment with implantable defibrillators, which will be discussed below.

The Role of Implantable Cardioverter Defibrillators

CORONARY ARTERY DISEASE

Three landmark trials investigated the use of prophylactic ICD implantation specifically in this patient group. The MUSTT investigators *(87)* randomized 704 patients to electrophysiologically guided antiarrhythmic therapy versus no antiarrhythmic therapy. Patients randomized to EP-guided therapy were started on antiarrhythmic drugs (class I, sotalol, or amiodarone) and retested. If a patient had at least one unsuccessful drug test after suitable loading period (four to five half-lives), a defibrillator could be implanted. Ultimately, 46% of patients randomized to EP-guided therapy received a defibrillator. In this trial, EP-guided therapy was associated with a significant reduction in cardiac arrest or death from arrhythmia at 5 years of 27% ($P = 0.04$). The overall 2- and 5-year mortality rates for the EP-guided group were 22% and 42%, compared with the no antiarrhythmic therapy group, which were 28% and 48% ($P = 0.06$). The benefit of EP-guided therapy was solely attributable to defibrillators. Five-year rates of cardiac arrest or arrhythmic death were 9% in EP-guided therapy with ICD versus 37% in the EP-guided therapy without ICD ($P < 0.001$). The 5-year mortality was 24% versus 55% in the same groups, respectively. The adjusted relative risk of arrhythmic events and overall mortality for patients with ICDs and without were 0.24 (95% CI 0.13–0.45) and 0.40 (95% CI 0.27–0.059), respectively. These results are consistent with those of the MADIT I trial *(123)*, which randomized 196 patients with previous myocardial infarction, LVEF $\leq 35\%$, documented NSVT, and inducible VT on EPS despite procainamide. The primary endpoint in this trial was total mortality, rather than sudden death. Patients randomized to defibrillator therapy in this trial experienced a 54% reduction in total mortality, compared to patients randomized to pharmacologic therapy. The 2-year total mortality of 32% in patients randomized to the conventional (pharmacologic) therapy arm was very similar to that of patients in the MUSTT study randomized to no antiarrhythmic therapy (28%).

The mortality of the control group in MADIT I was also similar to that observed in MUSTT patients randomized to EP-guided antiarrhythmic therapy who were not treated with a defibrillator – 33%.

Finally, the MADIT II Trial *(124)* subsequently dropped both NSVT and inducibility of VT using EPS from its entry criteria, and found that post-MI patients with LVEF $\leq$ 30% benefit from prophylactic ICD implantation (HR for death = 0.69; P = 0.016).

Based on these results, guidelines emerged suggesting it is reasonable to implant a defibrillator in patients with coronary artery disease after 40 days of a documented MI with class II–III heart failure and LVEF $\leq$ 35%. In patients with class I symptoms, the LVEF cutoff of 30% is utilized. On the other hand, patients with NSVT and LVEF between 35% and 40% should undergo an electrophysiologic study to further delineate their risks.

Nonischemic Dilated Cardiomyopathy

The DEFINITE trial enrolled patients with nonischemic cardiomyopathy, symptomatic CHF, LVEF $\leq$ 35%, and NSVT (or at least 10 PVCs/h) to empiric defibrillator therapy (with adequate background medical therapy) versus medical therapy along. This showed an 80% reduction in arrhythmic death, but a nonsignificant 35% reduction in overall mortality (P = 0.08) *(61)*. More recently, SCD-HeFT showed a statistically significant 23% relative mortality benefit favoring prophylactic ICD therapy over amiodarone and placebo in patients with class II or III heart failure (45% nonischemic) with an LVEF $\leq$ 35% *(62)*. Of note, this trial did not require NSVT for enrollment.

SPECIFIC DISORDER

Hypertrophic Cardiomyopathy

The benefit of antiarrhythmics in the setting of hypertrophic cardiomyopathy remains controversial. One study reported a possible benefit of amiodarone over conventional antiarrhythmics in patients with hypertrophic cardiomyopathy and ventricular tachycardia *(125)*. However, another study showed that amiodarone can cause conduction abnormalities and facilitate induction of VT in others *(126)*. Further, long-term use of amiodarone may be limited by the unacceptable side effects among younger patients with this disorder.

Implantable cardioverter-defibrillator therapy has emerged as an important component of care for this patient population. In patients with a history of syncope, a family history of sudden death, or NSVT, there was a 5% per year "appropriate" discharge rate for presumed ventricular tachycardia or ventricular fibrillation *(127)*. On the other hand, there was an 11% per year rate of "appropriate" discharges in patients who had defibrillators placed for secondary prevention after resuscitation from cardiac arrest (with documented ventricular fibrillation) or sustained ventricular tachycardia. By extrapolation, this suggests that 50% of patients at 10 years with a defibrillator would have an "appropriate discharge" (presumably preventing sudden death from ventricular tachycardia or ventricular fibrillation). More than a third of the patients who had an appropriate discharge of the defibrillator were on amiodarone, underscoring the imperfect protection of amiodarone in these patients.

Several important questions in this patient population remain unanswered. Precise identification of patients for whom the risk of sudden death is high enough to warrant intervention remains a central issue. For example, is a defibrillator warranted in a patient with hypertrophic cardiomyopathy and only NSVT as a risk factor? Advances in our understanding of the molecular basis of this disorder as well as genetic markers of increased risk of sudden cardiac death may play a role in identifying patients at highest risk. For now, it is clear that further prospective studies are needed to further clarify the role of electrophysiologic study and defibrillator therapy in this patient group.

CONCLUSIONS

The approach to patients with NSVT depends on the presence of symptoms and the underlying substrate. Treatment is sometimes needed for suppression of symptoms, and beta-adrenergic blocking agents are usually the first choice. However, NSVT is most commonly asymptomatic, especially in patients with significant ventricular dysfunction. In such cases the clinician must determine the prognostic significance, the role of EP study and other risk stratification tests, as well as defibrillator therapy. The role of such interventions depends largely on the underlying cardiac substrate.

REFERENCES

1. Denes P, Gillis AM, Pawitan Y et al (1991) Prevalence, characteristics and significance of ventricular premature complexes and ventricular tachycardia detected by 24-hour continuous electrocardiographic recording in the Cardiac Arrhythmia Suppression Trial. CAST Investigators. Am J Cardiol 68(9):887–896
2. Anderson KP, DeCamilla J, Moss AJ (1978) Clinical significance of ventricular tachycardia (3 beats or longer) detected during ambulatory monitoring after myocardial infarction. Circulation 57(5):890–897
3. Fleg JL, Lakatta EG (1984) Prevalence and prognosis of exercise-induced nonsustained ventricular tachycardia in apparently healthy volunteers. Am J Cardiol 54(7):762–764
4. Marinchak RA, Rials SJ, Filart RA et al (1997) The top ten fallacies of nonsustained ventricular tachycardia. Pacing Clin Electrophysiol 20(11):2825–2847
5. McHenry PL, Fisch C, Jordan JW et al (1972) Cardiac arrhythmias observed during maximal treadmill exercise testing in clinically normal men. Am J Cardiol 29(3):331–336
6. Sobotka PA, Mayer JH, Bauernfeind RA et al (1981) Arrhythmias documented by 24-hour continuous ambulatory electrocardiographic monitoring in young women without apparent heart disease. Am Heart J 101(6):753–759
7. Romhilt DW, Chaffin C, Choi SC et al (1984) Arrhythmias on ambulatory electrocardiographic monitoring in women without apparent heart disease. Am J Cardiol 54(6):582–586
8. Brodsky M, Wu D, Denes P et al (1977) Arrhythmias documented by 24 hour continuous electrocardiographic monitoring in 50 male medical students without apparent heart disease. Am J Cardiol 39(3):390–395
9. Califf RM, McKinnis RA, Burks J et al (1982) Prognostic implications of ventricular arrhythmias during 24 hour ambulatory monitoring in patients undergoing cardiac catheterization for coronary artery disease. Am J Cardiol 50(1):23–31
10. Hinkle LE, Jr., Carver ST, Stevens M (1969) The frequency of asymptomatic disturbances of cardiac rhythm and conduction in middle-aged men. Am J Cardiol 24(5):629–650
11. Kantelip JP, Sage E, Duchene-Marullaz P (1986) Findings on ambulatory electrocardiographic monitoring in subjects older than 80 years. Am J Cardiol 57(6):398–401
12. Pantano JA, Oriel RJ (1982) Prevalence and nature of cardiac arrhythmias in apparently normal well-trained runners. Am Heart J 104(4 Pt 1):762–768
13. Pilcher GF, Cook AJ, Johnston BL et al (1983) Twenty-four-hour continuous electrocardiography during exercise and free activity in 80 apparently healthy runners. Am J Cardiol 52(7):859–861
14. Hiss RG, Lamb LE (1962) Electrocardiographic findings in 122,043 individuals. Circulation 25:947–961
15. Wajngarten M, Grupi C, Bellotti GM et al (1990) Frequency and significance of cardiac rhythm disturbances in healthy elderly individuals. J Electrocardiol 23(2):171–176
16. Campbell RW, Murray A, Julian DG (1981) Ventricular arrhythmias in first 12 hours of acute myocardial infarction. Natural history study. Br Heart J 46(4):351–357
17. de Soyza N, Bennett FA, Murphy ML et al (1978) The relationship of paroxysmal ventricular tachycardia complicating the acute phase and ventricular arrhythmia during the late hospital phase of myocardial infarction to long-term survival. Am J Med 64(3):377–381
18. Bigger JT, Jr., Weld FM, Rolnitzky LM (1981) Prevalence, characteristics and significance of ventricular tachycardia (three or more complexes) detected with ambulatory electrocardiographic recording in the late hospital phase of acute myocardial infarction. Am J Cardiol 48(5):815–823
19. Cats VM, Lie KI, Van Capelle FJ et al (1979) Limitations of 24 hour ambulatory electrocardiographic recording in predicting coronary events after acute myocardial infarction. Am J Cardiol 44(7):1257–1262
20. Kleiger RE, Miller JP, Thanavaro S et al (1981) Relationship between clinical features of acute myocardial infarction and ventricular runs 2 weeks to 1 year after infarction. Circulation 63(1):64–70
21. Schulze RA, Jr., Strauss HW, Pitt B (1977) Sudden death in the year following myocardial infarction. Relation to ventricular premature contractions in the late hospitals phase and left ventricular ejection fraction. Am J Med 62(2):192–199

22. Vismara LA, Amsterdam EA, Mason DT (1975) Relation of ventricular arrhythmias in the late hospital phase of acute myocardial infarction to sudden death after hospital discharge. Am J Med 59(1):6–12

23. Heidbuchel H, Tack J, Vanneste L et al (1994) Significance of arrhythmias during the first 24 hours of acute myocardial infarction treated with alteplase and effect of early administration of a beta-blocker or a bradycardiac agent on their incidence. Circulation 89(3):1051–1059

24. Maggioni AP, Zuanetti G, Franzosi MG et al (1993) Prevalence and prognostic significance of ventricular arrhythmias after acute myocardial infarction in the fibrinolytic era. GISSI-2 results. Circulation 87(2):312–322

25. Moller M, Nielsen BL, Fabricius J (1980) Paroxysmal ventricular tachycardia during repeated 24-hour ambulatory electrocardiographic monitoring of postmyocardial infarction patients. Br Heart J 43(4):447–453

26. Maron BJ, Casey SA, Poliac LC et al (1999) Clinical course of hypertrophic cardiomyopathy in a regional United States cohort. JAMA 281(7):650–655

27. Maron BJ, Savage DD, Wolfson JK et al (1981) Prognostic significance of 24 hour ambulatory electrocardiographic monitoring in patients with hypertrophic cardiomyopathy: a prospective study. Am J Cardiol 48(2):252–257

28. McKenna WJ, Camm AJ (1989) Sudden death in hypertrophic cardiomyopathy. Assessment of patients at high risk. Circulation 80(5):1489–1492

29. Mulrow JP, Healy MJ, McKenna WJ (1986) Variability of ventricular arrhythmias in hypertrophic cardiomyopathy and implications for treatment. Am J Cardiol 58(7):615–618

30. Newman H, Sugrue D, Oakley CM et al (1985) Relation of left ventricular function and prognosis in hypertrophic cardiomyopathy: an angiographic study. J Am Coll Cardiol 5(5):1064–1074

31. Savage DD, Seides SF, Maron BJ et al (1979) Prevalence of arrhythmias during 24-hour electrocardiographic monitoring and exercise testing in patients with obstructive and nonobstructive hypertrophic cardiomyopathy. Circulation 59(5):866–875

32. Spirito P, Rapezzi C, Autore C et al (1994) Prognosis of asymptomatic patients with hypertrophic cardiomyopathy and nonsustained ventricular tachycardia. Circulation 90(6):2743–2747

33. Levy D, Anderson KM, Savage DD et al (1987) Risk of ventricular arrhythmias in left ventricular hypertrophy: the Framingham heart study. Am J Cardiol 60(7):560–565

34. Pringle SD, Dunn FG, Macfarlane PW et al (1992) Significance of ventricular arrhythmias in systemic hypertension with left ventricular hypertrophy. Am J Cardiol 69(9):913–917

35. Doval HC, Nul DR, Grancelli HO et al (1996) Nonsustained ventricular tachycardia in severe heart failure. Independent marker of increased mortality due to sudden death. GESICA-GEMA investigators. Circulation 94(12):3198–3203

36. Huang SK, Messer JV, Denes P (1983) Significance of ventricular tachycardia in idiopathic dilated cardiomyopathy: observations in 35 patients. Am J Cardiol 51(3):507–512

37. Neri R, Mestroni L, Salvi A et al (1986) Arrhythmias in dilated cardiomyopathy. Postgrad Med J 62(728):593–597

38. Olshausen KV, Stienen U, Schwarz F et al (1988) Long-term prognostic significance of ventricular arrhythmias in idiopathic dilated cardiomyopathy. Am J Cardiol 61(1):146–151

39. Singh SN, Fisher SG, Carson PE et al (1998) Prevalence and significance of nonsustained ventricular tachycardia in patients with premature ventricular contractions and heart failure treated with vasodilator therapy. Department of veterans affairs CHF STAT investigators. J Am Coll Cardiol 32(4):942–947

40. Suyama A, Anan T, Araki H et al (1986) Prevalence of ventricular tachycardia in patients with different underlying heart diseases: a study by Holter ECG monitoring. Am Heart J 112(1):44–51

41. Teerlink JR, Jalaluddin M, Anderson S et al (2000) Ambulatory ventricular arrhythmias in patients with heart failure do not specifically predict an increased risk of sudden death. PROMISE (prospective randomized milrinone survival evaluation) investigators. Circulation 101(1):40–46

42. Unverferth DV, Magorien RD, Moeschberger ML et al (1984) Factors influencing the one-year mortality of dilated cardiomyopathy. Am J Cardiol 54(1):147–152

43. Berger MD, Waxman HL, Buxton AE et al (1988) Spontaneous compared with induced onset of sustained ventricular tachycardia. Circulation 78(4):885–892

44. Thanavaro S, Kleiger RE, Miller JP et al (1983) Coupling interval and types of ventricular ectopic activity associated with ventricular runs. Am Heart J 106(3):484–491

45. Winkle RA, Derrington DC, Schroeder JS (1977) Characteristics of ventricular tachycardia in ambulatory patients. Am J Cardiol 39(4):487–492

46. Buxton AE, Marchlinski FE, Doherty JU et al (1984) Repetitive, monomorphic ventricular tachycardia: clinical and electrophysiologic characteristics in patients with and patients without organic heart disease. Am J Cardiol 54(8):997–1002

47. Buxton AE, Waxman HL, Marchlinski FE et al (1983) Right ventricular tachycardia: clinical and electrophysiologic characteristics. Circulation 68(5):917–927

48. Ritchie AH, Kerr CR, Qi A et al (1989) Nonsustained ventricular tachycardia arising from the right ventricular outflow tract. Am J Cardiol 64(10):594–598

49. Callans DJ, Menz V, Schwartzman D et al (1997) Repetitive monomorphic tachycardia from the left ventricular outflow tract: electrocardiographic patterns consistent with a left ventricular site of origin. J Am Coll Cardiol 29(5):1023–1027

50. Roden DM, Lazzara R, Rosen M et al (1996) Multiple mechanisms in the long-QT syndrome. Current knowledge, gaps, and future directions. The SADS foundation task force on LQTS. Circulation 94(8):1996–2012

51. el-Sherif N, Turitto G (1999) The long QT syndrome and torsade de pointes. Pacing Clin Electrophysiol 22(1 Pt 1): 91–110

52. Lerman BB, Stein K, Engelstein ED et al (1995) Mechanism of repetitive monomorphic ventricular tachycardia. Circulation 92(3):421–429

53. Pogwizd SM (1995) Nonreentrant mechanisms underlying spontaneous ventricular arrhythmias in a model of nonischemic heart failure in rabbits. Circulation 92(4):1034–1048

54. Pogwizd SM (1994) Focal mechanisms underlying ventricular tachycardia during prolonged ischemic cardiomyopathy. Circulation 90(3):1441–1458

55. Buxton AE, Kleiman RB, Kindwall KE et al (1993) Endocardial mapping during sinus rhythm in patients with coronary artery disease and nonsustained ventricular tachycardia. Am J Cardiol 71(8):695–698

56. Kennedy HL, Underhill SJ (1976) Frequent or complex ventricular ectopy in apparently healthy subjects: a clinical study of 25 cases. Am J Cardiol 38(2):141–148

57. Tada H, Ohe T, Yutani C et al (1996) Sudden death in a patient with apparent idiopathic ventricular tachycardia. Jpn Circ J 60(2):133–136

58. Holmes J, Kubo SH, Cody RJ et al (1985) Arrhythmias in ischemic and nonischemic dilated cardiomyopathy: prediction of mortality by ambulatory electrocardiography. Am J Cardiol 55(1):146–151

59. Gradman A, Deedwania P, Cody R et al (1989) Predictors of total mortality and sudden death in mild to moderate heart failure. Captopril-Digoxin study group. J Am Coll Cardiol 14(3):564–570; discussion 571–562

60. Wilson JR, Schwartz JS, Sutton MS et al (1983) Prognosis in severe heart failure: relation to hemodynamic measurements and ventricular ectopic activity. J Am Coll Cardiol 2(3):403–410

61. Kadish A, Dyer A, Daubert JP et al (2004) Prophylactic defibrillator implantation in patients with nonischemic dilated cardiomyopathy. N Engl J Med 350(21):2151–2158

62. Bardy GH, Lee KL, Mark DB et al (2005) Amiodarone or an implantable cardioverter-defibrillator for congestive heart failure. N Engl J Med 352(3):225–237

63. Meinertz T, Hofmann T, Kasper W et al (1984) Significance of ventricular arrhythmias in idiopathic dilated cardiomyopathy. Am J Cardiol 53(7):902–907

64. Zecchin M, Di Lenarda A, Gregori D et al (2008) Are nonsustained ventricular tachycardias predictive of major arrhythmias in patients with dilated cardiomyopathy on optimal medical treatment? Pacing Clin Electrophysiol 31(3):290–299

65. Rouleau JL, Talajic M, Sussex B et al (1996) Myocardial infarction patients in the 1990s–their risk factors, stratification and survival in Canada: the Canadian assessment of myocardial infarction (CAMI) study. J Am Coll Cardiol 27(5):1119–1127

66. Eldar M, Sievner Z, Goldbourt U et al (1992) Primary ventricular tachycardia in acute myocardial infarction: clinical characteristics and mortality. The SPRINT study group. Ann Intern Med 117(1):31–36

67. Cheema AN, Sheu K, Parker M et al (1998) Nonsustained ventricular tachycardia in the setting of acute myocardial infarction: tachycardia characteristics and their prognostic implications. Circulation 98(19):2030–2036

68. Bigger JT, Jr., Fleiss JL, Rolnitzky LM (1986) Prevalence, characteristics and significance of ventricular tachycardia detected by 24-hour continuous electrocardiographic recordings in the late hospital phase of acute myocardial infarction. Am J Cardiol 58(13):1151–1160

69. Bigger JT, Jr., Fleiss JL, Kleiger R et al (1984) The relationships among ventricular arrhythmias, left ventricular dysfunction, and mortality in the 2 years after myocardial infarction. Circulation 69(2):250–258

70. Gomes JA, Winters SL, Stewart D et al (1987) A new noninvasive index to predict sustained ventricular tachycardia and sudden death in the first year after myocardial infarction: based on signal-averaged electrocardiogram, radionuclide ejection fraction and Holter monitoring. J Am Coll Cardiol 10(2):349–357

71. Hallstrom AP, Bigger JT, Jr., Roden D et al (1992) Prognostic significance of ventricular premature depolarizations measured 1 year after myocardial infarction in patients with early postinfarction asymptomatic ventricular arrhythmia. J Am Coll Cardiol 20(2):259–264

72. Preliminary Report (1989) Effect of encainide and flecainide on mortality in a randomized trial of arrhythmia suppression after myocardial infarction. The cardiac arrhythmia suppression trial (CAST) investigators. N Engl J Med 321(6):406–412

73. Effect of the antiarrhythmic agent moricizine on survival after myocardial infarction (1992) The cardiac arrhythmia suppression trial II investigators. N Engl J Med 327(4):227–233

74. Das SK, Morady F, DiCarlo L Jr et al (1986) Prognostic usefulness of programmed ventricular stimulation in idiopathic dilated cardiomyopathy without symptomatic ventricular arrhythmias. Am J Cardiol 58(10):998–1000

75. Grimm W, Hoffmann J, Menz V et al (1998) Programmed ventricular stimulation for arrhythmia risk prediction in patients with idiopathic dilated cardiomyopathy and nonsustained ventricular tachycardia. J Am Coll Cardiol 32(3):739–745

76. Meinertz T, Treese N, Kasper W et al (1985) Determinants of prognosis in idiopathic dilated cardiomyopathy as determined by programmed electrical stimulation. Am J Cardiol 56(4):337–341

77. Poll DS, Marchlinski FE, Buxton AE et al (1986) Usefulness of programmed stimulation in idiopathic dilated cardiomyopathy. Am J Cardiol 58(10):992–997

78. Stamato NJ, O'Connell JB, Murdock DK et al (1986) The response of patients with complex ventricular arrhythmias secondary to dilated cardiomyopathy to programmed electrical stimulation. Am Heart J 112(3):505–508

79. Rolf S, Haverkamp W, Borggrefe M et al (2009) Induction of ventricular fibrillation rather than ventricular tachycardia predicts tachyarrhythmia recurrences in patients with idiopathic dilated cardiomyopathy and implantable cardioverter defibrillator for secondary prophylaxis. Europace 11(3):289–296

80. Fananapazir L, Chang AC, Epstein SE et al (1992) Prognostic determinants in hypertrophic cardiomyopathy. Prospective evaluation of a therapeutic strategy based on clinical, Holter, hemodynamic, and electrophysiological findings. Circulation 86(3):730–740

81. Saumarez RC, Slade AK, Grace AA et al (1995) The significance of paced electrogram fractionation in hypertrophic cardiomyopathy. A prospective study. Circulation 91(11):2762–2768

82. Watson RM, Schwartz JL, Maron BJ et al (1987) Inducible polymorphic ventricular tachycardia and ventricular fibrillation in a subgroup of patients with hypertrophic cardiomyopathy at high risk for sudden death. J Am Coll Cardiol 10(4):761–774

83. Buxton AE, Marchlinski FE, Flores BT et al (1987) Nonsustained ventricular tachycardia in patients with coronary artery disease: role of electrophysiologic study. Circulation 75(6):1178–1185

84. Klein RC, Machell C (1989) Use of electrophysiologic testing in patients with nonsustained ventricular tachycardia: prognostic and therapeutic implications. J Am Coll Cardiol 14(1):155–161; discussion 162–153

85. Wilber DJ, Olshansky B, Moran JF et al (1990) Electrophysiological testing and nonsustained ventricular tachycardia. Use and limitations in patients with coronary artery disease and impaired ventricular function. Circulation 82(2): 350–358

86. Kowey PR, Waxman HL, Greenspon A et al (1990) Value of electrophysiologic testing in patients with previous myocardial infarction and nonsustained ventricular tachycardia. Philadelphia arrhythmia group. Am J Cardiol 65(9):594–598

87. Buxton AE, Lee KL, Fisher JD et al (1999) A randomized study of the prevention of sudden death in patients with coronary artery disease. Multicenter unsustained tachycardia trial investigators. N Engl J Med 341(25):1882–1890

88. Buxton AE, Lee KL, DiCarlo L et al (2000) Electrophysiologic testing to identify patients with coronary artery disease who are at risk for sudden death. Multicenter unsustained tachycardia trial investigators. N Engl J Med 342(26): 1937–1945

89. Raviele A, Bongiorni MG, Brignole M et al (2005) Early EPS/ICD strategy in survivors of acute myocardial infarction with severe left ventricular dysfunction on optimal beta-blocker treatment. The BEta-blocker STrategy plus ICD trial. Europace 7(4):327–337

90. De Ferrari GM, Rordorf R, Frattini F et al (2007) Predictive value of programmed ventricular stimulation in patients with ischaemic cardiomyopathy: implications for the selection of candidates for an implantable defibrillator. Europace 9(12):1151–1157

91. Nalos PC, Gang ES, Mandel WJ et al (1987) The signal-averaged electrocardiogram as a screening test for inducibility of sustained ventricular tachycardia in high risk patients: a prospective study. J Am Coll Cardiol 9(3):539–548

92. Winters SL, Stewart D, Targonski A et al (1988) Role of signal averaging of the surface QRS complex in selecting patients with nonsustained ventricular tachycardia and high grade ventricular arrhythmias for programmed ventricular stimulation. J Am Coll Cardiol 12(6):1481–1487

93. Turitto G, Fontaine JM, Ursell SN et al (1988) Value of the signal-averaged electrocardiogram as a predictor of the results of programmed stimulation in nonsustained ventricular tachycardia. Am J Cardiol 61(15):1272–1278

94. Turitto G, Fontaine JM, Ursell S et al (1990) Risk stratification and management of patients with organic heart disease and nonsustained ventricular tachycardia: role of programmed stimulation, left ventricular ejection fraction, and the signal-averaged electrocardiogram. Am J Med 88(1N):35N–41N

95. Keeling PJ, Kulakowski P, Yi G et al (1993) Usefulness of signal-averaged electrocardiogram in idiopathic dilated cardiomyopathy for identifying patients with ventricular arrhythmias. Am J Cardiol 72(1):78–84

96. Mancini DM, Wong KL, Simson MB (1993) Prognostic value of an abnormal signal-averaged electrocardiogram in patients with nonischemic congestive cardiomyopathy. Circulation 87(4):1083–1092

97. Buxton AE, Simson MB, Falcone RA et al (1987) Results of signal-averaged electrocardiography and electrophysiologic study in patients with nonsustained ventricular tachycardia after healing of acute myocardial infarction. Am J Cardiol 60(1):80–85

98. Gomes JA, Cain ME, Buxton AE et al (2001) Prediction of long-term outcomes by signal-averaged electrocardiography in patients with unsustained ventricular tachycardia, coronary artery disease, and left ventricular dysfunction. Circulation 104(4):436–441

99. Carlson MD, White RD, Trohman RG et al (1994) Right ventricular outflow tract ventricular tachycardia: detection of previously unrecognized anatomic abnormalities using cine magnetic resonance imaging. J Am Coll Cardiol 24(3):720–727

100. Chimenti C, Calabrese F, Thiene G et al (2001) Inflammatory left ventricular microaneurysms as a cause of apparently idiopathic ventricular tachyarrhythmias. Circulation 104(2):168–173

101. Ouyang F, Cappato R, Ernst S et al (2002) Electroanatomic substrate of idiopathic left ventricular tachycardia: unidirectional block and macroreentry within the purkinje network. Circulation 105(4):462–469

102. O'Donnell D, Cox D, Bourke J et al (2003) Clinical and electrophysiological differences between patients with arrhythmogenic right ventricular dysplasia and right ventricular outflow tract tachycardia. Eur Heart J 24(9):801–810

103. Kienzle MG, Martins JB, Constantin L et al (1992) Effect of direct, reflex and exercise-provoked increases in sympathetic tone on idiopathic ventricular tachycardia. Am J Cardiol 69(17):1433–1438

104. Klein LS, Shih HT, Hackett FK et al (1992) Radiofrequency catheter ablation of ventricular tachycardia in patients without structural heart disease. Circulation 85(5):1666–1674

105. Effect of metoprolol CR/XL in chronic heart failure (1999) Metoprolol CR/XL Randomised Intervention Trial in Congestive Heart Failure (MERIT-HF). Lancet 353(9169):2001–2007

106. Krum H, Roecker EB, Mohacsi P et al (2003) Effects of initiating carvedilol in patients with severe chronic heart failure: results from the COPERNICUS Study. JAMA 289(6):712–718

107. The Cardiac Insufficiency Bisoprolol Study II (CIBIS-II) (1999) A randomised trial. Lancet 353(9146):9–13

108. Flather MD, Shibata MC, Coats AJ et al (2005) Randomized trial to determine the effect of nebivolol on mortality and cardiovascular hospital admission in elderly patients with heart failure (SENIORS). Eur Heart J 26(3):215–225

109. Effects of enalapril on mortality in severe congestive heart failure (1987) Results of the cooperative North Scandinavian enalapril survival study (CONSENSUS). The CONSENSUS trial study group. N Engl J Med 316(23):1429–1435

110. Effect of enalapril on survival in patients with reduced left ventricular ejection fractions and congestive heart failure (1991) The SOLVD investigators. N Engl J Med 325(5):293–302

111. Cleland JG, Erhardt L, Murray G et al (1997) Effect of ramipril on morbidity and mode of death among survivors of acute myocardial infarction with clinical evidence of heart failure. A report from the AIRE Study Investigators. Eur Heart J 18(1):41–51

112. Fletcher RD, Cintron GB, Johnson G et al (1993) Enalapril decreases prevalence of ventricular tachycardia in patients with chronic congestive heart failure. The V-HeFT II VA Cooperative Studies Group. Circulation 87(6 Suppl): VI49–VI55

113. Pfeffer MA, Braunwald E, Moye LA et al (1992) Effect of captopril on mortality and morbidity in patients with left ventricular dysfunction after myocardial infarction. Results of the survival and ventricular enlargement trial. The SAVE investigators. N Engl J Med 327(10):669–677

114. Pratt CM, Gardner M, Pepine C et al (1995) Lack of long-term ventricular arrhythmia reduction by enalapril in heart failure. SOLVD investigators. Am J Cardiol 75(17):1244–1249

115. Pitt B, Poole-Wilson PA, Segal R et al (2000) Effect of losartan compared with captopril on mortality in patients with symptomatic heart failure: randomised trial–the Losartan heart failure survival study ELITE II. Lancet 355(9215):1582–1587

116. Pitt B, Zannad F, Remme WJ et al (1999) The effect of spironolactone on morbidity and mortality in patients with severe heart failure. Randomized aldactone evaluation study investigators. N Engl J Med 341(10):709–717

117. Pitt B, Remme W, Zannad F et al (2003) Eplerenone, a selective aldosterone blocker, in patients with left ventricular dysfunction after myocardial infarction. N Engl J Med 348(14):1309–1321

118. The effect of digoxin on mortality and morbidity in patients with heart failure (1997) The digitalis investigation group. N Engl J Med 336(8):525–533

119. Singh SN, Fletcher RD, Fisher SG et al (1995) Amiodarone in patients with congestive heart failure and asymptomatic ventricular arrhythmia. Survival trial of antiarrhythmic therapy in congestive heart failure. N Engl J Med 333(2):77–82

120. Doval HC, Nul DR, Grancelli HO et al (1994) Randomised trial of low-dose amiodarone in severe congestive heart failure. Grupo de Estudio de la Sobrevida en la Insuficiencia Cardiaca en Argentina (GESICA). Lancet 344(8921): 493–498

121. Julian DG, Camm AJ, Frangin G et al (1997) Randomised trial of effect of amiodarone on mortality in patients with left-ventricular dysfunction after recent myocardial infarction: EMIAT. European myocardial infarct amiodarone trial investigators. Lancet 349(9053):667–674

122. Cairns JA, Connolly SJ, Roberts R et al (1997) Randomised trial of outcome after myocardial infarction in patients with frequent or repetitive ventricular premature depolarisations: CAMIAT. Canadian amiodarone myocardial infarction arrhythmia trial investigators. Lancet 349(9053):675–682

123. Moss AJ, Hall WJ, Cannom DS et al (1996) Improved survival with an implanted defibrillator in patients with coronary disease at high risk for ventricular arrhythmia. Multicenter automatic defibrillator implantation trial investigators. N Engl J Med 335(26):1933–1940

124. Moss AJ, Zareba W, Hall WJ et al (2002) Prophylactic implantation of a defibrillator in patients with myocardial infarction and reduced ejection fraction. N Engl J Med 346(12):877–883

125. McKenna WJ, Oakley CM, Krikler DM et al (1985) Improved survival with amiodarone in patients with hypertrophic cardiomyopathy and ventricular tachycardia. Br Heart J 53(4):412–416

126. Fananapazir L, Epstein SE (1991) Value of electrophysiologic studies in hypertrophic cardiomyopathy treated with amiodarone. Am J Cardiol 67(2):175–182

127. Maron BJ, Shen WK, Link MS et al (2000) Efficacy of implantable cardioverter-defibrillators for the prevention of sudden death in patients with hypertrophic cardiomyopathy. N Engl J Med 342(6):365–373

11

Ventricular Tachycardia and Fibrillation: Pharmacologic Therapy

Gerald V. Naccarelli and John Field

CONTENTS

Abstract

This chapter reviews the clinical pharmacology, electrophysiology, efficacy and safety, and current recommendations of use of class IA, IB, IC, II, and III antiarrhythmic agents in the acute and chronic treatment of ventricular tachycardia. In addition, the role of these drugs in patients with implantable cardioverter-defibrillators is discussed.

Key Words: Ventricular tachycardia; ventricular fibrillation; antiarrhythmic drugs; quinidine; procainamide; digoxin, disopyramide; lidocaine; amiodarone; ESVEM study; mexiletine; flecainide; propafenone; beta blockers; death in heart failure trial (SCD-HeFT); sotalol.

Although the implantable-cardioverter-defibrillator (ICD) has minimized the use of antiarrhythmic drugs in the treatment of sustained ventricular tachycardia (VT) and ventricular fibrillation (VF), intravenous (IV) antiarrhythmic drugs are still used in the acute setting and oral antiarrhythmic drugs are used in the suppression of symptomatic and life-threatening ventricular arrhythmias. We will review IV and oral antiarrhythmic drugs and their safety and efficacy in the treatment of VT and VF.

CLASS IA ANTIARRHYTHMIC DRUGS

The class IA antiarrhythmic drugs, quinidine, procainamide, and disopyramide, are used *(1)* uncommonly for the treatment of supraventricular and ventricular arrhythmias.

From: *Contemporary Cardiology: Management of Cardiac Arrhythmias*
Edited by: Gan-Xin Yan, Peter R. Kowey, DOI 10.1007/978-1-60761-161-5_11
© Springer Science+Business Media, LLC 2011

Table 1
Sicilian Gambit Classification of Antiarrhythmic Drugs *(2)*

Drug	Channel Blockers					Receptors			
	Na	Na	Na						
	Fast	Med	Slow	Ca	K	α	β	M2	P
Lidocaine	L								
Mexiletine	L								
Tocainide	L								
Moricizine	H,I								
Procainamide		H,A			M				
Disopyramide		H,A			M			L	
Quinidine		H,A			M			L	
Propafenone		H,A					L		
Flecainide			H,A	L					
Verapamil	L			H		M			
Diltiazem				M					
Bretylium					H	Ag/Ant	Ag/Ant		
Sotalol					H				
Amiodarone	L			L	H	M	M		
Ibutilide*					L				
Dofetilide					H				
Azimilide					H				
Propranolol	L						H		
Acebutolol							H		
Esmolol							H		
Adenosine							H		Ag

M2 Muscurinic, *P* purine, *L* low, *M* medium, *H* high, *O* open, *A* activated, *Ag* agonist, *Ant* antagonist, Na sodium, Ca calcium

*Ibutilide enhances Na flow into the cell during the plateau phase of the action potential

Quinidine blocks I_{Kr}, I_{Ks}, I_{to}, I_{Na} in addition to having alpha-blocking and vagolytic effects (Table 1) *(2)*. In addition, quinidine blocks muscarinic subtype 2 receptors. Quinidine reduces automaticity by raising threshold potential and decreasing the rate of rise of phase 4 depolarization and decreases the rate of rise of phase 0 of the action potential by blocking sodium influx predominantly in the activated state, thus slowing conduction. This action of quinidine is frequency dependent with depression of V_{max} being greater at faster heart rates. Quinidine prolongs action potential duration (APD), primarily by blocking the potassium channel, and also prolongs the effective refractory period (ERP) and the ERP/APD ratio.

Quinidine is metabolized by hydroxylation in the liver. 3-hydroxyquinidine and 2′-oxoquinidine appear to have some antiarrhythmic activity. Quinidine is a potent inhibitor of CYP2D6 and thus can cause increased plasma concentrations if used with drugs that are metabolized via this mechanism. Quinidine also inhibits P-glycoprotein and thus decreases digoxin clearance resulting in increased digoxin levels when used concomitantly (3).

Quinidine is effective for the long-term suppression of ventricular ectopic activity. Holter monitoring studies demonstrate that quinidine effectively suppresses premature ventricular complexes (PVCs), couplets, and non-sustained ventricular tachycardia (NSVT) in about 60% of patients (4). In patients with sustained VT/VF, efficacy rates as determined by programmed stimulation range from 16% in the Electrophysiologic Study Versus Electrocardiographic Monitoring (ESVEM) trial to 20–25% in uncontrolled trials (5, 6). Combination therapy with mexiletine, using lower maintenance doses of both drugs, achieves added efficacy and lower toxicity (7). Quinidine, by blocking Ito, may have some usefulness in suppressing VT associated with the Brugada syndrome (8).

Quinidine causes subjective adverse reactions including nausea, vomiting, anorexia, or diarrhea in up to 35% of patients. Fever, rash, and tinnitus can rarely occur. Rarely, the vasodilatory properties of quinidine can lead to orthostatic hypotension. End-organ toxicity includes the occurrence of a rare drug-induced thrombocytopenia and granulomatous hepatitis.

Quinidine may prolong the QT interval and cause drug-aggravated torsades de pointes in up to 5% of patients. There are no large controlled trials defining the safety of using quinidine in post-myocardial infarction (MI) or congestive heart failure (CHF) patients. One small study (9) suggests that quinidine increases mortality in patients with CHF.

Procainamide has electrophysiologic properties similar to quinidine but has less vagolytic effects (Table 1). Procainamide is acetylated in the liver by n-acetyl-transferase to an active metabolite, n-acetylprocainamide (NAPA), which is an I_{Kr} blocker and has 70% of the antiarrhythmic activity of the parent compound. In rapid acetylators, NAPA levels usually exceed the parent compound. Thirty to sixty percent of the drug is excreted unchanged in the urine and the remainder is excreted as NAPA.

Procainamide is available intravenously and orally. Oral procainamide is about 60% effective at suppressing PVCs, couplets, and NSVT as assessed by noninvasive techniques, and effective in 20–25% of cases in suppressing inducible sustained VT as assessed by programmed stimulation (10, 11).

IV procainamide requires loading doses of up to 17 mg/kg at 20 mg/min usually given over 25–30 min (12). The infusion should be decreased or stopped if hypotension occurs or the QRS duration widens by greater than 50%. Following loading, the drug is given in 1- to 4-mg/min IV infusions with reduced dosing in the presence of renal insufficiency (maximal total dose 12 mg/kg; maintenance infusion 1–2 mg/min). Studies have shown that intravenous procainamide will terminate VT more frequently than intravenous lidocaine (13). Procainamide has the additional benefit of being effective in the treatment of supraventricular arrhythmias by either affecting the retrograde limb of the AV node, the retrograde limb of the accessory pathway, or suppressing irritable atrial foci. In a wide QRS tachycardia of undetermined etiology, IV procainamide should be considered.

Procainamide may cause nausea, anorexia, vomiting, and rash. End-organ toxicity of concern is a rare agranulocytosis that usually occurs during the first three months of treatment.

The major limiting adverse reaction with procainamide has been the development of a systemic lupus-like reaction in 10–20% of patients. This is more likely to occur in slow acetylators. Similar to quinidine, procainamide can cause high-degree AV block and ventricular proarrhythmia including the new onset of sustained, monomorphic VT, or torsades de pointes, and has been associated with increased mortality when used in CHF patients (9).

Disopyramide has similar electrophysiologic and vagal effects as previously described with quinidine (Table 1). Fifty-five percent of a dose is recovered after renal excretion unchanged in the urine while 25% is recovered as the active n-monodealkylated metabolite. Disopyramide has nonlinear pharmacokinetics with decreasing plasma protein binding as serum concentrations increase.

Although rarely used, oral disopyramide is as effective as procainamide and quinidine in suppressing PVCs, ventricular couplets, and NSVT as assessed by Holter monitoring *(14)*. Because of the drug's significant negative inotropic effects, this drug is not recommended in patients with congestive heart failure *(15)*.

Disopyramide's subjective toxicity is primarily secondary to its anticholinergic activity and includes dry mouth, blurred vision, urinary retention, constipation, and worsening of glaucoma. No significant end-organ toxicity has been noted with disopyramide. Disopyramide's most important adverse reaction is worsening of CHF secondary to its significant negative inotropic activity and increase of peripheral vascular resistance. CHF occurs in 50% of patients with a prior history of CHF and only 5% of other patients *(15)*. Slowing of conduction and prolongation of QT interval can cause proarrhythmias such as monomorphic sustained VT and torsade de pointes.

Class Ia antiarrhythmics are rarely used today in the treatment of either ventricular or atrial tachyarrhythmias due to their risk of causing torsade de pointes *(16)* and having adverse effects including increased mortality in patients with structural heart disease *(9)*.

LIDOCAINE

IV lidocaine hydrochloride is a short-acting class Ib antiarrhythmic agent *(1, 2, 17)*. Electrophysiologically, lidocaine minimally blocks both open and inactivated fast sodium channels (Table 1) and minimally slows conduction in the His-Purkinje system and myocardium. Lidocaine has more conduction slowing properties in ischemic tissue interrupting reentry circuits. Lidocaine has little or no effect on atrial or AV nodal recessive pathway tissue. Lidocaine suppresses automaticity in Purkinje fibers and is efficacious in suppressing irritable ventricular foci. In addition to slowing conduction in cardiac tissue, lidocaine increases ERP/APD ratio which may help prevent reentrant ventricular arrhythmias.

Lidocaine has poor oral bioavailability since 90% of an administered dose is rapidly metabolized in the liver via the CYP3A4 system into two major metabolites, monoethylglycinexylidide (MEG) and glycinexylidide (GX) *(18)*. MEG is 80% and GX is 10% as potent as the parent compound. Because of rapid first-pass metabolism, lidocaine is not used orally. Lidocaine is administered intravenously as a bolus; it is rapidly distributed into the intravascular compartment with a half-life of 8 min.

Recommended dosing includes a loading bolus infusion of 1–1.5 mg/kg intravenously followed by a 1- to 4-mg/min infusion. Within 15 min of the first bolus, a second bolus of 0.5–0.75 mg/kg can be given to maintain levels *(12, 19)*. If maintenance infusions at higher doses are needed, patients should receive an additional bolus before the rate of the maintenance infusion is increased.

Lidocaine is used for suppression of ventricular arrhythmias. Meta analysis studies suggest that lidocaine should not be routinely used as a post-MI prophylactic antiarrhythmic *(20)*.

Intravenous lidocaine is an acceptable alternative drug to amiodarone for the treatment of persistent or recurrent VF/pulseless VT *(12)*. In this situation, lidocaine is considered for persistent VF/pulseless VT after at least two initial shocks and the administration of a vasoconstrictor agent (epinephrine or vasopressin) have failed to terminate the ventricular arrhythmia. Lidocaine has a class indeterminant recommendation for this indication *(12)* due to a lack of randomized controlled trials demonstrating improved survival to hospital discharge.

In one retrospective study, lidocaine improved rates of resuscitation and admission alive to the hospital *(21)*. In this study, lidocaine was given to out-of-hospital cardiac arrest patients caused by ventricular fibrillation. Among patients with sustained VF, those who received lidocaine had a return to spontaneous circulation more frequently ($p < 0.001$) and were hospitalized alive more frequently 38% vs. 18%, ($p < 0.01$) than patients who did not receive lidocaine. However, the rate of survival the hospital discharge was no different between the two groups. In addition, patients who were converted to a perfusing rhythm were more frequently admitted to the hospital if the patients received prophylactic lidocaine than if they did not (94% vs. 84%, $p < 0.05$). The rate of discharge did not differ significantly between the two groups. However, other trials of lidocaine and comparisons of lidocaine to bretylium and amiodarone found no statistical difference in outcomes (22–24). A randomized comparison of lidocaine and epinephrine demonstrated a higher incidence of asystole with lidocaine use and no difference in return or spontaneous circulation (25). Lidocaine has some practical advantage for the use in persistent VF and pulseless VT. The drug has a rapid onset of action with minimal serious hemodynamic adverse effects when administered rapidly.

Lidocaine has dose-related neurologic and gastrointestinal adverse effects. Neurologic side effects include numbness, tingling, seizures, tremors, paresthesias, disorientation, dulled sensorium, tinnitus, and drowsiness. GI side effects include nauseas and vomiting. Lidocaine is generally well-tolerated hemodynamically. Lidocaine also had minimal conduction slowing in the His-Purkinje system and is unlikely to aggravate Mobitz Type II AV Block. Metabolism of lidocaine is affected by liver blood flow and microsomal activity. A reduction in dosage is required with advanced age, liver disease, and in congestive heart failure (26).

MEXILETINE

Mexiletine is a Class Ib oral agent (1, 2) that chemically resembles lidocaine in structure. Electrophysiologically, it is similar to lidocaine and has minimal effects on slowing sodium channel (Table 1); and electrocardiographically, its only effect is to shorten the QT interval.

Mexiletine is well absorbed orally and has more than 90% bioavailability. Hepatic metabolism via the CYP2D6 enzyme is the major route of elimination with only 10–15% of the drug being excreted unchanged in the urine. The drug has an onset of action of 1–2 h and elimination half-life average is 10–12 h. No significant drug interactions have been reported with mexiletine. The usual dosing is to initiate 150 mg three times per day and increase the dose to 200, 250, 300 mg three times per day as needed.

In the ESVEM study, 67% of patients had suppression of their ventricular arrhythmia as assessed by Holter monitoring (6). Mexiletine has been shown to be comparable to quinidine in suppressing ventricular ectopic activity (27). Adding a type IA antiarrhythmic agent or amiodaorone to mexiletine is associated with added efficacy and decreased toxicity. Mexiletine was not found to reduce mortality in a post-MI population (IMPACT study), although it significantly reduced the frequency of PVCs (28). Mexiletine's effects on survival in CHF patients have not been studied. In patients with recurrent sustained VT studied in the electrophysiology laboratory, mexiletine appears to be effective in 10–15% of patients. Efficacy rates between 20–30% have been demonstrated in patients with ventricular fibrillation who survived an out-of-hospital cardiac arrest (29, 30). Mexiletine is very effective in treating pediatric patients who have ventricular arrhythmias after surgery for Tetralogy of Fallot (31). Mexiletine is effective in treating some patients with the prolonged QT syndrome (LGQT3) by blocking the plateau sodium current in patients who have an abnormal amino acid substitution in the sodium channel (32).

Mexiletine has dose-related central nervous system and GI side effects, most commonly causing nausea. Subjective side effects are minimized by giving the drug with meals. The drug is relatively free of end-organ toxicity and is well-tolerated hemodynamically.

Mexiletine's main use is in patients with prolonged QT syndrome (32) and also in some patients who have had ICD shocks in whom other antiarrhythmic drugs have failed to suppress the ventricular arrhythmias causing these shocks.

FLECAINIDE

Flecainide is a class Ic antiarrhythmic agent (Table 1) that prolongs refractoriness and slows conduction in the atria, AV node, His-Purkinje system, ventricles, and accessory pathways *(33)*. Flecainide is a potent sodium channel blocker with slow onset and offset kinetics. Flecainide minimally blocks I_{Kr}.

Flecainide has a bioavailability of 90% to 95% and a half-life average 12–27 h *(33)*. Flecainide is 70% metabolized hepatically and 30% excreted through the renal route. The drug is used on a twice daily dosing schedule. The usual starting dose is 100 mg twice a day and increased to 150 mg twice a day as necessary. The drug prolongs the PR and QRS interval when therapeutic plasma levels are achieved.

Flecainide is predominantly used in the treatment of supraventricular tachyarrhythmias not associated with any significant structural heart disease. However, flecainide has been shown to be extremely effective (>70%) in decreasing the frequency of PVCs in patients with frequent ventricular ectopy *(4)*. In comparative trials with quinidine and disopyramide, flecainide has been shown to be statistically superior in the suppression of PVCs, ventricular couplets, and runs of NSVT *(4)*. In patients with symptomatic ventricular arrhythmias in the post-myocardial infarction period, the Cardiac Arrhythmia Survival Trial (CAST) study demonstrated that both encainide- and flecainide-enhanced mortality compared to placebo despite effective PVC suppression *(34)*. In patients with sustained VT, the efficacy of flecainide (20%) has been comparable to type IA antiarrhythmic agents *(35)*. Efficacy rates are higher in patients with preserved left ventricular function. For ventricular arrhythmias, flecainide has predominantly been used in the treatment of VT in patients with no structural heart disease if beta blockers are ineffective and/or if the patient is not a good candidate for a catheter ablation procedure *(36)*. Flecainide can be used to unmask concealed Brugada syndrome.

Flecainide is very well-tolerated. Dose-related noncardiac side effects include dizziness, visual disturbances, and headache. Since the drug depresses left ventricular function, it should not be used in patients with depressed ejection fractions and, as noted above, is contraindicated in patients with coronary artery disease, especially if they have already had a myocardial infarction *(34)*. Flecainide is a potent sodium channel blocker and may aggravate preexisting His-Purkinje conduction disturbance and should be used cautiously if the patient has preexisting intraventicular conduction disturbances.

PROPAFENONE

Propafenone is a class Ic agent that has weak associated beta-blocking characteristics (Table 1) *(37)*. Propafenone's electrophysiology is very similar to flecainide.

Propafenone undergoes first-pass hepatic elimination through the CYP2D6 enzyme system which can be inhibited by quinidine *(37–39)*. There is a major active metabolite, 5-hydroxypropafenone. The recommended starting dose for propafenone is 150 mg three times per day, with increases to 225–300 mg three times per day, if needed. With the sustained release form, the drug is started at 225 mg twice per day and increased to 325 or 425 mg twice per day, as needed. The sustained release form of the drug has not been studied in ventricular arrhythmias.

Propafenone is efficacious in suppressing ventricular ectopic activity in more than 65% of patients based on Holter monitoring studies *(40)*. In patients with a history of sustained VT or VF, the drug is effective in about 20% of patients in suppressing inducible VT *(41)*. In the CASH Trial *(42)*, the propafenone arm of the study was prematurely discontinued since the drug was not as effective as metroprolol, amiodarone, or ICD in the survival of patients with sustained VT. Although propafenone was not a drug in CAST, the drug is not recommended for use in patients with significant structural heart disease *(43)*. Similar to flecainide, propafenone is recommended in patients with VT without structural heart disease.

BETA BLOCKERS

The only beta blockers that have Food and Drug Administration approval for treatment of ventricular arrhythmias are propanolol and acebutolol (44, 45). However, all of the currently available beta blockers have some use in the treatment of ventricular arrhythmias including in the acute situation.

In general, beta blockers suppress ventricular arrhythmias based on noninvasive monitoring in about 45–50% of patients. They are very unlikely to suppress inducible ventricular tachycardia in the electrophysiology lab, being effective in less than 5% of patients studied. Patients who have VT/VF storm, defined as two or more episodes of collapse and shock from VF or VT in 24 h and requiring defibrillation or cardioversion, have been studied with beta blockers (46). In one trial, patients with electrical storm had much better outcomes with intravenous beta blockade. This was when compared to a standard ACLS guideline for VF is being followed. However, beta blockers are the drug of choice in exercise-aggravated or exercise-induced ventricular tachycardia and in patients with prolonged QT syndromes (47, 48). In addition, beta blockers are very effective as adjunct therapy in combination with other antiarrhythmic drugs for the treatment of ventricular tachycardia. Since many of the beta blockers, including propanolol, timolol, and carvedilol, prolong survival in the post-myocardial infarction patient, and carvedilol, bisoprolol and long-acting metorprolol improve survival in patients with depressed left ventricular function, these drugs should be considered as frontline therapy of ventricular arrhythmias in these settings (43).

Beta blockers can provoke sinus node slowing and AV block. Beta blockers that are not cardioselective can exacerbate bronchospasm. Beta blockers do have some significant inotropic potential and can provoke worsening of heart failure in patients with depressed ejection fractions although they prolong survival and reduce sudden death in this setting (43).

BRETYLIUM

Bretylium is an intravenous class III agent that has been used in the past in the emergent treatment of sustained tachyarrhythmias (24, 49). However, bretylium is no longer recommended in the VF/pulseless VT algorithm (12). In addition, bretylium has been difficult to obtain commercially, and because of this, it has been pulled from most of the crash carts. Due to this, we will not discuss this drug further.

AMIODARONE

Amiodarone has a combination of class I, II, III, and IV mechanisms of antiarrhythmic action (Table 1) (50). Amiodarone prolongs refractoriness and slows conduction of the atria AV node, His-Purkinje system, and ventricles. It also slows sinus node automaticity and heart rate. Significant prolongation of action potential duration is noted, although due to a disproportionate prolongation of action potential duration in the epicardium, endocardium, and mesocardium, there is less dispersion of action potential duration and therefore the incidence of torsades de pointes is uncommon (51).

Intravenous amiodarone has complex pharmacokinetics (52, 53). Because of the rapid distribution of the drug, serum concentrations decrease to 19% of peak values within the 30–45 min of discontinuation. In cardiac arrest, an initial 300 mg dose is given IV push and can be followed by one additional 150 mg dose in 3–5 min (12). For recurrent life-threatening ventricular arrhythmias, intravenous dosing starts with a 150-mg bolus injection given over 10 min. This is followed by slow-loading infusion of 360 mg given over 6 h at 1 mg/min. This is then followed by 540 mg given at 0.5 mg/min over the remaining 18 h. Supplemental infusions of 150 mg bolus are given over 10 min for breakthrough arrhythmias and before an increase in the infusion is given, when needed. Usually amiodarone is run at 1–2 mg/min for continuous infusion. Intravenously amiodarone slows heart rate and prolongs AV node refractoriness and has some immediate effects on ventricular refractoriness. Initially given intravenously, amiodarone is not associated with any significant action potential duration, prolongation, or use-dependent sodium channel blockade. Its short-term effects may be partially explained by its sympatholytic and calcium channel-blocking effects *(53)*.

Oral amiodarone pharmacokinetics are complex and best represented by a three compartment model *(50)*. Its average half-life is 53 days. Because of high lipophilicity, amiodarone and its active metabolites extensively distributed into fat, muscle, liver, lungs, and spleen. Oral amiodarone dosing requires an oral load of 800–1400 mg a day for several weeks, with tapering loading doses down to 600 mg, then 400 mg/day. In an attempt to minimize toxicity, amiodarone is usually maintained at doses of under 400 mg/day. Therapeutic blood levels are in the 1.0–2.5 μg/mL range.

Amiodarone is approved for the treatment of life-threatening sustained ventricular tachyarrhythmias. It is effective in more than 60% of such patients *(54)*. Empiric amiodarone therapy has been demonstrated to be more effective than guided therapy with more conventional agents in the CASCADE trial *(55)*. Multiple trials, including AVID, have shown that the ICD is more effective at improving survival than amiodarone *(43, 56, 57)*. Although not approved for patients with less serious ventricular arrhythmias, amiodarone is effective in over 70% of patients in suppressing significant ventricular activity as assessed by Holter monitoring. In primary prevention studies such as MADIT, there was a 54% improvement in trial patients treated with an ICD compared with amiodarone or other antiarrhythmics in a post-MI population with a depressed left ventricular ejection fraction and NSVT, who also has inducible sustained VT that was not suppressed by intravenous procainamide *(58)*. Based on the guidelines and multiple studies, amiodarone is reasonably safe to use in the post-myocardial infarction and congestive heart failure populations which make it a popular drug to use in ventricular arrhythmias not responsive to beta blockers in this setting *(43, 59)*.

Intravenous amiodarone has been demonstrated to control life-threatening tachyarrhythmias *(60)* with an efficacy comparable to that of bretylium *(23)*. In the ALIVE trial intravenous amiodarone was effective with 23% of patients surviving to hospital admission compared to 11% on lidocaine *(61)*. Also in the ARREST trial intravenous amiodarone was effective in 44% of patients surviving to hospital admission compared to 34% on placebo *(62)*. Intravenous amiodarone has a class IIb recommendation for the treatment of persistent or recurrent VF/pulseless VT *(12)*. The drug is considered for persistent VF/pulseless VT after at least two initial shocks and the administration of a vasoconstrictor agent (epinephrine or vasopressin) have failed to terminate the ventricular arrhythmia *(63)*.

Adverse effects during amiodarone therapy are common *(50, 63)*. Minor side effects seldom requiring drug discontinuation include corneal microdeposits, asymptomatic transient elevation of hepatic enzymes, photosensitivity of the skin, bluish-gray skin discoloration, and subjective gastrointestinal side effects. Amiodarone-induced hypothyroidism occurs in about 8% of our patients and requires the addition of thyroid replacement. Drug-induced hyperthyroidism (2%) may require discontinuation of therapy. Other serious end-organ toxicities which may require discontinuation of amiodarone include interstitial pneumonitis (3–7%) and drug-induced hepatitis (2%). Neurologic side effects, including a peripheral neuropathy and myopathy, usually resolve on lowering the dose. Drug-induced bradycardia may require backup permanent pacing in up to 2% of patients. Low-dose amiodarone may minimize the frequency of the above adverse effects. The predominant adverse effect of intravenous amiodarone is drug-induced hypotension and venous sclerosis can be minimized if intravenous amiodarone is given through a central venous line.

Amiodarone has been shown to interact with digoxin, warfarin, quinidine, procainamide, flecainide, and simvastatin *(50)*. Concomitant use of these drugs requires lower doses and close monitoring.

Based on the above, the use of IV and oral amiodarone for malignant ventricular arrhythmias was summarized by a Heart rhythm Society consensus group *(63)*: "It is the consensus of this committee that amiodarone is the antiarrhythmic drug of choice, in combination with other appropriate therapies such as beta-blocking agents, in patients who have sustained ventricular tachyarrhythmias associated with structural heart disease, especially if associated with left ventricular dysfunction, who are not candidates for an implantable cardioverter-defibrillator (ICD). This recommendation is based on the following observations: (1) efficacy of amiodarone at 2 years to prevent sustained VT/VF or death is approximately 60%; (2) amiodarone has minimal negative inotropic effects; (3) amiodarone has low pro-arrhythmic potential; (4) prospective trial data demonstrate long-term neutral effects on survival and safety in patients with post-myocardial infarction left ventricular dysfunction, and in patients with either ischemic and nonischemic dilated cardiomyopathy; (5) the empiric use of amiodarone has been found to be more effective than the use of class I antiarrhythmic drugs even though these drugs had their efficacy guided by serial invasive or noninvasive tests; and (6) the efficacy of amiodarone is similar to ICD therapy inpatients with left ventricular ejection fractions greater than 35%. Because amiodarone is effective in suppressing ventricular arrhythmias and has had neutral effects on survival in patients with left ventricular dysfunction, the drug is often used to suppress symptomatic, nonsustained VT in these patients".

However, amiodarone adversely affected survival in NYHA III patients in the Sudden Cardiac Death in Heart Failure Trial (SCD-HeFT). Thus, amiodarone should be reserved for patients with nonsustained VT that is symptomatic, refractory to beta-blocker therapy, and concerning enough to warrant treatment. IV amiodarone is approved by the FDA for treatment and prophylaxis of recurrent VF and hemodynamically unstable VT in patients who are refractory to other antiarrhythmic therapy. IV amiodarone is also approved to treat (suppress and prevent) VF or VT in patients who are candidates for oral amiodarone but are unable to take the oral preparation. IV amiodarone has a "class IIb" indication in the Advanced Cardiac Life Support (ACLS) guidelines. Based on two prospective randomized parallel dose–response studies, IV amiodarone is now the antiarrhythmic drug of first choice for persistent VF or pulseless VT if standard (non-antiarrhythmic) resuscitative measures are ineffective. Amiodarone has also been advocated for treatment of VT/VF refractory to lidocaine after acute myocardial infarction and as an adjunct for "electrical storm," defined as multiple episodes of recurrent rapid poorly tolerated VT or VF requiring multiple defibrillation attempts over a short period of time (24 h or less) in which recurrent VT/VF can be only transiently terminated. Although not tested prospectively, IV amiodarone has been used to suppress recurrent, symptomatic, non-sustained (<30 sec) VT and recurrent episodes of VT in patients with ICDs who have frequent device activations (shock or anti-tachycardia pacing therapies).

SOTALOL

Sotalol is a nonselective beta blocker (L-stereoisomer) with class III antiarrhythmic properties (D-stereoisomer) (Table 1) *(64)*. Sotalol prolongs repolarization (QT interval) by blocking I_{Kr} in a dose-dependent fashion, although the drug displays reverse use dependence with loss of effects at faster heart rates. Sotalol slows sinus node cycle and lengthens AV node refractoriness and refractory periods of the atrium, ventricle, and accessory pathway. No effect has been demonstrated on the H-V interval. Electrocardiographically, sotalol prolongs PR and the QT interval. Sotalol's beta-blocking properties predominate at lower doses and its class III antiarrhythmic agents predominate at higher doses. Sotalol is nearly completely absorbed and is predominately excreted through the kidney with minimal metabolic breakdown. Elimination half-life average is about 10 h *(65)*. Dosing with sotalol starts at 80 mg twice per day and increased 120–160 mg twice per day as needed.

Sotalol is effective in suppressing ventricular ectopic activities as assessed by Holter monitoring in 50–60% of patients. In ESVEM *(6)*, sotalol was as effective as quinidine, procainamide, mexiletine, and propafenone in achieving suppression of ventricular arrhythmias as assessed by serial Holter monitoring. In sustained VT, as assessed by programmed stimulation, sotalol has been demonstrated to be effective in suppressing VT induction up to 30% of patients and was as effective as or more effective than any of the other class I drugs studied in the ESVEM trial *(6)*. In a post-MI study *(66)*, sotalol reduced mortality by 18% (*p* NS) and reduced reinfarction rate by 41% (*p* < 0.05).

Sotalol's predominant adverse effects are those associated with beta blockade including bradycardia and AV block. The drug prolongs the QT interval in torsades de pointes, the most common proarrhythmia that occurs in up to 2% of patients. This is minimized by using a peak daily dosage of 320 mg/day and decreasing the dose if the QTc is longer than 520 msec. Given its safety in the post-myocardial infarction setting, sotalol is commonly used in patients with coronary artery disease and symptomatic ventricular arrhythmias.

ANTIARRHYTHMIC DRUGS IN PATIENTS WITH ICDS

Over 50% of patients with ICDs have concomitant use of antiarrhythmic drugs *(67)*. Antiarrhythmic drugs are commonly used to eliminate therapy from triggering non-sustained ventricular tachycardia, supraventricular arrhythmias, or to slow ventricular tachycardia to a hemodynamically tolerated rate to increase the efficacy of anti-tachycardia pacing *(67)*. ICD antiarrhythmic drug interactions including alteration of the defibrillation threshold, slowing of the ventricular tachycardia rate below the tachycardia detection interval, causing a drug-induced proarrhythmia, and more incessant ventricular tachycardia requiring even higher amounts of ICD therapy, drug-induced aggravation of bradycardia requiring more anti-bradycardia pacing, and alteration of pacing thresholds *(67)*.

In general, class I drugs and amiodarone have all been demonstrated to increase defibrillation thresholds. Class III agents, such as sotalol, have been shown to decrease the defibrillation threshold. There are mixed results in studies with drugs such as procainamide, which has a class I and class III agent, and propafenone, which in one study *(68)* showed to have no significant increase in defibrillation thresholds at lower doses compared to placebo. Data from several controlled studies showed that sotalol, dronedarone, azimilide, and amiodarone, in conjunction with the beta blocker, all reduce the frequency of ICD therapies *(69)*. Parentally, we would recommend starting with a beta blocker and using drugs, such as sotalol or amiodarone, to follow as needed in patients who have frequent ICD shocks from sustained ventricular tachycardia. In cases where drug therapy is ineffective, catheter ablation of ventricular tachycardia has been shown to suppress the need for ICD therapies *(70)*.

REFERENCES

1. Vaughn Williams EM (1984) A classification of antiarrhythmic actions reassessed after a decade of new drugs. J Clin Pharmacol 24:129–147
2. Task Force of the Working Group on Arrhythmias of the European Society of Cardiology (1991) The Sicilian Gambit. A new approach to the classification of antiarrhythmic drugs based on their actions on arrhythmogenic mechanisms. Circulation 84:1831–1851
3. Fromm MF, Kim RB, Stein CM et al (1999) Inhibition of P-glycoprotein-mediated drug transport: A unifying mechanism to explain the interaction between digoxin and quinidine. Circulation 99:552–557
4. Salerno DM (1988) Review: Antiarrhythmic drugs; 1987. Part I-J Electrophysiology 1:217, 1987; Part II-1:300–319, 1987, Part III-1:435–465, 1987; Part IV-2:55–87
5. DiMarco JP, Garan H, Ruskin JN (1983) Quinidine for ventricular arrhythmias. Value of electrophysiologic testing. Am J Cardiol 51:90–95
6. Mason JW and the ESVEM Investigators (1993) A comparison of seven antiarrhythmic drugs in patients with ventricular tachyarrhythmias. N Engl J Med 329:452–458
7. Duff HJ, Kolodgie FD, Roden DM, Woosley RL (1986) Electropharmacologic synergism with mexiletine and quinidine. J Cardiovasc Pharmacol 8:840–846
8. Antzelevitch C, Brugada P, Borggrefe M, Brugada J, Brugada R, Corrado D, Gussak I, LeMarec H, Nademanee K, Perez Riera AR, Shimizu W, Schulze-Bahr E, Tan H, Wilde A (2005) Brugada syndrome: report of the second consensus conference. Endorsed by the heart rhythm society and the European heart rhythm association. Circulation 111:659–670
9. Flaker GC, Blackshear JL, McBride R et al (1992) Antiarrhythmic drug therapy and cardiac mortality in atrial fibrillation. J Am Coll Cardiol 20:527–532

10. Greenspan AM, Horowitz LN, Spielman SR, Josephson ME (1980) Large-dose procainamide therapy for ventricular tachyarrhythmia. Am J Cardiol 46:453–462

11. Waxman HL, Buxton AE, Sadowski LM, Josephson ME (1982) Resposne to procainamide during electrophysiologic study for sustained ventricular tachycardia predicts response to other drugs. Circulation 67:30–37

12. ACLS-The Reference Textbook (2003) Cummins RO (ed), Field JM, Hazinski MF (associate eds), ACLS principles and practice, pp 57–70

13. Gorgels APM, van den Dool A, Hofs A, Mullenerrs R, Smeets JLRM, Vos MA, Wellens HJJ (1996) Comparison of procainamide and lidocaine in terminating sustained monomorphic ventricular tachycardia. Am J Cardiol 78:43–46

14. Lermann BB, Waxman HL, Buxton AE, Josephson ME (1983) Disopyramide: evaluation of electrophysiologic effects and clinical efficacy in patients with sustained ventricular tachycadia or ventricular fibrillation. Amer J Cardiol 51: 759–764

15. Podrid PJ, Schoeneberger A, Lown B (1980) Congestive heart failure caused by oral disopyramide. N Engl J Med 302:614–617

16. Roden DM, Woosley RL, Primm K (1986) Incidence and clinical features of the quinidine-associated long QT syndrome: implications for patient care. Am Heart J 111:1088–1093

17. Grant AO, Wendt DJ (1991) Blockade of ion channels by antiarrhythmic drugs. J Cardiovasc Electrophysiol 2: 5153–5158

18. Collingsworth KA, Kalman SN, Harrison DC (1974) The clinical pharmacology of lidocaine as an antiarrhythmic drug. Circulation 50:1217–1230

19. Harrison DC (1975) Practical guidelines for the use of lidocaine. Prevention and treatment of cardiac arrhythmias. JAMA 233:1202–1204

20. Hine LK, Laird N, Hewitt P et al (1989) Meta-analytic evidence against prophylactic use of lidocaine in acute myocardial infarction. Arch Intern Med 149:2694–2698

21. Lie KI, Wellens HJJ, VanCapelle FJ, Durrer D (1974) Lidocaine in the prevention of ventricular fibrillation. N Engl J Med 291:1324–1326

22. Herlitz J, Ekstrom L, Wennerblom B, Axelsson A, Bang A, Lindkvist J, Persson NG, Holmberg S (1997) Lidocaine in out-of-hospital ventricular fibrillation. Does it improve survival? Resuscitation 33:199–205

23. Kowey PR, Levine JH, Herre JM, Pacifico A, Lindsay BD, Plumb VJ, Janosik DL, Kopelman HA, Scheinman MM (1994) Randomized, double-blind comparison of intravenous amiodarone and bretylium in the treatment of patients with recurrent, hemodynamically destabilizing ventricular tachycardia or fibrillation. The intravenous amiodarone multicenter investigators group. Circulation 92:3255–3263

24. Haynes RE, Chinn TL, Capass MK, Cobb LA (1981) Comparison of bretylium tosylate and lidocaine in management of out-of-hospital ventricular fibrillation. A randomized clinical trial. Am J Cardiol 48:353–356

25. Weaver WD, Fahrenbruch CE, Johnson DD, Hallstrom AP, Cobb LA, Copass MK (1990) Effect of epinephrine and lidocaine therapy on outcome after cardiac arrest due to ventricular fibrillation. Circulation 82:2027–2034

26. Thompson PD et al (1973) Lidocaine pharmcokinetics in advanced heart failure, liver disease and renal failure in humans. Ann Int Med 78:499–508

27. Campbell RWF (1987) Mexiletine. N Engl J Med 316:29–34

28. Impact Research Group (1984) International mexiletine and placebo antiarrhythmic coronary trial. I. Report on arrhythmia and other findings. J Am Coll Cardiol 4:1148–1163

29. DiMarco JP, Garan H, Ruskin JN (1981) Mexiletine for refractory ventricular arrhythmias: Results using serial electrophysiologic testing. Am J Cardiol 47:131–140

30. Berns E, Naccarelli GV, Dougherty AH, Povia C, Rinkenberger RL (1988) Mexiletine: Lack of predictors of clinical response in patients treated for life-threatening tachyarrhythmias. J Electrophysiol 2:201–206

31. Garson A, Randall DC, Gillette PC, Smith RT, Moak JP, McVey JP, McNamara DG (1985) Prevention of sudden death after repair of Tetralogy of Fallot: treatment of ventricular arrhythmias. J Am Coll Cardiol 6:221–227

32. Ruan Y, Liu N, Bloise R, Napolitano C, Prior SG (2007) Gating properties of SCN5A mutations and the response to mexiletine in long-QT syndrome type 3 patients. Circulation 116:1137–1144

33. Roden DM, Woosley RL (1986) Drug therapy: flecainide. N Engl J Med 315:36–41

34. The Cardiac Arrhythmia Suppression Trial Investigators (1989) Preliminary report: Effect of encainide and flecainide on mortality in a randomized trial of arrhythmia suppression after myocardial infarction. N Engl J Med 321:406–412

35. Flecainide ventricular tachycardia study group (1986) Treatment of resistant ventricular tachycardia with flecainide acetate. Amer J Cardiol 57:1299–1304

36. Gill JS, Mehta D, Ward DE, Camm AJ (1992) Efficacy of flecainide, sotalol, and verapamil in the treatment of right ventricular tachycardia in patients without overt cardiac abnormality. Br Heart J 68:392–397

37. Podrid PJ, Lown B (1984) Propafenone: a new agent for ventricular arrhythmias. J Am Coll Cardiol 4:117–125

38. Connally SJ, Kates RE, Lebsack CS, Harrison DC, Winkle RA (1983) Clinical pharmacology of propafenone. Circulation 68:589–596

39. Siddoway LA, Thompson EA, McAllister CB et al (1987) Polymorphism propafenone metabolism and disposition in man: clinical and pharmacokinetic consequences. Circulation 75:785–791

40. Naccarella F, Bracchetti D, Palmieri M, Cantinelli I, Bertaccini P, Ambrosioni E (1985) Comparison of propafenone and disopyramide for treatment of chronic ventricular arrhythmias: placebo-controlled, double-blind, randomized crossover study. Am Heart J 109:833–839

41. Chilson DA, Heger JJ, Zipes DP, Browne KF, Prystowsky EN (1985) Electrophysiologic effects and clinical efficacy of oral propafenone therapy in patients with ventricular tachycardia. J Am Coll Cardiol 5:1407

42. Siebels J, Cappato R, Ruppel R, Schneider MAE, Kuck KH, and the CASH Investigators (1993) Preliminary results of the cardiac arrest study hamburg (CASH). Am J Cardiol 72:109F–113F

43. Naccarelli GV, Wolbrette DL, Dell'Orfano JT, Patel HM, Luck JC (1998) A decade of clinical trial developments in postmyocardial infarction, congestive heart failure, and sustained ventricular tachyarrhymia patients: from CAST to AVID and beyond. J Cardiovasc Electrophysiol 9:864–891

44. Singh SN, DiBianco R, Davidson ME, Gottdeiner JS, Johnson WL, Laddu AR, Fletcher RD (1982) Comparison of acebutolol and propranolol for treatment of chronic ventricular arrhythmia: a placebo-controlled, double-blind, randomized crossover study. Circulation 65:1356–1364

45. DeSoyza N, Shapiro W, Chandraratna PAN, Aronow WS, Laddu AR, Thompson CH (1982) Acebutolol therapy for ventricular arrhythmias. A randomized, placebo-controlled double-blind multicenter study. Circulation 65:1129–1133

46. Nademanee, K, Taylor, R, Bailey WE et al (2000) Treating electrical storm. Sympathetic blockade versus advanced cardiac life support-guided therapy. Circulation 102:742

47. Morgera T, Pivotti F, Gori P, Maras P (1987) Mechanism of action and efficacy of verapamil and beta-blockers in exercise-induced ventricular tachycardia. Eur Heart J 8: D99–D105

48. Vincent GM, Schwartz PJ, Denjoy I, Swan H, Bithell C, Spazzolini C, Crotti L, Piippo K, Lupoglazoff JM, Villain E, Priori SG, Napolitano C, Zhang L (2009) High efficacy of beta-blockers in long-QT syndrome type 1: contribution of noncompliance and QT-prolonging drugs to the occurrence of beta-blocker treatment "failures". Circulation 119: 215–221

49. Hanyok JJ, Chow MS, Kluger J, Fieldman A (1988) Antifibrillatory effects of high dose bretylium and a lidocaine-bretylium combination during cardiopulmonary resuscitation. Crit Care Med 16:691–694

50. Naccarelli GV, Rinkenberger RL, Dougherty AH, Giebel RA (1985) Amiodarone: pharmacology and antiarrhythmic and adverse effects. Pharmacotherapy 5:298–313

51. Hohnloser SH, Klingenhebe T, Singh BN (1994) Amiodarone-associated proarrhythmic effects: a review with special reference to Torsade de Pointes tachycardia. Ann Intern Med 121:529–535

52. Desai AD, Chun S, Sung RJ (1997) The role of intravenous amiodarone in the management of cardiac arrhythmias. Ann Intern Med 127:294–303

53. Naccarelli GV, Jalal S (1995) Intravenous amiodarone: Another option in the acute management of sustained ventricular tachyarrhythmias. Circulation 92:3154–3155

54. Herre JM, Sauve MJ, Malone P et al (1989) Long-term results of amiodarone therapy in patients with recurrent sustained ventricular tachycardia or ventricular fibrillation. J Am Coll Cardiol 13:442–449

55. The CASCADE Investigators (1993) Randomized antiarrhythmic drug therapy in survivors of cardiac arrest (the CASCADE study). Am J Cardiol 72:280–287

56. The Antiarrhythmics Versus Implantable Defibrillators (AVID) Investigators (1997) A comparison of antiarrhythmic drug therapy with implantable defibrillators in patients resuscitated from near fatal ventricular arrhythmias. N Engl J Med 337:1576–1583

57. Connolly S, Gent M, Roberts R et al (1993) Canadian implantable defibrillator study (CIDS): study design and organization. Am J Cardiol 72:103F–108F

58. Moss AJ, Hall WJ, Cannom DS et al for the Multicenter Automatic Defibrillator Implantation Trial Investigators (1996) Improved survival with an implanted defibrillator in patients with coronary disease at high risk for ventricular arrhythmia. N Engl J Med 335:1933–1940

59. Bardy GH, Lee KL, Mark DB, Poole JE, Packer DL, Boineau R, Domanski M, Troutman C, Anderson J, Johnson G, McNulty SE, Clapp-Channing N, Davidson-Ray LD, Fraulo ES, Fishbein DP, Luceri RM, Ip JH for the Sudden Cardiac Death in Heart Failure Trial (SCD-HeFT) Investigators (2005) Amiodarone or an implantable-cardioverter-defibrillator for congestive heart failure. N Engl J Med 352:225–237

60. Levine JH, Massumi A, Scheinman MM, Winkle RA, Platia EV, Chilson DA, Gomes A, Woosley RL (1996) Intravenous amiodarone for recurrent sustained hypotensive ventricular tachyarrhythmias. Intravenous amiodarone multicenter trial group. J Am Coll Cardiol 27:67–75

61. Dorian P, Cass D, Schwartz B, Cooper R, Gelaznikas R, Barr A (2002) A randomized, blinded trial of intravenous amiodarone versus lidocaine in shock resistant ventricular fibrillation. N Engl J Med 346:884–890

62. Kudenchuk PJ, Cobb LA, Copass MK, Cummins RO, Doherty AM, Fahrenbruch CE et al (1999) Amiodarone for resuscitation after out-of-hospital cardiac arrest due to ventricular fibrillation. N Eng J Med 341:871–878

63. Goldschlager N, Epstein AE, Naccarelli GV, Olshansky B, Singh B, Collard HR, Murphy E (2007) A Practical Guide for clinicians who treat patients with amiodarone: 2007. Heart Rhythm 4:1250–1259

64. Singh BN (1993) Electrophysiologic basis for the antiarrhythmic actions of sotalol and comparison with other agents. Am J Cardiol 72:8A–18A

65. Hanyok JJ (1993) Clinical pharmacokinetics of sotalol. Am J Cardiol 72:19A–26A

66. Julian DG, Jackson FS, Prescott RJ, Szekely P (1982) Controlled trial of sotalol for one year after myocardial infarction. Lancet 1:1142–1147

67. Naccarelli GV, Dougherty AH, Wolbrette D (1995) Antiarrhythmic drug-implantable cardioverter/defibrillator interactions. In: Zipes DP, Jalife J (eds) Cardiac electrophysiology: from cell to bedside. W.B. Saunders Co., Philadelphia, pp 1426–1433

68. Stevens SK, Haffajee CI, Naccarelli GV, Schwartz KM, Luceri RM, Packer DL, Kowey PR, Rubin AM, and the Propafenone DFT Investigators (1996) The effects on defibrillation and pacing thresholds of oral propafenone in patients receiving permanent pacer-cardioverter-defibrillator devices. J Am Coll Cardiol 28:418–422

69. Connolly SJ, Dorian P, Roberts RS, Gent M, Bailin S, Fain ES, Thorpe K, Champagne J, Talajic M, Coutu B, Gronefeld GC, Hohnloser SH, Optimal Pharmacological Therapy in Cardioverter Defibrillator Patients (OPTIC) Investigators (2006) Comparison of beta-blockers, amiodarone plus beta-blockers, or sotalol for prevention of shocks from implantable cardioverter defibrillators: the OPTIC Study: a randomized trial. JAMA 295(2):165–171

70. Stevenson WG, Soejima K (2007) Catheter ablation for ventricular tachycardia. Circulation 115:2750–2760

12 Ablation for Ventricular Tachycardia

Dusan Kocovic

CONTENTS

Abstract

Sustained ventricular tachycardia (VT) is an important cause of morbidity and mortality in patients with heart disease and an important cause of morbidity in patients with normal heart. It is most common in patients with coronary artery disease with a history of myocardial infarction but it can develop in patients with other heart diseases. Since the advent and introduction of implantable cardioverter-defibrillators, the therapeutic approach to recurrent sustained VT in patients with heart disease significantly changed. Advances over the past decade now allow ablation of multiple, hemodynamically unstable, epicardial, and polymorphic VTs, formerly considered unmappable. Specific locations for the origins of idiopathic VT outside of the RVOT have been defined. These procedures are often difficult and are best approached by experienced operators in experienced laboratories. When the expertise is available, catheter ablation should be considered earlier in the therapeutic armamentarium for treatment of recurrent VT.

Key Words: Ventricular tachycardia; radiofrequency ablation; coronary artery disease; idiopathic tachycardia; right ventricular outflow tract; epicardial mapping; endocardial mapping; entrainment mapping; pace mapping; scar mapping; scar-related reentry; VT isthmus; VT exit; outflow tract ventricular tachycardia; LV fascicular idiopathic VT.

From: *Contemporary Cardiology: Management of Cardiac Arrhythmias*
Edited by: Gan-Xin Yan, Peter R. Kowey, DOI 10.1007/978-1-60761-161-5_12
© Springer Science+Business Media, LLC 2011

INTRODUCTION

Sustained ventricular tachycardia (VT) is an important cause of morbidity and mortality in patients with heart disease and an important cause of morbidity in patients with normal heart *(1)*. It is most common in patients with coronary artery disease with a history of myocardial infarction but it can develop in patients with other heart diseases. Since the advent and introduction of implantable cardioverter-defibrillators (ICDs), the therapeutic approach to recurrent sustained VT in patients with heart disease significantly changed. ICDs reliably terminate VT and VF episodes, reducing the risk of sudden death. Recurrent VT develops in 40–60% of patients who receive an ICD after an episode of spontaneous sustained VT, and in high-risk population a first episode of VT occurs in 20% of patients within 3–5 years after ICD implantation for primary prevention of sudden death *(2–4)*. Despite life-saving effects of ICD's ICD shocks reduce quality of life and is associated with an increased risk of death and post-traumatic stress disorder *(2–4)*. Antiarrhythmic drug therapy with amiodarone or sotalol reduces number of VT episodes but with high incidence of side effects and low efficacy *(2)*. Catheter ablation remains as useful tool for reducing VT episodes and can be life saving when VT is incessant *(1, 5, 6)*.

In patients without a structural heart disease, idiopathic VTs can occur but rarely cause sudden death. Electrophysiological study with catheter ablation is often warranted to confirm the diagnosis, to provide further evidence for the absence of ventricular scar or other disease, and often to cure the arrhythmia. Ablation is also an option for symptomatic non-sustained VT and frequent ventricular ectopy in these patients *(1)*.

DEFINITIONS

Ventricular tachycardia: a tachycardia (rate >100/min) with three or more consecutive beats that originates from the ventricles independent of atrial or AV nodal conduction.

Idioventricular rhythm: is three or more consecutive beats at a rate of <100/min that originate from the ventricles independent of atrial or AV nodal conduction.

Definitions in relation to VT morphologies: Monomorphic VT has a similar QRS configuration from beat to beat (Fig. 1 a–d). Some variability in QRS morphology at initiation is not uncommon, followed by stabilization of the QRS morphology. *Multiple monomorphic VTs* refer to more than one morphologically distinct monomorphic VT, occurring as different episodes or induced at different times. *Polymorphic VT* has a continuously changing QRS configuration from beat to beat indicating a changing ventricular activation sequence (Fig. 1e). *Pleomorphic VT* has more than one morphologically distinct QRS complex occurring during the same episode of VT, but the QRS is not continuously changing. *Right and left bundle branch block-like VT configurations*: terms used to describe the dominant deflection in V1, with a dominant R wave described as "right bundle branch block-like" (Fig. 1b) and a dominant S wave as "left bundle branch block-like" (Fig. 1a) configurations. This terminology is potentially misleading as the VT may not show features characteristic of the same bundle branch block-like morphology in other leads (Fig. 1c). *Ventricular flutter* is a term that has been applied to rapid VT that has a sinusoidal QRS configuration that prevents identification of the QRS morphology. It is preferable to avoid this term, in favor of monomorphic VT with indeterminant QRS morphology *(1, 7, 8)*.

Definitions in relation to VT hemodynamic stability: Hemodynamically unstable VT causes hemodynamic compromise requiring prompt termination. *Unmappable VT* does not allow interrogation of multiple sites to define the activation sequence or perform entrainment mapping; this may be due to: hemodynamic intolerance that necessitates immediate VT termination, spontaneous or pacing-induced transition to other morphologies of VT, or repeated termination during mapping.

Definitions in relation to VT duration: Incessant VT is continuous sustained VT that recurs promptly despite repeated intervention for termination over several hours. *Non-sustained VT* terminates spontaneously within 30 sec. *Repetitive monomorphic VT* has continuously repeating episodes of self-terminating non-sustained VT. *Sustained VT* is continuous VT for ≥30 sec or that requires an intervention for termination

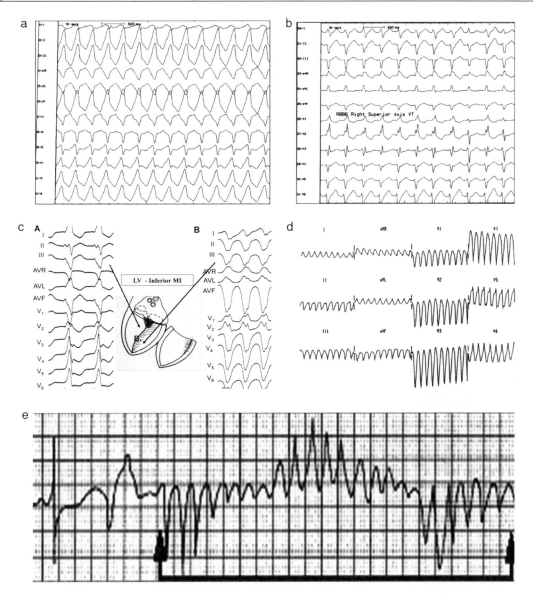

Fig. 1. ECG types of VT and most common causes are shown with characteristic ECG features of selected VTs. LBBB indicates left bundle branch block; RBBB, right bundle branch block; L, left; and R, right. (**a**) Sustained monomorphic ventricular tachycardia with LBBB and inferior axis suggesting origin from RVOT. This tachycardia is idiopathic in origin. (**b**) Sustained monomorphic ventricular tachycardia with RBBB and right superior axis, suggesting origin in the left ventricular septum. This type of tachycardia is commonly idiopathic in origin. (**c**) Two different ventricular tachycardias originating in the left ventricle long after an inferior wall myocardial infarct. This type of VT is related to scars that form after myocardial infarct. (**d**) Fast ventricular tachycardia with LBBB and left superior axis. Morphology and rate are suggestive of bundle branch reentry ventricular tachycardia. This type of VT is related to nonischemic cardiomyopathy. (**e**) Polymorphic ventricular tachycardia. This type of tachycardia is frequently related to electrolyte abnormalities, ischemia, or drug toxicity.

(such as cardioversion). *VT storm* is considered three or more separate episodes of sustained VT within 24 h, each requiring termination by an intervention.

Definitions in relation to mechanisms: Scar-related reentry describes arrhythmias that have characteristics of reentry and originate from an area of myocardial scar identified from electrogram characteristics or myocardial imaging. Large reentry circuits that can be defined over several centimeters are commonly referred to as "macroreentry" (Fig. 2). *Focal VT* has a point source of earliest ventricular activation with a spread of activation away in all directions from that site. The mechanism can be automaticity, triggered activity, or microreentry. *Idiopathic VT* is a term that has been used to indicate VT that is known to occur in the absence of a clinically apparent structural heart disease.

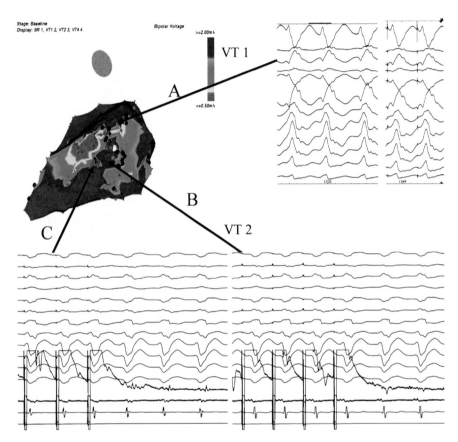

Fig. 2. LV mapping data from a patient with VT due to prior myocardial infarction. A voltage map of the LV is present in the middle of the panel. Purple indicates normal bipolar electrogram amplitude >1.55 mV. The amplitude diminished from *blue* to *green* to *yellow* to *red*. A large lateral basal wall low-voltage infarct area was present. Panel A shows VT-1, which had a right bundle branch block right inferior axis configuration. Pacing at the superior aspect of the infarct A (*arrow*) reproduced the VT-1 QRS morphology, indicating that the exit for VT-1 was near the pacing site. B shows pacing at a site in the middle of the infarct that was a channel for VT-2. During entrainment mapping (B), the long delay from the pacing stimulus to the QRS indicates slow conduction through the scar to the margin of the infarct. The paced QRS had a right bundle branch block inferior axis configuration that matched VT-2. Pacing at the site during VT (B) entrained (reset) tachycardia with a long stimulus-to-QRS interval without changing the QRS morphology and with a postpacing interval that matched the VT cycle length. C shows that the exit for VT-2 was at the inferior margin of the infarct. Potential ablation targets are the site B and C.

MECHANISMS

Mechanisms and Basis for Catheter Ablation of Ventricular Tachycardia

Monomorphic VT can occur in individuals with or without structural heart disease. The underlying heart disease and clinical characteristics of the VT often suggest a potential mechanism and origin. Ventricular tachycardias that are due to automaticity are expected to have a focal origin, making them susceptible to ablation with discrete radiofrequency (RF) lesions *(8–15)*. Triggered activity or automaticity is likely causes of focal origin VTs, although small reentry circuits can not be excluded. Idiopathic outflow tract (OT)-VTs have a focal origin. Relatively large reentry circuits are common in VT associated with ventricular scar, such as prior infarction, but VT may appear focal if the reentry circuit is small or due to a focal endocardial breakthrough from an epicardial reentry circuit (Figs. 2 and 3). Automaticity can occur in some patients with ventricular scars.

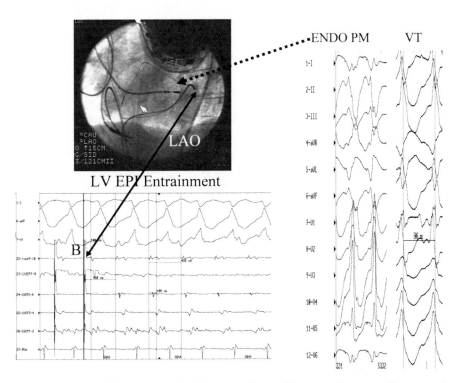

Fig. 3. Epicardial and endocardial mapping data from a patient with nonischemic cardiomyopathy are shown. *Top left*, left anterior oblique (LAO) fluoroscopic image of a mapping catheter placed retrograde through the aorta into the LV (*white arrow*) at the earliest endocardial site for VT. An epicardial catheter had been inserted by a subxiphoid puncture into the pericardial space (*black arrow*). During entrainment mapping (B), the long delay from the pacing stimulus to the QRS indicates slow conduction through the scar. The paced QRS has a right bundle branch block right inferior axis configuration that matched VT. Pacing at the site during VT entrained (reset) tachycardia with a long stimulus-to-QRS interval without changing the QRS morphology and with a postpacing interval that matched the VT cycle length. Epicardial recording showed that presystolic activity was recorded during VT. Endocardial pacing across the epicardial site produced a different QRS morphology that did not match VT. Ablation through the epicardial site abolished the inducible VT.

Triggered Activity and Automaticity

Triggered activity arises from oscillations in membrane potential during (early afterdepolarizations) or following (delayed afterdepolarizations) an action potential. Experimental evidence implicates early afterdepolarizations in the initiation of polymorphic tachycardias in the long QT syndromes *(16)*. However, the mechanism of the premature ventricular beats targeted for ablation in these syndromes is unknown *(8)*.

Delayed afterdepolarizations can be caused by intracellular calcium overload which activates the Na^+/Ca^{2+} exchanger resulting in the transient inward current I_{ti} *(1, 10, 15)*. Factors that increase intracellular calcium include increases in heart rate, β-adrenergic stimulation, and digitalis. β-Adrenergic effects are mediated through a cAMP-induced increase in intracellular calcium and are antagonized by adenosine, which effects a decrease in cAMP. Termination of idiopathic right ventricular outflow tract (RVOT) tachycardias by an intravenous bolus of adenosine or infusion of calcium channel blockers or by vagotonic maneuvers is consistent with triggered activity as the likely mechanism for some of these tachycardias *(15)*. These tachycardias can be difficult to induce at electrophysiology (EP) testing; rapid burst pacing and/or isoproterenol infusion is often required. Aminophylline, calcium infusion, and atropine may also be useful *(12, 13)*.

Less commonly, focal VT may be due to automaticity that is provoked by adrenergic stimulation that is not triggered *(12, 13, 17)*. This type of VT may become incessant under stress or during isoproterenol administration, but cannot be initiated or terminated by programmed electrical stimulation; it can sometimes be suppressed by calcium channel blockers or β-blockers. In contrast to its effects on triggered RVOT tachycardia, adenosine transiently *suppresses* the arrhythmia but does not *terminate* it *(12, 17)*. Automaticity from damaged Purkinje fibers has been suggested as a mechanism for some catecholamine sensitive, focal origin VTs *(7, 18)*. Whether these VTs are due to abnormal automaticity, originating from partially depolarized myocytes, as has been shown for VTs during the early phase of myocardial infarction (MI), is not clear.

Although automaticity is often implicated as a mechanism of VT in the absence of overt structural heart disease, disease processes that diminish cell-to-cell coupling are likely to facilitate automaticity *(19, 20)*. Automatic VTs can occur in structural heart disease *(20)*, and automatic premature beats may initiate reentrant VTs.

Scar-Related Reentry

The majority of sustained monomorphic VTs (SMVTs) in patients with structural heart disease are due to reentry associated with areas of scar, designated as *scar-related reentry*. Evidence supporting reentry includes initiation and termination by programmed stimulation (although this does not exclude triggered activity), demonstrable entrainment or resetting with fusion, and continuous electrical activity that cannot be dissociated from VT by extrastimuli. Myocardial scar is identified from: low-voltage regions on ventricular voltage maps, areas with fractionated electrograms, unexcitability during pace mapping, evidence of scar on myocardial imaging, or from an area of known surgical incision. Prior MI is the most common cause, but scar-related VT also occurs in other myocardial diseases including arrhythmogenic right ventricular cardiomyopathy (ARVC), sarcoidosis, Chagas disease, dilated cardiomyopathy, and after cardiac surgery for congenital heart disease (particularly tetralogy of Fallot) or valve replacement (Figs. 2, 3, 4, 5, and 6) *(21–28)*.

The substrate supporting scar-related reentry is characterized by (i) regions of slow conduction, (ii) unidirectional conduction block at some point in the reentry path that allows initiation of reentry, and (iii) areas of conduction block that often define parts of the reentry path *(29–33)*. Ventricular tachycardia after MI has been extensively studied in canine models and in humans *(29–33)*. Reentry occurs through surviving muscle bundles, commonly located in the subendocardium, but that can also occur in the mid-myocardium and epicardium. There is evidence of ongoing ion channel

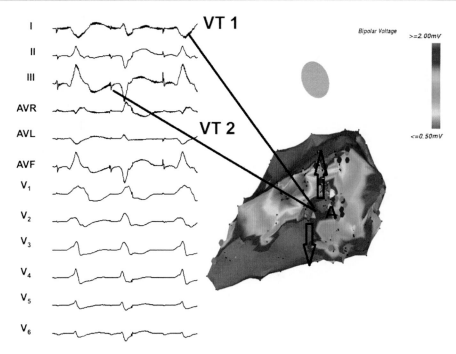

Fig. 4. LV mapping data from a patient with VT due to prior infarction. A voltage map of the LV was present in the middle of the panel. Purple color indicates normal bipolar electrogram amplitude >1.55 mV. The amplitude diminished from *blue* to *green* to *yellow* to *red*. A large lateral basal wall low-voltage infarct area was present. Panel shows VT-1, which has a right bundle branch block right inferior axis configuration and VT-2 right bundle branch block left superior axis configuration. Pacing at the inferior aspect of the infarct A reproduced both VT morphologies that were alternating. VT-1 QRS morphology has a long Stim-QRS interval indicating that the exit for VT-1 is far from the pacing site. VT-2 QRS morphology has a short Stim-QRS interval indicating that the exit is close to the pacing site. Pacing site is the ablation target for both VTs.

remodeling within scar, at least early after MI, resulting in regional reductions in I_{Na} and I_{Ca} *(34)*, although late after infarction action potential characteristics of surviving myocytes can be near normal *(35)*. Coupling between myocyte bundles and myocytes is reduced by increased collagen and connective tissue, diminished gap junction density, and alterations in gap junction distribution, composition, and function. Surviving fibers can be connected side to side in regions where the collagenous sheathes are interrupted, resulting in a zigzag pattern of transverse conduction along a pathway lengthened by branching and merging bundles of surviving myocytes *(34–36)*. The pattern of fibrosis may be important in determining the degree of conduction delay; patchy fibrosis between strands of surviving muscle produces greater delay than diffuse fibrosis *(30)*. These aspects of scar remodeling contribute to the formation of channels and regions where conduction time is prolonged, facilitating reentry *(35, 36)*.

Unidirectional conduction block may occur after a properly timed extra-beat and is probably functional rather than fixed in most instances. Regions of conduction block can be anatomically fixed such that they are present during tachycardia and sinus rhythm; dense, non-excitable fibrosis, or valve annuli create these types of anatomical boundaries for reentry. Alternatively, conduction block can be functional and present only during tachycardia when the refractory period of the tissue exceeds the tachycardia cycle length or is maintained by collision of excitation waves *(34–37)*. Functional conduction block can occur in figure of eight type of reentry circuits *(37, 38)*.

Many reentry circuits contain a protected isthmus or channel of variable length, isolated by arcs of conduction block. Depolarization of the small mass of tissue in a channel is not detectable in the

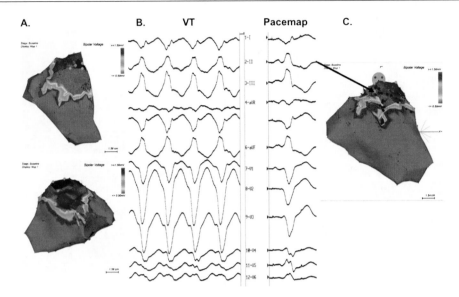

Fig. 5. RV mapping data from a patient with VT due to RV dysplasia. A voltage map of the RV is presented in two projections. The *upper panel* is AP and the *lower panel* is modified PA projection. *Purple color* indicates normal bipolar electrogram amplitude >1.55 mV. Amplitude diminished from *blue* to *green* to *yellow* to *red*. A large low-voltage scar area in RVOT around pulmonary valves was present. Panel shows VT-1, which has a left bundle branch block right inferior axis configuration. Pacing at the superior aspect of the scar (arrow) reproduced the VT-1 QRS morphology, indicating that the exit for VT-1 is near the pacing site and that is the potential ablation target site.

body surface ECG; thus catheter-recorded electrograms in this region are manifest during "electrical diastole" between QRS complexes. At the exit from the channel, the wavefront propagates across the ventricles establishing the QRS complex. To return to the entrance to the channel, the reentry wavefront may propagate along the border of the scar in an outer loop or may propagate through the scar in an inner loop. Multiple potential loops may be present. There are a variety of potential reentry circuit configurations and locations that vary from patient to patient *(29–39)*. Often VT isthmus sites span a few centimeters at the border zone of scars. Larger macroreentry circuits spanning several centimeters can also be encountered. In cardiomyopathies and inferior wall infarcts, reentry circuits are often located adjacent to a valve annulus, suggesting that the valve annulus often helps to define a reentry path (Figs. 2, 3, 4, and 5) *(39)*.

Multiple VT morphologies are usually inducible in the same patient, often related to multiple reentry circuits. Two different reentry circuits may share the same exit with functional block changing the QRS morphology, may have the same or similar common isthmus with a different exit, or may have two different isthmuses in different areas of the same scar or in different scars (Figs. 2 and 4). The presence of multiple potential reentry circuit paths and the anatomic complexity of scars that support reentry complicate mapping and ablation. It can be difficult to distinguish bystander regions that are not part of the reentry circuit from a critical isthmus *(29–31)*. A bystander region for one VT may participate in a different VT. Further complicating assessment is the potential three-dimensional configuration of circuits, which can involve the endocardium, epicardium, or mid-myocardium (Fig. 3) *(40–42)*.

It is possible that other reentry mechanisms cause some VTs. Spiral wave reentry can be induced in excitable tissue in the absence of tissue discontinuities and could cause ventricular fibrillation (VF) or polymorphic VT (PMVT); anchoring to a discontinuity or region of slow conduction could theoretically cause monomorphic VT *(33)*. Whether this type of functional reentry causes VT in humans and whether it would be susceptible to ablation is not known.

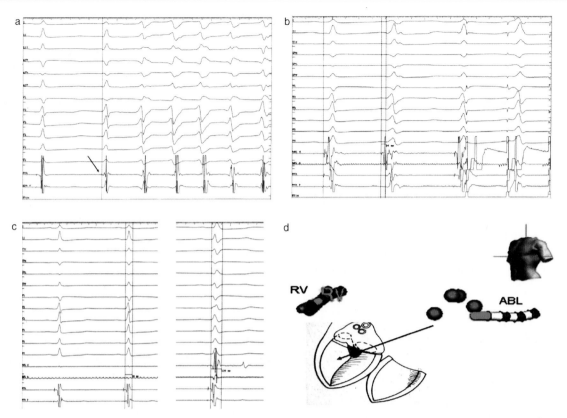

Fig. 6. Recordings from a patient with idiopathic ventricular fibrillation and electrical storm are shown. **Panels a, b, c** show recordings from the electrophysiology laboratory. Frequent premature ventricular contractions were present. LV mapping identified sites with early potentials preceding the onset of the premature ventricular contractions (*arrow* at the onset of endocardial signal). Ablation at these sites abolished ventricular ectopy and episodes of ventricular fibrillation. Panel **c**: post-ablation ECG demonstrates widening of QRS complex, a result of ablation of a part of His–Purkinje network in the LV. **Panel d** shows the position of the RF ablation catheter in the LV at the time of ablation.

Reentry in the Purkinje System

Reentry within the Purkinje fibers and the specialized conduction system causes ˜5% of all sustained monomorphic VTs encountered in patients undergoing catheter ablation. Macroreentry through the bundle branches occurs in patients with slowed conduction through the His–Purkinje system and is usually associated with severe left ventricular (LV) dysfunction due to dilated cardiomyopathy, valvular heart disease, and less often ischemic heart disease (Fig. 1d) *(43)*.

Left ventricular intrafascicular verapamil-sensitive VT occurs in patients without structural heart disease. The mechanism is reentry that appears to involve a portion of the LV Purkinje fibers, most often in the region of the left posterior fascicle, giving rise to a characteristic right bundle branch block (RBBB) superior axis QRS configuration and a QRS duration that is only slightly prolonged (Fig. 1b) *(44)*.

ELECTROPHYSIOLOGICAL BASIS FOR CATHETER ABLATION

The mechanism of VT is a key determinant for selection of mapping strategies to identify ablation target sites. For idiopathic VT, the focal origin or critical portion of the reentry path is usually contained in a very small area such that discrete lesions can abolish VT; therefore, mapping targets a precise region. For scar-related VTs, ablation is aimed at transecting the critical VT isthmus. Ventricular tachycardia isthmuses may be narrow, allowing a discrete lesion to abolish VT, or broad, requiring larger ablation areas. In addition, in patients with unmappable VTs and multiple VTs, larger ablation areas targeting putative critical reentry sites, often in or near the border zone of scars, are often employed. In post-MI VT, selection of catheter ablation for an individual patient should consider risks and benefits that are determined by patient characteristics, as well as the availability of appropriate facilities with technical expertise. In patients with structural heart disease, episodes of sustained VT are a marker for increased mortality and reduce quality of life in patients who have implanted defibrillators and structural heart disease. Antiarrhythmic medications can reduce the frequency of ICD therapies, but have disappointing efficacy and side effects *(1–4)*. Advances in technology and understanding of VT substrates now allow ablation of multiple and unstable VTs with acceptable safety and efficacy, even in patients with advanced heart disease. In the past, ablation was often not considered until pharmacological options had been exhausted, often after the patient had suffered substantial morbidity from recurrent episodes of VT and ICD shocks. At this point of time catheter ablation for VT should generally be considered early in the treatment of patients with recurrent VT.

INDICATIONS FOR VT ABLATION

Patients with Structural Heart Diseases Including Prior MI, Dilated Cardiomyopathy, and Arrhythmogenic Right Ventricular Cardiomyopathy/Dysplasia (ARVC/D)

CATHETER ABLATION OF VT IS RECOMMENDED

1. for symptomatic sustained monomorphic VT (SMVT), including VT terminated by an ICD, that recurs despite antiarrhythmic drug therapy or when antiarrhythmic drugs are not tolerated or not desired;
2. for control of incessant SMVT or VT storm that is not due to a transient reversible cause;
3. for patients with frequent PVCs, NSVTs, or VT that is presumed to cause ventricular dysfunction;
4. for bundle branch reentrant or interfascicular VTs;
5. for recurrent sustained polymorphic VT and VF that is refractory to antiarrhythmic therapy when there is a suspected trigger that can be targeted for ablation *(1)*.

CATHETER ABLATION SHOULD BE CONSIDERED

1. in patients who have one or more episodes of SMVT despite therapy with one of more class I or III antiarrhythmic drugs;
2. in patients with recurrent SMVT due to prior MI who have LV ejection fraction >0.30 and expectation for >1 year of survival and is an acceptable alternative to amiodarone therapy;
3. in patients with hemodynamically tolerated SMVT due to prior MI who have reasonably preserved LV ejection fraction (>0.35) even if they have not failed antiarrhythmic drug therapy.

Patients Without Structural Heart Disease

CATHETER ABLATION OF VT IS RECOMMENDED FOR PATIENTS WITH IDIOPATHIC VT

1. for monomorphic VT that is causing severe symptoms;
2. for monomorphic VT when antiarrhythmic drugs are not effective, not tolerated, or not desired;
3. for recurrent sustained polymorphic VT and VF (electrical storm) that is refractory to antiarrhythmic therapy when there is a suspected trigger that can be targeted for ablation.

VT CATHETER ABLATION IS CONTRAINDICATED

1. in the presence of a mobile ventricular thrombus (epicardial ablation may be considered);

2. for asymptomatic PVCs and/or NSVT that are not suspected of causing or contributing to ventricular dysfunction;
3. for VT due to transient, reversible causes, such as acute ischemia, hyperkalemia, or drug-induced Torsades de Pointes.

This recommendation for ablation stands regardless of whether VT is stable or unstable or multiple VTs are present *(1)*.

TECHNICAL CONSIDERATIONS

Ablative therapy is directed at destroying arrhythmogenic tissue or a critical part of the presumed focus or reentrant circuit responsible for the genesis and maintenance of VT. Previous work in animal models of sustained VT and in human VT that follows myocardial infarction has demonstrated the presence of certain types of electrical endocardial activity. Techniques that have been used to localize the site of origin of tachycardia follow the concept that majority of VTs develop subendocardially. Methods for localization of VT include analysis of the ECG morphology during VT, endocardial activation mapping during VT, endocardial pace mapping, mapping of ventricular activation during VT, scar mapping, and isolated potential mapping.

Analysis of the standard 12-lead ECG QRS morphology during VT can regionalize, narrow down the possible sites of origin. With knowledge of the location of myocardial infarction, bundle branch block pattern of VT, frontal plane QRS axis, and precordial R wave progression pattern, the area of origin can be narrowed down significantly. Initial 12-lead ECG analysis allows for ablation procedure to narrow at least to left-or right-sided approach. The ablation procedure then proceeds in four main steps. The first is a vascular access, venous for ablation in the right ventricle, arterial for retrograde approach to the left ventricle, or transseptal if the arterial approach is compromised, dependent on

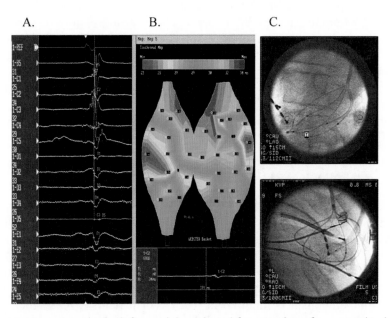

Fig. 7. Basket catheter was present in the left ventricle and used for mapping of non-sustained ventricular tachycardia or a single VPD. Electrode pair with the earliest endocardial electrogram is represented with the *red color* on the isochrone color map in the *middle panel*. Position of the basket catheter is given in two different projections RAO and LAO on the panel on the *right*.

initial presentation of arrhythmia. The second is arrhythmia induction and the third is mapping and ablation. The fourth is testing – attempt to reinduce the arrhythmia at the end of the procedure.

Mapping for Localization of VT Origin

When VT is hemodynamically stable, mapping can be performed during VT. Many patients with heart disease have VTs that are "unmappable" or "unstable" because they require immediate termination because of hemodynamic intolerance, they cannot be reliably induced, or they frequently change from one VT to another. Substrate mapping or multielectrode mapping approaches have been developed to guide ablation of these VTs (Figs. 6 and 7).

Mapping systems that recreate the geometry of the ventricles from point-by-point sampling while providing continuous display of catheter position are in common use *(45, 46)*. Electrophysiological data such as the activation time and electrogram amplitude are color coded for display (Figs. 2, 4, and 5). Cardiac motion introduces some error. Papillary muscles and other fine anatomic details are not visible. Registration of pre-acquired computed tomographic or magnetic resonance images on mapping systems shows promise for improving anatomic definition.

Balloon or basket electrode arrays sample from multiple sites simultaneously, potentially allowing activation to be defined from a single beat or brief run of VT (Fig. 7). A "noncontact" mapping system mathematically reconstructs potentials from adjacent sites *(45, 46)*.

ABLATION TECHNOLOGIES

The simplicity and safety of radiofrequency (RF) current make it the most common ablation energy. Solid 4- or 5-mm electrodes are used for ablation of idiopathic VTs, but scar-related VTs often require repeated RF applications and larger, deeper lesions that are facilitated by irrigated RF ablation or larger (e.g., 8 mm) electrodes. Large electrodes are convenient but reduce mapping precision and have a greater risk of coagulum formation because of the greater temperature disparities across the electrode compared with smaller electrodes *(47, 48)*. Irrigated and large-tip electrodes are prone to deep heating within the tissue (Fig. 8), sometimes causing steam formation that can explode through the tissue ("steam pops"). Tamponade can occur but is rare during ablation of scar-related left ventricular (LV) tachycardias. The risk is likely greater in the thin-walled right ventricle (RV) and with power >40 W. External irrigation has been suggested to reduce the risk of thrombus formation, but administration of intravascular saline requires monitoring volume status and often diuresis *(47–51)*.

Experience with catheter cryoablation is limited, but it may pose less risk of injury to adjacent coronary arteries for epicardial ablation than RF ablation *(52)*.

ENDOCARDIAL MAPPING AND ABLATION

Access to the LV for endocardial mapping is commonly achieved retrogradely across the aortic valve. Damage to the aortic valve or coronary artery ostia is possible but rare *(20)*. Significant vascular access complications, including arterial dissection, significant bleeding, and femoral atrioventricular fistulas, occurred in 2.1% of patients in one multicenter study *(51)*. A transseptal approach to the left atrium allows access to the LV through the mitral valve for patients with peripheral vascular disease or a mechanical aortic valve or for insertion of multiple mapping catheters.

Cerebral or systemic embolism is reported in 0–2.7% of patients *(51)*. Echocardiography should be performed before the procedure to detect mobile LV thrombus, which is a contraindication to LV mapping. If laminated thrombus is suspected, a several week period of anticoagulation with warfarin may be considered in the hope of reducing the presence of friable thrombus, but no data exist assessing this approach.

During LV mapping and ablation, patients are systemically anticoagulated with heparin. After ablation, continued anticoagulation with aspirin or warfarin is recommended depending on the extent of ablation performed. Atrioventricular block can occur with either RV or LV ablation and may be unavoidable when VT originates from the septum.

EPICARDIAL MAPPING AND ABLATION

Endocardial ablation fails if VT originates from a deep intramural or epicardial source. Percutaneous epicardial mapping and ablation are performed as described by Sosa and colleagues (53, 54). The pericardial space is entered with an epidural needle under fluoroscopic imaging with contrast injection, followed by placement of a guidewire and introducer sheath for the mapping catheter. In the absence of adhesions, the catheter moves freely in the pericardial space for mapping (Fig. 3) (53). Epicardial ablation with standard solid RF ablation electrodes can be successful, but absence of cooling from circulating blood often results in low-power heating with limited lesion creation, requiring irrigated RF ablation (55, 56).

The risk of injury to epicardial coronary arteries is a major concern and is dependent on proximity to the vessel, overlying fat, and vessel diameter, with smaller vessels more susceptible to thermal injury. Proximity to the coronary arteries is assessed from angiography while the ablation catheter is at the target site; ablation directly on major vessels is avoided (51, 56).

Pericardial bleeding can occur but rarely requires prolonged drainage or surgical treatment. Rarely, puncture of a subdiaphragmatic vessel can cause significant abdominal bleeding. The left phrenic nerve is potentially susceptible to injury as it courses down the lateral aspect of the LV but can be identified by pacing from the ablation catheter. After ablation, symptoms of pericarditis are common but generally resolve within a few days.

Pericardial adhesions after cardiac surgery often prevent percutaneous access, although limited access to the inferior wall may be possible. A direct surgical approach to the pericardial space via a subxiphoid pericardial window or thoracotomy in the electrophysiology laboratory can be used for mapping and ablation (57).

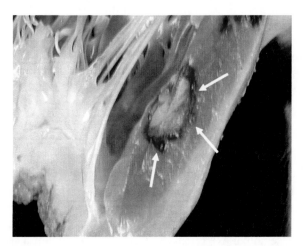

Fig. 8. One-week old radiofrequency lesion in a patient with nonischemic cardiomyopathy. Lesion was created with the "Chilli" closed irrigation catheter. There was a clear hemorrhagic delineation of the lesion that was 8 mm deep and about 16 mm wide. There was some endocardial sparing as well.

ABLATION OF MONOMORPHIC VT IN STRUCTURAL HEART DISEASES

Patients with VT and structural heart diseases often have depressed ventricular function, heart failure, and coronary artery disease. Induced VT is often poorly tolerated, requiring prompt restoration of sinus rhythm, rendering VT unmappable with catheter techniques. Inability to tolerate long episodes of VT was a deterrent to ablation in the past but is now commonly addressed with substrate mapping approaches or multielectrode catheter mapping. Even so, induction of VT is generally needed to confirm the type of VT and to assess the effect of ablation, placing the patient at risk of hemodynamic deterioration and ischemia during periods of tachycardia and hypotension. Assessment and management of these risks begin before the procedure. Intravascular volume status should be optimized. A recent assessment of potential myocardial ischemia with perfusion imaging or angiography is helpful to guide management decisions if hypotension or pulmonary edema occurs during the procedure. Before the procedure, it is desirable to discontinue antiarrhythmic drugs that may interfere with initiation of VTs, but this may not be safe or necessary when VT occurs despite therapy.

Consideration of risks and benefits should be individualized. Procedural risks are likely to be increased in the elderly and in patients with severe underlying heart disease. In many patients, VT recurrences are acceptably reduced by antiarrhythmic drug therapy, and ablation is not required. Recurrent VT episodes can be a marker for deterioration of heart failure and mortality risk despite an ICD. Some patients warrant assessment for cardiac transplantation or LV assist device placement so that the eligibility of these options is known in the event of further deterioration.

Scar-Related Sustained Monomorphic VT

Scar-related reentry is the most common cause of sustained monomorphic VT in patients with structural heart disease. Causes include old myocardial infarction, cardiomyopathies, and surgical incisions. Ventricular scars are composed of variable regions of dense fibrosis that create conduction block and surviving myocyte bundles with interstitial fibrosis and diminished coupling, which produce circuitous slow-conduction paths that promote reentry *(36, 37)*.

Many scar-related reentry circuits can be modeled as having an isthmus or channel composed of a small mass of tissue that does not contribute to the surface ECG. The QRS complex is inscribed when the excitation wavefront emerges from an exit along the border of the scar and spreads across the ventricles (Fig. 9). Reentry circuit configurations and locations vary from patient to patient. Large macroreentry circuits spanning several centimeters are common causes of slow VTs. Scars causing VT often border a valve annulus that forms a border segment for part of the reentry circuit *(35–39)*.

Repeated programmed stimulation typically induces >1 monomorphic VT. Multiple VTs can be due to different circuits in widely disparate areas of scar, different exits from the same region of scar, or changes in activation remote from the circuit due to functional regions of block. Ablation at one region often abolishes >1 VTs (Fig. 4) *(59, 60)*.

QRS Morphology as a Guide to the VT Exit

The QRS morphology of VT is an indication of the location of the circuit exit. VTs with a left bundle branch block-like configuration in lead V1 have an exit in the RV or interventricular septum; dominant R waves in V1 indicate an LV exit. The frontal plane axis indicates whether the exit is on the inferior wall, which produces a superiorly directed axis, or on the anterior (cranial) wall, which produces an inferiorly directed axis. The mid precordial leads, V3 and V4, provide an indication of exit location between the base and apex; apical exits generate dominant S waves; basal exits generate dominant R waves. VTs that originate in the subepicardium generally have a longer QRS duration and slower QRS upstrokes in the precordial leads than those with an endocardial exit *(61, 62)*.

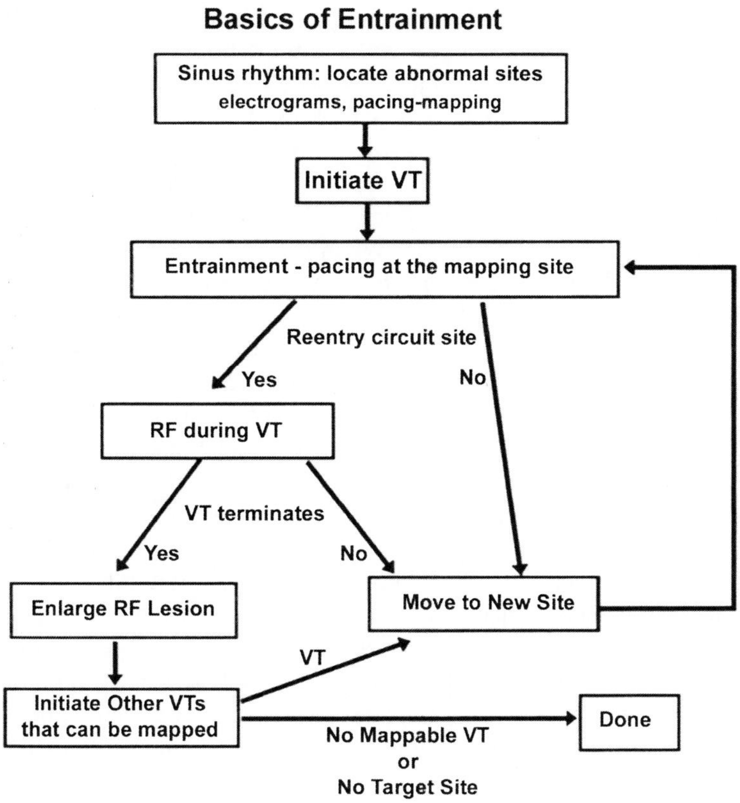

Basics of Entrainment

```
┌─────────────────────────────────────┐
│  Sinus rhythm: locate abnormal sites │
│     electrograms, pacing-mapping     │
└─────────────────────────────────────┘
                  │
                  ▼
            ┌───────────┐
            │Initiate VT│
            └───────────┘
                  │
                  ▼
┌─────────────────────────────────────┐
│ Entrainment - pacing at the mapping site │◄──────┐
└─────────────────────────────────────┘          │
         Reentry circuit site                     │
   Yes ◄                    No ▼                   │
      ┌──────────────┐                             │
      │ RF during VT │                             │
      └──────────────┘                             │
         VT terminates                             │
   Yes ▼          No ▼                             │
┌──────────────┐   ┌──────────────────┐           │
│Enlarge RF Lesion│  │ Move to New Site │──────────┘
└──────────────┘   └──────────────────┘
      │          VT ▲
      ▼             │
┌──────────────────┐  No Mappable VT   ┌──────┐
│Initiate Other VTs│        or         │ Done │
│that can be mapped │───────────────────►└──────┘
└──────────────────┘  No Target Site
```

Fig. 9. Schematics used for entrainment mapping in hemodynamically stable patient.

Mapping During VT

When VT is stable for mapping, an isthmus can be targeted during VT *(59, 61)*. In activation sequence maps, the circuit exit and isthmus are identified from presystolic (before the QRS onset) and diastolic (earlier than presystolic) activation, respectively, and are confirmed with pacing maneuvers such as entrainment (Figs. 2, 4, and 9) *(29, 35, 60, 62)*.

Multielectrode and noncontact mapping systems identify endocardial exit regions of presystolic electric activity in >90% of VTs. Some diastolic activity is identified in approximately two-thirds of patients, but complete reentry circuits are defined in <20% *(29, 35, 60)*.

Because of heterogeneity of scars with multiple potential conduction paths and channels, electrogram timing alone is not a reliable guide for targeting a specific reentry circuit isthmus *(29, 35)*. Confirmation that a site is involved in the reentry circuit can be obtained by pacing at the site (entrainment mapping; Figs. 2, 4, and 9) or reproducible VT termination by mechanical pressure at the site *(29, 35, 62–64)*. It is not necessary to define the entire circuit if an isthmus can be identified for ablation.

Substrate Mapping

For multiple and unstable VTs, substrate mapping can be used to identify regions of scar and potential reentry circuit channels during stable sinus or paced rhythm. Voltage maps are created from three-dimensional anatomic plots of electrogram amplitude (Figs. 2, 3, and 4). Low-voltage regions (<0.55 mV in bipolar recordings) identify areas of scar *(65–67)*.

The low-voltage region contains the reentry circuit but is usually too large for ablation of the entire region or its circumference. Additional markers of the circuit exit or isthmus are sought for ablation. During sinus rhythm the exit can often be located by pace mapping along the scar border. Pacing in the exit region replicates the QRS morphology of VT. (Figs. 2 and 4) *(68, 69)*.

A potential isthmus or channel within low-voltage regions can also be identified during sinus rhythm, suggested by low-amplitude isolated potentials and late potentials inscribed after the end of the QRS complex. Pacing in a channel produces a QRS that emerges after a delay due to slow conduction through the channel (Figs. 2 and 4). When the stimulated wavefront propagates through a reentry circuit exit region, the paced QRS morphology resembles VT, strongly suggesting that the pacing site is in a reentry circuit isthmus. If the wavefront leaves the scar by another path, the paced QRS morphology may differ from VT or resemble a different VT. Absence of channels may indicate that functional block is present during VT or that the channels are not endocardial *(69, 70)*.

Areas of dense fibrosis that form some reentry circuit borders can be detected as electrically unexcitable scar, where pacing does not capture (pacing threshold >10 mA at 2-ms pulse width). Marking electrically unexcitable scar areas creates a visual map of potential channels, which can then be investigated for ablation. Not all scars have large electrically unexcitable scar areas; narrow bands of normal tissue within fibrosis likely escape detection on the basis of pacing threshold. Areas of block can also be indicated by very low-amplitude regions on either side of a larger amplitude channel *(66, 68–70)*.

Most recent ablation series include patients with multiple and unstable VTs targeted by these techniques. When VT is stable, substrate mapping during sinus rhythm can be used to identify regions for further evaluation during VT, minimizing the time spent in VT. Brief entrainment is often possible, even for unstable VTs, to confirm the location of a reentry circuit, potentially allowing ablation with a smaller number of RF lesions than when ablation is guided only by substrate mapping.

Inducible VTs and Ablation End Points

On average, three different monomorphic VTs are usually inducible with repeated programmed stimulation. VTs that have been observed to occur spontaneously are often referred to as "clinical VTs"; the others are often designated "nonclinical," implying that they are unlikely to occur spontaneously. This distinction can be problematic; nonclinical VTs may subsequently occur spontaneously *(71, 72)*. In many patients, the ECG morphology of spontaneous VT is not known because an ICD promptly terminates VT.

Abolishing incessant VT and inducible clinical VT is generally the minimum end point that defines a successful procedure. Some centers attempt to abolish all inducible VTs or all inducible mappable VTs, aiming to reduce recurrences. These different end points have not been compared directly. After ablation, at least one VT is no longer inducible in 73–100% of patients, and all inducible VTs are abolished in 38–95% of patients. Remaining inducible VTs are often faster and are induced by aggressive stimulation *(72–75)*.

When the targeted VT remains inducible after ablation, the recurrence risk exceeds 60% *(71, 74)*. Absence of inducible VT has been associated with a lower but still significant incidence of recurrence, ranging from <3 to 27% in single-center reports *(73–75)*. Inducible, nonclinical VTs are associated with increased risk of recurrence in some studies *(75)*. Healing of initial ablation lesions and reduction of antiarrhythmic medications likely contribute to recurrences, and some patients benefit from a repeat procedure. Even when VT recurs, the frequency of episodes is often reduced. In a multicenter trial in 146 patients, the immediate effect on inducible VT did not predict outcomes; VT recurred in 44% of patients who had no inducible VT and 46% of those who had inducible VT *(51)*. The frequency of spontaneous VT during short-term follow-up was reduced by >75% in the majority of patients.

Purkinje System VT

A diseased Purkinje system causes VT in 8% of patients with structural heart disease referred for catheter ablation *(13)*. VT can be due to macroreentry or focal automaticity that is catecholamine sensitive. VT has an ECG appearance of typical left or right bundle branch block and is often associated with severely depressed LV function.

In bundle branch reentrant VT, the circulating wavefront propagates up the left bundle branch and antegrade down the right bundle branch, producing VT with a QRS configuration of typical left bundle branch block (Fig. 1d). Less frequently, the circuit revolves in the opposite direction, producing a right bundle branch block configuration. Ablation of the right or left bundle branch is curative, but ablation of the right bundle is generally preferred to avoid hemodynamic consequences of left bundle branch block. Associated infranodal conduction delay and the frequent presence of other, scar-related VTs in approximately a third of patients warrant pacemaker or ICD implantation as well.

ABLATION IN SPECIFIC DISEASES

Prior Myocardial Infarction

Patients have generally been referred after failed drug therapy and ICD implantation. Ablation is initially successful, abolishing one or more VTs in 77–95% of patients. During follow-up, previously ineffective antiarrhythmic drugs, frequently amiodarone, are often continued. VT recurs in 19–50% of patients, although the frequency is reduced in the majority. Multiple morphologies of VT and unstable VTs are associated with a higher recurrence risk. Failure of endocardial ablation can be due to intramural or epicardial reentry circuits. Epicardial circuits are present in 10–30% of patients, more often in inferior wall as opposed to anterior wall infarctions *(28, 41, 42)*.

Major complications occur in 5–10% of patients including cardiac tamponade, shock, stroke, aortic valve injuries, and vascular injuries. Procedure mortality, 2.7% in one trial, is often due to failure to control VT rather than complications *(51)*.

The annual mortality after catheter ablation ranges from 5 to >20%, with death from progressive heart failure being the most common cause *(75, 76)*. The substantial mortality is consistent with the severity of heart disease and association of spontaneous VT with mortality and heart failure even when VT is treated effectively by an ICD *(4)*. Older age and greater LV size and dysfunction increase mortality *(75, 76)*. The potential for ablation to adversely affect LV function is cause for concern, although assessment of LV ejection fraction after ablation has not shown deterioration *(77)*. Confining ablation lesions to regions of low-amplitude scar and attention to appropriate medical therapy beneficial to patients with LV dysfunction are prudent.

Dilated Cardiomyopathy Without Coronary Artery Disease

Sustained monomorphic VT is not common in nonischemic dilated cardiomyopathies, but 80% of those that occur are due to scar-related reentry, with the remainder due to bundle branch reentry or a focal origin. Myocardial scar has been demonstrated with magnetic resonance imaging and is frequently abutting a valve annulus *(77, 78)*. Progressive replacement fibrosis is a likely cause. VT ablation is often more difficult than in coronary artery disease, but recurrent arrhythmias are controlled in >60% of patients *(23, 24)*. Reentry circuits require epicardial ablation in a third or more of patients (Figs. 3 and 8). Occasionally, incessant idiopathic VT or ventricular ectopy causes a tachycardia-induced cardiomyopathy that improves after ablation *(79)*.

RV Cardiomyopathies

Scar-related RV tachycardias occur in idiopathic cardiomyopathy, arrhythmogenic RV dysplasia/cardiomyopathy, and cardiac sarcoidosis. VT has a left bundle branch block configuration. Reentry circuits are often in scars adjacent to the tricuspid or pulmonic annulus. Focal origin VTs or epicardial reentry with a focal endocardial breakthrough also occurs. Areas of scar associated with VT can also be identified from delayed enhancement on magnetic resonance imaging. Ablation is often successful in the short term, but late arrhythmia recurrences are common, suggesting disease progression. Cardiac perforation is the major complication but is infrequent *(55, 58, 61, 67, 79, 82, 84)*.

Repaired Congenital Heart Diseases

Scar-related VT involving RV regions of repair also occur late after surgical correction of congenital heart disease, notably tetralogy of Fallot. Catheter ablation is feasible and can reduce recurrences, but in a small series only 43% of 14 patients with tetralogy of Fallot remained free of VT *(84)*. Dense fibrosis or synthetic patches used in the repair may hinder ablation in some patients.

IDIOPATHIC MONOMORPHIC VTS

Idiopathic monomorphic VTs tend to present in young, healthy individuals, often precipitated by exertion or emotion. The most common forms have a focal origin in the RV or LV outflow regions *(13, 15, 17, 81–85)*. Up to 12% are due to reentry involving LV Purkinje fascicles. Initial evaluation should exclude structural heart disease, particularly arrhythmogenic RV dysplasia, cardiac sarcoidosis, and other cardiomyopathies. Any sinus rhythm ECG abnormality should increase suspicion for underlying structural disease. Areas of delayed enhancement consistent with fibrosis on magnetic resonance imaging suggest scar-related VT. Magnetic resonance imaging in patients with idiopathic RV outflow tract (RVOT) VTs often shows focal areas of thinning, fatty infiltration, and diminished wall motion that can be normal variants *(83)*.

The prognosis is good and the risk of sudden death is remote provided that underlying heart disease is excluded. Rarely, an RVOT focus is the trigger for idiopathic ventricular fibrillation or polymorphic VT in the presence of an inherited arrhythmia syndrome *(86)*. Incessant VT or extremely frequent ectopy can cause depressed LV function that improves after the arrhythmia is controlled *(80)*.

Ventricular Tachycardia
Ablation in RVOT

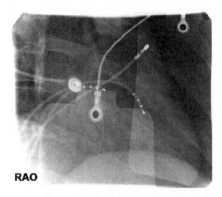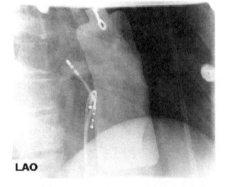

Fig. 10. Typical catheter positions for ablation of idiopathic ventricular tachycardia originating in RVOT.

Long-term therapy with β-adrenergic blockers, calcium channel blockers, or both or with a membrane active antiarrhythmic drug is often effective. Catheter ablation is an accepted therapy for sustained or symptomatic arrhythmias when medications are ineffective or not desired *(1)*.

Outflow-Type Idiopathic VT

Outflow-type VTs have an inferiorly directed frontal plane axis (Figs. 1a and 10). Most originate in the RV and have a left bundle branch block configuration in V1. VT is often induced with isoproterenol infusion and burst pacing and can be terminated with high-dose adenosine, consistent with cAMP-mediated delayed afterdepolarizations and triggered activity as the mechanism *(82, 89)*. An acquired somatic cell mutation in the inhibitory G protein Gi2 has been found in the RV in some patients *(87)*.

Clinical presentations include paroxysmal exercise-induced VT, repetitive monomorphic VT, with bursts of non-sustained VT separated by one or more sinus beats, and frequent premature ventricular beats. The location of the discrete VT focus is suggested by the ECG, but the close anatomic relations of the RVOT, LV outflow tract, and their great vessels preclude definitive localization from the ECG alone *(88)*. Success rates for catheter ablation range from 85 to 97% *(82, 89)*. Long-term follow-up is limited, but recurrence rates are generally low.

The variety of potential locations makes it desirable to perform mapping and ablation during VT. Inability to initiate the arrhythmia in the laboratory, likely related to sedation and systemic absorption of local anesthetic, is a major cause of ablation failure. The first step is to induce VT, confirm the diagnosis, and obtain a 12-lead ECG to allow pace mapping to guide ablation if VT becomes quiescent.

RVOT Tachycardia

The free wall of the RVOT is oriented diagonally from posterior to anterior as a catheter moves from right to left. The side of the RVOT that is opposite the free wall sits anterior to the aorta and superior to the LV outflow tract. VT originating from the RVOT has a left bundle branch block configuration in V1 with a transition to more positive QRS by V4. A free wall origin is suggested by QRS duration >140 ms and notches in the inferior leads (II, III, AVF). Deeper S waves in aVL than in aVR suggest a leftward superior focus, and this ratio decreases with sites located more rightward and inferior in RVOT *(90, 91)*.

Precise localization relies on combined use of pace mapping and activation mapping. In most patients, a site with a pace map QRS that exactly matches that of VT can be identified at or very close to the VT focus, but excellent pace maps may be obtained several millimeters distant from the earliest activation *(92)*. Earliest activation during VT or premature ventricular contractions from the focus typically precedes the QRS onset by 15–45 ms, with a characteristic QS complex in the unipolar signal *(92)*. RF application often produces acceleration followed by termination of VT and renders it no longer inducible.

Successful ablation is achieved in 65–97% of patients *(90, 93)*. Serious complications are infrequent but include perforation of the RV free wall. Although the left main coronary artery can be in close proximity to the posterior aspect of the RVOT (Fig. 10), we are not aware of any cases of recognized coronary injury *(88)*. Infrequently, the focus is adjacent to the His bundle, where heart block is a risk of ablation *(94)*.

Pulmonary Artery VTs

VT can originate from sleeves of myocardium extending along the pulmonary artery, above the pulmonary valve, requiring ablation from within the pulmonary artery *(95, 96)*. VT typically has large R waves in the inferior leads and greater R/S ratio in lead V2 than in RVOT VT. Ablation risks are not well defined for these infrequent VTs.

LV Outflow Tract VTs

LV outflow tract VT can originate from the superior basal region of the left interventricular septum or LV free wall, aortic sinuses of Valsalva, or LV epicardium. The QRS has an inferior axis, but the precordial transition to positive R waves is earlier, with prominent R waves often present in V1 or V2 compared with RVOT tachycardia.

LV endocardial VTs can originate from foci below the aortic valve *(97–99)*. Heart block and aortic valve and coronary artery injury are potential risks for ablation but are reported rarely.

Aortic Cusp VTs

VT originating from extension of ventricular myocardium above the aortic annulus, requiring ablation from the left or right sinus of Valsalva, caused 21% of idiopathic VTs in one series *(64)*. Pace mapping in the aortic sinus may require high output and may not exactly reproduce the VT QRS. Activation mapping is required and typically shows a two-component electrogram with the earliest deflection preceding the QRS complex by an average of 39 ms *(97, 98)*.

The potential for acute occlusion of the left main or right coronary arteries is a major risk consideration. Coronary angiography and intracardiac ultrasound imaging have been used to define the proximity of the coronary ostia to the ablation site. RF ablation has been performed safely at sites >8 mm below the coronary artery ostia with careful continuous monitoring of catheter position during the RF application. Standard RF ablation with tip temperature maintained at <55°C has been suggested to prevent aortic valve damage observed in animal studies *(99)*.

Epicardial Outflow Tract VTs

Epicardial foci cause VTs with a QRS onset that is often slurred, creating a pseudo-delta wave appearance. The interval from the onset of the QRS to earliest maximal deflection in the precordial leads is delayed, consistent with late access of the wavefront to the endocardial Purkinje system *(100)*. The VT focus may be adjacent to an epicardial vein that can be cannulated via the coronary sinus, and successful ablation has been performed via this route as well as via percutaneous pericardial access. When proximity to a epicardial coronary artery precludes catheter ablation, a direct surgical approach can be an option *(100)*.

Mitral Annulus VT

Focal VTs from the mitral annulus accounted for 5% of 352 idiopathic VTs in one series. VT has a right bundle branch block or RS pattern in V1 and monophasic R or RS pattern in leads V2–V6. The QRS axis depends on the location on the annulus. Endocardial ablation is usually successful; ablation from within the coronary sinus may be required occasionally *(101)*.

LV Fascicular Idiopathic VT

Verapamil-sensitive idiopathic LV tachycardia typically presents as exercise-related VT between the ages of 15 and 40 years; 60–80% of patients are male *(102–104)*. VT has a right bundle branch block configuration, most commonly with a superiorly directed frontal plane axis (Fig. 1b).

VT is due to reentry involving fascicles of the left bundle and an abnormal region, possibly also in the Purkinje system, with slow conduction that is sensitive to verapamil and that is depolarized early in diastole in VT and in sinus rhythm. More than 80% of these VTs involve the posterior fascicles of the left bundle, identified along the inferoseptal aspect of the LV *(105, 106)*.

Ablation targets the anterograde Purkinje potentials or diastolic potentials during VT, avoiding the proximal Purkinje system to avoid causing left bundle branch block. Mechanical trauma from catheter manipulation often terminates VT and prevents reinitiation. Ablation then targets the site of mechanical termination, low amplitude, or diastolic sinus rhythm potentials or creates a line of lesions through this region *(102, 103)*. Efficacy is >80%. Complications are infrequent.

ABLATION FOR POLYMORPHIC VT AND VENTRICULAR FIBRILLATION

Recurrent polymorphic VT causing "electrical storm" not due to ongoing acute ischemia is rare but is seen in idiopathic ventricular fibrillation, long QT syndromes, Brugada syndrome, and myocardial infarction *(1, 86, 105–107)*. VT is often initiated by premature beats from one or a few foci that can be ablated if they occur with enough frequency to be located (Fig. 6a–d). Most appear to originate from the Purkinje system and have sharp presystolic potentials recorded from the focus. Less frequently, an RVOT focus is a trigger *(86)*. Successful ablation requires the presence of spontaneous ectopic beats for mapping. Electrical storms can wax and wane with long periods of quiescence. Immediate transport of the patient to the laboratory when the arrhythmia is active is warranted if ablation is to be attempted. In selected patients, excellent outcomes can be achieved, with 90% of patients free from recurrent arrhythmias during follow-up, but the number of patients reported is small *(1, 86, 106)*.

Advances over the past decade now allow ablation of multiple, hemodynamically unstable, epicardial, and polymorphic VTs, formerly considered unmappable. Specific locations for the origins of idiopathic VT outside of the RVOT have been defined that can be expected to improve overall success for ablation of these arrhythmias. These procedures are often more difficult than ablation of many supraventricular tachycardias and are best approached by experienced operators in experienced laboratories. The field continues to benefit from technological developments (Fig. 11). When the expertise is available, catheter ablation should be considered earlier in the therapeutic armamentarium for treatment of recurrent VT.

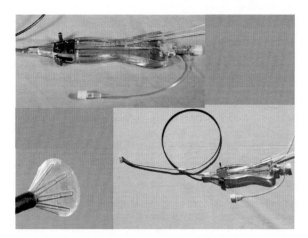

Fig. 11. New and emerging catheter technologies may offer better visualization and contact within the mapping area in the ventricles. This is the catheter that would allow direct visualization of the ventricular wall by injecting small stream of saline through the center of the small hood at the end of the catheter. The same saline stream may be used for ablation.

DISCLOSURES

Dr Kocovic has received speaking honoraria from Medtronic, Inc, Boston Scientific, Inc, St Jude, Inc, and is a consultant to and has received research support from Medtronic, Boston Scientific Inc Guidant and St Jude.

REFERENCES

1. Aliot EM, Stevenson WG, Almendral-Garrote JM, Bogun F, Calkins CH, Delacretaz E, Della Bella P, Hindricks G, Jaïs P, Josephson ME, Kautzner J, Kay GN, Kuck KH, Lerman BB, Marchlinski F, Reddy V, Schalij MJ, Schilling R, Soejima K, Wilber D (2009) EHRA/HRS expert consensus on catheter ablation of ventricular arrhythmias: developed in a partnership with the European heart rhythm association (EHRA), a registered branch of the European society of cardiology (ESC), and the heart rhythm society (HRS); in collaboration with the American college of cardiology (ACC) and the American heart association (AHA). European heart rhythm association (EHRA); registered branch of the European society of cardiology (ESC); heart rhythm society (HRS); American college of cardiology (ACC); American heart association (AHA). Heart Rhythm 6(6):886–933

2. Connolly SJ, Dorian P, Roberts RS, Gent M, Bailin S, Fain ES, Thorpe K, Champagne J, Talajic M, Coutu B, Gronefeld GC, Hohnloser SH (2006) Comparison of beta-blockers, amiodarone plus beta-blockers, or sotalol for prevention of shocks from implantable cardioverter defibrillators: the OPTIC Study: a randomized trial. JAMA 295:165–171

3. Schron EB, Exner DV, Yao Q, Jenkins LS, Steinberg JS, Cook JR, Kutalek SP, Friedman PL, Bubien RS, Page RL, Powell J (2002) Quality of life in the antiarrhythmics versus implantable defibrillators trial: impact of therapy and influence of adverse symptoms and defibrillator shocks. Circulation 105:589–594

4. Moss AJ, Greenberg H, Case RB, Zareba W, Hall WJ, Brown MW, Daubert JP, McNitt S, Andrews ML, Elkin AD (2004) Long-term clinical course of patients after termination of ventricular tachyarrhythmia by an implanted defibrillator. Circulation 110:3760–3765

5. Brugada J, Berruezo A, Cuesta A, Osca J, Chueca E, Fosch X, Wayar L, Mont L (2003) Nonsurgical transthoracic epicardial radiofrequency ablation: an alternative in incessant ventricular tachycardia. J Am Coll Cardiol 41:2036–2043

6. Bansch D, Oyang F, Antz M, Arentz T, Weber R, Val-Mejias JE, Ernst S, Kuck KH (2003) Successful catheter ablation of electrical storm after myocardial infarction. Circulation 108:3011–3016

7. Lopera G, Stevenson WG, Soejima K, Maisel WH, Koplan B, Sapp JL, Satti SD, Epstein LM (2004) Identification and ablation of three types of ventricular tachycardia involving the His-Purkinje system in patients with heart disease. J Cardiovasc Electrophysiol 15:52–58

8. Haissaguerre M, Extramiana F, Hocini M, Cauchemez B, Jais P, Cabrera JA, Farre G, Leenhardt A, Sanders P, Scavee C, Hsu LF, Weerasooriya R, Shah DC, Frank R, Maury P, Delay M, Garrigue S, Clementy J (2003) Mapping and ablation of ventricular fibrillation associated with long-QT and Brugada syndromes. Circulation 108:925–928

9. Buxton AE, Waxman HL, Marchlinski FE, Simson MB, Cassidy D, Josephson ME (1983) Right ventricular tachycardia: clinical and electrophysiologic characteristics. Circulation 68:917–927

10. Ito S, Tada H, Naito S, Kurosaki K, Ueda M, Hoshizaki H et al (2003) Development and validation of an ECG algorithm for identifying the optimal ablation site for idiopathic ventricular outflow tract tachycardia. J Cardiovasc Electrophysiol 14:1280–1286

11. Kamakura S, Shimizu W, Matsuo K, Taguchi A, Suyama K, Kurita T et al (1998) Localization of optimal ablation site of idiopathic ventricular tachycardia from right and left ventricular outflow tract by body surface ECG. Circulation 98:1525–1533

12. Lerman BB, Belardinelli L, West GA, Berne RM, DiMarco JP (1986) Adenosine-sensitive ventricular tachycardia: evidence suggesting cyclic AMP-mediated triggered activity. Circulation 74:270–280

13. Lerman BB, Stein K, Engelstein ED, Battleman DS, Lippman N, Bei D et al (1995) Mechanism of repetitive monomorphic ventricular tachycardia. Circulation 92:421–429

14. Sung RJ, Keung EC, Nguyen NX, Huycke EC (1988) Effects of beta-adrenergic blockade on verapamil-responsive and verapamil-irresponsive sustained ventricular tachycardias. J Clin Invest 81:688–699

15. Tada H, Tadokoro K, Miyaji K, Ito S, Kurosaki K, Kaseno K et al (2008) Idiopathic ventricular arrhythmias arising from the pulmonary artery: prevalence, characteristics, and topography of the arrhythmia origin. Heart Rhythm 5:419–426

16. Antzelevitch C, Shimizu W (2002) Cellular mechanisms underlying the long QT syndrome. Curr Opin Cardiol 17:43–51

17. Lerman BB (2007) Mechanism of outflow tract tachycardia. Heart Rhythm 4:973–976

18. Damle RS, Landers M, Kelly PA, Reiter MJ, Mann DE (1998) Radiofrequency catheter ablation of idiopathic left ventricular tachycardia originating in the left anterior fascicle. Pacing Clin Electrophysiol 21:1155–1158

19. Huelsing DJ, Spitzer KW, Pollard AE (2003) Spontaneous activity induced in rabbit Purkinje myocytes during coupling to a depolarized model cell. Cardiovasc Res 59:620–627

20. Spitzer KW, Pollard AE, Yang L, Zaniboni M, Cordeiro JM, Huelsing DJ (2006) Cell-to-cell electrical interactions during early and late repolarization. J Cardiovasc Electrophysiol 17(Suppl 1):S8–S14

21. Belhassen B, Caspi A, Miller H, Shapira I, Laniado S (1984) Extensive endocardial mapping during sinus rhythm and ventricular tachycardia in a patient with arrhythmogenic right ventricular dysplasia. J Am Coll Cardiol 4:1302–1306

22. Delacretaz E, Stevenson WG, Ellison KE, Maisel WH, Friedman PL (2000) Mapping and radiofrequency catheter ablation of the three types of sustained monomorphic ventricular tachycardia in nonischemic heart disease. J Cardiovasc Electrophysiol 11:11–17

23. Eckart RE, Hruczkowski TW, Tedrow UB, Koplan BA, Epstein LM, Stevenson WG (2007) Sustained ventricular tachycardia associated with corrective valve surgery. Circulation 116:2005–2011

24. Ellison KE, Friedman PL, Ganz LI, Stevenson WG (1998) Entrainment mapping and radiofrequency catheter ablation of ventricular tachycardia in right ventricular dysplasia. J Am Coll Cardiol 32:724–728

25. Josephson ME, Horowitz LN, Farshidi A, Kastor JA (1978) Recurrent sustained ventricular tachycardia. 1. Mechanisms. Circulation 57:431–440

26. Josephson ME, Almendral JM, Buxton AE, Marchlinski FE (1987) Mechanisms of ventricular tachycardia. Circulation 75(Pt 2):III41–III47

27. Koplan BA, Soejima K, Baughman K, Epstein LM, Stevenson WG (2006) Refractory ventricular tachycardia secondary to cardiac sarcoid: electrophysiologic characteristics, mapping, and ablation. Heart Rhythm 3:924–929

28. Sosa E, Scanavacca M, D'Avila A, Piccioni J, Sanchez O, Velarde JL et al (1998) Endocardial and epicardial ablation guided by nonsurgical transthoracic epicardial mapping to treat recurrent ventricular tachycardia. J Cardiovasc Electrophysiol 9:229–239

29. Stevenson WG, Khan H, Sager P, Saxon LA, Middlekauff HR, Natterson PD et al (1993) Identification of reentry circuit sites during catheter mapping and radiofrequency ablation of ventricular tachycardia late after myocardial infarction. Circulation 88(Pt 1):1647–1670

30. Dillon SM, Allessie MA, Ursell PC, Wit AL (1988) Influences of anisotropic tissue structure on reentrant circuits in the epicardial border zone of subacute canine infarcts. Circ Res 63:182–206

31. Downar E, Harris L, Mickleborough LL, Shaikh N, Parson ID (1988) Endocardial mapping of ventricular tachycardia in the intact human ventricle: evidence for reentrant mechanisms. J Am Coll Cardiol 11:783–791

32. Downar E, Kimber S, Harris L, Mickleborough L, Sevaptsidis E, Masse S et al (1992) Endocardial mapping of ventricular tachycardia in the intact human heart. II. Evidence for multiuse reentry in a functional sheet of surviving myocardium. J Am Coll Cardiol 20:869–878

33. Kleber AG, Rudy Y (2004) Basic mechanisms of cardiac impulse propagation and associated arrhythmias. Physiol Rev 84:431–488

34. Baba S, Dun W, Cabo C, Boyden PA (2005) Remodeling in cells from different regions of the reentrant circuit during ventricular tachycardia. Circulation 112:2386–2396

35. Kocovic DZ, Harada T, Friedman PL, Stevenson WG (1999) Characteristics of electrograms recorded at reentry circuit sites and bystanders during ventricular tachycardia after myocardial infarction. J Am Coll Cardiol 34:381–388

36. de Bakker JM, van Capelle FJ, Janse MJ, Wilde AA, Coronel R, Becker AE et al (1988) Reentry as a cause of ventricular tachycardia in patients with chronic ischemic heart disease: electrophysiologic and anatomic correlation. Circulation 77:589–606

37. de Bakker JM, van Capelle FJ, Janse MJ, Tasseron S, Vermeulen JT, de JN et al (1993) Slow conduction in the infarcted human heart. 'Zigzag' course of activation. Circulation 88:915–926

38. El-Sherif N, Mehra R, Gough WB, Zeiler RH (1983) Reentrant ventricular arrhythmias in the late myocardial infarction period. Interruption of reentrant circuits by cryothermal techniques. Circulation 68:644–656

39. Hadjis TA, Stevenson WG, Harada T, Friedman PL, Sager P, Saxon LA (1997) Preferential locations for critical reentry circuit sites causing ventricular tachycardia after inferior wall myocardial infarction. J Cardiovasc Electrophysiol 8:363–370

40. Brugada P, Abdollah H, Wellens HJ (1985) Continuous electrical activity during sustained monomorphic ventricular tachycardia. Observations on its dynamic behavior during the arrhythmia. Am J Cardiol 55:402–411

41. Kaltenbrunner W, Cardinal R, Dubuc M, Shenasa M, Nadeau R et al (1991) Epicardial and endocardial mapping of ventricular tachycardia in patients with myocardial infarction. Is the origin of the tachycardia always subendocardially localized? Circulation 84:1058–1071

42. de Bakker JM, Stein M, van Rijen HV (2005) Three-dimensional anatomic structure as substrate for ventricular tachycardia/ventricular fibrillation. Heart Rhythm 2:777–799

43. Caceres J, Jazayeri M, McKinnie J, Avitall B, Denker ST, Tchou P et al (1989) Sustained bundle branch reentry as a mechanism of clinical tachycardia. Circulation 79:256–270

44. Nakagawa H, Beckman KJ, McClelland JH, Wang X, Arruda M, Santoro I et al (1993) Radiofrequency catheter ablation of idiopathic left ventricular tachycardia guided by a Purkinje potential. Circulation 88:2607–2617

45. Reddy VY, Malchano ZJ, Holmvang G, Schmidt EJ, d'Avila A, Houghtaling C, Chan RC, Ruskin JN (2004) Integration of cardiac magnetic resonance imaging with three-dimensional electroanatomic mapping to guide left ventricular catheter manipulation: feasibility in a porcine model of healed myocardial infarction. J Am Coll Cardiol 44:2202–2213

46. Della Bella P, Pappalardo A, Riva S, Tondo C, Fassini G, Trevisi N (2002) Non-contact mapping to guide catheter ablation of untolerated ventricular tachycardia. Eur Heart J 23:742–752

47. Soejima K, Delacretaz E, Suzuki M, Brunckhorst CB, Maisel WH, Friedman PL, Stevenson WG (2001) Saline-cooled versus standard radiofrequency catheter ablation for infarct-related ventricular tachycardias. Circulation 103: 1858–1862

48. Matsudaira K, Nakagawa H, Wittkampf FH, Yamanashi WS, Imai S, Pitha JV, Lazzara R, Jackman WM (2003) High incidence of thrombus formation without impedance rise during radiofrequency ablation using electrode temperature control. Pacing Clin Electrophysiol 26:1227–1237

49. Yokoyama K, Nakagawa H, Wittkampf FH, Pitha JV, Lazzara R, Jackman WM (2006) Comparison of electrode cooling between internal and open irrigation in radiofrequency ablation lesion depth and incidence of thrombus and steam pop. Circulation 113:11–19

50. Cooper JM, Sapp JL, Tedrow U, Pellegrini CP, Robinson D, Epstein LM, Stevenson WG (2004) Ablation with an internally irrigated radiofrequency catheter: learning how to avoid steam pops. Heart Rhythm 1:329–333

51. Calkins H, Epstein A, Packer D, Arria AM, Hummel J, Gilligan DM, Trusso J, Carlson M, Luceri R, Kopelman H, Wilber D, Wharton JM, Stevenson W (2000) Catheter ablation of ventricular tachycardia in patients with structural heart disease using cooled radiofrequency energy: results of a prospective multicenter study. J Am Coll Cardiol 35:1905–1914

52. Lustgarten DL, Bell S, Hardin N, Calame J, Spector PS (2005) Safety and efficacy of epicardial cryoablation in a canine model. Heart Rhythm 2:82–90

53. Sosa E, Scanavacca M, d'Avila A, Oliveira F, Ramires JA (2000) Nonsurgical transthoracic epicardial catheter ablation to treat recurrent ventricular tachycardia occurring late after myocardial infarction. J Am Coll Cardiol 35:1442–1449

54. Sosa E, Scanavacca M, D'Avila A, Antonio J, Ramires F (2004) Nonsurgical transthoracic epicardial approach in patients with ventricular tachycardia and previous cardiac surgery. J Interv Card Electrophysiol 10:281–288

55. Soejima K, Stevenson WG, Sapp JL, Selwyn AP, Couper G, Epstein LM (2004) Endocardial and epicardial radiofrequency ablation of ventricular tachycardia associated with dilated cardiomyopathy: the importance of low-voltage scars. J Am Coll Cardiol 43:1834–1842

56. Sosa E, Scanavacca M (2007) Percutaneous pericardial access for mapping and ablation of epicardial ventricular tachycardias. Circulation 115:e542–e544

57. Soejima K, Couper G, Cooper JM, Sapp JL, Epstein LM, Stevenson WG (2004) Subxiphoid surgical approach for epicardial catheter-based mapping and ablation in patients with prior cardiac surgery or difficult pericardial access. Circulation 110:1197–1201

58. Bansch D, Bocker D, Brunn J, Weber M, Breithardt G, Block M (2000) Clusters of ventricular tachycardias signify impaired survival in patients with idiopathic dilated cardiomyopathy and implantable cardioverter defibrillators. J Am Coll Cardiol 36:566–573

59. de Chillou C, Lacroix D, Klug D, Magnin-Poull I, Marquie C, Messier M, Andronache M, Kouakam C, Sadoul N, Chen J, Aliot E, Kacet S (2002) Isthmus characteristics of reentrant ventricular tachycardia after myocardial infarction. Circulation 105:726–731

60. Soejima K, Suzuki M, Maisel WH, Brunckhorst CB, Delacretaz E, Blier L, Tung S, Khan H, Stevenson WG (2001) Catheter ablation in patients with multiple and unstable ventricular tachycardias after myocardial infarction: short ablation lines guided by reentry circuit isthmuses and sinus rhythm mapping. Circulation 104:664–669

61. Berruezo A, Mont L, Nava S, Chueca E, Bartholomay E, Brugada J (2004) Electrocardiographic recognition of the epicardial origin of ventricular tachycardias. Circulation 109:1842–1847

62. Delacretaz E, Stevenson WG (2001) Catheter ablation of ventricular tachycardia in patients with coronary heart disease, part I: mapping. Pacing Clin Electrophysiol 24:1261–1277

63. Bogun F, Good E, Han J, Tamirisa K, Reich S, Elmouchi D, Igic P, Lemola K, Oral H, Chugh A, Pelosi F, Morady F (2005) Mechanical interruption of postinfarction ventricular tachycardia as a guide for catheter ablation. Heart Rhythm 2:687–691

64. El-Shalakany A, Hadjis T, Papageorgiou P, Monahan K, Epstein L, Josephson ME (1999) Entrainment/mapping criteria for the prediction of termination of ventricular tachycardia by single radiofrequency lesion in patients with coronary artery disease. Circulation 99:2283–2289

65. Marchlinski FE, Callans DJ, Gottlieb CD, Zado E (2000) Linear ablation lesions for control of unmappable ventricular tachycardia in patients with ischemic and nonischemic cardiomyopathy. Circulation 101:1288–1296

66. Arenal A, del Castillo S, Gonzalez-Torrecilla E, Atienza F, Ortiz M, Jimenez J, Puchol A, Garcia J, Almendral J (2004) Tachycardia-related channel in the scar tissue in patients with sustained monomorphic ventricular tachycardias: influence of the voltage scar definition. Circulation 110:2568–2574

67. Cesario DA, Vaseghi M, Boyle NG, Fishbein MC, Valderrabano M, Narasimhan C, Wiener I, Shivkumar K (2006) Value of high-density endocardial and epicardial mapping for catheter ablation of hemodynamically unstable ventricular tachycardia. Heart Rhythm 3:1–10

68. Kottkamp H, Wetzel U, Schirdewahn P, Dorszewski A, Gerds-Li JH, Carbucicchio C, Kobza R, Hindricks G (2003) Catheter ablation of ventricular tachycardia in remote myocardial infarction: substrate description guiding placement of individual linear lesions targeting noninducibility. J Cardiovasc Electrophysiol 14:675–681

69. Arenal A, Glez-Torrecilla E, Ortiz M, Villacastin J, Fdez-Portales J, Sousa E, del Castillo S, Perez de Isla L, Jimenez J, Almendral J (2003) Ablation of electrograms with an isolated, delayed component as treatment of unmappable monomorphic ventricular tachycardias in patients with structural heart disease. J Am Coll Cardiol 41:81–92

70. Soejima K, Stevenson WG, Maisel WH, Sapp JL, Epstein LM (2002) Electrically unexcitable scar mapping based on pacing threshold for identification of the reentry circuit isthmus: feasibility for guiding ventricular tachycardia ablation. Circulation 106:1678–1683

71. van der Burg AE, de Groot NM, van Erven L, Bootsma M, van der Wall EE, Schalij MJ (2002) Long-term follow-up after radiofrequency catheter ablation of ventricular tachycardia: a successful approach? J Cardiovasc Electrophysiol 13:417–423

72. Segal OR, Chow AW, Markides V, Schilling RJ, Peters NS, Davies DW (2005) Long-term results after ablation of infarct-related ventricular tachycardia. Heart Rhythm 2:474–482

73. Della Bella P, Riva S, Fassini G, Giraldi F, Berti M, Klersy C, Trevisi N (2004) Incidence and significance of pleomorphism in patients with postmyocardial infarction ventricular tachycardia: acute and long-term outcome of radiofrequency catheter ablation. Eur Heart J 25:1127–1138

74. O'Donnell D, Bourke JP, Furniss SS (2003) Standardized stimulation protocol to predict the long-term success of radiofrequency ablation of postinfarction ventricular tachycardia. Pacing Clin Electrophysiol 26:348–351

75. Della Bella P, De Ponti R, Uriarte JA, Tondo C, Klersy C, Carbucicchio C, Storti C, Riva S, Longobardi M (2002) Catheter ablation and antiarrhythmic drugs for haemodynamically tolerated post-infarction ventricular tachycardia; long-term outcome in relation to acute electrophysiological findings. Eur Heart J 23:414–424

76. Nabar A, Rodriguez LM, Batra RK, Timmermans C, Cheriex E, Wellens HJ (2002) Echocardiographic predictors of survival in patients undergoing radiofrequency ablation of postinfarct clinical ventricular tachycardia. J Cardiovasc Electrophysiol 13:S118–S121

77. Khan HH, Maisel WH, Ho C, Suzuki M, Soejima K, Solomon S, Stevenson WG (2002) Effect of radiofrequency catheter ablation of ventricular tachycardia on left ventricular function in patients with prior myocardial infarction. J Interv Card Electrophysiol 7:243–247

78. Hsia HH, Callans DJ, Marchlinski FE (2003) Characterization of endocardial electrophysiological substrate in patients with nonischemic cardiomyopathy and monomorphic ventricular tachycardia. Circulation 108:704–710

79. Nazarian S, Bluemke DA, Lardo AC, Zviman MM, Watkins SP, Dickfeld TL, Meininger GR, Roguin A, Calkins H, Tomaselli GF, Weiss RG, Berger RD, Lima JA, Halperin HR (2005) Magnetic resonance assessment of the substrate for inducible ventricular tachycardia in nonischemic cardiomyopathy. Circulation 112:2821–2825

80. Yarlagadda RK, Iwai S, Stein KM, Markowitz SM, Shah BK, Cheung JW, Tan V, Lerman BB, Mittal S (2005) Reversal of cardiomyopathy in patients with repetitive monomorphic ventricular ectopy originating from the right ventricular outflow tract. Circulation 112:1092–1097

81. Miljoen H, State S, de Chillou C, Magnin-Poull I, Dotto P, Andronache M, Abdelaal A, Aliot E (2005) Electroanatomic mapping characteristics of ventricular tachycardia in patients with arrhythmogenic right ventricular cardiomyopathy/dysplasia. Europace 7:516–524

82. O'Donnell D, Cox D, Bourke J, Mitchell L, Furniss S (2003) Clinical and electrophysiological differences between patients with arrhythmogenic right ventricular dysplasia and right ventricular outflow tract tachycardia. Eur Heart J 24:801–810

83. Tandri H, Saranathan M, Rodriguez ER, Martinez C, Bomma C, Nasir K, Rosen B, Lima JA, Calkins H, Bluemke DA (2005) Noninvasive detection of myocardial fibrosis in arrhythmogenic right ventricular cardiomyopathy using delayed-enhancement magnetic resonance imaging. J Am Coll Cardiol 45:98–103

84. Morwood JG, Triedman JK, Berul CI, Khairy P, Alexander ME, Cecchin F, Walsh EP (2004) Radiofrequency catheter ablation of ventricular tachycardia in children and young adults with congenital heart disease. Heart Rhythm 1: 301–308

85. Tada H, Ito S, Naito S, Kurosaki K, Kubota S, Sugiyasu A, Tsuchiya T, Miyaji K, Yamada M, Kutsumi Y, Oshima S, Nogami A, Taniguchi K (2005) Idiopathic ventricular arrhythmia arising from the mitral annulus: a distinct subgroup of idiopathic ventricular arrhythmias. J Am Coll Cardiol 45:877–886

86. Noda T, Shimizu W, Taguchi A, Aiba T, Satomi K, Suyama K, Kurita T, Aihara N, Kamakura S (2005) Malignant entity of idiopathic ventricular fibrillation and polymorphic ventricular tachycardia initiated by premature extrasystoles originating from the right ventricular outflow tract. J Am Coll Cardiol 46:1288–1294

87. Lerman BB, Dong B, Stein KM, Markowitz SM, Linden J, Catanzaro DF (1998) Right ventricular outflow tract tachycardia due to a somatic cell mutation in G protein subunitalphai2. J Clin Invest 101:2862–2868

88. Vaseghi M, Cesario DA, Mahajan A, Wiener I, Boyle NG, Fishbein MC, Horowitz BN, Shivkumar K (2006) Catheter ablation of right ventricular outflow tract tachycardia: value of defining coronary anatomy. J Cardiovasc Electrophysiol 17:632–637

89. Iwai S, Cantillon DJ, Kim RJ, Markowitz SM, Mittal S, Stein KM, Shah BK, Yarlagadda RK, Cheung JW, Tan VR, Lerman BB (2006) Right and left ventricular outflow tract tachycardias: evidence for a common electrophysiologic mechanism. J Cardiovasc Electrophysiol 17:1052–1058

90. Vestal M, Wen MS, Yeh SJ, Wang CC, Lin FC, Wu D (2003) Electrocardiographic predictors of failure and recurrence in patients with idiopathic right ventricular outflow tract tachycardia and ectopy who underwent radiofrequency catheter ablation. J Electrocardiol 36:327–332

90. Tanner H, Hindricks G, Schirdewahn P, Kobza R, Dorszewski A, Piorkowski C, Gerds-Li JH, Kottkamp H (2005) Outflow tract tachycardia with R/S transition in lead V3: six different anatomic approaches for successful ablation. J Am Coll Cardiol 45:418–423

91. Yoshida Y, Hirai M, Murakami Y, Kondo T, Inden Y, Akahoshi M, Tsuda M, Okamoto M, Yamada T, Tsuboi N, Hirayama H, Ito T, Toyama J, Saito H (1999) Localization of precise origin of idiopathic ventricular tachycardia from the right ventricular outflow tract by a 12-lead ECG: a study of pace mapping using a multielectrode "basket" catheter. Pacing Clin Electrophysiol 22:1760–1768

92. Azegami K, Wilber DJ, Arruda M, Lin AC, Denman RA (2005) Spatial resolution of pacemapping and activation mapping in patients with idiopathic right ventricular outflow tract tachycardia. J Cardiovasc Electrophysiol 16:823–829

93. Krittayaphong R, Sriratanasathavorn C, Dumavibhat C, Pumprueg S, Boonyapisit W, Pooranawattanakul S, Phrudprisan S, Kangkagate C (2006) Electrocardiographic predictors of long-term outcomes after radiofrequency ablation in patients with right-ventricular outflow tract tachycardia. Europace 8:601–606

94. Yamauchi Y, Aonuma K, Takahashi A, Sekiguchi Y, Hachiya H, Yokoyama Y, Kumagai K, Nogami A, Iesaka Y, Isobe M (2005) Electrocardiographic characteristics of repetitive monomorphic right ventricular tachycardia originating near the His-bundle. J Cardiovasc Electrophysiol 16:1041–1048

95. Sekiguchi Y, Aonuma K, Takahashi A, Yamauchi Y, Hachiya H, Yokoyama Y, Iesaka Y, Isobe M (2005) Electrocardiographic and electrophysiologic characteristics of ventricular tachycardia originating within the pulmonary artery. J Am Coll Cardiol 45:887–895

96. Timmermans C, Rodriguez LM, Crijns HJ, Moorman AF, Wellens HJ (2003) Idiopathic left bundle branch block-shaped ventricular tachycardia may originate above the pulmonary valve. Circulation 108:1960–1967

97. Ouyang F, Fotuhi P, Ho SY, Hebe J, Volkmer M, Goya M, Burns M, Antz M, Ernst S, Cappato R, Kuck KH (2002) Repetitive monomorphic ventricular tachycardia originating from the aortic sinus cusp: electrocardiographic characterization for guiding catheter ablation. J Am Coll Cardiol 39:500–508

98. Tada H, Naito S, Ito S, Kurosaki K, Ueda M, Shinbo G, Hoshizaki H, Oshima S, Taniguchi K, Nogami A (2004) Significance of two potentials for predicting successful catheter ablation from the left sinus of Valsalva for left ventricular epicardial tachycardia. Pacing Clin Electrophysiol 27:1053–1059

99. Hoachiya H, Aonuma K, Yamauchi Y, Igawa M, Nogami A, Iesaka Y (2002) How to diagnose, locate, and ablate coronary cusp ventricular tachycardia. J Cardiovasc Electrophysiol 13:551–556

100. Daniels DV, Lu YY, Morton JB, Santucci PA, Akar JG, Green A, Wilber DJ (2006) Idiopathic epicardial left ventricular tachycardia originating remote from the sinus of Valsalva: electrophysiological characteristics, catheter ablation, and identification from the 12-lead electrocardiogram. Circulation 113:1659–1666

101. Kumagai K, Yamauchi Y, Takahashi A, Yokoyama Y, Sekiguchi Y, Watanabe J, Iesaka Y, Shirato K, Aonuma K (2005) Idiopathic left ventricular tachycardia originating from the mitral annulus. J Cardiovasc Electrophysiol 16:1029–1036

102. Nogami A, Naito S, Tada H, Taniguchi K, Okamoto Y, Nishimura S, Yamauchi Y, Aonuma K, Goya M, Iesaka Y, Hiroe M (2000) Demonstration of diastolic and presystolic Purkinje potentials as critical potentials in a macroreentry circuit of verapamil-sensitive idiopathic left ventricular tachycardia. J Am Coll Cardiol 36:811–823

103. Ouyang F, Cappato R, Ernst S, Goya M, Volkmer M, Hebe J, Antz M, Vogtmann T, Schaumann A, Fotuhi P, Hoffmann-Riem M, Kuck KH (2002) Electroanatomic substrate of idiopathic left ventricular tachycardia: unidirectional block and macroreentry within the Purkinje network. Circulation 105:462–469

104. Arya A, Haghjoo M, Emkanjoo Z, Fazelifar AF, Dehghani MR, Heydari A, Sadr-Ameli MA (2004) Comparison of presystolic Purkinje and late diastolic potentials for selection of ablation site in idiopathic verapamil sensitive left ventricular tachycardia. J Interv Card Electrophysiol 11:135–141

105. Haissaguerre M, Shoda M, Jais P, Nogami A, Shah DC, Kautzner J, Arentz T, Kalushe D, Lamaison D, Griffith M, Cruz F, de Paola A, Gaita F, Hocini M, Garrigue S, Macle L, Weerasooriya R, Clementy J (2002) Mapping and ablation of idiopathic ventricular fibrillation. Circulation 106:962–967

106. Szumowski L, Sanders P, Walczak F, Hocini M, Jais P, Kepski R, Szufladowicz E, Urbanek P, Derejko P, Bodalski R, Haissaguerre M (2004) Mapping and ablation of polymorphic ventricular tachycardia after myocardial infarction. J Am Coll Cardiol 44:1700–1706

107. Marrouche NF, Verma A, Wazni O, Schweikert R, Martin DO, Saliba W, Kilicaslan F, Cummings J, Burkhardt JD, Bhargava M, Bash D, Brachmann J, Guenther J, Hao S, Beheiry S, Rossillo A, Raviele A, Themistoclakis S, Natale A (2004) Mode of initiation and ablation of ventricular fibrillation storms in patients with ischemic cardiomyopathy. J Am Coll Cardiol 43:1715–1720

13 Indications for Implantable Cardioverter-Defibrillators

Gustavo Lopera and Robert J. Myerburg

CONTENTS

Abstract

Ventricular fibrillation (VF) and hemodynamically unstable ventricular tachycardia (VT) likely remain the most common initiating and potentially reversible mechanisms of out-of-hospital cardiac arrest and sudden cardiac death (SCD). Defibrillation is the only predictably effective therapy for reverting VF and pulseless VT to an effective rhythm for restoration of blood flow. Current indications for implantation of implantable cardioverter-defibrillators are the result of risk stratification strategies that can be divided as follows: (1) secondary prevention indications; (2) primary prevention in high-risk groups with acquired diseases; and (3) SCD prevention in selected patients with specific inherited arrhythmogenic syndromes or less common acquired diseases. Further improvement and understanding of different risk stratification strategies will eventually identify individuals at specific risk for SCD and, hence, determine the type of preventive intervention required for small, high-risk subsets of individuals, who are currently diluted within larger population groups or the general population that account for the majority of SCD victims.

Key Words: Sudden cardiac death; implantable cardioverter-defibrillators; indications; risk stratification.

Ventricular fibrillation (VF) and hemodynamically unstable ventricular tachycardia (VT) likely remain the most common initiating and potentially reversible mechanisms of out-of-hospital cardiac arrest (CA) and sudden cardiac death (SCD). Data from King County, Washington, from 1990 to 1999 identified VF or VT as the initial rhythm in 65% of witnessed CA compared to 28% in non-witnessed CA *(1, 2)*. In European communities, VF was the reported rhythm in 42% (7758 of 18,105) of CA treated by the Emergency Medical Systems (EMS) *(3)*. Despite data from EMS systems suggesting

From: *Contemporary Cardiology: Management of Cardiac Arrhythmias*
Edited by: Gan-Xin Yan, Peter R. Kowey, DOI 10.1007/978-1-60761-161-5_13
© Springer Science+Business Media, LLC 2011

that the proportion of CA caused by VF and VT is decreasing (61% in 1980 to 41% in 2000) *(4)*, an undetermined number of events spontaneously evolve from VT/VF to asystole or pulseless electrical activity (PEA) before EMS arrival.

Among US communities, reported survival rates range from 0% to 46%, clustering around 5–10% for most communities *(1, 2)*. In European communities, the mean survival is 10.7% (1907/17,761) for all mechanisms of CA, and 21.2% (989/4668) for VF arrest treated by the EMS *(3)*. Survival from VF remains low despite programs of bystander cardiopulmonary resuscitation (CPR) and early defibrillation. The time to initiation of CPR and to defibrillation are both critical to patient survival. Delay of CPR for >10 min renders defibrillation ineffective and largely eliminates the potential benefit of prompt CPR *(5, 6)*. Treatment delays of more than 10 min result in a 95% mortality *(7)* (Fig. 1).

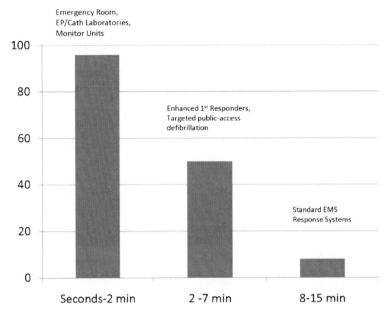

Fig. 1. Expected survival according to the interval between collapse and the administration of the first shock by the defibrillator. Modified from Ref. *(7)*.

Because of the importance of time to defibrillation as a determinant of survival, the impact of community-based strategies on cumulative SCD statisitics is limited by delays in contacting EMS, unavailability for AEDs for early defibrillation, and arrival time delays because of traffic and locations. Accordingly, while EMS responders are an important element for survival from unexpected CAs in out-of-hospital settings, the continuous monitoring and responses provided by implantable cardioverter-defibrillators (ICDs) provide a higher order of protection based upon nearly "immediate" response times. The challenge is to identify specific individual candidates for the efficient and effective prescription of ICD therapy.

DEFIBRILLATION THERAPY

Defibrillation is the only predictably effective therapy for reverting VF and pulseless VT to an effective rhythm for restoration of blood flow. The first documentation of successful termination of VF in dogs with alternating current shock was reported in 1899 by Prevost and Batelli *(8)*. Beck et al. reported the first successful termination of VF with alternating current (AC) shock in humans. In this case, a 14-year-old boy developed VF during sternal resection for correction of severe funnel chest, termination of VF required direct application of AC to the open heart, a technique that was developed by Wiggers and Hooker *(9)*. Zoll et al. reported the first successful termination of VF with

AC transthoracic countershock *(10)*. Lown et al. reported in 1962 successful termination ventricular arrhythmias with transthoracic synchronized direct current (DC) shock *(11)*, which is the preferred energy configuration for cardioversion and defibrillation.

EVOLVING INDICATIONS OF IMPLANTABLE DEFIBRILLATORS

Current indications for implantation of ICD are the result of risk stratification strategies that can be divided as follows: (1) secondary prevention indications; (2) primary prevention in high-risk groups with acquired diseases; and (3) SCD prevention in patients with well-identified inherited arrhythmogenic syndromes or less common acquired disease.

Current recommendations for indications for a diagnostic procedure, a particular therapy, or an intervention for management of patients with ventricular arrhythmias and prevention of sudden cardiac death (SCD) summarize both clinical evidence and expert opinion. A concise summary of the basis for the ACC/AHA/ESC classification of recommendations and definitions of levels of supporting evidence are provided in Table 1 *(12)*.

Table 1
Overview of Classifications of Recommendations and Levels of Evidence

Indication classification	Class I	Class IIa	Class IIb	Class III
	Benefit >>> Risk Procedure/ treatment should be performed/ administered	*Benefit >> Risk* It is *reasonable* to performed procedure/ administer treatment	*Benefit ≥ Risk* Procedure/ treatment *may be* considered	*Risk ≥ Benefit* Procedure/ treatment *should not* be performed/ administered
Level of evidence	Level A Multiple populations evaluated; Data derived from *multiple randomized trials*	Level B *Limited populations evaluated;* Data derived from a single randomized trial or multiple nonrandomized trials	Level C *Consensus opinion* of experts based on case studies, experimental data, and generally accepted practices	

Modified from Ref. *(12)*

SECONDARY PREVENTION INDICATIONS

ICD therapy was initially evaluated in survivors of VT/VF due to the known high risk of recurrence of events in this patient population, with 3-year mortality as high as 50% *(13)*. Three subsequent randomized clinical trials evaluated the role of ICD therapy among VT/VF survivors. Based on the results of these trials, ICD therapy became a class I indication in this patient population.

The AVID Trial was a multicenter, randomized clinical trial comparing anti-arrhythmic therapy vs. ICD among 1016 patients with a history of resuscitated VF, VT with syncope, or VT with LVEF 40% and symptoms suggesting severe hemodynamic compromise due to the arrhythmia (near-syncope, congestive heart failure, and angina). The mean follow-up was 18.2±12.2 months, the mean LVEF was 32% in the ICD arm and 31% in anti-arrhythmic group. At 2 years follow-up, amiodarone and sotalol were used in 82.4% and 8.5% in the anti-arrhythmic group as compared to 9.3% and 3.1% in

Table 2
Secondary Prevention Trials

Trial {f/u analysis} Year published	Study group Defined entry criteria	Time from diagnosis of qualifying condition to randomization	Ejection fraction Enrolled patients	All-cause mortality (%)		Benefit (%)	
				Control	ICD	Rel R R	Abs R R
AVID {2 year analysis} 1997	VFib, VT with syncope, VT with EF≤40%	Entry criterion: Undefined Actual: Not reported EF: 3 days post-qualifying event (median)	32% (SD = ±13%)	25	18	−27	−7
CIDS {2 year analysis} 2000	VFib, out-of-hospital cardiac arrest due to V Fib or VT, VT with syncope, VT with symptoms and EF≤35%, unmonitored syncope with subsequent spontaneous or induced VT	Entry criterion: Undefined Actual: Time from qualifying event to randomization not reported. Median time from randomization to ICD 7 days (>90% in ≤21 days) EF: Not reported	34% (SD = ±14%)	21	15	−30	−6
CASH {9 year analysis} 2000	VFib, VT	Entry criteria: Not defined Actual: Not reported EF: Not reported	46% (SD = ±18%)	44	36	−23	−8

EF ejection fraction, *AbsRR* absolute risk reduction, *RelRR* relative risk reduction, *f/u* follow-up, *VFib* ventricular fibrillation, *VT* ventricular tachycardia
From Ref. (*15*), with permission of publisher

the ICD group, respectively. Patients in the ICD arm achieved a 2-year relative risk reduction (RRR) of 27%, corresponding to an absolute mortality risk reduction (ARR) of 7% *(14, 15)* (Table 2).

In the AVID trial, the post-arrest EF and/or a history of congestive heart failure (CHF) significantly influenced the patient outcomes. All-cause mortality was significantly greater (*P*<0.0001) in patients with history of CHF compared with those without history of CHF. Survival in the group without prior CHF who received ICDs *(16)*, or with EF greater than 35%, was no different than in those treated with anti-arrhythmic therapy. In contrast, patients with history of CHF or EFs less than 35% had a substantially better outcome when they received an ICD, compared with those treated with anti-arrhythmic therapy (*P*<0.0001) *(16, 17)*.

The CIDS trial was randomized clinical study comparing ICD vs. amiodarone among 659 patients with documented VF; documented sustained VT causing syncope; documented sustained VT at a rate 150 beats/min, causing presyncope or angina in a patient with a LVEF 35%; or unmonitored syncope with subsequent documentation of either spontaneous VT 10 sec or sustained (30 sec) monomorphic VT induced by programmed ventricular stimulation. The mean follow-up was 3 year, the mean age was 63, and the mean LVEF was 34%. CIDS was stopped early after the results of AVID were reported and therefore demonstrated only a nonsignificant reduction in the risk of death and arrhythmic death in the ICD group, with a 2-year RRR of 30%, corresponding to an ARR of 6% *(18)*, a trend similar to the pattern observed in AVID (Table 2).

CASH trial was a randomized comparison of ICD vs. antiarrhythmic drugs among 288 patients resuscitated from CA secondary to documented sustained ventricular arrhythmias. Patients were randomized to an ICD, amiodarone, propafenone, or metoprolol. The primary end point was all-cause mortality. The propafenone arm was discontinued early due to a higher all-cause mortality rate than the ICD group. The mean follow-up was of 57±34 months, the mean age was 58 years, and the mean LVEF was 46% in the three groups. Therapy with an ICD was associated with a 23% (nonsignificant) reduction of all-cause mortality rates when compared with outcomes in the combined amiodarone and metoprolol arms *(19)*.

A meta-analysis of these trials showed a 28% RRR in all-cause mortality (*P*=0.0006) with ICD therapy that was due almost entirely to a 50% RRR in arrhythmic death (*P* < 0.0001) (Fig. 2). Patients with LVEF >35% had significantly less benefit from the ICD than those with LVEF ≤35% (*P*=0.011)

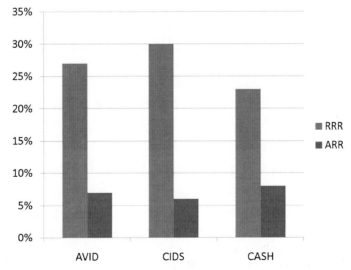

Fig. 2. Survival benefit of ICD therapy in secondary prevention trials. Definitions: RRR = relative risk reduction; ARR = absolute risk reduction.

Table 3
Secondary Prevention Indications 2008 ACC/AHA/HRS Guidelines

Class I
- ICD therapy is indicated in patients who are survivors of cardiac arrest due to VF or hemodynamically unstable sustained VT after evaluation to define the cause of the event and to exclude any completely reversible causes. *(Level of Evidence: A)*
- ICD therapy is indicated in patients with structural heart disease and spontaneous sustained VT, whether hemodynamically stable or unstable. *(Level of Evidence: B)*
- ICD therapy is indicated in patients with syncope of undetermined origin with clinically relevant, hemodynamically significant sustained VT or VF induced at electrophysiological study. *(Level of Evidence: B)*

CLASS IIa
- ICD implantation is reasonable for patients with unexplained syncope, significant LV dysfunction, and nonischemic DCM.*(Level of Evidence: C)*
- ICD implantation is reasonable for patients with sustained VT and normal or near-normal ventricular function. *(Level of Evidence:C)*

CLASS IIb
- ICD therapy may be considered in patients with syncope and advanced structural heart disease in whom thorough invasive and noninvasive investigations have failed to define a cause. *(Level of Evidence: C)*

CLASS III
- ICD therapy is not indicated for patients who do not have a reasonable expectation of survival with an acceptable functional status for at least 1 year, even if they meet ICD implantation criteria specified in the Class I, IIa, and IIb recommendations above. *(Level of Evidence: C)*
- ICD therapy is not indicated for patients with incessant VT or VF. *(Level of Evidence: C)*
- ICD therapy is not indicated in patients with significant psychiatric illnesses that may be aggravated by device implantation or that may preclude systematic follow-up. *(Level of Evidence: C)*
- ICD therapy is not indicated for syncope of undetermined cause in a patient without inducible ventricular tachyarrhythmias and without structural heart disease. *(Level of Evidence: C)*
- ICD therapy is not indicated when VF or VT is amenable to surgical or catheter ablation (e.g., RV or LV outflow tract VT, idiopathic VT, or fascicular VT in the absence of structural heart disease). *(Level of Evidence: C)*
- ICD therapy is not indicated for patients with ventricular tachyarrhythmias due to a completely reversible disorder in the absence of structural heart disease (e.g., electrolyte imbalance, drugs, or trauma). *(Level of Evidence: B)*

Modified from: Ref. *(12)*

(20). The recommendations from ACC/AHA/HRS 2008 Guidelines for ICD therapy for secondary prevention are shown in Table 3 *(12)*.

PRIMARY PREVENTION INDICATIONS IN HIGH-RISK POPULATIONS

Reliable identification of patients at risk of SCD remains challenging. Based on data from the Resuscitation Outcomes Consortium, 294,851 emergency medical services-treated out-of-hospital CA occur annually in the United States *(21)*. The majority of potential SCD victims come from larger populations groups, such as the general population, those with coronary risk factors without clinically evident disease, or those with known disease who either have either normal or mildly depressed LVEFs without functional limitations (see Fig. 3) *(22)*. These subpopulations are characterized by low-risk calculations, based on large denominators that dilute out large cumulative numbers in the denominators.

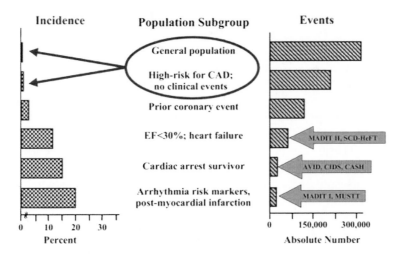

Fig. 3. Estimates of incidence and total annual population burden for general adult population and increasingly high-risk subgroups. Modified from Ref. *(15)*, with permission of publisher.

Risk stratification to identified potential SCD victims have been extensively studied in the past three decades. Four distinct types of SCD risk stratifiers can be identified:

(1) Markers of abnormal substrate or structural heart disease: LVEF, nonsustained ventricular tachycardia (NSVT), frequent ventricular ectopy, QRS duration;
(2) Markers of abnormal repolarization or electrical instability: electrophysiologic studies (EPS), T wave alternans (TWA), signal averaged ECG (SAECG), QT dispersion;
(3) Markers of abnormal autonomic balance: heart rate variability (HRV) and baroreceptor sensitivity (BRS).
(4) Genetic markers

Incorporation of a risk marker into clinical practice will depend on its power to predict adverse clinical outcomes if positive (positive predictive value, PPV) and/or their power to predict lack of adverse outcomes if negative (negative predictive value, NPV).

The practice of medicine is largely based on the application of a therapy or intervention in many individuals to prevent or avoid an adverse outcome in some. For example, data from 16 individual trials of subjects treated with HMG-CoA reductase inhibitors (statin drugs) demonstrated a 28% RRR in cardiovascular mortality, but only a 1.7% decrease in ARR of cardiovascular mortality, during an average follow-up of 3.3 years. In the GISSI trial, thrombolytic therapy was associated with a RRR in mortality of 18%, but the ARR in mortality was 2.3% *(23)*. Yet, both these therapies are well accepted in the care of patients with cardiovascular disease, with lesser effects on mortality than most of the ICD trials.

As predicted by Miroski and Mower, in addition to use in survivors of potentially fatal arrhythmias, ICD therapy has expanded to include the implantation of prophylactic ICDs in individuals with high risk of SCD, but no prior history of VT/VF. At present, the results of seven major primary prevention trials have been reported. These trials used LVEF, NSVT, EPS, TWA, and SAECG as their risk stratification tools in different degrees as follow.

The Multicenter Automatic Defibrillator Implantation Trial (MADIT) I was a randomized clinical study among 196 patients in New York Heart Association functional class I, II, or III with prior myocardial infarction; LVEF < 35%; a documented episode of asymptomatic NSVT (a run of 3–30 ventricular ectopic beats at a rate >120 beats/min); and inducible, nonsuppressible ventricular tachyarrhythmia on EPS. Patients were randomly assigned to ICD or medical therapy. The mean follow-up was 27 months, the mean age was 63, and the mean LVEF was 26%. ICD therapy was associated with a 59% RRR and a 19% ARR in mortality (Table 4) *(15, 24).*

In the CABG PATCH trial 900 patients scheduled for coronary bypass surgery, LVEF < 36%, and abnormal SAECG (duration of the filtered QRS complex, >114 msec; root-mean-square voltage in the terminal 40 msec of the QRS complex, <20 μV; or duration of the terminal filtered QRS complex at <40 μV, >38 msec) were prospectively randomized to ICD or medical therapy. The primary end point of the study was overall mortality. The mean follow-up was 32 months, the mean age was 63, and the mean LVEF was 27%. There were no significant differences in overall mortality in the two groups (HR = 1.07, $P = 0.64$) *(25).*

In the Multicenter Unsustained Tachycardia Trial (MUSTT) 704 patients with coronary artery disease, LEVF <40%, asymptomatic NSVT ($\geq$ 3 beats and onset $\geq$ 4 days after myocardial infarction or revascularization procedure), and inducible, sustained ventricular tachyarrhythmias were randomly assigned to electrophysiologically guided therapy (drugs and/or ICD) or no antiarrhythmic therapy. Among the 351 patients assigned to electrophysiologically guided therapy, 158 (45%) were discharged with antiarrhythmic drugs (class I agents, 26%; amiodarone, 10%; and sotalol, 9%). After discharge, 12% switched from antiarrhythmic drugs to ICD. The mean follow-up was 39 months, the mean age was 66, and the mean LVEF was 30%. The primary end point of CA or death from arrhythmia were 25% among those receiving electrophysiologically guided therapy and 32%, representing a reduction in risk of 27%. The lower rates of arrhythmic events among the patients assigned to electrophysiologically guided therapy were largely attributable to the use of defibrillators. The 5-year rate of CA or death from arrhythmia was 9% among the patients assigned to electrophysiologically guided therapy who received an ICD, as compared with 37% among those in this group who did not receive an ICD ($P<0.001$). In other words, the ICD subgroup achieved a 58% RRR and 31 ARR of death over 5 years of observation (Table 4) *(15, 26).*

The Defibrillators in Non-Ischemic Cardiomyopathy Treatment Evaluation (DEFINITE) trial was a prospective randomized clinical trial of medical therapy for HF vs. medical therapy for HF and ICD among 458 patients with nonischemic dilated cardiomyopathy, LVEF <36%, and premature ventricular complexes or NSVT. The mean follow-up was 29 months, the mean age was 58, and the mean LVEF was 21%. There were 28 in the ICD group, as compared to 40 in the medical therapy group (HR=0.65, P=0.08). There were 17 sudden deaths from arrhythmia: 3 in the ICD group, as compared with 14 in the medical therapy group (HR, 0.20; P=0.006) *(28).*

The Sudden Cardiac Death in Heart Failure Trial (SCD-HeFT) evaluated the role of medical therapy for HF plus placebo vs. medical therapy plus amiodarone vs. medical therapy for HF plus shock-only, single-lead ICD on 2521 patients with ischemic and non-ischemic HF, New York Heart Association class II or III HF, and LVEF $\leq$ 35%. The primary end point was death from any cause. The mean follow-up was 45 months, the mean age was 60 and the mean LVEF was 25%. There were 244 deaths (29%) in the placebo group, 240 (28%) in the amiodarone group, and 182 (22%) in the ICD group. As compared with placebo, amiodarone was associated with a similar risk of death (HR=1.06, P=0.53) and ICD therapy was associated with a RRR of death of 23% and an ARR in mortality of 7.2% after 5 years in the overall population. Results did not vary according to either ischemic or nonischemic causes of CHF. Among patients with NYHA class III CHF, there was a relative 44% increase in the risk of death among patients in the amiodarone group, as compared with those in the placebo group (HR=1.44) *(29).*

The Defibrillator in Acute Myocardial Infarction Trial (DINAMIT) was a randomized, open-label comparison of ICD therapy and no ICD therapy in 674 patients 6–40 days after a myocardial infarction, LVEF $\leq$ 35%, and impaired cardiac autonomic function (manifested as depressed HRV, standard deviation of normal-to-normal RR intervals of $\leq$70 msec, or an elevated average 24-h heart rate on

Table 4
Primary Prevention ICD Trials

Trial [f/u analysis] Year published	Study group Defined entry criteria	Time from diagnosis of qualifying condition to randomization	Ejection fraction Enrolled patients	All-cause mortality (%) Control	ICD	Benefit (%) Rel RR	Abs RR
MADIT {2 year analysis} 1996	Prior MI, EF ≤35%, N-S VT, Inducible VT, Failed I.V. PA	Entry criterion: ≥3 weeks Actual: 75% ≥6 months Qualifying EF: Interval not reported	26% (SD = ±7%)	32%	13%	-59%	19%
CABG-Patch {2 year analysis} 1997	Coronary bypass surgery, EF<36%, SAECG (+)	Diagnosis of CAD: Interval not reported Qualifying EF: Interval not reported SAECG: Day of randomization	27% (SD = ±6%)	18%	18%	N/A	N/A
MUSTT {5 year analysis} 1999	CAD (Prior MI ~95%), EF ≤40%, N-S VT, Inducible VT	Qualifying N-S VT: ≥4 days from MI Time from MII: 17% ≤1 month 50% ≥3 years Qualifying EF: Interval not reported	30% (21%, 35%) [median (25th, 75th percentile)]	55% [E-P guided arm: AAD]	24%	-58% [vs. ICD @ 60 m]	-31%
MADIT-II {2 year analysis} 2002	Prior MI (> 1 month), EF ≤30%	Entry criteria: ≥1 month Actual: 88% ≥6 months Qualifying EF: Interval not reported	23% (SD = ±5%)	22%	16%	-28%	-6%
DEFINITE {2½ year analysis} 2004	Nonischemic CM, Hx HF, EF≤35%, ≥10 PVCs/h or N-S VT	Heart failure onset [mean]: – Controls = 3.27 years –ICD group = 2.39 years	21% (range = 7-35%)	14%	8%	-44%	-6%
DINAMIT {2½ year analysis} 2004	Recent MI (6-40 days), EF ≤35%, abnormal HRV or mean 24 heart rate ≥80/min	Entry criteria: 6-40 days Actual: Mean = 18 days	28% (SD = ±5%)	17%	19%	N/A	N/A
SCD-HeFT {5 year analysis} 2005	Class II-III CHF, EF≤35%	Entry criteria: Interval not reported Qualifying EF: Interval not reported	25% (20%, 30%) [median (25th, 75th percentile)]	36%	29%	-23%	-7%

MI myocardial infarction, *EF* ejection fraction, *AbsRR* absolute risk reduction, *RelRR* relative risk reduction, *f/u* follow-up, *PVCs* premature ventricular complexes, *VT* ventricular tachycardia, *N-S* non-sustained, *CHF* congestive heart failure, *AAD* antiarrhythmic drug, *E-P* electrophysiologically, *I.V. PA* intravenous procainamide, *SAECG* (+) positive signal-averaged ECG, *CAD* coronary artery disease, *CM* cardiomyopathy, (*C*)*HF* (congestive) heart failure, *HRV* heart rate variability

From Ref. (*15*), with permission of publisher

Holter monitoring, ≥80 beats/min). The primary outcome was mortality from any cause. Death from arrhythmia was a secondary endpoint. The mean follow-up was 30 months, the mean age was 61, and the mean LVEF was 28%. There was no difference in overall mortality between the two treatment groups (HR=1.08, P=0.66). There were 12 deaths due to arrhythmia in the ICD group, as compared with 29 in the control group (HR=0.42, P=0.009). This benefit was offset by an increased in nonarrhythmic mortality in the ICD group (HR=1.75. P=0.02) *(30)*.

Although the overall average HR of all 7 primary prevention trials depicted in Fig. 4 was 0.72, indicating a 28% reduction in the risk of death in the ICD-treated patients as compared with the conventionally treated patients, the overall absolute 2-year mortality reduction was 3% (17.3% in the conventionally treated patients vs. 14.3% in the ICD-treated patients) *(31)*. However, within this group, CABG PATCH and DINAMIT, studies which had potentially confounding design features (anti-ischemic surgical intervention in CABG-Patch and earlier ICD intervention in DINAMITE) did not show any significant mortality benefits.

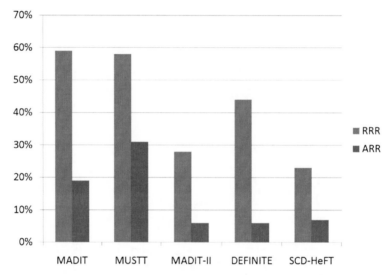

Fig. 4. Survival benefit of ICD therapy in primary prevention trials. Definitions: RRR = relative risk reduction; ARR = absolute risk reduction.

POTENTIAL STRATIFYING TOOLS FOR ICD TRIALS

Left Ventricular Ejection Fraction

The mean LVEF in the ICD trials for secondary prevention of SCD was 32% (AVID), 33%, (CIDS) and 46% (CASH). Consequently, most patients in these trials had an LVEF >30% *(14, 15, 18, 19)*. In these trials, an average relative risk reduction of death of 35% was observed, combined with an absolute risk reduction of 7.5% in ICD-treated patients as compared to medical therapy. While a meta-analysis suggested that benefit clustered primarily among patients with EFs <35%, it is likely that there are population subgroups within the overall subgroup of patients with LVEF >35% that achieve greater benefit. Nonetheless, present guidelines do not define indications for ICDs for secondary prevention on the basis of EF (Fig. 2) *(31)*.

Primary prevention trials of ICD therapy have focused on depressed left ventricular ejection fraction (LVEF) as the most strongly emphasized risk stratification tool to identify individuals with a high risk of SCD *(32, 33)*. However, risk stratification strategies based predominantly on severely depressed LVEF may fail to identify up to two-thirds of SCD victims who could potentially benefit from prophylactic ICDs and/or other therapeutic interventions *(33)*. In the Maastricht circulatory arrest registry, 56.5% of the SCD victims had an LVEF >30 and 20% had a LVEF >50% *(34)*.

In the Oregon Sudden Unexpected Death Study, the LVEF was severely (<35%) reduced in 36 patients (30%), mildly to moderately (36–54% LVEF) reduced in 27 patients (22%), and normal in 58 patients (48%). Those with normal LVEF were younger and had a lower prevalence of established coronary artery disease *(35)*.

The prognostic value of a depressed LVEF appears to be influenced by other factors. Analysis of data from 674 patients enrolled in the MUSTT study who did not receive antiarrhythmic or ICD therapy revealed that other variables, such as functional class, history of heart failure, NSVT, age, left ventricular conduction abnormalities, inducible sustained ventricular tachycardia, and atrial fibrillation influence arrhythmic death and total mortality risk. Patients with an LVEF ≤30%, but no other risk factors had a low predicted mortality risk. Patients with LVEF >30% and other risk factors may have a higher mortality and a higher risk of sudden death than some patients with LVEF ≤30%. Thus, the risk of SCD depends on multiple variables in addition to EF *(36)*.

Subgroup analyses from primary prevention trials had reported greater benefits from ICD therapy among subgroups with the more severely depressed LVEF and marginal or uncertain benefit from ICD therapy among patients with LVEF close to the enrollment inclusion cutoff. This is partly due the differences between the entry criteria cutoff and the mean or median values for patients who were actually enrolled in these trials. For example, patients with LVEF >30% in SCD-HeFT trial had no apparent benefit from ICD therapy *(29)*. Similarly, in MADIT, patients with LVEF >26% had no significant benefit from ICD therapy *(37, 38)*. Both of these examples are based on post hoc subgroup analyses, and therefore still require future prospective confirmation.

Current primary prevention recommendations for are based on the upper limit entry criteria cutoff LVEF of patients enrolled in primary prevention trials *(12)* (Table 4). This is in part due to the inherent limitations of subgroup analysis, which sometimes can lead to misleading interpretations. However, subgroup analysis do raise important clinical questions that should be validated in prospective clinical trials *(39)*.

Programmed Electrical Stimulation Studies and Risk Stratification

The predictive value of inducing sustained VT/VF during EPS (positive EPS) was tested in two large prospective multicenter trials (MADIT, MUSTT). These trials demonstrated that a positive EPS in patients with prior MI, LVEF ≤35% or ≤40%, and NSVT identifies populations with a substantial benefit from prophylactic ICD therapy, with a 56% and 76% RRR of overall mortality and cardiac arrest and arrhythmic death, respectively *(24, 26, 40)*.

More specifically, the prognostic value of positive EPS in 353 MUSTT patients who were randomized not to receive antiarrhythmic therapy was compared to that of negative EPS among 1397 patients who were followed in the MUSTT registry. The primary endpoint was CA or death from arrhythmia. The 2-year and 5-year rates of CA or death due to arrhythmia were 12% and 24%, respectively, among the patients in the registry, as compared with 18% and 32% among the patients with inducible tachyarrhythmias who were assigned to no antiarrhythmic therapy (adjusted *P*< 0.001). Overall mortality after 5 years was 48% among the patients with inducible tachyarrhythmias, as compared with 44% among the patients in the registry (adjusted *P* = 0.005) *(26)*. However, even patients without inducible tachyarrhythmias had a relatively high risk of death, indicating that patients with negative EPS still had high mortality rates and could potentially benefit from prophylactic ICD therapy.

The presence of inducible sustained ventricular tachycardia proved to be a relatively specific predictor of death from arrhythmia in this group of patients. The proportion of deaths classified as due to arrhythmia was greater among the patients with inducible tachyarrhythmias who were randomly assigned to no antiarrhythmic therapy than among the patients in the registry in whom sustained tachyarrhythmias could not be induced. In the MUSTT registry, the 2-year negative predictive value of EPS for CA or death due to arrhythmia was 88%. However, the negative predictive value of EPS may diminish with time as coronary artery disease and LV dysfunction worsen (40).

In the MADIT II study, 593 (82%) of 720 patients randomized to the ICD arm also underwent EPS. Inducible patients had a greater likelihood of experiencing ICD therapy for spontaneous VT than non-inducible patients ($P = 0.023$). However, ICD therapy for spontaneous VF was less frequent in inducible patients. Therefore, the 2-year event rate for combined VT/VF was 29.4% for inducible patients and 25.5% for noninducible patients. ($P = 0.280$). In other words, a positive EPS is a good predictor of VT, but not a good predictor of VF (41).

The combination of NSVT, positive EPS, and depressed LVEF in the MADIT I and MUSTT trial showed that four ICDs needed to be implanted to save a life during the mean follow-up of 33 month, whereas in the MADIT II 18 ICDs would need to be implanted to save a life during the mean follow-up of 20 months. In other words, as the indications for prophylactic ICDs are expanded and the risk stratification strategies are simplified, the NNT to save a life increases (42, 43).

Today, EPS still has a role in the risk stratification of asymptomatic patients with NSVT, coronary artery disease, and LVEF between ≤35%. It also has a potential role in risk stratification of coronary heart disease patients with unexplained syncope and better preserved LVEFs.

Microvolt T Wave Alternans (TWA)

Results from clinical studies suggest that TWA have similar prognostic value in ischemic and non-ischemic cardiomyopathy, adds predictive value to the other risk markers (LVEF, EPS and NSVT) and could identify different populations at risk of arrhythmic events to those identified with LVEF, nonsustained VT, and EPS (44).

Results from the most recent and larger population studies confirm that result of a TWA test cannot identify or exclude benefit from prophylactic ICD therapy among patients with LVEF ≤35% (44), but patients with negative TWA and LVEF ≤35% seems to have less benefit from prophylactic ICD therapy. This could be clinically relevant when patients are informed about risks and benefits of pro-phylactic ICD therapy. Chow et al. reported that among MADIT II-like patients the results of TWA testing could be used to determine future benefit of ICD therapy. They reported that the NNT with an ICD for 2 years to save one life was 9 among non-negative TWA patients and 76 among negative TWA patients. However, this data is derived from a relative small population group (45).

The recommendations from ACC/AHA/HRS 2008 Guidelines for ICD therapy for primary pre-vention in patient with depressed LVEF are summarized in Table 5 (12). These guidelines state that "it would be best to have ICDs offered to patients with clinical profiles as similar to those included in the trials as possible". These guidelines also acknowledge that the determination of LVEF lacks a "gold standard" and that there may be variation among the commonly used clinical techniques of LVEF determination. All clinical methods of LVEF determination lack precision and the accuracy of techniques varies amongst laboratories and institutions. Based on these considerations, this writ-ing committee recommends that the clinician use the LVEF determination that they feel is the most clinically accurate and appropriate in their institution.

Signal Averaged Electrocardiography

The predictive value of SAECG was evaluated in 1268 patients (66%) out of 1925 patients enrolled in the MUSTT trial who had a baseline SAECG. In subjects with an abnormal SAECG, the 5-year rates of the primary endpoint of arrhythmic death or cardiac arrest (28% vs. 17%, $P = 0.0001$), cardiac death (37% vs. 25%, $P = 0.0001$), and total mortality (43% vs. 35%, $P = 0.0001$) were significantly higher (46).

In the CABG Patch Trial, 900 patients scheduled for elective coronary bypass surgery with an LVEF 35%, and an abnormal SAECG were randomly assigned to therapy with an ICD (446 patients) or to the control group (454 patients). The primary endpoint of the study was overall mortality. During an

Table 5
Primary Prevention Indications 2008 ACC/AHA/HRS Guidelines

Class I
- ICD therapy is indicated in patients with LVEF less than 35% due to prior MI who are at least 40 days post-MI and are in NYHA functional Class II or III. *(Level of Evidence: A)*
- ICD therapy is indicated in patients with nonischemic DCM who have an LVEF less than or equal to 35% and who are in NYHA functional Class II or III. *(Level of Evidence: B)*
- ICD therapy is indicated in patients with LV dysfunction due to prior MI who are at least 40 days post-MI, have an LVEF less than 30%, and are in NYHA functional Class I. *(Level of Evidence: A)*
- ICD therapy is indicated in patients with NSVT due to prior MI, LVEF < 40%, and inducible VF or sustained VT at electrophysiological study. *(Level of Evidence: B)*

Class IIa
- ICD implantation is reasonable for nonhospitalized patients awaiting transplantation. *(Level of Evidence: C)*

Class IIb
- ICD therapy may be considered in patients with nonischemic heart disease who have an LVEF of less than or equal to 35% and who are in NYHA functional Class I. *(Level of Evidence: C)*

Class III
- ICD therapy is not indicated for patients who do not have a reasonable expectation of survival with an acceptable functional status for at least 1 year, even if they meet ICD implantation criteria specified in the Class I, IIa, and IIb recommendations above.*(Level of Evidence: C)*
- ICD therapy is not indicated in patients with significant psychiatric illnesses that may be aggravated by device implantation or that may preclude systematic follow-up. *(Level of Evidence: C)*
- ICD therapy is not indicated for NYHA Class IV patients with drug-refractory congestive heart failure who are not candidates for cardiac transplantation or CRT-D. *(Level of Evidence: C)*

Modified from Ref. *(12)*

average follow-up of 32±16 months, there were 101 deaths in the defibrillator group and 95 in the control group (hazard ratio = 1.07; P = 0.64). Revascularization may have altered the immediate prognosis irrespective of the SAECG and EF. On the other hand, in many patients, EF may have improved after revascularization, or the substrate for arrhythmogenesis could have been substantially altered. Further analysis of the CABG Patch study showed that ICD use reduced arrhythmic death by 45%, although total mortality was not reduced because of an increase in nonarrhythmic deaths *(25)*.

Observations from these studies are not necessarily contradictory, since they compared different patient populations and different definitions of an abnormal SAECG were used (filtered QRS duration >114 msec in MUSTT vs. filtered QRS duration >114 msec; root-mean-square voltage in the terminal 40 msec of the QRS complex <20 μV; or duration of the terminal filtered QRS complex at <40 μV >38 msec in the CABG Patch Trial). Hence, the SAECG might still have a role in risk stratification for arrhythmic death.

ICD INDICATIONS IN PATIENTS WITH INHERITED ARRHYTHMOGENIC SYNDROMES

In the general population, there is a subgroup of individuals that exhibit a great propensity to develop lethal cardiac arrhythmias. These individuals are affected by channelopathies (long/short QT syndrome, Brugada syndrome, early repolarization syndrome) or structural heart disease with preserve LVEF (hypertrophic cardiomyopathies, cardiac sarcoidosis, and arrhythmogenic right ventricular dysplasia). The therapeutic alternatives are limited in this population and, often times, ICD represents the only therapeutic alternative (Table 6).

Table 6
ICD Indications in Genetic Disorders Associated with SCD Risk

Diagnosis guidelines	ICD indication	Primary source of data	Risk indicators	Classification	Evidence
HCM	Secondary SCA protection	Registries; cohorts	Prior SCA, pulseless VT	Class I	Level B
			Sustained VT, unexplained syncope	Class II a	Level C
	Primary SCA protection	Registries; cohorts	LV thickness >30 mm, high LV outflow gradient, family history of SCD, N-S VT, blunted BP response to exercise	Class II a	Level C
ARVD/RVCM	Secondary SCA protection	Registry; case series	Prior SCA, sustained VT	Class I	Level B,C
			Unexplained syncope	Class IIa	Level C
	Primary SCA protection	Registry; case series	Induced VT, ambient N-S VT, extensive disease	Class IIa	Level C
Congenital LQT	Secondary SCA protection	Registry; cohorts	Prior SCA, symptomatic VT	Class I	Level B
	Primary SCA protection	Registry; cohorts	VT or syncope on β-blocker, QTc >500 msec, family history premature SCA(?)	Class IIa,b	Level B
Familial SQT	Secondary SCA protection	Small case series	Prior SCA, "idiopathic" VF	Class I	Level C
	Primary SCA protection	Small case series	Unknown; family history of SCD (?)	Class IIb, III	Level C
Brugada syndrome	Secondary SCA protection	Case cohorts	Prior SCA, pulseless VT	Class I	Level B
	Primary SCA protection	Case cohorts	Symptomatic VT, unexplained syncope, family history of premature SCA with Type I ECG pattern	Class IIa	Level C
CPVT/F	Secondary SCA protection	Small case series	Prior SCA, pulseless VT	Class I	Level C
	Primary SCA protection	Small case series	Syncope or VT while receiving β-blockers, family history premature SCA(?)	Class II a	Level C

HCM hypertrophic cardiomyopathy, *ARVD/RVCM* arrhythmogenic right ventricular dysplasia/cardiomyopathy, *LQT* long QT syndrome, *SQT* short QT syndrome, *CPVT/F* catecholaminergic polymorphic ventricular tachycardia/"idiopathic" ventricular fibrillation, *SCA* sudden cardiac arrest, *VT* ventricular tachycardia, *N–S* nonsustained, *PVT* polymorphic ventricular tachycardia, *VA* ventricular arrhythmias, (?)=uncertain

Guideline classifications and levels of evidence are derived from an amalgamation of narrative and tabular statements in two recent Guideline documents (see references) with variations in the documents adjudicated by the authors. Definitions are the standard usages provided in Guidelines documents

From Ref. *(15)*, with permission of publisher

Long QT Syndrome (LQTS)

LQTS is a genetic channelopathy with variable penetrance that is associated with increased propensity for polymorphic ventricular tachyarrhythmias (torsades de pointes) and SCD. QT prolongation is the hallmark of LQTS and may arise from a reduction in the outward potassium current ("loss of function") or an augmented late entry of sodium or calcium ions ("gain of function"). Beta-blockers constitute the mainstay therapy for LQTS, but beta-blockers appear to be less effective in LQT2 and are without value in LQT3.

The incidence of cardiac events is higher among LQT1, but lethality of events is higher in LQT3. During childhood, male patients display a higher event rate than females, whereas after this time period, females exhibit higher event rates than males.

Data from the International LQTS Registry demonstrated genotype information do not contribute significantly to outcome after adjustment for clinical risk factors. This may be related to variable penetrance among patients carrying the same genotype. The same data also demonstrated that syncope is the most powerful predictor of subsequent life-threatening events. Interestingly, the risk associated with a history of syncope is significantly higher in females than in males and most pronounced when the event occurred within the past 2 years.

Duration of QT prolongation has also been consistently demonstrated to be a major risk factor. Priori et al. reported a 70% cumulative incidence of first cardiac event from birth to age 40 in patients with QTc >500 msec.

Data analysis from the International LQTS Registry among 1915 LQTS probands and first- and second-degree relatives from birth through age 40 years showed that sibling death is not significantly associated with an increase in the rate of subsequent life-threatening cardiac events (CA or SCD), which might also be related to variable penetrance among relatives.

Data analysis from the International LQTS Registry also indicated that the risk of cardiac events remains elevated after the age of 40 among LQTS subjects. In this population, QTc duration 470 msec was associated with a twofold increase in the risk of CA or death compared with unaffected subjects with QTc <440 msec.

Currently, clinical risk factors constitute the main tool for patient selection for ICD therapy. LQTS risk groups are categorized as high (history of CA and/or documented torsades de pointes), intermediate (history of syncope and/or QTc prolongation >0.50 sec), and low (No prior syncope and with QTc duration ≤0.50 sec) risk.

ICD therapy is recommended for the high-risk (secondary prevention) and the intermediate risk groups (primary prevention). Early therapy with an ICD should also be considered in high-risk Jervell and Lange-Nielsen patients, because the efficacy of beta-blocker therapy was found to be limited in this population (47–52).

Hypertrophic Cardiomyopathy (HCM)

HCM is a complex disease that is relatively common among the genetic cardiac disorders (about 1:500 in the general adult population). There is a clear consensus that secondary prevention of SCD with ICDs for those patients HCM who have survived a CA or documented sustained VT due to their high risk of recurrence rates. Current risk stratification strategies for primary prevention utilizes five clinical markers that have been defined in several retrospective and observational studies (49–57). These primary-prevention high-risk factors are (1) family history of SCD; (2) history of syncope, inconsistent with neurocardiogenic syncope; (3) multiple and/or prolonged runs of nonsustained VT on serial 24-h Holter monitoring at heart rates ≥120 beats/min; (4) hypotensive or attenuated blood pressure response to exercise; and (5) massive left ventricular hypertrophy (maximum wall thickness ≥30 mm).

In largest cohort of patients with HCMP ($N = 506$) treated with ICDs, 35% of the primary prevention patients who received appropriate device therapy for potentially lethal ventricular arrhythmias had been implanted with ICDs based on the presence of single high-risk factor *(58)*.

The routine use of prophylactic ICD after alcohol septal ablation for symptomatic obstructive HCM remains unclear. A recent prospective study in 123 patients with obstructive HCM who underwent alcohol septal ablation and had an ICD implanted for primary prevention of SCD for known risk factors. During a mean follow-up of 2.9 years, septal ablation was not associated with an increased risk of ventricular arrhythmias *(59)*.

The Brugada Syndrome

This entity is characterized by ST-segment elevation in the right precordial ECG leads and high incidence of SCD. The syndrome typically manifests during adulthood, with a mean age of SCD of 41 years. The syndrome is estimated to be responsible for at least 20% of SCD in patients with structurally normal hearts. The prevalence of the disease is estimated to be 5/10,000 inhabitants *(60)*. Amiodarone and beta-blockers have been shown to be ineffective, and class I antiarrhythmic drugs are contraindicated *(61)*. Currently, an ICD is the only proven effective treatment for the disease. The Second Consensus Conference on Brugada syndrome recommends ICD therapy for patients with type 1 Brugada ECG (either spontaneously or after sodium channel blockade) with history of SCD or cardiac syncope (class I, secondary prevention).

EPS is recommended for asymptomatic patients with type 1 Brugada ECG (either spontaneously or after sodium channel blockade) and family history of SCD. EPS is also recommended if the type 1 ECG occurs spontaneously, even in the absence of family history of SCD. If inducible for ventricular arrhythmia, then the patient should receive an ICD (class II, primary prevention). Asymptomatic patients without family history of SCD who develop a type 1 ECG only after sodium channel blockade should be followed up closely *(60)*.

Arrhythmogenic Right Ventricular Dysplasia (ARVD)

ARVD is an inherited cardiomyopathy characterized by ventricular arrhythmias and structural abnormalities of the right ventricle that result from progressive replacement of right ventricular myocardium with fatty and fibrous tissue. The precise prevalence of ARVD in the United States has been estimated to be 1 in 5000 of the general population. ARVD accounts for approximately 10% of SCD in individuals <35 years of age *(62)*.

Patients with ARVD who are at the highest risk for arrhythmic death include (1) history of SCD/syncope, (2) younger age, (3) marked right ventricular involvement, and (4) left ventricular involvement *(63, 64)*. EPS was not a good predictor of appropriate ICD shocks in two large clinical trials *(65)*.

Centers with the largest experience recommend prophylactic ICD to all patients that meet the Task Force criteria for ARVD/C due to their high risk for SCD.

At the present time, catheter ablation is best used as a palliative measure for patients with refractory VT/frequent ICD shocks.

Short QT Syndrome (SQTS)

SQTS is an apparently inherited channelopathy characterized by a short QT interval (QTc $\leq$320 msec) associated with atrial fibrillation, syncope, and/or SCD in patients with no underlying structural heart disease. Five forms of SQTS are currently recognized, SQTS 1–3 are due to mutations causing gain of function on potassium currents and SQTS 4–5 are due to mutations causing loss of function of calcium channels. ICD implantation is recommended in all patients due to the high risk of SCD. Quinidine can prolong the QT interval significantly in this patient population and can be used as an alternative treatment when ICD implantation is not feasible, especially in very young patients *(50, 66, 67)*.

Early Repolarization Syndrome (ERS)

Early repolarization is a common electrocardiographic finding that is generally considered to be benign. The prevalence of ERS varies between 1% and 2%, especially in young men. Although considered benign manifestation for long time, recent experimental studies suggest that that depression of the epicardial action potential plateau creates a transmural gradient that manifests as a ST-segment elevation which might be prone to development of large transmural dispersion of repolarization, that might be proarrhythmic *(68)*. Haïssaguerre et al. reported a high incidence of ERS among 206 CA survivors due to idiopathic VF compared to controls (31% vs. 5%, P<0.001) *(69)*.

Therefore, ERS is potentially relevant in patients with family history of SCD or syncope. Recently, a variant of KCNJ8/K ATP was reported in a patient with idiopathic VF and ERS *(70)*. The role of EPS for risk stratification is not clear in this patient population *(65)*, Quinidine and isoproterenol do have antiarrhythmic effects in this patient group in the chronic and acute setting, respectively *(71)*.

There is no clear risk stratification strategy that could identify patient that could benefit from implantable defibrillator, except perhaps patients with family history of SCD or syncope.

Catecholaminergic Polymorphic Ventricular Tachycardia (CPVT)

CPVT is a rare inherited disorder that predominantly affects childldren or adolescents with structurally normal hearts. It is characterized by bidirectional VT, monomorphic, and polymorphic VT induced by physical or emotional stress, and a high risk for sudden cardiac death (30–50% by age 20–30 years). Mutations in genes encoding the cardiac ryanodine receptor 2 (RyR2) or calsequestrin 2 in patients have been associated with this condition. Beta-blockers, nadolol in particular, are considered the best therapeutic option in CPVT *(72)*.

ICD therapy is indicated in patients with history of CA, patients with syncope or ventricular arrhythmias despite adequate beta-blocker therapy, and patient intolerant or not complain with beta-blockers.

Left cardiac sympathetic denervation could also be considered for patients having recurrent symptoms despite blocker therapy, intolerant or not complain with beta-blockers, and patients with frequent ICD shocks *(73)*.

ICD INDICATIONS IN PATIENTS UNCOMMON WITH ACQUIRED DISORDERS

Myocarditis

Subclinical myocarditis is common in benign viral infections, but it may be associated with cardiac arrhythmias, including potentially lethal arrhythmias, with or without significant ventricular dysfunction. SCD can occur in myocarditis in the absence of clinical evidence of left ventricular dysfunction. In a study of SCD among previously screened military recruits, myocarditis-observed post-mortem was determined to be the cause of death in 42% of the victims, and in a study from Sweden, 68% of SCDs due to myocarditis had no pre-mortem symptoms. However, among survivors of CA or VT due to acute myocarditis, risk does not persist in the absence of chronic post-myocarditis cardiomyopathy and ICDs are generally not indicated. With chronic heart failure or markedly reduced EF after healing, however, indications follow the same pattern as other nonischemic cardiomyopathies *(12, 74)*.

Infiltrative Disorders

Cardiac sarcoidosis is a multisystem disorder of unknown etiology characterized by the accumulation of T lymphocytes, phagocytes, and noncaseating granulomas in involved tissue. Cardiac involvement is usually manisfested with heart block, ventricular tachycardia, and left ventricular dysfunction. ICD therapy is indicated in patients with cardiac sarcodosis and syncope or VT (sustained and possibly nonsustained), and patients with LVEF <35%. EPS could be used for risk stratification in patients with significant scars detected with MRI, high-grade PVCs, or LVEF >35%. Due to its progressive progressive nature, ICD is also recommended in patients with cardiac sarcoidosis requiring pacing for heart block *(75, 76)*.

Other infiltrative disorders have indication criteria that are variable and not well defined, as outlined in the 2008 ACC/AHA/HRS guidelines *(12)*. However, the data are not extensive, and to a significant degree, indications are determined by life expectancy.

The recommendations from ACC/AHA/HRS 2008 Guidelines for ICD therapy in arrhythmogenic syndromes are summarized in Table 6 *(12)*.

FUTURE STRATEGIES FOR REFINING INDICATIONS FOR ICDs

The majority of potential SCD victims come from larger populations groups, such as those with coronary risk factors or the general population who either have preserved LVEFs or unrecognized LV dysfunction *(22)*. Future risk stratification strategies will probably concentrate in the identification of individuals with high risk among subjects with LVEF > 40%. However, risk stratification strategies in the population are limited by the relative lower incidence of events in this population group. Hence, successful risk stratification strategies that could eventually identify most of the potential victims of SCD probably require the combination of multiple risk stratification tools, such as TWA, EPS, and genetic profiling.

The implementation of prophylactic ICD therapy and/or other therapeutic intervention in these larger population groups is, at least partially, limited by their cost, risk-benefit ratio (NNT), impact on quality of life, the lack of reliable risk stratification tools in larger population groups, and lack of scientific evidence that ICD therapy improves survival in these lower risk populations.

Large multicenter clinical trials are needed before this suggested approach could be implemented in clinical practice.

REFERENCES

1. Becker L, Gold LS, Eisenberg M, White L, Hearne T, Rea T (2008) Ventricular fibrillation in King County, Washington: a 30-year perspective. Resuscitation 79:22–27
2. Eisenberg MS, Mengert TJ (2001) Cardiac resuscitation. N Engl J Med 344:1304–1313
3. Atwood C, Eisenberg MS, Herlitz J, Rea TD (2005) Incidence of EMS-treated out-of-hospital cardiac arrest in Europe. Resuscitation 67:75–80
4. Cobb LA, Fahrenbruch CE, Olsufka M, Copass MK (2002) Changing incidence of out-of-hospital ventricular fibrillation, 1980–2000. JAMA 288:3008–3013
5. Valenzuela TD, Roe DJ, Cretin S, Spaite DW, Larsen MP (1997) Estimating effectiveness of cardiac arrest interventions: a logistic regression survival model. Circulation 96:3308–3313
6. Marenco JP, Wang PJ, Link MS, Homoud MK, Estes NA 3rd (2001) Improving survival from sudden cardiac arrest: the role of the automated external defibrillator. JAMA 285:1193–1200
7. Weaver WD, Peberdy MA (2002) Defibrillators in public places – one step closer to home. N Engl J Med 347:1223–1224
8. Passman R, Kadish A (2007) Sudden death prevention with implantable devices. Circulation 116:561–571
9. Beck CS, Pritchard WH, Feil HS (1947) Ventricular Fibrillation of Long Duration Abolished by Electric Shock. JAMA 135:985–986
10. Zoll PM, Linenthal AJ, Gibson W, Paul MH, Norman LR (1956) Termination of ventricular fibrillation in man by externally applied electric countershock. N Engl J Med 254:727–732
11. Lown B, Amarasingham R, Neuman J (1962) New method for terminating cardiac arrhythmias. Use of synchronized capacitor discharge. JAMA 182:548–555
12. ACC/AHA/HRS (2008) Guidelines for Device-Based Therapy of Cardiac Rhythm Abnormalities: a report of the American College of Cardiology/American Heart Association Task Force on Practice Guidelines (Writing Committee to

Revise the ACC/AHA/NASPE 2002 Guideline Update for Implantation of Cardiac Pacemakers and Antiarrhythmia Devices) developed in collaboration with the American Association for Thoracic Surgery and Society of Thoracic Surgeons. J Am Coll Cardiol 51:e1–e62

13. Goldstein S, Landis JR, Leighton R, Ritter G, Vasu CM, Wolfe RA, Acheson A, VanderBrug Medendorp S (1985) Predictive survival models for resuscitated victims of out-of-hospital cardiac arrest with coronary heart disease. Circulation 71:873–880

14. A comparison of antiarrhythmic-drug therapy with implantable defibrillators in patients resuscitated from near-fatal ventricular arrhythmias (1997) The antiarrhythmics versus implantable defibrillators (AVID) investigators. N Engl J Med 337:1576–1583

15. Myerburg RJ, Reddy V, Castellanos A (2009) Indications for implantable cardioverter-defibrillators based on evidence and judgment. J Am Coll Cardiol 54:747–763

16. Brodsky MA, McAnulty J, Zipes DP, Baessler C, Hallstrom AP, AVID Investigators (2006) A history of heart failure predicts arrhythmia treatment efficacy: data from the Antiarrythmics versus Implantable Defibrillators (AVID) study. Am Heart J 152:724–730

17. Domanski MJ, Sakseena S, Epstein AE, Hallstrom AP, Brodsky MA, Kim S, Lancaster S, Schron E (1999) Relative effectiveness of the implantable cardioverter-defibrillator and antiarrhythmic drugs in patients with varying degrees of left ventricular dysfunction who have survived malignant ventricular arrhythmias. AVID investigators. Antiarrhythmics versus implantable defibrillators. J Am Coll Cardiol 34:1090–1095

18. Connolly SJ, Gent M, Roberts RS, Dorian P, Roy D, Sheldon RS, Mitchell LB, Green MS, Klein GJ, O'Brien B (2000) Canadian implantable defibrillator study (CIDS): a randomized trial of the implantable cardioverter defibrillator against amiodarone. Circulation 101:1297–302

19. Kuck KH, Cappato R, Siebels J, Rüppel R (2000) Randomized comparison of antiarrhythmic drug therapy with implantable defibrillators in patients resuscitated from cardiac arrest: the cardiac arrest study hamburg (CASH). Circulation 102(7):748–754

20. Connolly SJ, Hallstrom AP, Cappato R, Schron EB, Kuck KH, Zipes DP, Greene HL, Boczor S, Domanski M, Follmann D, Gent M, Roberts RS (2000) Meta-analysis of the implantable cardioverter defibrillator secondary prevention trials. AVID, CASH and CIDS studies. Antiarrhythmics vs implantable defibrillator study. Cardiac Arrest Study Hamburg . Canadian implantable defibrillator study. Eur Heart J 21:2071–2078

21. American Heart Association (2009) Heart disease and stroke statistics – 2009 update. American Heart Association, Dallas, Texas

22. Huikuri HV, Castellanos A, Myerburg RJ (2001) Sudden death due to cardiac arrhythmias. N Engl J Med 345: 1473–1482

23. Myerburg RJ, Mitrani R, Interian A Jr, Castellanos A (1998) Interpretation of outcomes of antiarrhythmic clinical trials: design features and population impact. Circulation 97:1514–1s521

24. Moss AJ, Hall WJ, Cannom DS, Daubert JP, Higgins SL, Klein H, Levine JH, Saksena S, Waldo AL, Wilber D, Brown MW, Heo M (1996) Improved survival with an implanted defibrillator in patients with coronary disease at high risk for ventricular arrhythmia. Multicenter automatic defibrillator implantation trial investigators. N Engl J Med 335: 1933–1940

25. Bigger JT Jr (1997) Prophylactic use of implanted cardiac defibrillators in patients at high risk for ventricular arrhythmias after coronary-artery bypass graft surgery. Coronary Artery Bypass Graft (CABG) Patch Trial Investigators. N Engl J Med 337:1569–1575

26. Buxton AE, Lee KL, Fisher JD, Josephson ME, Prystowsky EN, Hafley G (1999) A randomized study of the prevention of sudden death in patients with coronary artery disease. Multicenter unsustained tachycardia trial investigators. N Engl J Med 341:1882–1890

27. Moss AJ, Zareba W, Hall WJ, Klein H, Wilber DJ, Cannom DS, Daubert JP, Higgins SL, Brown MW, Andrews ML (2002) Multicenter automatic defibrillator implantation trial II investigators prophylactic implantation of a defibrillator in patients with myocardial infarction and reduced ejection fraction. N Engl J Med 346:877–883

28. Kadish A, Dyer A, Daubert JP, Quigg R, Estes NA, Anderson KP, Calkins H, Hoch D, Goldberger J, Shalaby A, Sanders WE, Schaechter A, Levine JH (2004) Defibrillators in Non-Ischemic Cardiomyopathy Treatment Evaluation (DEFINITE) Investigators. Prophylactic defibrillator implantation in patients with nonischemic dilated cardiomyopathy. N Engl J Med 350:2151–2158

29. Bardy GH, Lee KL, Mark DB et al (2005) for the Sudden Cardiac Deathin Heart Failure Trial (SCD-HeFT) Investigators. Amiodarone or an implantable cardioverter-defibrillator for congestive heart failure. N Engl J Med 352:225–237

30. Hohnloser SH, Kuck KH, Dorian P et al (2004) for the DINAMIT Investigators. Prophylactic use of an implantable cardioverter-defibrillator after acute myocardial infarction. N Engl J Med 351:2481–2488

31. Moss AJ (2005) Should everyone with an ejection fraction less than or equal to 30% receive an implantable cardioverter-defibrillator? Everyone with an ejection fraction < or = 30% should receive an implantable cardioverter-defibrillator. Circulation 111:2537–2549

32. Al-Khatib SM, Sanders GD, Mark DB et al (2005) Expert panel participating in a Duke Clinical Research Institute-sponsored conference. Implantable cardioverter defibrillators and cardiac resynchronization therapy in patients with left ventricular dysfunction: randomized trial evidence through 2004. Am Heart J 149:1020–1034

33. Kusmirek SL, Gold MR (2007) Sudden cardiac death: the role of risk stratification. Am Heart J 153(Suppl):25–33

34. Gorgels AP, Gijsbers C, de Vreede-Swagemakers J, Lousberg A, Wellens HJ (2003) Out-of-hospital cardiac arrest–the relevance of heart failure. The Maastricht Circulatory Arrest Registry. Eur Heart J 24:1204–1209

35. Stecker EC, Vickers C, Waltz J et al (2006) Population-based analysis of sudden cardiac death with and without left ventricular systolic dysfunction: two-year findings from the Oregon sudden unexpected death study. J Am Coll Cardiol 47:1161–1166

36. Buxton AE, Lee KL, Hafley GE et al (2007) Limitations of ejection fraction for prediction of sudden death risk in patients with coronary artery disease: lessons from the MUSTT study. J Am Coll Cardiol 50:1150–1157

37. Myerburg RJ (2008) Implantable cardioverter-defibrillators after myocardial infarction. N Engl J Med 359:2245–2253

38. Moss AJ, Fadl Y, Zareba W, Cannom DS, Hall WJ (2001) Defibrillator Implantation Trial Research Group. Survival benefit with an implanted defibrillator in relation to mortality risk in chronic coronary heart disease. Am J Cardiol 88:516–520

39. Wang R, Lagakos SW, Ware JH, Hunter DJ, Drazen JM (2007) Statistics in medicine – reporting of subgroup analyses in clinical trials. N Engl J Med 357(21):2189–2194

40. Buxton AE, Lee KL, DiCarlo L, Gold MR, Greer GS, Prystowsky EN, O'Toole MF, Tang A, Fisher JD, Coromilas J, Talajic M, Hafley G (2000) Electrophysiologic testing to identify patients with coronary artery disease who are at risk for sudden death. Multicenter unsustained tachycardia trial investigators. N Engl J Med 342:1937–1945

41. Daubert JP, Zareba W, Hall WJ et al (2006) MADIT II Study Investigators. Predictive value of ventricular arrhythmia inducibility for subsequent ventricular tachycardia or ventricular fibrillation in Multicenter automatic defibrillator implantation trial (MADIT) II patients. J Am Coll Cardiol 47:98–107

42. Lopera G, Curtis AB (2009) Risk stratification for sudden cardiac death: current approaches and predictive value. Curr Cardiol Rev 5(1)

43. Hohnloser SH, Ikeda T, Bloomfield DM, Dabbous OH, Cohen RJ (2003) T-wave alternans negative coronary patients with low ejection and benefit from defibrillator implantation. Lancet 362:125–126

44. Lopera G, Curtis AB (2009) Role of T wave alternans testing in risk stratification for sudden cardiac death. J Med 2(1):34–40

45. Chow T, Kereiakes DJ, Bartone C et al (2007) Microvolt T-wave alternans identifies patients with ischemic cardiomyopathy who benefit from implantable cardioverter-defibrillator therapy. J Am Coll Cardiol 49:50–58

46. Gomes JA, Cain ME, Buxton AE, Josephson ME, Lee KL, Hafley GE (2001) Prediction of long-term outcomes by signal-averaged electrocardiography in patients with unsustained ventricular tachycardia, coronary artery disease, and left ventricular dysfunction. Circulation 104:436–441

47. Goldenberg I, Moss AJ (2008) Long QT syndrome. J Am Coll Cardiol 51:2291–2300

48. Goldenberg I, Zareba W, Moss AJ (2008) Long QT syndrome. Curr Probl Cardiol 33:629–694

49. Daubert JP, Zareba W, Rosero SZ, Budzikowski A, Robinson JL, Moss AJ (2007) Role of implantable cardioverter defibrillator therapy in patients with long QT syndrome. Am Heart J 153(4 Suppl):53–58

50. Zareba W, Cygankiewicz I (2008) Long QT syndrome and short QT syndrome. Prog Cardiovasc Dis 51:264–278

51. Goldenberg I, Moss AJ, Bradley J, Polonsky S, Peterson DR, McNitt S, Zareba W, Andrews ML, Robinson JL, Ackerman MJ, Benhorin J, Kaufman ES, Locati EH, Napolitano C, Priori SG, Qi M, Schwartz PJ, Towbin JA, Vincent GM, Zhang L (2008) Long-QT syndrome after age 40. Circulation 117:2192–2201

52. Priori SG, Schwartz PJ, Napolitano C, Bloise R, Ronchetti E, Grillo M, Vicentini A, Spazzolini C, Nastoli J, Bottelli G, Folli R, Cappelletti D (2003) Risk stratification in the long-QT syndrome. N Engl J Med 348:1866–1874

53. Maron BJ, Spirito P (2008) Implantable defibrillators and prevention of sudden death in hypertrophic cardiomyopathy. J Cardiovasc Electrophysiol 19:1118–1126

54. Begley DA, Mohiddin SA, Tripodi D, Winkler JB, Fananapazir L (2003) Efficacy of implantable cardioverter defibrillator therapy for primary and secondary prevention of sudden cardiac death in hypertrophic cardiomyopathy. Pacing Clin Electrophysiol 26:1887–1896

55. Maron BJ, Shen WK, Link MS, Epstein AE, Almquist AK, Daubert JP, Bardy GH, Favale S, Rea RF, Boriani G, Estes NA 3rd, Spirito P (2000) Efficacy of implantable cardioverter-defibrillators for the prevention of sudden death in patients with hypertrophic cardiomyopathy. N Engl J Med 342:365–373

56. Almquist AK, Montgomery JV, Haas TS, Maron BJ (2005) Cardioverter-defibrillator implantation in high-risk patients with hypertrophic cardiomyopathy. Heart Rhythm 2:814–819

57. Maron BJ, McKenna WJ, Danielson GK, Kappenberger LJ, Kuhn HJ, Seidman CE, Shah PM, Spencer WH 3rd, Spirito P, Ten Cate FJ, Wigle ED (2003) Task force on clinical expert consensus documents. American College of Cardiology; Committee for Practice Guidelines. European Society of Cardiology. American College of Cardiology/European Society of Cardiology clinical expert consensus document on hypertrophic cardiomyopathy. A report of the American College

of Cardiology Foundation Task Force on Clinical Expert Consensus Documents and the European Society of Cardiology Committee for Practice Guidelines. J Am Coll Cardiol 42:1687–1713

58. Maron BJ, Spirito P, Shen WK, Haas TS, Formisano F, Link MS, Epstein AE, Almquist AK, Daubert JP, Lawrenz T, Boriani G, Estes NA 3rd, Favale S, Piccininno M, Winters SL, Santini M, Betocchi S, Arribas F, Sherrid MV, Buja G, Semsarian C, Bruzzi P (2007) Implantable cardioverter-defibrillators and prevention of sudden cardiac death in hypertrophic cardiomyopathy. JAMA 298:405–412

59. Cuoco FA, Spencer WH 3rd, Fernandes VL, Nielsen CD, Nagueh S, Sturdivant JL, Leman RB, Wharton JM, Gold MR (2008) Implantable cardioverter-defibrillator therapy for primary prevention of sudden death after alcohol septal ablation of hypertrophic cardiomyopathy. J Am Coll Cardiol 52:1718–1723

60. Antzelevitch C, Brugada P, Borggrefe M, Brugada J, Brugada R, Corrado D, Gussak I, LeMarec H, Nademanee K, Perez Riera AR, Shimizu W, Schulze-Bahr E, Tan H, Wilde A (2005) Brugada syndrome: report of the second consensus conference: endorsed by the Heart rhythm society and the European heart rhythm association. Circulation 111:659–670

61. Brugada J, Brugada R, Brugada P (1998) Right bundle-branch block and ST-segment elevation in leads V1 through V3: a marker for sudden death in patients without demonstrable structural heart disease. Circulation 97:457–460

62. Muthappan P, Calkins H (2008) Arrhythmogenic right ventricular dysplasia. Prog Cardiovasc Dis 51:31–43

63. Wichter T, Paul M, Wollmann C, Acil T, Gerdes P, Ashraf O, Tjan TD, Soeparwata R, Block M, Borggrefe M, Scheld HH, Breithardt G, Böcker D (2004) Implantable cardioverter/defibrillator therapy in arrhythmogenic right ventricular cardiomyopathy: single-center experience of long-term follow-up and complications in 60 patients. Circulation 109:1503–1508

64. Corrado D, Leoni L, Link MS, Della Bella P, Gaita F, Curnis A, Salerno JU, Igidbashian D, Raviele A, Disertori M, Zanotto G, Verlato R, Vergara G, Delise P, Turrini P, Basso C, Naccarella F, Maddalena F, Estes NA 3rd, Buja G, Thiene G (2003) Implantable cardioverter-defibrillator therapy for prevention of sudden death in patients with arrhythmogenic right ventricular cardiomyopathy/dysplasia. Circulation 108:3084–3091

65. Piccini JP, Dalal D, Roguin A, Bomma C, Cheng A, Prakasa K, Dong J, Tichnell C, James C, Russell S, Crosson J, Berger RD, Marine JE, Tomaselli G, Calkins H (2005) Predictors of appropriate implantable defibrillator therapies in patients with arrhythmogenic right ventricular dysplasia. Heart Rhythm 2:1188–1194

66. Giustetto C, Di Monte F, Wolpert C, Borggrefe M, Schimpf R, Sbragia P, Leone G, Maury P, Anttonen O, Haissaguerre M, Gaita F (2006) Short QT syndrome: clinical findings and diagnostic-therapeutic implications. Eur Heart J 27:2440–2447

67. Gaita F, Giustetto C, Bianchi F, Schimpf R, Haissaguerre M, Calò L, Brugada R, Antzelevitch C, Borggrefe M, Wolpert C (2004) Short QT syndrome: pharmacological treatment. J Am Coll Cardiol 43:1494–1499

68. Gussak I, Antzelevitch C (2000) Early repolarization syndrome: clinical characteristics and possible cellular and ionic mechanisms. J Electrocardiol 33:299–309

69. Haïssaguerre M, Derval N, Sacher F, Jesel L, Deisenhofer I, de Roy L, Pasquié JL, Nogami A, Babuty D, Yli-Mayry S, De Chillou C, Scanu P, Mabo P, Matsuo S, Probst V, Le Scouarnec S, Defaye P, Schlaepfer J, Rostock T, Lacroix D, Lamaison D, Lavergne T, Aizawa Y, Englund A, Anselme F, O'Neill M, Hocini M, Lim KT, Knecht S, Veenhuyzen GD, Bordachar P, Chauvin M, Jais P, Coureau G, Chene G, Klein GJ, Clémenty J (2008) Sudden cardiac arrest associated with early repolarization. N Engl J Med 358:2016–2023

70. Haïssaguerre M, Chatel S, Sacher F, Weerasooriya R, Probst V, Loussouarn G, Horlitz M, Liersch R, Schulze-Bahr E, Wilde A, Kääb S, Koster J, Rudy Y, Le Marec H, Schott JJ (2009) Ventricular fibrillation with prominent early repolarization associated with a rare variant of KCNJ8/KATP channel. J Cardiovasc Electrophysiol 20:93–98

71. Haïssaguerre M, Sacher F, Nogami A, Komiya N, Bernard A, Probst V, Yli-Mayry S, Defaye P, Aizawa Y, Frank R, Mantovan R, Cappato R, Wolpert C, Leenhardt A, de Roy L, Heidbuchel H, Deisenhofer I, Arentz T, Pasquié JL, Weerasooriya R, Hocini M, Jais P, Derval N, Bordachar P, Clémenty J (2009) Characteristics of recurrent ventricular fibrillation associated with inferolateral early repolarization role of drug therapy. J Am Coll Cardiol 53:612–619

72. Antzelevitch C (2007) Heterogeneity and cardiac arrhythmias: an overview. Heart Rhythm 4:964–972

73. Collura CA, Johnson JN, Moir C, Ackerman MJ (2009) Left cardiac sympathetic denervation for the treatment of long QT syndrome and catecholaminergic polymorphic ventricular tachycardia using video-assisted thoracic surgery. Heart Rhythm 6:752–759

74. Diaz FJ, Loewe C, Jackson A (2006) Death caused by myocarditis in WayneCounty, Michigan: a 9-year retrospective study. Am J Forensic Med Pathol 27:300–303

75. Soejima K, Yada H (2009) The work-up and management of patients with apparent or subclinical cardiac sarcoidosis: with emphasis on the associated heart rhythm abnormalities. J Cardiovasc Electrophysiol 20(5):578–583

76. Kim JS, Judson MA, Donnino R, Gold M, Cooper LT Jr, Prystowsky EN, Prystowsky S (2009) Cardiac sarcoidosis. Am Heart J 157(1):9–21

14 Bradyarrhythmias

*Ernest Matthew Quin, J. Marcus Wharton,
and Michael R. Gold*

CONTENTS

Abstract

Bradyarrhythmias are due to a variety of disorders leading to a reduction of heart rate below that which is required to meet physiologic demand. The limitation of heart rate can be related to impaired impulse formation, blocked impulses, or a combination of these. Bradycardia related to sinus node dysfunction most frequently results from a reduction in the number of pacemaker impulses, while bradycardia related to the atrioventricular node most often is due to impaired conduction. Regardless of the cause, the diagnostic algorithm for bradycardia is straightforward and includes an electrocardiogram with use of ambulatory electrocardiographic monitoring when needed. For special situations, exercise testing or electrophysiologic testing can be useful. Therapy of bradyarrhythmias consists of removing aggravating factors and permanent pacemaker implantation when necessary.

Key Words: Chronotropy; dromotropy; sinoatrial node; atrioventricular node; chronotropic incompetence; atrioventricular node; sinus node dysfunction; sick sinus syndrome; pacemaker; AV delay; first-degree AV block (f); second-degree AV block type I (f); second-degree AV block type II (f); third-degree AV block (f); pacemaker syndrome; high-grade AV block; junctional rhythm; ventricular rhythm; isorhythmic AV dissociation; congenital heart block; Lev's disease; Lenègre's disease; endocarditis; Lyme disease; infiltrative diseases; Chagas disease; neuromuscular disorders; obstructive sleep apnea; electrophysiological study (f); Holter monitor.

From: *Contemporary Cardiology: Management of Cardiac Arrhythmias*
Edited by: Gan-Xin Yan, Peter R. Kowey, DOI 10.1007/978-1-60761-161-5_14
© Springer Science+Business Media, LLC 2011

INTRODUCTION

Bradyarrhythmias are due to either a decrease in the number (frequency) of impulses generated or a block of the impulse once generated. A reduction in the frequency of stimulus generation is called reduced chronotropy; impairment in stimulus conduction is referred to as reduced dromotropy. While many disorders affect both chronotropy and dromotropy, it is useful to discriminate between the two for a discussion of mechanisms.

Pacemaker cells within the sinoatrial (SA) node are capable of spontaneous action potential generation due to slow diastolic depolarization during phase 4 of the action potential, which is due largely to an inward transmembrane current termed I_f, or "funny" current. Numerous mechanisms affect the slope of I_f; in particular, modulation of the cyclic AMP (cAMP) cascade by β (beta) blockers has provided a useful method for reducing phase 4 depolarization in the SA node to reduce heart rate. Regardless of cause, the clinical correlate of impaired chronotropy is bradycardia.

Unlike the mechanism of impaired chronotropy, reduced dromotropy has more complex and varied origins. Conduction block occurs at sites that exhibit impaired or absent conduction, either functional and/or structural in origin. Slowed, or decremental, conduction is due to entry of the action potential into tissue that has slower conduction. This property is normal and even protective in the atrioventricular (AV) node. The relative paucity of gap junctions and slowly activating calcium-dependent action potentials in this structure permits conduction of impulses at physiologic rates, but restricts conduction at high rates (such as during atrial fibrillation). Similar functional impairment of impulse conduction can occur as a result of drug administration or endocrine abnormalities. Structural abnormalities within myocardium leading to fibrosis, as a consequence of infarction, aging, or other mechanisms, can lead to complete blockade of impulses at high or low rates. For example, impaired conduction out of the SA node by fibrosis of nodal cells or by drugs can lead to failure of an SA nodal impulse to depolarize the atria, called sinoatrial block. Structural disease of the AV junction, AV node, and His-Purkinje systems can lead to intermittent or complete block of atrial impulses to the ventricles (AV block).

By convention, the range of normal heart rates is from 60 to 100 beats per minute (bpm), with bradycardia by definition less than 60 bpm, although population averages are slightly slower *(1)*. The first distinction that must be made for heart rates in the bradycardic range is whether or not the etiology represents a pathological state. There are numerous reports of well-conditioned athletes with average heart rates in the 40s *(2–4)*, and in the era of aggressive β blockade for ischemic heart disease, it is common to encounter heart rates between 40 and 60 bpm. The differentiating factor between normal

Table 1
Causes of Bradycardia

Cause	Affected site
Congenital	AV node
Post-surgical	SA node, AV node
Ischemic heart disease	SA node, AV node
Ageing	SA node, AV node
Endocarditis	AV node, His-Purkinje system
Hyperkalemia	SA node, AV node, His-Purkinje system
Hypothyroidism	SA node
Neurocardiogenic syndromes	SA node, AV node
Neuromuscular diseases	AV node
Obstructive sleep apnea	SA node, AV node
Infiltrative diseases (amyloidosis, sarcoidosis)	AV node
Drugs	SA node, AV node

or functional bradycardia and pathological bradycardia is the presence of symptoms which reflect the inability to meet the metabolic need or cardiac output in that situation. Although the absolute heart rate is the most commonly used measure to determine bradycardia, a heart rate that is inappropriately low for a given level of exertion, or chronotropic incompetence, can also lead to functional limitation (5, 6). The differential diagnosis of bradyarrhythmia is broad, and can be logically divided into dysfunction of the SA node or AV node. SA nodal disease or sick sinus syndrome encompasses a spectrum from sinus bradycardia and sinus pauses to sinoatrial exit block and junctional rhythm. Heart rate is regulated by modulation of the autonomic nervous system; high parasympathetic (or vagal) tone may underly episodes of sinus bradycardia or AV block. AV nodal dysfunction can be due to multiple causes including congenital block, endocarditis, or fibrosis of the conduction system and/or surrounding tissue due to aging or ischemic heart disease. Medical therapies, either pharmacologic or surgical, can affect both SA node and AV node (see Table 1).

SINUS NODE DYSFUNCTION

Symptomatic sinus bradycardia, often associated with sinus pauses, is related to impaired automaticity within the sinus node or to lack of conduction of sinus impulses to atrial tissue due to block in the perinodal tissue. Typical symptoms include fatigue, exercise intolerance, dizziness, dyspnea, and syncope in the most severely affected. Sinus node dysfunction predominantly affects the elderly, and is the primary diagnosis in approximately 48% of pacemaker implants (7). In the majority of cases, SA nodal dysfunction is caused by progressive fibrosis of SA nodal cells as a result of aging; however, any process that results in damage to the SA node, such as collagen vascular diseases, atherosclerosis of the SA nodal artery, infiltrative diseases, or surgical trauma, can be a contributing factor (5, 8). Fibrotic tissue in or around the damaged SA node may act to slow intrinsic activity, or can act as a barrier to prevent conduction of sinus impulses, leading to sinoatrial block (9, 10). Clinical "sinus pauses" may actually represent episodes of sinoatrial block in a significant fraction of patients (11).

A subset of sick sinus syndrome associated with paroxysmal atrial fibrillation or other atrial tachycardia is the "tachy-brady" syndrome. Highly symptomatic patients are characterized by long recovery times for the sinus node after conversion of atrial fibrillation to sinus rhythm, due either to sinoatrial block or overdrive suppression of the SA node (12, 13). Attempts to control tachycardia associated with atrial fibrillation are frequently frustrated by symptomatic bradyarrhythmias when atrial fibrillation is absent. In affected individuals permanent pacing is often indicated, either to ameliorate resting bradycardia or to allow more aggressive titration of rate-controlling and antiarrhythmic medications (5).

Some patients with asymptomatic resting bradycardia have exercise intolerance or lightheadedness with activity due to a less than normal increase in heart rate with exertion. While diagnostic criteria are imperfect, a commonly held metric is that patients who achieve less than 80% of their age-predicted maximum heart rate with maximal activity have chronotropic incompetence (5, 6). The best exercise protocol to assess chronotropic response remains controversial. For some patients with chrontopic incompetence, implanted pacemaker therapy is indicated and has been shown to mimic normal heart rate responses with activity, although objective improvements in quality of life have been more difficult to document in this situation (14, 15).

The clinical course of sick sinus syndrome is typically progressive, with 57% of patients experiencing symptoms over a 4 year period if untreated, and a 23% prevalence of syncope over the same time frame (16). Among patients treated with pacemakers, mortality is determined by underlying comorbidities rather than complications related to the bradyarrhythmia itself (17).

Whereas implanted pacemakers are currently the only therapy for symptomatic sinus node dysfunction, the type of pacing therapy utilized remains varied. Atrial pacing only is safe and effective, but the rate of development of high-grade AV block in patients with pacemakers for sinus node disease is 1.8% per year *(18)*, prompting many to implant dual chamber systems in these patients. However, right ventricular pacing is associated with higher rates of atrial fibrillation, increased heart failure, and decreased quality of life *(19–21)*. Therefore, in sinus node dysfunction, minimizing or eliminating ventricular pacing is a key goal. It is interesting that with newer pacemaker algorithms, or atrial pacing only, marked prolongation of the AV delay can occur with pacing. Whether there are limits where very long AV delays are more deleterious than right ventricular pacing is an area of current debate.

AV NODE DYSFUNCTION

Disease of the AV node also exists along a spectrum. Mild degrees of impulse slowing in the AV node leads to slight prolongation of the P–R segment, causing first-degree AV block (1st-degree AVB), which is defined as prolongation of the P–R interval to greater than 0.20 sec. More significant dysfunction of the AV node can lead to second-degree AV block (2nd-degree AVB), which is subclassified as Mobitz type I and type II. A distinctive electrocardiographic finding in patients with 2nd-degree AVB is "group beating", in which QRS complexes tend to cluster (see Fig. 1). Mobitz type I 2nd-degree AVB (Wenckebach block) demonstrates progressive P–R interval prolongation with an eventual non-conducted beat, with return to a shorter P–R interval on the first beat following the nonconducted beat.

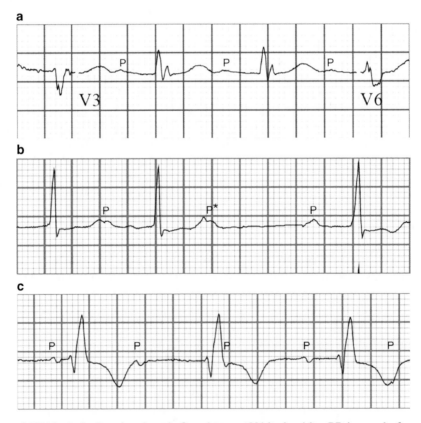

Fig. 1. Spectrum of AV block. In *Panel a*, there is first-degree AV block with a PR interval of approximately 280 msec (P waves are noted). *Panel b* shows second-degree AV block, with conduction block following the second P wave. *Panel c* shows third-degree (complete) AV block, with dissociation between atrial and ventricular beats and a wide complex ventricular escape rhythm.

Mobitz type II 2nd-degree AVB is characterized by a fixed P–R interval before and after a dropped beat. Type I 2nd-degree AVB is more commonly due to dysfunction of the AV node itself, whereas type II 2nd-degree AVB usually implies disease of the His bundle (intra-Hisian block) or bundle branches (infra-Hisian block). Among patients exhibiting 2:1 AV block, identification of the type of block cannot be assumed; however, since type II 2nd-degree AVB involves the distal conduction system, it is more commonly associated with QRS prolongation or bundle branch block. Advanced, or high-grade, 2nd-degree AV block is present when there is more than one consecutive nonconducted beat; in the setting of AV node disease, AV conduction is severely affected, but some degree of function is maintained (an important exception is neurally mediated AV block in the setting of high parasympathetic tone). The diagnosis of high-grade AV block should be considered when there are prolonged pauses in ventricular activation exceeding 5 sec during atrial fibrillation *(5)*. Third-degree, or complete, AV block (3rd-degree AVB) implies a complete lack of conduction from atrium to ventricle; usually an escape rhythm is present from the AV junction or within the ventricle. Electrocardiography in this situation demonstrates dissociated atrial and ventricular activation, often with a wide QRS complex (Fig. 1). The lack of a consistent relationship between atrial and ventricular activity does not always represent block, however. Atrioventricular dissociation (including *isorhythmic* AV dissociation) can occur in the setting of accelerated junctional or ventricular rhythms, in which a lower focus paces the ventricles at a rate faster than the sinus node; this does not typically represent block, as AV conduction is usually intact.

Disease of the cardiac conduction system can be detected, even without heart block, in the presence of left or right bundle branch block. Poor conduction in both the right and the left bundle branches (e.g., concomitant right bundle branch block and left anterior fascicular block), or bifascicular block, is associated with increased risk of complete heart block. Alternating bundle branch block is diagnosed when disease of both bundle branches are present on serial ECG monitoring.

First-degree AVB is not associated with bradycardia except in the setting of sinus bradycardia. While it is commonly associated with damage and/or fibrosis of the AV node, it can also be physiologic in healthy individuals and during sleep *(2–4, 22)*. The prevalence of 1st-degree AVB is approximately 1% in the general population *(23)*. Mild 1st-degree AVB (less than 0.30 sec) is typically asymptomatic and does not warrant specific therapy. More severe AV block has been associated with loss of AV synchrony and symptoms similar to pacemaker syndrome *(24)*. Anecdotal reports indicate pacing can alleviate symptoms, and current guidelines support the use of dual chamber pacing in this setting, although there are no large randomized studies of pacing for marked first-degree AV block *(5)*. Pacing for 1st-degree AVB is a very unusual indication for pacemaker implantation.

Like 1st-degree AVB, type I 2nd-degree AVB can occur in normal individuals and is common during sleep in 4–6% *(25)*. It may be particularly prevalent among patients with obstructive sleep apnea, in which therapy with positive airway pressure often alleviates the finding *(26)*. Type I 2nd-degree AVB can lead to loss of AV synchrony, although this is typically not problematic unless a substantial 1st-degree AVB is also present *(5)*. Pacing is indicated in these patients in the setting of symptomatic bradycardia, and is reasonable when there is concomitant disease at the level of the His bundle or at infra-His levels *(5)*. In select patients with symptoms suggesting more severe conduction system disease, electrophysiologic study may be warranted as infra-Hisian conduction disease can occasionally be associated with a Wenckebach pattern *(27)*; in the setting of bundle branch block a Wenckebach pattern is related to infra-Hisian block and AV nodal block with similar frequencies *(28)*.

Type II 2nd-degree AV block is associated with disease of the conduction system below the AV node *(28)*, and as such has a higher likelihood of progression to complete AV block *(29, 30)*. The characteristic finding in patients with type II 2nd-degree AV block is prolonged conduction in the His-Purkinje system, which is demonstrated during electrophysiology study by an abnormally long H–V interval (Fig. 2). However, the surface electrocardiogram is usually sufficient to make a diagnosis and invasive study is not often required. Exercise treadmill testing can be used diagnostically as well, since type I 2nd-degree AVB generally improves with exercise, whereas type II 2nd-degree AVB often worsens. For patients with symptomatic 2nd-degree AVB, dual chamber pacemaker is warranted; pacemaker implantation is reasonable for 2nd-degree AVB at His or infra-His levels in asymptomatic individuals. Asymptomatic patients exhibiting type II 2nd-degree AVB who have atrial fibrillation and pauses in ventricular activation with 5 sec or longer pauses are also thought to benefit from dual chamber pacing *(5)*.

High-grade AV block and complete heart block represent the most severe forms of AV nodal disease, and are associated with substantial risk of syncope and death *(31)*. The prevalence of 3rd-degree AVB in the general population is low (0.04%), and usually associated with underlying heart disease *(32)*. Electrocardiography shows independently activated atria and ventricles, with the ventricular rate slower than the atrial. The ventricular rate is dependent on the level of the pacemaker driving the ventricles. A junctional pacemaker typically leads to a narrow complex QRS with a ventricular rate from 40 to 60 bpm; ventricular pacemakers result in a wide QRS complex with rates generally less than 40 bpm. Individuals with high-grade AV block (not related to parasympathetic tone) and complete heart block often benefit from pacemaker implantation (see below).

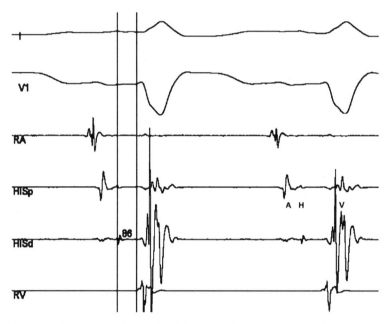

Fig. 2. Prolonged H–V interval noted on electrophysiologic testing. From *top* to *bottom* are surface ECG leads I and V1, followed by intracardiac electrograms from the right atrium (RA), proximal and distal His bundle (HISp and HISd, respectively), and the right ventricle (RV). The HV interval is 86 msec.

PATHOPHYSIOLOGY OF SINUS AND ATRIOVENTRICULAR NODE DYSFUNCTION

Although the causes of sinus and AV nodal dysfunction are quite diverse, a majority of instances are explained by relatively few diagnoses. Ageing is the most common cause of bradyarrhythmia and is due to chronic fibrotic changes in the cardiac conduction system *(9, 10)*. Progressive senescence of the SA node leads to sick sinus syndrome; degeneration of the proximal bundle branches (Lev's disease) or distal bundle branches (Lenègre's disease) is the most common cause of AV block *(33)*. As these disorders are related to scarring and fibrosis of the cardiac connective tissue or degeneration of His-Purkinje cells, they are irreversible *(34)*, and pacemaker therapy is often required.

The most common reversible cause of AV nodal disease remains myocardial ischemia. Bradyarrhythmias, including complete heart block, are common in the setting of acute myocardial ischemia. Ischemia or infarction of the artery to the SA node can lead to chronic sinus bradycardia. Myocardial infarction with ST-segment elevation is associated with a 30–40% rate of sinus bradycardia and heart block in 6–14% *(35)*. These bradyarrhythmias are usually transient, lasting 2–3 days, and prognosis is determined by the degree of myocardial injury rather than the effects of AV block. However, in a minority of patients there is permanent damage to the conduction system. Pacemaker implantation is indicated for patients with sustained 2nd- or 3rd-degree AVB in the setting of bilateral bundle branch block and conduction block in the distal conduction system (within the His-Purkinje system), or for symptomatic patients with persistent 2nd- or 3rd-degree AVB regardless of the location of block *(35)*. In general, heart block or bradycardia associated with an inferior myocardial infarction is more likely to resolve, so permanent pacemaker implantation is delayed. Indications for pacing in chronic ischemic heart disease follow general guidelines for pacemaker use in conduction system disease of any type.

Congenital heart disease, both unrepaired and repaired, comprises an increasing number of patients with bradyarrhythmias presenting to adult cardiology clinics. In patients with congenital complete AV block who have remained asymptomatic to the age of 15 years, there is a 5% mortality risk before the age of 50 years, and 30% will experience syncope or heart failure over the same time frame *(36)*. Symptoms may appear at any age, as there is a progressive decline in ventricular rates with increasing age. Permanent pacemaker implantation is now performed routinely typically as a teenager after puberty, but before the age of 18 rather than waiting for symptoms or slowing of mean heart rate. AV block in the setting of repaired congenital heart disease represents a particular problem, as AV block occurs in 1–3%; greater than 90% of those with postoperative complete heart block do not recover AV conduction *(37, 38)*. Compounding the issue is the late occurrence of AV block, which can be delayed several years following surgical intervention *(39)*. While recommendations for pacemaker implantation in adults with congenital heart disease generally mirror standard indications, these patients represent a high-risk group for development of AV conduction abnormalities and merit close follow-up.

Endocarditis often affects the cardiac conduction system, although the sensitivity of ECG abnormalities to detect patients with endocarditis is poor. Defects of AV conduction often imply perivalvular extension of infection, and as such portend a poor prognosis; new 1st-degree AV or bundle branch block imply high risk of complete heart block and sometimes warrant temporary pacing or surgery *(40)*. Whereas the decision for permanent pacemaker therapy is made on the same clinical grounds as for other diagnoses, implantation is made more difficult by the possibility of persistent infection at the time of implant. Certain infectious etiologies, such as Lyme disease, have a predilection for cardiac involvement. Whereas only 4–10% of affected patients have cardiac involvement *(41)*, of these 98% have 1st degree AVB, 40% have 2nd degree AVB (Mobitz type I), and temporary pacing for complete heart block is necessary in 38% *(42)*. Although some patients with Lyme disease will require permanent pacing, a significant proportion of patients have return of normal conduction with antibiotic therapy *(42, 43)*. In South America, both brady- and tachyarrhythmias are often associated with chronic Chagasic myocarditis. Typically this occurs late in the course of disease at a stage tachyarrhythmias often dominate the clinical picture *(44)*.

Metabolic disorders, endocrinopathies, infiltrative diseases, and collagen vascular disorders can also affect cardiac conduction. While hyperkalemia is often associated with sinus bradycardia, profoundly high potassium levels impair AV conduction as well *(45, 46)*. Hypothyroidism has been implicated in both sinus bradycardia and AV block *(47)*. Cardiac involvement in sarcoidosis, amyloidosis, and hemochromatosis has been associated with a variety of bradyarrhythmias *(5, 8, 48)*.

Bradycardia or milder forms of conduction system disease has been found across the spectrum of rheumatologic disorders, including Wegener's granulomatosis *(49)*, rheumatoid arthritis *(50)*, systemic sclerosis *(50, 51)*, systemic lupus erythematosus *(50, 52)*, psoriatic arthritis *(53)*, Reiter's syndrome *(54)*, ankylosing spondylitis *(55)*, and polymyositis-dermatomyositis *(56)*.

Neuromuscular diseases such as myotonic dystrophy and Emery Dreifuss muscular dystrophy have been associated with significant conduction system disease, including the sudden development of complete AV block *(57)*. Kearns-Sayre syndrome, or chronic progressive external opthalmoplegia, is a mitochondrial myopathy characterized by a clinical triad of progressive external opthalmoplegia, pigmentary retinopathy, and AV block. As with the neuromuscular diseases, development of AV block can be sudden and devastating. In patients with these diagnoses, consideration should be given early to pacemaker placement in the setting of conduction system disease on ECG or electrophysiologic testing *(5)*.

Finally, sinus bradycardia and 1st-degree AVB are common during sleep and are normal findings *(25)*. Obstructive sleep apnea is associated with more profound bradyarrhythmias, including sinus pauses and type II 2nd-degree AVB *(58, 59)*; fortunately, these rhythms respond favorably to standard therapy with continuous positive airway pressure *(60)*.

DIAGNOSTIC EVALUATION

Initial evaluation of patients suspected to have bradycardia begins with an electrocardiogram. Whereas sinus bradycardia and 1st-degree AVB are relatively apparent, higher degrees of block can be intermittent, and may not be apparent on preliminary evaluation. Electrocardiographic clues can suggest the possibility of more severe block, however; greater conduction impairment (as with severe 1st-degree AVB, right or left bundle branch block) often suggests advanced block. In the setting of sinus bradycardia with complete heart block, atrial and ventricular rates can be similar; diagnosis is frequently aided by an extended rhythm strip so that a lack of relationship between atria and ventricles is more easily recognized.

Sinus bradycardia often accompanies chronotropic incompetence, although resting heart rates can also be normal. When clinical suspicion is high due to symptoms of exertional fatigue, exercise testing can aid diagnosis. As noted previously, in the setting of poor exercise tolerance, the inability to raise heart rate above 80% of the age predicted maximum strongly suggests chronotropic incompetence *(61, 62)*.

For patients who have frequent symptoms that may be related to bradycardia, diagnoses can be facilitated with ambulatory rhythm monitoring (Holter monitor), although the yield for definitive diagnosis is only approximately 7.5% *(63)*. Patients should be encouraged to maintain a diary of symptoms; correlating symptoms with rhythm tracings can provide information useful for determination of cardiac cause in as many as 26% *(64)*. Unfortunately, due to the poor sensitivity of this approach owing to infrequency of symptoms, other diagnostic methods are often necessary *(65)*.

When resting and ambulatory electrocardiography have been unrevealing, formal electrophysiologic (EP) testing is sometimes useful to assess conduction, although sensitivity is poor for unexplained syncope or near syncope in the setting of an otherwise normal evaluation *(66)*. EP study is particularly effective in patients with some degree of underlying conduction system disease to assess the level at which impaired conduction occurs (see Fig. 2 and Table 2) *(67)*. In patients suspected of having sinus node dysfunction, assessment of the sinus node can be performed; atrial, AV nodal, and His-Purkinje conduction times are easily assessed. In selected patients with high clinical suspicion of severe conduction disease or borderline findings on EP testing, pharmacologic challenge with a class I antiarrhythmic drug, such as procainamide, can improve sensitivity *(68)*.

Table 2
Normal Conduction Times

Interval	Range of normal (msec)
SNRT	<1500
cSNRT	<550
PA	25–55
AH	55–125
HV	35–55
PR	120–200
QRS	≤ 100
R–R	≤ 1000

SNRT sinus node recovery time, cSNRT corrected SNRT, PA interval is time from earliest measured atrial activity to atrial depolarization noted on His catheter, AH interval is time from atrial to His depolarization on His catheter, HV is time from His depolarization to earliest recorded ventricular depolarization

Patients who experience only intermittent symptoms and/or have had nondiagnostic testing with the above modalities are candidates for long-term rhythm monitoring with a cutaneous or implanted rhythm monitor, also known as an implantable loop recorder (ILR). ILRs are placed entirely subcutaneously and can provide continuous assessment of heart rate for more than 2 years. Several manufacturers have models available; with some vendors the option of physician alerts for significant events is available. In selected patients experiencing intermittent syncope, use of an implanted rhythm monitor results in definitive diagnosis in 45–50% *(69)*. Although surgical implantation is necessary, these devices have proven not only to be clinically useful but cost-effective as well *(70)*.

INDICATIONS FOR PACEMAKER THERAPY

As mentioned above, indications for pacemaker therapy with sinus node dysfunction hinge on the presence of symptoms. Given the risk of abrupt and life-threatening bradycardia or asystole with AV nodal disease, the decision for permanent pacing relies not only on symptoms but also on the results of diagnostic testing. The decision to implant a pacemaker is a complex one, and should involve the patient in a discussion of the risks of implantation as well as the long-term risks of device malfunction, infection, and pulse generator replacement. In general, however, a reasonable approach suggests absolute and relative indications for pacing as well as situations in which pacing is not likely to be helpful. Pacing indications are summarized in Table 3, and guidelines for pacemaker implantation as set forth by the joint committee representing the American College of Cardiology, American Heart Association, and Heart Rhythm Society are included below as well *(5)*.

ACC/AHA/HRS GUIDELINES FOR DEVICE-BASED THERAPY (2008)

Recommendations for Permanent Pacing in Sinus Node Dysfunction

CLASS I

1. Permanent pacemaker implantation is indicated for sinus node dysfunction with documented symptomatic bradycardia, including frequent sinus pauses that produce symptoms.
2. Permanent pacemaker implantation is indicated for symptomatic chronotropic incompetence.

Table 3
Indications for Implanted Pacemaker

Absolute	Relative
Sinus node dysfunction	Sinus node dysfunction
• Symptomatic bradycardia	• Symptoms consistent with bradycardia and HR < 40 bpm
• Chronotropic incompetence	
• Symptomatic bradycardia due to required drug therapy	• Syncope presumed to be due to sinus bradycardia
AV node dysfunction	AV node dysfunction
• Symptomatic 2nd- or 3rd-degree AV block	• 3rd-degree AV block with heart rate > 40 bpm
• 2nd- or 3rd-degree block and escape rate < 40 bpm	• Asymptomatic 2nd-degree AV block at level of His or lower
• 2nd- or 3rd-degree AV block with atrial fibrillation and ventricular pauses ≥5 sec	• Syncope with bifascicular block and no other identified cause
• 2nd- or 3rd-degree AV block associated with neuromuscular diseases	• HV interval ≥ 5.0 sec with bifascicular block
• 2nd-degree AV block with symptomatic bradycardia	• Neuromuscular diseases with any degree of AV block
• 3rd-degree AV block with structural heart disease	• Neuromuscular diseases with bifascicular block
• Exercise-induced 2nd- or 3rd-degree AV block	
• 2nd-degree AV block with bifascicular block	
• Mobitz II 2nd-degree AV block with bifascicular block	
• Alternating bundle branch block	
• Carotid hypersensitivity with pauses > 3.0 sec	

3. Permanent pacemaker implantation is indicated for symptomatic sinus bradycardia that results from required drug therapy for medical conditions.

CLASS IIA

1. Permanent pacemaker implantation is reasonable for sinus node dysfunction with heart rate less than 40 bpm when a clear association between significant symptoms consistent with bradycardia and the actual presence of bradycardia has not been documented.
2. Permanent pacemaker implantation is reasonable for syncope of unexplained origin when clinically significant abnormalities of sinus node function are discovered or provoked in electrophysiological studies.

CLASS IIB

1. Permanent pacemaker implantation may be considered in minimally symptomatic patients with chronic heart rate less than 40 bpm while awake.

CLASS III

1. Permanent pacemaker implantation is not indicated for sinus node dysfunction in asymptomatic patients.
2. Permanent pacemaker implantation is not indicated for sinus node dysfunction in patients for whom the symptoms suggestive of bradycardia have been clearly documented to occur in the absence of bradycardia.
3. Permanent pacemaker implantation is not indicated for sinus node dysfunction with symptomatic bradycardia due to nonessential drug therapy.

Recommendations for Acquired Atrioventricular Block in Adults

CLASS I

1. Permanent pacemaker implantation is indicated for third-degree and advanced second-degree AV block at any anatomic level associated with bradycardia with symptoms (including heart failure) or ventricular arrhythmias presumed to be due to AV block.
2. Permanent pacemaker implantation is indicated for third-degree and advanced second-degree AV block at any anatomic level associated with arrhythmias and other medical conditions that require drug therapy that results in symptomatic bradycardia.
3. Permanent pacemaker implantation is indicated for third-degree and advanced second-degree AV block at any anatomic level in awake, symptom-free patients in sinus rhythm, with documented periods of asystole greater than or equal to 3.0 sec or any escape rate less than 40 bpm, or with an escape rhythm that is below the AV node.
4. Permanent pacemaker implantation is indicated for third-degree and advanced second-degree AV block at any anatomic level in awake, symptom-free patients with atrial fibrillation and bradycardia with 1 or more pauses of at least 5 sec or longer.
5. Permanent pacemaker implantation is indicated for third-degree and advanced second-degree AV block at any anatomic level after catheter ablation of the AV junction.
6. Permanent pacemaker implantation is indicated for third-degree and advanced second-degree AV block at any anatomic level associated with postoperative AV block that is not expected to resolve after cardiac surgery.
7. Permanent pacemaker implantation is indicated for third-degree and advanced second-degree AV block at any anatomic level associated with neuromuscular diseases with AV block, such as myotonic muscular dystrophy, Kearns-Sayre syndrome, Erb dystrophy (limb-girdle muscular dystrophy), and peroneal muscular atrophy, with or without symptoms.
8. Permanent pacemaker implantation is indicated for second-degree AV block with associated symptomatic bradycardia regardless of type or site of block.
9. Permanent pacemaker implantation is indicated for asymptomatic, persistent, third-degree AV block at any anatomic site with average awake ventricular rates of 40 bpm or faster if cardiomegaly or LV dysfunction is present or if the site of block is below the AV node.
10. Permanent pacemaker implantation is indicated for second- or third-degree AV block during exercise in the absence of myocardial ischemia.

CLASS IIA

1. Permanent pacemaker implantation is reasonable for persistent third-degree AV block with an escape rate greater than 40 bpm in asymptomatic adult patients without cardiomegaly.
2. Permanent pacemaker implantation is reasonable for asymptomatic second-degree AV block at intra- or infra-His levels found at electrophysiological study.
3. Permanent pacemaker implantation is reasonable for first- or second-degree AV block with symptoms similar to those of pacemaker syndrome or hemodynamic compromise.
4. Permanent pacemaker implantation is reasonable for asymptomatic type II second-degree AV block with a narrow QRS. When type II second-degree AV block occurs with a wide QRS, including isolated right bundle-branch block, pacing becomes a class I recommendation.

CLASS IIB

1. Permanent pacemaker implantation may be considered for neuromuscular diseases such as myotonic muscular dystrophy, Erb dystrophy (limb-girdle muscular dystrophy), and peroneal muscular atrophy with any degree of AV block (including first-degree AV block), with or without symptoms, because there may be unpredictable progression of AV conduction disease.

2. Permanent pacemaker implantation may be considered for AV block in the setting of drug use and/or drug toxicity when the block is expected to recur even after the drug is withdrawn.

CLASS III

1. Permanent pacemaker implantation is not indicated for asymptomatic first-degree AV block.
2. Permanent pacemaker implantation is not indicated for asymptomatic type I second-degree AV block at the supra-His (AV node) level or that which is not known to be intra- or infra-Hisian.
3. Permanent pacemaker implantation is not indicated for AV block that is expected to resolve and is unlikely to recur (e.g., drug toxicity, Lyme disease, or transient increases in vagal tone or during hypoxia in sleep apnea syndrome in the absence of symptoms).

Recommendations for Permanent Pacing in Chronic Bifascicular Block

CLASS I

1. Permanent pacemaker implantation is indicated for advanced second-degree AV block or intermittent third-degree AV block.
2. Permanent pacemaker implantation is indicated for type II second-degree AV block.
3. Permanent pacemaker implantation is indicated for alternating bundle branch block.

CLASS IIA

1. Permanent pacemaker implantation is reasonable for syncope not demonstrated to be due to AV block when other likely causes have been excluded, specifically ventricular tachycardia.
2. Permanent pacemaker implantation is reasonable for an incidental finding at electophysiological study of a markedly prolonged HV interval (greater than or equal to 100 msec) in asymptomatic patients.
3. Permanent pacemaker implantation is reasonable for an incidental finding at electrophysiological study of pacing-induced infra-His block that is not physiological.

CLASS IIB

1. Permanent pacemaker implantation may be considered in the setting of neuromuscular diseases such as myotonic muscular dystrophy, Erb dystrophy (limb-girdle muscular dystrophy), and peroneal muscular atrophy with bifascicular block or any fascicular block, with or without symptoms.

CLASS III

1. Permanent pacemaker implantation is not indicated for fascicular block without AV block or symptoms.
2. Permanent pacemaker implantation is not indicated for fascicular block with first-degree AV block without symptoms.

Recommendations for Permanent Pacing After the Acute Phase of Myocardial Infarction

CLASS I

1. Permanent ventricular pacing is indicated for persistent second-degree AV block in the His-Purkinje system, with alternating bundle branch block or third-degree AV block within or below the His-Purkinje system after ST-segment elevation MI.
2. Permanent ventricular pacing is indicated for transient advanced second- or third-degree infranodal AV block and associated bundle-branch block. If the site of block is uncertain, electrophysiological study may be necessary.
3. Permanent ventricular pacing is indicated for persistent and symptomatic second- or third-degree AV block.

CLASS IIA

1. Permanent ventricular pacing may be considered for persistent second- or third-degree AV block at the AV node level, even in the absence of symptoms.

CLASS III

1. Permanent ventricular pacing is not indicated for transient AV block in the absence of intraventricular conduction defects.
2. Permanent ventricular pacing is not indicated for transient AV block in the presence of isolated left anterior fascicular block.
3. Permanent ventricular pacing is not indicated for new bundle-branch block or fascicular block in the absence of AV block.
4. Permanent ventricular pacing is not indicated for persistent asymptomatic first-degree AV block in the presence of bundle-branch or fascicular block.

REFERENCES

1. Spodick DH, Raju P, Bishop RL et al (1992) Operational definition of normal sinus heart rate. Am J Cardiol 69:1245–1246
2. Viitasalo MT, Kala R, Eisalo A (1982) Ambulatory electrocardiographic recording in endurance athletes. Br Heart J 47:213–220
3. Northcote RJ, Canning GP, Ballantyne D (1989) Electrocardiographic findings in male veteran endurance athletes. Br Heart J 61:267–278
4. Link MS, Homoud MK, Wang PJ et al (2002) Cardiac arrhythmias in the athlete: the evolving role of electrophysiology. Curr Sports Med Rep 1:75–85
5. Epstein AE, DiMarco JP, Estes NA 3rd et al (2008) ACC/AHA/HRS 2008 Guidelines for device-based therapy of cardiac rhythm abnormalities. J Am Coll Cardiol 51:e1–e62
6. Katritsis D, Camm AJ (1993) Chronotropic incompetence: a proposal for definition and diagnosis. Br Heart J 70:400–402
7. Bernstein AD, Parsonnet V (2001) Survey of cardiac pacing and implanted defibrillator practice patterns in the United States in 1997. Pacing Clin Electrophysiol 24:842–855
8. Mangrum JM, DiMarco JP (2000) The evaluation and management of bradycardia. N Engl J Med 342:703–708
9. Kohl P, Camelliti P, Burton FL, Smith GL (2005) Electrical coupling of fibroblasts and myocytes: relevance for cardiac propagation. J Electrocardiol 38(Suppl 4):45–50
10. Jones SA, Lancaster MK, Boyett MR (2004) Ageing-related changes of connexins and conduction within the sinoatrial node. J Physiol 560:429–437
11. Thery C, Gosselin B, LeKieffre J, Warembourg H (1977) Pathology of the sinoatrial node: correlations with electrocardiographic findings in 111 patients. Am Heart J 93:735–740
12. Asseman P, Berzin B, Desry D et al (1983) Persistent sinus nodal electrograms during abnormally prolonged postpacing atrial pauses in sick sinus syndrome in humans: sinoatrial block vs. overdrive suppression. Circulation 68:33–41
13. Wu D, Yeh SJ, Lin FC et al (1992) Sinus automaticity and sinoatrial conduction in severe symptomatic sick sinus syndrome. J Am Coll Cardiol 19:355–364
14. Israel CW, Hohnloser SH (2000) Current status of dual-sensor pacemaker systems for correction of chronotropic incompetence. Am J Cardiol 86:86 K–94 K
15. Lamas GA, Knight JD, Sweeney MO et al (2007) Impact of rate-modulated pacing on quality of life and exercise capacity—evidence from the advanced elements of pacing randomized controlled trial (ADEPT). Heart Rhythm 4:1125–1132
16. Menozzi C, Brignole M, Alboni P et al (1998) The natural course of untreated sick sinus syndrome and identification of the variables predictive of unfavorable outcome. Am J Cardiol 82:1205–1209
17. Simon AB, Janz N (1982) Symptomatic bradyarrhythmias in the adult: natural history following ventricular pacemaker implantation. Pacing Clin Electrophysiol 5:372–383
18. Brandt J, Anderson H, Fahraeus T, Schuller H (1992) Natural history of sinus node disease treated with atrial pacing in 213 patients: implications for selection of stimulation mode. J Am Coll Cardiol 20:633–639
19. Sweeney MO, Bank AJ, Nsah E et al (2007) Minimizing ventricular pacing to reduce atrial fibrillation in sinus-node disease. N Engl J Med 357:1000–1008

20. Lamas GA, Lee KL, Sweeney MO et al (2002) Ventricular pacing or dual-chamber pacing for sinus-node dysfunction. N Engl J Med 346:1854–1862

21. Andersen HR, Nielsen JC, Thomsen PE et al (1997) Long-term follow-up of patients from a randomized trial of atrial versus ventricular pacing for sick-sinus syndrome. Lancet 350:1210–1216

22. Durham D, Worthley LI (2002) Cardiac arrhythmias: diagnosis and management. The bradycardias. Crit Care Resusc 4:54–60

23. Bexton RS, Camm AJ (1984) First degree atrioventricular block. Eur Heart J 5(Suppl A):107–109

24. Hayes DL (1999) Evolving indications for permanent pacing. Am J Cardiol 83:161D–165D

25. Adlakha A, Shepard JW (1998) Cardiac arrhythmias during normal sleep and in obstructive sleep apnea syndrome. Sleep Med Rev 2:45–60

26. Somers VK, White DP, Amin R et al (2008) Sleep apnea and cardiovascular disease: an American heart association/American college of cardiology foundation scientific statement from the American heart association council for high blood pressure research professional education committee, council on clinical cardiology, stroke council, and council on cardiovascular nursing. J Am Coll Cardiol 52:686–717

27. Zipes DP (1979) Second-degree atrioventricular block. Circulation 60:465–472

28. Puech P (1975) Contribution of the his bundle recording to the diagnosis of bilateral bundle branch conduction defects. Adv Cardiol 14:178–188

29. Dhingra RC, Denes P, Wu D et al (1974) The significance of second degree atrioventricular block and bundle branch block. Observations regarding site and type of block. Circulation 49:638–646

30. Bexton RS, Camm AJ (1984) Second degree atrioventricular block. Eur Heart J 5:111–114

31. Edhag O, Swahn A (1976) Prognosis of patients with complete heart block or arrhythmic syncope who were not treated with artificial pacemakers. A long-term follow-up study of 101 patients. Acta Med Scand 200:457–463

32. Kojic EM, Hardarson T, Sigfusson N, Sigvaldason H (1999) The prevalence and prognosis of third-degree atrioventricular conduction block: the Reykjavik study. J Intern Med 246:81–86

33. Davies MJ (1976) Pathology of chronic A-V block. Acta Cardiol Suppl 21:19–30

34. Katz AM (2006) Arrhythmias. In: Physiology of the heart, 4th edn. Lippincott Williams & Wilkins, Philadelphia, PA, pp 483–489

35. Antman EM, Anbe DT, Armstrong PW et al (2004) ACC/AHA guidelines for the management of patients with ST-elevation myocardial infarction: a report of the American college of cardiology/American heart association task force on practice guidelines (committee to revise the 1999 guidelines for the management of patients with acute myocardial infarction). J Am Coll Cardiol 44:E1–E211

36. Michaelsson M, Riesenfeld T, Jonzon A (1997) Natural history of congenital complete atrioventricular block. Pacing Clin Electrophysiol 20:2098–2101

37. Gross GJ, Chiu CC, Hamilton RM et al (2006) Natural history of postoperative heart block in congenital heart disease: implications for pacing intervention. Heart Rhythm 3:601–604

38. Batra AS, Wells WJ, Hinoki KW et al (2003) Late recovery of atrioventricular conduction after pacemaker implantation for complete heart block associated with surgery for congenital heart disease. J Torac Cardiovasc Surg 125: 1291–1293

39. Liberman L, Pass RH, Hordof AJ, Spotnitz HM (2008) Late onset of heart block after open heart surgery for congenital heart disease. Pediatr Cardiol 29:56–59

40. Carpenter JL (1991) Perivalvular extension of infection in patients with infectious endocarditis. Rev Infect Dis 13:127–138

41. Haywood GA, O'Connell S, Gray HH (1993) Lyme carditis: a United Kingdom perspective. Br Heart J 70:15–16

42. van der Linde MR, Crijns JH, de Koning J et al (1990) Range of atrioventricular conduction disturbances in Lyme borreliosis: a report of four cases and review of other published reports. Br Heart J 63:162–168

43. McAlister HF, Klementowicz PT, Andrews C et al (1989) Lyme carditis: an important cause of reversible heart block. Ann Intern Med 110:339–345

44. Elizari MV (2002) Arrhythmias associated with Chagas' heart disease. Card Electrophysiol Rev 6:115–119

45. Noble K, Isles C (2006) Hyperkalaemia causing profound bradycardia. Heart 92:1063

46. Michaeli J, Bassan MM, Brezis M (1986) Second degree type II and complete atrioventricular block due to hyperkalemia. J Electrocardiol 19:393–396

47. Gammage M, Franklyn J (1997) Hypothyroidism, thyroxine treatment, and the heart. Heart 77:189–190

48. Prochorec-Sobieszek M, Szufladowicz E, Szaroszyk W et al (2005) Clinical and morphological diagnosis of cardiac AL amyloidosis: a review of findings and difficulties as illustrated in one case. Med Sci Monit 11:CS45–CS48

49. Ghaussy NO, Du Clos TW, Ashley PA (2004) Limited Wegener's granulomatosis presenting with complete heart block. Scand J Rheumatol 33:115–118

50. Seferović PM, Ristić AD, Maksimović R et al (2006) Cardiac arrhythmias and conduction disturbances in autoimmune rheumatic diseases. Rheumatology (Oxford) 45:iv39–iv42

51. Janosik DL, Osborn TG, Moore TL et al (1989) Heart disease in systemic sclerosis. Semin Arthritis Rheum 19:191–200
52. Huo AP, Su KC, Liao HT et al (2005) Second-degree atrioventricular block as an early manifestation of adult systemic lupus erythematosis. J Microbiol Immunol Infect 38:296–299
53. Feld J, Weiss G, Rosner I et al (2008) Electrocardiographic findings in psoriatic arthritis: a case-controlled study. J Rheumatol 35:2379–2382
54. Haverman JF, van Albada-Kuipers GA, Dohmen HJ et al (1988) Atrioventricular conduction disturbance as an early feature of Reiter's syndrome. Ann Rheum Dis 47:1017–1020
55. Alves MG, Espirito-Santo J, Queiroz MV et al (1988) Cardiac alterations in ankylosing spondylitis. Angiology 39:567–571
56. Lundberg IE (2006) The heart in dermatomyositis and polymyositis. Rheumatology (Oxford) 45:iv18–iv21
57. Lazarus A, Varin J, Babuty D et al (2002) Long-term follow-up of arrhythmias in patients with myotonic dystrophy treated by pacing: a multicenter diagnostic pacemaker study. J Am Coll Cardiol 40:1645–1652
58. Guilleminault C, Connolly SJ, Winkle RA (1983) Cardiac arrhythmia and conduction disturbances during sleep in 400 patients with sleep apnea syndrome. Am J Cardiol 52:490–494
59. Becker HF, Koehler U, Stammnitz A, Peter JH (1998) Heart block in patients with sleep apnoea. Thorax 53:S29–S32
60. Grimm W, Koehler U, Fus E et al (2000) Outcome of patients with sleep apnea-associated severe bradyarrhythmias after continuous positive airway pressure therapy. Am J Cardiol 86:688–692
61. Brubaker PH, Kitzman DW (2007) Prevalence and management of chronotropic incompetence in heart failure. Curr Cardiol Rep 9:229–235
62. Wilkoff BL, Miller RE (1992) Exercise testing for chronotropic assessment. Cardiol Clin 10:705–717
63. Maloney JD (1980) An approach to the management of outpatients with cardiac arrhythmias. Cardiovas Clin 10:19–32
64. Ward DE, Camm AJ, Darby N (1980) Assessment of the diagnostic value of 24-hour ambulatory electrocardiographic monitoring. Biotelem Patient Monit 7:57–66
65. DiMarco JP, Philbrick JT (1990) Use of ambulatory electrocardiographic (Holter) monitoring. Ann Intern Med 113:53–68
66. Gulamhusein S, Naccarelli GV, Ko PT et al (1982) Value and limitations of clinical electrophysiologic study in assessment of patients with unexplained syncope. Am J Med 73:700–705
67. Hammill SC (1989) Overview of the clinical electrophysiology study. J Electrocardiol 22(Suppl):209–217
68. Englund A, Bergfeldt L, Rosenqvist M (1998) Pharmacological stress testing of the His-Purkinje system in patients with bifascicular block. Pacing Clin Electrophysiol 21:1979–1987
69. Pezawas T, Stix G, Kastner J et al (2008) Implantable loop recorder in unexplained syncope: classification, mechanism, transient loss of consciousness and role of major depressive disorder in patients with and without structural heart disease. Heart 94:e17
70. Krahn AD, Klein GJ, Skanes AC, Yee R (2004) Insertable loop recorder use for detection of intermittent arrhythmias. Pacing Clin Electrophysiol 27:657–664

V ARRHYTHMIAS IN SPECIFIC POPULATIONS

15 Arrhythmias in the Athlete

John A. Kalin, Mark S. Link,
and N.A. Mark Estes III

CONTENTS

Abstract

While athletes are symbols of the healthiest segments of our society, they are occasionally affected by cardiovascular conditions and arrhythmias that come to the attention of the clinician. Evaluation and management of the athlete with cardiovascular disease and arrhythmias represent a unique challenge. Despite the best available evaluation and testing diagnostic uncertainty occurs with considerable frequency. The cardiovascular conditions predisposing to arrhythmias and the arrhythmias that can occur in the absence of any structural heart disease in the athlete are reviewed in this chapter from multiple perspectives. These include clinical evaluation of the athlete with arrhythmias, screening strategies for cardiovascular conditions that predispose to arrhythmias and guidelines for athletic participation.

Key Words: Arrhythmia; athlete; athletics; supraventricular arrhythmia; ventricular arrhythmia; bardycardia; exercise.

While athletes are symbols of the healthiest segments of our society, they are occasionally affected by cardiovascular conditions and arrhythmias that come to the attention of the clinician. Evaluation and management of the athlete with cardiovascular disease and arrhythmias represents a unique challenge. Despite the best available evaluation and testing, diagnostic uncertainty occurs with considerable frequency. Clinical judgment commonly is the basis for recommendations for therapy and athletic participation. In this setting, there is the real risk of failing to detect an arrhythmia or cardiac condition that may result in serious or even life-threatening consequences. At the same time, there is the risk of unnecessarily treating and restricting athletic participation in an athlete misdiagnosed as having a

From: *Contemporary Cardiology: Management of Cardiac Arrhythmias*
Edited by: Gan-Xin Yan, Peter R. Kowey, DOI 10.1007/978-1-60761-161-5_15
© Springer Science+Business Media, LLC 2011

cardiovascular condition or arrhythmia. The cardiovascular conditions that predispose to life-threatening complications of athletic participation are well characterized *(1)*. Guidance is available for the clinician related to athletic participation for those with cardiovascular conditions and arrhythmias *(2–6)*. Recommendations for management of athletes with arrhythmias based on expert consensus also are available *(5, 6)*. The cardiovascular conditions predisposing to arrhythmias and the arrhythmias that can occur in the absence of any structural heart disease in the athlete are reviewed in this chapter from multiple perspectives. These include clinical evaluation of the athlete with arrhythmias, screening strategies for cardiovascular conditions that predispose to arrhythmias and guidelines for athletic participation.

BRADYARRHYTHMIAS

Athletes of all ages typically maintain a high level of cardiovascular conditioning and commonly develop an increase in vagal tone manifesting in a spectrum of bradycardias *(7–17)*. (Table 1) This physiologic adaptation of autonomic tone accompanying physical training influences the vagal and sympathetic modulation of the sinus and atrioventricular (AV) nodes. As such, bradyarrhythmias involving these anatomic structures are common. Sinus bradycardia is associated with a higher degree of cardiovascular fitness and is more commonly observed in endurance sports *(10, 11)*. In athletes, resting heart rates <40 beats/min are common and occasionally can be 30 beats/min or less during sleep *(7–17)*. With exercise and competition, vagal tone decreases and sympathetic tone increases. At rest, vagal tone predominates with slowing of the sinus node and a negative chronotropic effect at the level of the AV node. While influencing resting heart rates and AV conduction, conditioning has no effect on peak heart rate attainable for the athlete. Thus the resting heart rate does not bear a relation to the peak heart rates with exertion. Sinus bradycardia and first-degree AV block (PR $\geq$ 200 msec) are common in athletes and generally do not require evaluation or therapy *(7–17)*. As is the case in the nonathlete, symptomatic slow resting heart rates resulting in symptoms such as lightheadedness, dizziness, or syncope may occasionally require therapy. Typically, physical deconditioning is sufficient to eliminate symptomatic sinus bradycardia in the athlete.

Table 1
Bradycardias

Condition	Symptoms	ECG	Diagnosis	Treatment options
Sinus bradycardia	Asymptomatic, LH, syncope	Sinus rate less than 50 bpm	ECG	Reassurance, PPM if symptoms
Second-degree Mobitz I (Wenckebach) AV block	Asymptomatic, LH, syncope	Grouped beating, progressive PR prolongation	ECG	Reassurance, PPM if symptoms
Second-degree Mobitz II AV block	Asymptomatic, LH, syncope	Grouped beating, stable PR, dropped QRS	ECG, EP study in some cases	PPM
Third-degree AV block (complete heart block)	Asymptomatic, fatigue, LH, syncope	Dissociation of p-waves and QRS	ECG	PPM

PPM permanent pacemaker, *LH* light headedness, *BPM* beats/min

Generally, maximum heart rates attainable are approximately 220 minus the individual's age. Athletes should be able to achieve their predicted maximal heart rate for age although it may require longer duration and intensity of exercise compared to the nonathlete. Chronotropic incompetence, which by definition is the inability to raise the heart rate appropriately with exercise, is rare in the younger athlete (aged less than 35), but can be seen in older athletes with primary sinus node dysfunction *(7–17)*. Invasive electrophysiologic studies are of no clinical utility in patients with this sinus node dysfunction as such testing is neither sensitive nor specific for bradyarrhythmias. Evaluation and management of bradycardias are guided by clinical assessment of symptoms and their relationship to clinically documented arrhythmias.

At present, there are no medications that effectively treat sinus node dysfunction on a long-term basis. The definitive therapy for symptomatic bradycardia is a permanent pacemaker. It is evident that discontinuation of pharmacologic agents that slow sinus node function should be the initial approach to any athlete or other individual with symptomatic sinus bradycardia. Rarely it becomes necessary to implant a permanent pacemaker. Virtually all available pacemakers have the ability to enhance heart rate based on sensed activity. With the placement of a permanent pacemaker, there are sport specific recommendations regarding participation. Contact sports with risk of impact are not advisable in patients with a permanent pacemaker *(5, 6)*. Activities that involve repetitive movement of the upper extremity and movement of the clavicle over the ribs, like weightlifting, freestyle swimming, and pitching in baseball, are also associated with a greater risk of damage to leads. Accordingly, they should be avoided.

HEART BLOCK

Like sinus bradycardia, 2nd-degree heart block Mobitz type I (Wenckebach) is a common finding in athletes at rest due to the influence of enhanced vagal tone *(7–17)*. With exercise, vagal tone is withdrawn and Wenckebach generally resolves, as does sinus bradycardia. Wenckebach type AV block that occurs during sleep does not warrant treatment. Symptoms of syncope or lightheadedness, however, are concerning in the athlete with Wenckebach rhythm. Wenckebach not resolving with exercise is abnormal and suggests underlying pathology of the AV node. Under such circumstances, like symptomatic sinus bradycardia, a permanent pacemaker is the only effective treatment *(18)*.

More advanced heart block such as 2nd-degree Mobitz type II heart block or 3rd-degree heart block (complete heart block) are generally considered abnormal, even in the highly trained athlete. Findings of Mobitz II or complete heart block indicate that the site of block is below the AV node and not under vagal influence. Generally, Mobitz II and complete heart block are an indication for permanent pacemaker, particularly when occurring in the setting of structural heart disease or symptoms *(18)*.

Occasionally, 2:1 AV block is seen with two P-waves for every QRS complex. It can be difficult to determine whether the block is at the level of the AV node or below. This distinction assumes clinical importance, as the former is typically benign and not treated. By contrast, the latter typically warrants a pacemaker as it commonly progresses to a higher degree of heart block. The width of the QRS complex is useful in making assumptions regarding the level of block when 2:1 AV conduction is noted clinically. A narrow QRS complex (<120 msec) suggests block at the level of the AV node and an intact His-Purkinje system. A wide QRS complex ($\geq$120 msec) more commonly signifies disease in the His-Purkinje system. In patients in whom the level of block cannot be determined, invasive electrophysiologic studies can provide useful prognostic information and guide decisions regarding the need for a pacemaker. Block at the level of the AV node (Wenckebach) and is generally benign and not progressive. Block in the His-Purkinje system or below generally requires permanent pacing *(18)*.

SUPRAVENTRICULAR TACHYCARDIAS

Supraventricular tachycardia (SVT) typically occurs with the same frequency in athletes as in the general population. Classification of SVTs is based on the electrophysiologic mechanism of the arrhythmia as noted in Table 2 *(19, 20)*. With understanding of the fundamental mechanisms of SVT and development of techniques of mapping and ablation of most SVTs, it is now possible to cure most athletes with this spectrum of arrhythmias.

Table 2
Supraventricular Tachycardia

Condition	Symptoms	ECG	Diagnosis	Treatment
APCs	Palpitations	Often normal	Monitor	Reassurance, BB or CCB if highly symptomatic
Atrial fibrillation	Palpitations	Often normal	Monitor	Rate control, anticoagulation, antiarrhythmics, ablation
Atrial flutter	Palpitations	Often normal	Monitor	Rate control, anticoagulation, antiarrhythmics, ablation
AVNRT	Palpitations, LH, syncope	Often Normal	Monitor, EP study	BB or CCB, digoxin, RFA
AVRT (WPW)	Asymptomatic	Short PR, delta wave	ECG, EP study	No therapy, ablation if high risk
AVRT (WPW)	Symptomatic (palpitations, syncope, LH)	Short PR, delta wave	ECG, EP study	Antiarrhythmics, ablation

ECG electrocardiogram, *APC* atrial premature complex, *AVNRT* atrioventricular nodal reentrant tachycardia, *AVRT* atrioventricular reentrant tachycardia, *BB* beta blockers, *CCB* calcium channel blockers, *WPW* Wolfe-Parkinson-White syndrome

A common tachycardia in athletes is sinus tachycardia that is a normal response of the sinus node to physiologic demands. Sympathetic tone increases and vagal tone is withdrawn with exercise, fear, pain and other physiologic states of increased oxygen demand. Sinus tachycardia can occasionally mimic other SVTs, particularly in young athletes who are capable of high sinus rates. Typically sinus tachycardia has a gradual onset and termination in contrast to atrioventricular nodal reentrant tachycardia (AVNRT) or atrioventricular reciprocating tachycardia (AVRT), discussed in prior chapters. Characteristically the P-wave morphology on the ECG is similar to that at rest with the P-wave vector oriented inferiorly and leftward. Sinus tachycardia, however, is a normal response to physiologic stimuli and does not require therapy. Atrial premature contractions (APCs) are common in adults including trained athletes and also do not require therapy *(17)*. In the minority of patients, these APCs may be symptomatic, manifesting as palpitations, skipped beats, or extra beats in the heart. APCs can be treated with medications such as beta-blockers which may suppress the extra-systoles and improve symptoms. Typically beta-blocker therapy is not well tolerated with side effects of fatigue and a decrease in exercise capacity noted by many athletes. Additionally, beta-blockers are banned in some types of athletic competition.

ATRIOVENTRICULAR NODAL REENTRANT TACHYCARDIA (AVNRT)

AVNRT is the most common SVT representing approximately 60–70% of all SVTs. Mechanistically it occurs when a reentrant circuit is present involving the AV node *(19, 20)*. The circuit typically requires dual AV nodal physiology with an anterior "fast" pathway and a posterior "slow" pathway. With the common type of AVNRT, the antegrade refractory period of the fast pathway is longer than that of the slow pathway. An appropriately timed atrial premature beat can block antegrade in the fast pathway, travel through the slow pathway and "echo" retrograde via the fast pathway to initiate and perpetuate this tachycardia. Under the proper conditions, a reentrant arrhythmia can be sustained with antegrade conduction via the slow pathway and retrograde conduction via the fast. AVNRT is characterized by rates between 130 and 240 beats/min with abrupt onset and termination *(19, 20)*. The resting ECG is generally normal. The ECG during the tachycardia usually demonstrates a narrow QRS complex tachycardia that is regular with atrial activity manifesting with a small R′ wave in lead V1 and shallow S waves in leads II, III, and aVF. This rhythm can occasionally be terminated with vagal maneuvers. However, definitive acute therapy is intravenous adenosine. Preventative pharmacologic therapy involves the use of beta-blockers, calcium channel blockers, or other antiarrhythmic agents. However, AVNRT is safely and successfully cured in the vast majority of patients with catheter-based ablation of the slow pathway. Ablation is considered to be first-line therapy over medications for this reason *(19, 20)*.

ATRIOVENTRICULAR REENTRANT TACHYCARDIA (AVRT)

Wolfe-Parkinson-White syndrome (WPW) was first described in the 1930s in young, otherwise healthy subjects with abnormal ECG findings of a short PR interval and a widened QRS complex and paroxysmal tachycardia. This syndrome is now well understood to be cause by accessory pathways of myocardial tissue bridging the atrioventricular groove. This accessory pathway, or bundle of Kent, allows conduction between the atrium and ventricle. Accessory pathways, also known as a bypass tract, typically do not have decremental conduction like the AV node. When bypass tracts have the ability to conduct antegrade and result in a pattern of short PR interval with a delta wave on the ECG they are classified as "manifest" pre-excitation *(19, 20)*. Commonly, bypass tracts only have the ability to conduct retrograde and allow conduction between the ventricle and atrium during AVRT. Such bypass tracts that only conduct retrograde cannot be identified on the resting ECG in sinus rhythm and are labeled "concealed" *(19, 20)*.

Both manifest and concealed bypass tracts can serve as the anatomic substrate for a reentrant circuit that involving the AV node antegrade and the bypass tract retrograde. This reentrant arrhythmia is the second most common type of SVT and is classified as orthodromic reciprocating tachycardia *(19, 20)*. Less commonly, the reentrant circuit involves antegrade conduction via a manifest bypass tract and retrograde conduction via the AV node. This results in a wide complex tachycardia classified as antedromic reciprocating tachycardia. While antiarrhythmic agents can reduce symptoms by slowing or blocking conduction in the bypass tract or AV node in many patients, the preferred approach to cure with radiofrequency ablation of the bypass tract. When an athlete has symptomatic WPW, ablation therapy is curative and should be the recommended first-line therapy. Restriction from athletics is reasonable for a period of several weeks to allow vascular heeling *(5, 6)*.

Manifest bypass tracts typically lack decremental conduction and atrial fibrillation can be transmitted to the ventricle at rapid rates. Very rarely, individuals may be at risk of sufficiently high rates of ventricular response to cause hemodynamic instability or ventricular fibrillation. This unusual clinical circumstance occurs more commonly with physical exertion. WPW is commonly detected in asymptomatic athletes on ECG, as the condition is present in approximately 1/3000 individuals. Athletes who present with evidence of preexcitation on ECG but without symptoms have a very low risk of developing life-threatening arrhythmias. Based on this consideration, most experts do not recommend routine electrophysiologic evaluation of asymptomatic patients with ventricular preexcitation (5, 6). Some experts take the approach of performing electrophysiologic evaluation of asymptomatic athletes with preexcitation to characterize the properties and location of the bypass tract. If there are indications of high risk, such as multiple bypass tracts, antegrade refractory period of the bypass tract < 250 msec, or induction of sustained arrhythmias, ablation is felt to be reasonable (5, 6). For asymptomatic patients with preexcitation, and those symptomatic or those asymptomatic patients who have undergone successful ablation of their bypass tract, there are no limitations on competitive sports once there is an appropriate period of recovery from the procedure (5, 6).

ATRIAL TACHYCARDIA

Another common SVT is atrial tachycardia, which refers to an area in the atrium that has enhanced automaticity (19, 20). Typically, the sinus node acts to initiate the cardiac cycle through a property of automaticity that produces regular impulses from that are of the myocardium. In atrial tachycardia, an abnormal tract of atrial myocardium will depolarize and initiate localized and progressive activation of the myocardium. The rates of atrial tachycardia vary, but typically are fast enough to suppress sinus node activity and can be highly symptomatic, typically manifesting as palpitations. This SVT frequently has a "warm-up" period with progressively shortening cycle lengths with each beat and on ECG or electrocardiographic monitoring, this appears as a narrow complex tachycardia that is faster with each beat until the maximum tachycardia rate is reached. Atrial tachycardia can be suppressed by use of beta-blockers or calcium channel blockers, but is also amenable to catheter-based ablation, which is typically curative treatment.

ATRIAL FIBRILLATION AND FLUTTER

Atrial fibrillation likely occurs more commonly in athletes when compared to non-athletes due to adaptation of the autonomic nervous system with heightened vagal tone (21–26). This type of vagally mediated atrial fibrillation frequently occurs in the setting of nocturnal bradycardia (21–26). Bradycardia may allow for altered dispersion of atrial repolarization creating the electrophysiologic substrate for atrial fibrillation (21–26). Atrial fibrillation is a common arrhythmia in adults who are not athletes and is commonly related to systemic hypertension, congestive heart failure or coronary artery disease (27). In the athlete without these predisposing factors, atrial fibrillation is likely related to heightened vagal tone or the result of another SVT degenerating into atrial fibrillation (21–26).

Paroxysmal atrial fibrillation generally originates in the muscular sleeves that extend into the pulmonary veins from the left atrium and form a continuous transition between the left atrial tissue and the endothelium of the pulmonary veins (21–26). Electrophysiologic observations related to ablation of the tissue in the pulmonary veins support the notion that this location is the origin of most paroxysmal atrial. The principles of evaluation and management of atrial fibrillation in the athlete are similar to those that guide evaluation and management of this arrhythmia in the non-athlete (5, 6, 27). Every patient with atrial fibrillation should have a complete history, physical examination, ECG, and echocardiogram. Routine laboratory test should include a TSH to exclude hyper or hypothyroidism. Evaluation includes determination of the ventricular response during athletic activity or an exercise test comparable to the intended athletic competition.

The decision to take a rate control versus rhythm control strategy is largely driven by symptoms (27). Typically, when the arrhythmia is symptomatic, a rhythm control strategy is used with antiarrhythmic agents selected based on the presence or absence of structural heart disease (27). Curative approach with catheter ablation is typically reserved for symptomatic individuals who have failed at least one antiarrhythmic drug (27–29). Based on risks, benefits, and patient preference, it is reasonable to consider AF ablation as first-line therapy in selected symptomatic athletes (27–29). In less symptomatic or asymptomatic athletes, rate control with beta-blockers or calcium channel blockers is generally recommended (27, 28). Anticoagulation with aspirin or warfarin is selectively initiated based on the athlete's risk of thromboembolic events (27, 28). It should be noted that in athletes or other individuals undergoing a curative approach to atrial fibrillation with ablation, anticoagulation is recommended long term if the patient's $CHADS_2$ score is 2 or greater even if there is an apparent cure of the arrhythmia (27, 28).

Recommendations regarding participation in athletics for individuals with atrial fibrillation are based on the best available data and expert opinion (5, 6). In the absence of WPW syndrome, athletes with asymptomatic atrial fibrillation without structural heart disease who maintain a ventricular rate that increases and slows appropriately and is comparable to that of a normal sinus response in relation to the level of activity, while receiving no therapy or therapy with AV nodal blocking drugs, can participate in all competitive sports (5, 6). Athletes who have atrial fibrillation in the presence of structural heart disease who maintain a ventricular rate comparable to that of an appropriate sinus tachycardia during physical activity while receiving no therapy or therapy with AV nodal-blocking drugs can participate in sports consistent with the limitations of the structural heart disease (5, 6). It is evident that athletes who require anticoagulation should not participate in sports with danger of bodily collision (5, 6). Athletes without structural heart disease who have elimination of atrial fibrillation by an ablation technique, including surgery, may participate in all competitive sports after several weeks with an arrhythmia recurrence (5, 6).

Atrial flutter is another form of SVT that results from a macro-reentrant circuit in the right atrial myocardium (30). In the absence of an acute, limiting illness, sustained atrial flutter is an uncommon rhythm disturbance in athletes without structural heart disease. This arrhythmia typically rotates in a counterclockwise direction through the isthmus of tissue between the os of the coronary sinus and the annulus of the tricuspid valve, along the intra-atrial septum, and over the roof and lateral wall of the right atrium (30). Athletes developing atrial flutter should have the same standard evaluation as those presenting with atrial fibrillation. The typical form of atrial flutter manifests with the classic saw-toothed pattern with inverted flutter waves in the inferior leads of the ECG and a variable ventricular response (30).

Like atrial fibrillation, therapy for atrial flutter is guided by the presence or absence of symptoms (27). Because the potential for very rapid ventricular rates exists if the atrial flutter conducts 1:1 to the ventricles, ECG determination of the ventricular response during an exercise test or athletic event during treatment is essential (5, 6). Antiarrhythmic drugs can be effective in restoring and maintaining normal sinus rhythm (27). However, given the high efficacy of flutter ablation by creating a line of block along the cavo-tricuspid isthmus, many experts consider ablation to be the first-line approach (5, 6, 27). This ablation procedure is also accompanied by a very low complication rate given the right atrial location (29). When the strategy of rate control is taken, beta-blockers or calcium channel blockers can be used (27). Anticoagulation is selectively used based on the $CHADS_2$ score in a fashion similar to atrial fibrillation (27, 28). In some patients atrial flutter degenerates to atrial fibrillation. In such case, patient's ablation of the atrial flutter can prevent development of this secondary arrhythmia.

Athletes with atrial flutter in the absence of structural heart disease who maintain a ventricular rate that increases and slows appropriately comparable to that of a normal sinus response in relation to the level of activity, while receiving no therapy or therapy with AV nodal blocking drugs, can participate in competitive sports with the warning that rapid 1:1 conduction still may occur (5, 6). However, full participation in all competitive sports should not be allowed unless the athlete has been without atrial flutter for two to three months with or without drug treatment (5, 6). It is recommended that athletes with structural heart disease who have atrial flutter participate in competitive sports only after two to four weeks have elapsed without an episode of atrial flutter *(5, 6)*. Athletes without structural heart disease who have elimination of the atrial flutter by an ablation technique or surgery can participate in all competitive sports after two to four weeks without a recurrence, or in several days after an electrophysiologic study showing noninducibility of the atrial flutter in the presence of bidirectional isthmus block *(5, 6, 30)*. As with atrial fibrillation, athletes in whom anticoagulation is deemed necessary cannot participate in competitive sports where the danger of bodily collision is present *(5, 6)*.

PRE-PARTICIPATION SCREENING

Most athletes at risk for sudden cardiac death (SCD) with athletic activity have preexisting and underlying heart disease *(1)*. The conditions associated with an increased risk of SCD in association with exercise have been identified and many of them can be detected by cardiovascular screening (Table 3). It has been determined that systematic screening for these underlying cardiovascular conditions allows for identification of athletes at risk for SCD *(2, 3, 31–33)*. The strategy of withdrawing those identified at high risk for SCD from vigorous training or competition is felt to reduce the risk of SCD *(31–33)*. Most experts accept the notion that the risk for SCD increases with vigorous training *(31–33)*. The best available evidence for the efficacy of screening athletes and selectively restricting athletic participation comes from Italy *(31–33)*. Through a national program all athletes engaged in organized sports must undergo yearly screening. This systematic approach served as the impetus for a proposal in 2005 by the European Society of Cardiology (ESC) for a common European protocol for pre-participation athlete screening *(31–33)*.

Fundamental to these recommendations are pre-participation athletic screenings by specially trained sports medicine physicians *(31–33)*. This evaluation consists of personal and family history, physical

Table 3
Cardiovascular Conditions Associated with Sudden Death in the Athlete

Structural heart diseases

Hypertrophic cardiomyopathy
Coronary artery anomalies
Left ventricular hypertrophy of indeterminate causation
Myocarditis
Ruptured aortic aneurysm (Marfan's syndrome)
Arrhythmogenic right ventricular cardiomyopathy
Tunneled (bridged) coronary artery
Aortic-valve stenosis
Atherosclerotic coronary artery disease
Dilated cardiomyopathy
Myxomatous mitral-valve degeneration
Asthma (or other pulmonary condition)
Heat stroke

Channelopathies

Long QT syndrome
Short QT Syndrome
Catecholaminergic polymporphic ventricular tachycardia
Brugada syndrome
Idiopathic ventricular fibrillation

examination, and 12-lead electrocardiogram *(31–33)*. These European guidelines recommend repeated screening for the duration of exposure to athletic activity every 2 years to identify any cardiovascular conditions that may manifest following the previous evaluation *(31–33)*. Selective use of more advanced cardiovascular testing is utilized as appropriate. If cardiovascular conditions that are associated with an increased risk of SCD are detected, recommendations for exclusion of the individual from athletic activity are similar to the Bethesda 36 guidelines *(5, 6, 31–33)*.

In the United States, with a heterogeneous and diverse population, pre-participation evaluation of high school and college athletes has traditionally included only a history and physical examination *(33)*. This screening has been traditionally limited to a history and physical exam reflecting the larger and more diverse background of American athletes and the broader spectrum of normal ECGs that can be difficult to distinguish from abnormal *(33)*. Athletes in the United Stated are typically screened at the high school and collegiate level, and routine evaluation does not involve an ECG based on the best available data which remains incomplete *(33)*.

A study in 2005 suggested that this standard screening at US colleges may have a low sensitivity with regards to SCD *(33)*. A 2000 survey of 879 American colleges and universities reported that 97% did participate in screening of their student-athletes, but only 25% used at least 9 of 12 AHA recommended screening guidelines and 24% included less than or equal to 4 of 12 *(33)*. Screening is performed by a range of providers depending on the individual institution and to date, the screening system for competitive athletes in the United States remains highly variable and inconsistent. While many have called for a more uniform and standardized approach to American athletes, the complexity of the American health care system makes this a challenging endeavor. A wide range of complex medical, legal, and ethical issues remain unresolved related to athletic screening for cardiovascular conditions and athletic restrictions *(33, 34)*.

The American College of Cardiology and the American Heart Association recommend screening high school athletes every 2 years and college athletes initially and then every 4 years *(33, 34)*. Recommended aspects of this screening included personal and familial historical data and a physical examination. ECGs and echocardiograms are not recommended in all individuals, but rather that they be used selectively based on symptoms, family history, or findings on physical exam *(33, 34)*.

Whether ECGs should be performed in all athletes remains a controversial issue. Electrocardiograms are frequently abnormal in the competitive athlete and distinguishing normal variants from abnormal is not possible without further cardiovascular evaluation in many athletes (Table 4). Up to 50% of athletes, mostly men and endurance athletes, will have some abnormal finding on ECG *(35–38)*. Early repolarization patterns, deep Q-waves, high QRS voltage, and T-Wave inversions are most common. Endurance athletes may have findings on ECG of increases P-wave amplitude, incomplete right bundle branch block, and high QRS voltages suggestive of left and right ventricular hypertrophy *(35–38)*. Some elite athletes have highly abnormal or bizarre findings that in the presence of a negative workup are felt to be the limit of physiological change with the athlete's heart *(35–38)*. Criteria for LV hypertrophy and even ST changes consistent with ischemia frequently are present in the well-trained athlete *(35–38)*.

The cardiac diseases that can be identified or suspected by an ECG include HCM, the long QT syndromes, ARVD, and WPW syndrome. Hypertrophic cardiomyopathy can be suspected by interventricular conduction delays, septal or inferior Q waves, LV hypertrophy, and ST abnormalities on a 12-lead ECG *(35–38)*. With the LQTS, the diagnosis is made by the ECG, but up to 6% of gene carriers will have a QTc of 0.44 or less. Patients with ARVD may have RV conduction delays (epsilon wave), right bundle-branch blocks, and inverted T waves in the pre-cordial leads. Unfortunately, none of these ECG findings (other than a long QT) are sensitive or specific for ascertaining abnormal from normal findings in the athlete. Whether ECGs will become standard in the United States for screening athletes is not yet determined; however, at present, the American Heart Association guidelines do not advocate an ECG in the routine screening of athletes *(33, 34)*.

Table 4
ECG Abnormalities

Diagnosis of heart disease	ECG abnormalities
Hypertrophic cardiomyopathy	Left ventricular hypertrophy
	Anterior pseudoinfarct, Q-waves
	Rarely normal
Arrhythmogenic right ventricular dysplasia	Anterior T-wave inversions
	Epsilon wave
	RBBB (complete or incomplete)
	Rarely normal
Wolff–Parkinson–White	Short PR
	Delta Waves
	Pseudoinfarct patterns
Long QT syndrome	Prolonged QT
	Abnormal ST segment
Short QT syndrome	Shortened QT
	Tall T-waves
Catecholaminergic polymorphic ventricular tachycardia	Usually normal
	Prominent U-wave
Idiopathic dilated cardiomyopathy	LBBB
	Prolonged QT
	Can be normal
Anomalous coronary artery	Usually normal
Brugada syndrome	RBBB (complete or incomplete)
	ST elevation anteriorly
	Variable ECG

RBBB right bundle branch block, *LBBB* left bundle branch block

EVALUATION OF THE ATHLETE

The evaluation of the athlete with suspected cardiac arrhythmia is fundamentally different from routine screening for athletes recommended by the American Heart Association. The evaluation of these athletes is, however, similar to those members of the general population with suspected arrhythmia. The key elements of the evaluation include the history with detailed evaluation of symptoms. Syncope, while less serious than previous sudden death, is more ominous when occurring suddenly or occurring in the setting of intense exercise. Sudden syncope may be associated with significant bodily injury as it may have no premonitory symptoms to warn the patient. Presyncope and lightheadedness are frequent presentations, but are less likely to be associated with malignant ventricular arrhythmia than true syncope though they still require investigation Many of the cardiac syndromes associated with SCD have a genetic component including HCM, long QT, idiopathic cardiomyopathy, and ARVD to some degree. Accordingly, a detailed family history is warranted.

Initial evaluation following a thorough history and physical exam should include 12-lead ECG and transthoracic echocardiogram. In those patients over age 35, an evaluation for cardiac ischemia is warranted with an exercise nuclear stress test. Outpatient electrocardiographic monitoring including Holter monitors, or loop type of ambulatory monitoring in patients with infrequent or intermittent symptoms, aid in the evaluation by capturing the clinical arrhythmia in various settings including sleep, exercise, and varied times through the day. In patients with high risk features such as sudden syncope, additional imaging testing such as cardiac CT or MRI should be selectively done as appropriate to best define the presence or absence of structural heart disease. Invasive testing with cardiac catheterization, coronary angiography, and electrophysiologic study should be pursued selectively as clinically indicated *(36)*.

TREATMENT

The presence or absence of structural heart disease and symptoms related to ventricular arrhythmias are two key factors guiding evaluation and management of the athlete with ventricular arrhythmias (Table 5). The justification for and benefits of treatment of ventricular arrhythmias in the athlete are reducing symptoms or reducing the risk of sudden death. In those patients without structural heart disease, the risk of sudden death is generally considered to be low.

In athletes with documented ventricular arrhythmias without structural heart disease, exercise-induced or resting non-sustained ventricular tachycardia and frequent premature ventricular contractions generally do not increase including the risk of sudden death *(5, 6, 36)*. If the athlete's heart is completely normal neither treatment nor restriction from athletics is warranted *(5, 6, 36)*. Treatment is reasonable for clinically significant symptoms such as palpitations. Beta-blockers are the preferred initial agent. Treatment options for symptomatic ventricular arrhythmias in athletes without structural heart disease include beta-blockers, antiarrhythmic agents, and ablation. In athletes without structural heart disease, symptomatic sustained ventricular tachycardias originating from the right or left ventric-

Table 5
Ventricular Arrhythmia in the Athlete

Condition	Symptoms	ECG	VT morphology	Treatment options	Competitive athletics
HCM	Palpitations, syncope, SCD	LVH, anterior Q-waves	PMVT, VF	BB, AAD, myomectomy, ICD	Low intensity
ARVD	Palpitations, syncope, SCD	Anterior T-inversions, RBBB, Epsilon wave	Left bundle, inferior axis	Sotolol, Amio, ICD, RFA	Only low intensity
CAD	Palpitations, syncope, SCD	Infarcts, ischemic ST changes	RB or LB	Amio, ICD	Only low intensity
IDCM	Palpitations, syncope, SCD	Often LBBB	RB or LB	Amio, ICD	Only low intensity
LQTS	Palpitations, syncope, SCD	Long QTc	PMVT	BB, PPM, ICD	Only low intensity
Anomalous coronary	Exertional chest pain, syncope, SCD	Normal	VF	CABG	No restrictions post CABG with negative stress
Idiopathic RVOT VT	Palpitations, LH, syncope	Normal	LB, inferior axis	RFA	No restrictions post-RFA
Idiopathic LV VT	Palpitations, LH, syncope	Normal	RB, left axis	RFA	No restrictions post-RFA
Idiopathic VF	Syncope, SCD	Normal	VF	ICD	Only Low intensity

ECG electrocardiogram, *VT* ventricular tachycardia, *LV* left ventricle, *LH* lightheadedness, *Nl* normal, *RB* right bundle, *RFA* radiofrequency ablation, *RVOT* right ventricle outflow tract VT, *LB* left bundle, *HCM* hypertrophic cardiomyopathy, *SCD* sudden cardiac death, *BB* beta-blockers, *AAD* antiarrhythmic drugs, *ICD* implantable cardioverter defibrillator, *ARVD* arrhythmogenic right ventricular dysplasia, *RBBB* right bundle branch block, *LBBB* left bundle branch block, *sot* sotalol, *amio* amiodarone, *PPM* permanent pacemaker, *CABG* coronary artery bypass surgery, *PMVT* polymorphic VT (torsades de point)

ular outflow tracts or the left posterior fascicle of the left bundle can be safely and successfully cured with mapping and radiofrequency ablation *(5, 6, 36)* (Table 5). Once the ablation has been successfully performed, such athletes can return to athletic activities without restrictions *(5, 6, 36)*. When structural heart disease is identified in the athlete, recommendations for treatment and athletic restriction are considerably different from those that are relevant to athletes without structural heart disease *(5, 6, 36)* (Table 3). With most types of structural heart disease that predisposes to sudden death the presence or absence of symptoms is not a factor in clinical decision regarding treatment or athletic restriction *(5, 6, 36)* (Table 5).

The Bethesda Guidelines related to ventricular arrhythmias provide the best available guidance for evaluation, management, and athletic restriction of athletes with ventricular arrhythmias *(4, 5)*. Athletes without structural heart disease who have premature ventricular complexes at rest and during exercise, including exercise testing that is comparable to the sport in which they compete, can participate in all competitive sports without restrictions *(5)*. If the premature ventricular complexes increase during with exercise testing and produce symptoms produce symptoms of impaired consciousness, significant fatigue, or dyspnea, the athlete can participate low intensity sports such as bowling, billiards or golf *(4–6, 36)*. Athletes with structural heart disease who are in high-risk groups based on the presence of structural heart disease that predisposes to sudden death as noted in Table 3 and have premature ventricular complexes should only participate in low intensity sports regardless of treatment *(5)*. It is also recommended that such athletes with premature ventricular complexes that are suppressed by drug therapy as assessed by ambulatory ECG recordings during participation in the sport only participate in low-intensity sports *(4–6, 36)*.

Nonsustained or sustained monomorphic or polymorphic VT requires careful evaluation and should be considered a potentially serious occurrence particularly when occurring the setting of structural heart diseases that predispose to sudden death *(4–6, 36)*. Routinely, noninvasive tests should be performed including an ECG, exercise test, and echocardiogram *(5, 36)*. Ambulatory monitoring may be appropriate in selected patients. Cardiac catheterization and electrophysiologic study should be considered to exclude otherwise undetected heart disease and establish the location and mechanism VT. Patients with accelerated idioventricular rhythm in whom the arrhythmia rate is similar to the sinus rate should be treated in a fashion similar to athletes with premature ventricular complexes *(5, 36)*.

Athletes with a structurally normal heart and monomorphic nonsustained or sustained VT that can be localized to a specific site are candidates for a catheter ablation procedure that may potentially offer a cure *(5, 36)*. Following such a successful ablation procedure, with subsequent failure to induce VT during electrophysiologic study (EPS) with/without isoproterenol when the VT was reproducibly induced before ablation, the athlete can resume full competitive activity within a few weeks *(4–6, 36)*.

A more conservative approach is recommended for the athlete in whom antiarrhythmic drug suppression is used as therapy because catecholamines released during athletic activity can counter the suppressive effects of the drug, and the VT can reemerge *(5, 36)*. It is recommended that the athlete should not compete in any sports for at least two to three months after the last VT episode *(5–6, 36)*. In the absence of clinical recurrences, and inducibility of VT by testing and EPS, all competitive sports may be permitted in the athlete with no structural heart disease *(5)*. Occasionally, deconditioning can result in the loss or lessening of ventricular arrhythmias *(4–6, 36)*. Accordingly, a period of deconditioning and reevaluation is reasonable in some athletes.

For the athlete with structural heart disease and VT, moderate- and high-intensity competition is contraindicated regardless of whether the VT is suppressed or ablated. Generally, only low-intensity sports are sports are permitted for such athletes *(4–6, 36)*. An exception to this general recommendation is the asymptomatic athlete with brief episodes of nonsustained monomorphic VT (generally less than 8–10 consecutive ventricular beats), rates generally less than 150 beats/min, and no structural heart disease *(5, 36)*. Such athletes do not appear to be at increased risk for sudden cardiac death *(5)*. If exercise testing and ambulatory ECG recording during the specific competitive activity demonstrates suppression of the VT, there is no need for athletic restriction *(4–6, 36)*.

The Bethesda Guidelines specify that the desire of the athlete to continue athletic competition should not represent the primary indication for use of an implantable cardioverter-defibrillator (ICD) *(5)*. The efficacy with which these devices will terminate a potentially lethal arrhythmia under the extreme conditions of competitive sports, with the associated metabolic and autonomic changes, and possible myocardial ischemia, is unknown *(5, 6, 36)*. In addition, sports with physical contact may result in damage to the ICD and/or lead, preventing normal function *(5, 6, 36)*. For athletes with ICDs, all moderate and high-intensity sports are contraindicated. Class IA sports are permitted *(4–6, 36)*.

Athletes with cardiovascular disease that result in a predisposition to a cardiac arrest in the presence or absence of structural heart disease generally are treated with an ICD and cannot participate in any moderate or high-intensity competitive sports *(4–6, 36)*. However, athletes with ICDs and who have had no episodes of ventricular flutter or ventricular fibrillation requiring device therapy for six months may engage in low-intensity competitive sports *(4–6, 36)*.

CONCLUSION

Evaluation and management of the athlete with cardiovascular conditions including structural heart disease and inherited arrhythmia syndromes represents a challenge for the clinician. Among the factors that need to be carefully considered are the presence or absence of symptoms or cardiovascular conditions predisposing to sudden cardiac death. Since screening strategies for detecting and preventing sudden death on the athletic field have not been shown to have sufficient sensitivity, specificity, and cost-effectiveness in the United States, it is likely that initial manifestation of cardiovascular conditions predisposing to sudden death will continue to be cardiac arrest in a considerable number of athletes. Based on this, recommendations for automatic external defibrillation, training in cardiopulmonary resuscitation, and an emergency response planning have been developed for athletic activities *(39)*. With ongoing research, it is likely that evidence based medicine will guide strategies for identification, evaluation, and therapy of athletes with cardiac arrhythmia in the future. In the meantime, the clinician should consider the best available information and expert opinion and consensus to guide clinical management.

REFERENCES

1. Maron BJ (2003) Sudden death in young athletes. N Engl J Med 349:1064–1075
2. Heidbüchel H, Corrado D, Biffi A, Hoffmann E, Panhuyzen-Goedkoop N et al (2006) Recommendations for participation in leisure-time physical activity and competitive sports of patients with arrhythmias and potentially arrhythmogenic conditions. Part II: ventricular arrhythmias, channelopathies and implantable defibrillators. Study group on sports cardiology of the European association for cardiovascular prevention and rehabilitation. Eur J Cardiovasc Prev Rehabil 13(5):676–686
3. Maron BJ, Chaitman BR, Ackerman MJ, Bayés de Luna A, Corrado D et al (2004) Recommendations for physical activity and recreational sports participation for young patients with genetic cardiovascular diseases. Working groups of the American heart association committee on exercise, cardiac rehabilitation, and prevention; councils on clinical cardiology and cardiovascular disease in the young. Circulation 109(22):2807–2816
4. Maron BJ, Zipes DP et al (2005) 36th Bethesda conference: eligibility recommendations for competitive athletes with cardiovascular abnormalities. J Am Coll Cardiol 45:1318–1321
5. Zipes DP, Ackerman MJ, Estes NA 3rd, Grant AO, Myerburg RJ, Van Hare G (2005) Task Force 7: arrhythmias. J Am Coll Cardiol 45:1354–1363
6. Estes NA 3rd, Link MS, Cannom D et al (2001) Report of the NASPE policy conference on arrhythmias and the athlete. J Cardiovasc Electrophysiol 12:1208–1219
7. Balady GJ, Cadigan JB, Ryan TJ (1984) Electrocardiogram of the athlete: an analysis of 289 professional football players. Am J Cardiol 53:1339–1343

8. Smith ML, Hudson DL, Graitzer HM, Rave PB (1989) Exercise training bradycardia: the role of autonomic balance. Med Sci Sports Exerc 21:40–44

9. Foote CB, Michaud G (1998) The athletes electrocardiogram: distinguishing normal from abnormal. In: Estes NI, Salem D, Wang PJ (eds) Sudden cardiac death in the athlete. Futura Publishing Company, Armonk, NY, pp 101–114

10. Baldesberger S, Bauersfeld U, Candinas R, Seifert B, Zuber M et al (2008) Sinus node disease and arrhythmias in the long-term follow-up of former professional cyclists. Eur Heart J 29(1):71–78

11. Bjørnstad HH, Bjørnstad TH, Urheim S, Hoff PI, Smith G, Maron BJ (2009) Long-term assessment of electrocardiographic and echocardiographic findings in Norwegian elite endurance athletes. Cardiology 112(3):234–241

12. Zehender M, Meinertz T, Keul J, Just H (1990) ECG variants and cardiac arrhythmias in athletes: clinical relevance and prognostic importance. Am Heart J 119:1378–1391

13. Gillette PC, Shannon C, Garson A et al (1983) Pacemaker treatment of sick sinus syndrome in children. J Am Coll Cardiol 1:1325–1329

14. Zeppilli P, Fenici R, Sassasra M et al (1980) Wenckebach second degree AV block in top-ranking athletes: an old problem revisited. Am Heart J 100:281–294

15. Crouse SF, Meade T, Hansen BE, Green JS, Martin SE. Electrocardiograms of collegiate football athletes. Clin Cardiol. 2009 Jan; 32(1):37–42

16. Serra-Grima R, Puig T, Doñate M, Gich I, Ramon J. Long-term follow-up of bradycardia in elite athletes. Int J Sports Med. 2008 Nov;29(11):934–7

17. Talan DA, Bauernfeind RA, Ashley WW et al (1982) Twenty-four hour continuous ECG recordings in long-distance runners. Chest 82:19–24

18. Epstein AE, DiMarco JP, Ellenbogen KA, Estes NA 3rd, Freedman RA et al (2008) ACC/AHA/HRS 2008 guidelines for device-based therapy of cardiac rhythm abnormalities: a report of the American College of Cardiology/American Heart Association Task Force on Practice Guidelines (Writing Committee to Revise the ACC/AHA/NASPE 2002 Guideline Update for Implantation of Cardiac Pacemakers and Antiarrhythmia Devices): developed in collaboration with the American Association for Thoracic Surgery and Society of Thoracic Surgeons. American College of Cardiology/American Heart Association Task Force on Practice Guidelines (Writing Committee to Revise the ACC/AHA/NASPE 2002 Guideline Update for Implantation of Cardiac Pacemakers and Antiarrhythmia Devices); American Association for Thoracic Surgery; Society of Thoracic Surgeons. Circulation 117(21):e350–e408

19. Manolis AS, Wang PJ, Estes NA 3rd (1994) Radiofrequency catheter ablation for cardiac tachyarrhythmias. Ann Intern Med 121(6):452–461

20. Naccarelli GV, Shih H, Jalal S (1995) Catheter ablation for the treatment of paroxysmal supraventricular tachycardia. J Cardiovasc Electrophysiol 6:951–961

21. Pelliccia A, Maron BJ, Di Paolo FM, Biffi A, Quattrini FM, Pisicchio C, Roselli A, Caselli S, Culasso F (2005) Prevalence and clinical significance of left atrial remodeling in competitive athletes. J Am Coll Cardiol 46(4):690–696

22. Mont L, Elosua R, Brugada J (2009) Endurance sport practice as a risk factor for atrial fibrillation and atrial flutter. Europace 11(1):11–17

23. Aizer A, Gaziano JM, Cook NR, Manson JE, Buring JE, Albert CM (2009) Relation of vigorous exercise to risk of atrial fibrillation. Am J Cardiol 103(11):1572–1577

24. Furlanello F, Bertoldi A, Dallago M, Galassi A, Fernando F, Biffi A, Mazzone P, Pappone C, Chierchia S (1998) Atrial fibrillation in elite athletes. J Cardiovasc Electrophysiol 9(8 Suppl):S63–S68

25. Coumel P (1996) Autonomic influences in atrial tachyarrhythmias. J Cardiovasc Electrophysiol 7:999–1007

26. Haïssaguerre M, Jaïs P, Shah DC, Takahashi A, Hocini M, Quiniou G, Garrigue S, Le Mouroux A, Le Métayer P, Clémenty J (1998) Spontaneous initiation of atrial fibrillation by ectopic beats originating in the pulmonary veins. New Engl J Med 339(10):659–666

27. Fuster V, Rydén LE, Cannom DS, Crijns HJ, Curtis AB et al (2006) ACC/AHA/ESC 2006 Guidelines for the management of patients with atrial fibrillation: a report of the American College of Cardiology/American Heart Association Task Force on Practice Guidelines and the European Society of Cardiology Committee for Practice Guidelines (Writing Committee to Revise the 2001 Guidelines for the Management of Patients With Atrial Fibrillation): developed in collaboration with the European Heart Rhythm Association and the Heart Rhythm Society. American College of Cardiology/American Heart Association Task Force on Practice Guidelines; European Society of Cardiology Committee for Practice Guidelines; European Heart Rhythm Association; Heart Rhythm Society. Circulation 114(7):e257–354

28. Calkins H, Brugada J, Packer DL, Cappato R, Chen SA et al (2007) HRS/EHRA/ECAS expert consensus statement on catheter and surgical ablation of atrial fibrillation: recommendations for personnel, policy, procedures and follow-up. A report of the Heart Rhythm Society (HRS) Task Force on Catheter and Surgical Ablation of Atrial Fibrillation developed in partnership with the European Heart Rhythm Association (EHRA) and the European Cardiac Arrhythmia Society (ECAS); in collaboration with the American College of Cardiology (ACC), American Heart Association (AHA), and the Society of Thoracic Surgeons (STS). Endorsed and approved by the governing bodies of the American

College of Cardiology, the American Heart Association, the European Cardiac Arrhythmia Society, the European Heart Rhythm Association, the Society of Thoracic Surgeons, and the Heart Rhythm Society. Heart Rhythm Society; European Heart Rhythm Association; European Cardiac Arrhythmia Society; American College of Cardiology; American Heart Association; Society of Thoracic Surgeons. Europace 9(6):335–379

29. Haissaguerre M, Jais P, Shah DC et al (2000) Electrophysiological endpoint for catheter ablation of atrial fibrillation initiated from multiple pulmonary venous foci. Circulation 101:1409–1417

30. Fischer B, Haissaguerre M, Garrigues S et al (1995) Radiofrequency catheter ablation of common atrial flutter in 80 patients. J Am Coll Cardiol 25:1365–1372

31. Corrado D, Basso C, Schiavon M, Thiene G (1998) Screening for hypertrophic cardiomyopathy in young athletes. N Engl J Med 339(6):364–369

32. Corrado D, Pelliccia A, Bjørnstad HH et al (2005) Cardiovascular pre-participation screening of young competitive athletes for prevention of sudden death: proposal for a common European protocol: consensus statement of the study group of sport cardiology of the working group of cardiac rehabilitation and exercise physiology and the working group of myocardial and pericardial diseases of the European society of cardiology. Eur Heart J 26(5):516–524

33. Pfister GC, Puffer JC, Maron BJ (2000) Preparticipation cardiovascular screening for US collegiate student-athletes. JAMA 283:1597–1599

34. Paterick TE, Paterick TJ, Fletcher GF, Maron BJ (2005) Medical and legal issues in the cardiovascular evaluation of competitive athletes. JAMA 294(23):3011–3018

35. Estes NAM III, Link MS, Homoud MK, Wang PJ (2000) Electrocardiographic variants and cardiac rhythm and conduction disturbances in the athlete. In: Thompson PD (eds) Exercise and sports cardiology. McGraw Hill, New York, NY

36. Link MS, Wang PJ, Estes NAM III (1999) Cardiac arrhythmias and electrophysiologic observations in the athlete. In: Williams RA (eds) The athlete and heart disease: diagnosis, evaluation & management. Lippincott Williams & Wilkins, Philadelphia, PA, p 2196

37. Serra-Grima R, Estorch M, Carrio I, Subirana M, Berna L, Prat T (2000) Marked ventricular repolarization abnormalities in highly trained athletes' electrocardiograms: clinical and prognostic implications. J Am Coll Cardiol 36:1310–1316

38. Biffi A, Pelliccia A, Verdile L et al (2002) Long-term clinical significance of frequent and complex ventricular tachyarrhythmias in trained athletes. J Am Coll Cardiol 40:446–452

39. Myerburg RJ, Estes NA 3rd, Fontaine JM, Link MS, Zipes DP (2005) Task force 10: automated external defibrillators. J Am Coll Cardiol 45(8):1369–1371

16   Arrhythmias in Pregnancy and Postpartum

Kristen K. Patton and Richard L. Page

Contents

Abstract

The significant physiologic adaptations of pregnancy predispose to arrhythmias, while concurrent changes in pharmacokinetics and concerns for fetal health and well-being complicate management. An increased incidence of both atrial and ventricular arrhythmias has been reported in population-based Holter studies, yet most incident pregnancy-related arrhythmias are benign and do not require intervention. Pharmacologic absorption, distribution, metabolism, and elimination are altered, as are gut absorption, protein binding, and hepatic and renal blood flow. This chapter will review antiarrhythmic drug therapy by Vaughn Williams classification, nonpharmacologic arrhythmia therapy (cardiovascular implanted electronic devices and ablation), as well as management of specific cardiovascular conditions during pregnancy, labor, and postpartum.

Key Words: Pregnancy; hemodynamic; adaptation; cardiac output; arrhythmia; pharmacologic; pharmacokinetics; antiarrhythmic drugs; digoxin; adenosine; quinidine; procainamide; disopyramide; lidocaine; mexiletine; flecainide; propafenone; beta-blockers; sotalol; dofetalide; ibutilide; amiodarone; verapamil; diltiazem; cardiversion; cardiac arrest; cardiopulmonary resuscitation; pacemaker; implantable cardioverter

From: *Contemporary Cardiology: Management of Cardiac Arrhythmias*
Edited by: Gan-Xin Yan, Peter R. Kowey, DOI 10.1007/978-1-60761-161-5_16
© Springer Science+Business Media, LLC 2011

defibrillator; radiofrequency ablation; premature atrial contractions; premature ventricular contractions; atrioventricular nodal reentrant tachycardia; atrioventricular reentrant tachycardia; atrial tachycardia; atrial flutter; atrial fibrillation; ventricular tachycardia; congenital heart disease; long QT syndrome; Wolff-Parkinson-White syndrome; hypertrophic cardiomyopathy; structural heart disease; syncope; Marfan syndrome; labor and delivery; postpartum; and lactation.

INTRODUCTION

Pregnancy causes remarkable physiologic alterations, resulting in hemodynamic changes that predispose to arrhythmia generation. These adaptations occur in the setting of pregnancy-induced changes in maternal drug metabolism and concerns regarding the effect of antiarrhythmic therapies on the developing fetus. As a consequence, management of arrhythmias in pregnancy is complex, particularly in the setting of maternal heart disease.

PHYSIOLOGIC ADAPTATIONS OF PREGNANCY

The massive increase in total body water (average of 7 L) sustained during pregnancy results in a condition comparable to chronic volume overload (1, 2). Sodium and water retention is mediated by arginine vasopressin and the renin-angiotensin-aldosterone system, and results in a 30–50% increase in cardiac output and a dilutional anemia of pregnancy (1, 3, 4). The marked increase in cardiac output from 5 L/min to 7.3 L/min is due to an increase in both heart rate and stroke volume. Although there is some variation in human studies, the rise in cardiac output begins early, and by 12 weeks is nearly 40% of pre-gravid levels (5, 6). Cardiac output appears to peak between 25 and 30 weeks. Maternal heart rate also begins to rise early in pregnancy, paralleling the rise in cardiac output, and peaks at 15–20 beats/min above the pre-pregnancy state (1, 7). Stroke volume begins its rise slightly later, at approximately 8 weeks, reaching a peak 20–30% above pre-pregnancy levels at 20 weeks. In later pregnancy, cardiac output is dependent on maternal position. Blood return and stroke volume are reduced by both standing and lying supine; in the latter position, this is caused by uterine compression of the inferior vena cava (8).

Despite significantly increased cardiac output during pregnancy, maternal blood pressure falls due to a decrease in systemic vascular resistance (9). This fall occurs despite renin-angiotensin-aldosterone system activation in pregnancy; in normal pregnancy, the gravid woman is less responsive to angiotensin II-mediated vasoconstriction due to increased nitric oxide production and gestational hormones (10). Blood pressure falls to a nadir at mid-pregnancy and gradually increases to near pre-pregnancy levels at term (9).

Cardiac hypertrophy occurs during pregnancy; ultrasound studies have shown an increase in left ventricular mass of 52%, as well as an increase in left ventricular end-diastolic and end-systolic diameters (12 and 20%, respectively) (11). Left ventricular diastolic function, as demonstrated by changes in mitral valve flow velocities, increases in the first two trimesters but declines in the third trimester (12). Left atrial dimension also gradually increases during pregnancy, peaking at 40% at 30 weeks gestation (5).

During labor, cardiac output increases even further (7–10.6 L/min) (1), resulting from the increased stroke volume and the increased venous return that occurs during uterine contractions. Mean arterial pressure also increases in labor and during contractions. Cardiac output reaches its peak immediately post-partum and returns to pre-pregnancy levels in 2–4 weeks (5).

EPIDEMIOLOGY

An increase in arrhythmia during pregnancy has been documented in the literature. Holter studies showed a similar and high prevalence of premature atrial and ventricular contractions among both symptomatic and asymptomatic pregnant subjects (56% and 59%, respectively) *(13)*. The frequency of ventricular arrhythmias was higher in symptomatic patients (3235 ± 6397 vs. 678 ± 3358 beats/24 h p <0.05). Follow-up Holter monitoring in a subset of patients with frequent premature ventricular contractions during pregnancy revealed a substantial reduction in arrhythmia burden postpartum (9073 ± 9210/24 h to 1345 ± 1997/24 h (p <0.05)) *(13)*. In asymptomatic pregnant patients, a high incidence of arrhythmias was reported *(13)*.

A large retrospective review of over 136,000 pregnancy-related admissions to Parkland hospital in Dallas, TX, revealed 226 admissions with concurrent arrhythmia diagnosis (0.17%) *(14)*. The most frequently reported arrhythmias (sinus tachycardia, sinus bradycardia, and sinus arrhythmia) were benign and did not require intervention. Premature atrial and ventricular contractions were the second most common arrhythmia seen. Supraventricular tachycardia was less commonly noted (24/100,000), and either terminated spontaneously or responded well to adenosine. Episodes associated with Wolff-Parkinson-White syndrome responded to procainamide. The vast majority of episodes were the first presentation with an arrhythmia. Serious arrhythmias, such as high-degree atrioventricular block, ventricular arrhythmias, and cardiac arrest, were very rare (Fig. 1) *(14)*.

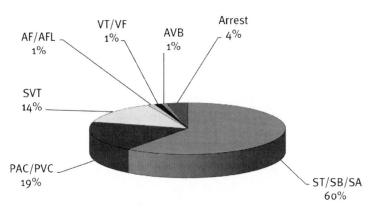

Fig. 1. Distribution of arrhythmias diagnosed during pregnancy (expressed as the percentage of total arrhythmia occurrence) (from Li et al., with permission) *(14)*. AF: atrial fibrillation; AFL: atrial aflutter; AVB: atrioventricular block; PAC: premature atrial contraction; PVC: premature ventricular contraction; SA: sinus arrhythmia; SB: sinus bradycardia; ST: sinus tachycardia; SVT: supraventricular tachycardia; VF: ventricular fibrillation; VT: ventricular tachycardia.

THERAPY OF ARRHYTHMIAS DURING PREGNANCY

Conservative, nonpharmacologic measures are generally preferred since antiarrhythmic therapy is complicated by concerns for potential risk to the fetus. Teratogenic risk is highest early in the first trimester; after eight weeks, organogenesis is largely completed *(15)*. Nonsustained episodes with mild symptomatology that do not compromise fetal well-being may best be treated with reassurance. Sustained episodes of supraventricular tachycardia may terminate with vagal maneuvers. Triggers of specific episodes may be avoided by hydration, avoidance of caffeine, and rest.

PHARMACOLOGIC CHANGES OF PREGNANCY

The substantial physiologic adaptions of pregnancy result in changes to each aspect of drug pharmacokinetics: absorption, distribution, metabolism, and elimination *(16)*. Determining antiarrhythmic dosage requirements of a pregnant patient is complex: changes in clearance affect the maintenance dose; increases in the volume of distribution modify loading dose; and changes in metabolism affect half-life, varying the time to steady state and the dosage interval. Drug concentrations are also affected by gut absorption, decreased protein binding, and changes in hepatic and renal blood flow, all of which vary throughout the course of pregnancy. Hepatic and intestinal CYP3A and renal *P*-glycoprotein activity are both increased during pregnancy *(17)*. Creatinine clearance increases by 45% during the first trimester, but returns to normal by term *(18)*.

SPECIFIC DRUGS IN PREGNANCY BY VAUGHN WILLIAMS CLASSIFICATION

Lidocaine and sotalol are category B: "Either animal-reproduction studies have not demonstrated a fetal risk but there are no controlled studies in pregnant women, or animal-reproduction studies have shown an adverse effect (other than a decrease in fertility) that was not confirmed in controlled studies in women in the first trimester (and there is no evidence of a risk in later trimesters). Most antiarrhythmic drugs are in Food and Drug Administration pregnancy category C; which states: "Animal reproduction studies have shown an adverse effect on the fetus and there are no adequate and well-controlled studies in humans, but potential benefits may warrant the use of the drug in pregnant women despite potential risks." Amiodarone, atenolol, and phenytoin are labeled pregnancy class D: "There is positive evidence of human fetal risk based on adverse reaction data from investigational or marketing experience or studies in humans, but potential benefits may warrant use of the drug in pregnant women despite potential risks" (Table 1).

Table 1
Antiarrhythmic Drugs During Pregnancy and Lactation

Vaughn Williams classification	Drug	FDA	Comments	Potential adverse effects	AAP lactation compatible
IA	Quinidine	C	Long history of use in pregnancy, now less common due to the availability of alternative agents	Mild uterine contractions, premature labor, fetal thrombocytopenia, and cranial nerve VIII toxicity	Yes
IA	Procainamide	C	Used for maternal and fetal tachyarrhythmia	Lupus-like syndrome	Yes
IA	Disopyramide	C	Negative inotrope, anticholinergic side effects	Uterine contractions, pre-term labor, abruptio placentae	Yes
IB	Lidocaine	B	Common anesthetic agent	Fetal acidosis	Yes
IB	Mexiletine	C	Limited data available	Fetal bradycardia, small size for gestational age, and low Apgar scores	Yes
IC	Flecainide	C	Most commonly used IC agent in pregnancy. Used for fetal arrhythmia.		Yes

(Continued)

Table 1
(Continued)

Vaughn Williams classification	Drug	FDA	Comments	Potential adverse effects	AAP lactation compatible
IC	Propafenone	C	Limited data available		Unknown
II	General class effect	C	Commonly used for maternal hypertension	Intrauterine growth retardation, fetal bradycardia, apnea, hypoglycemia, hyperbilirubinemia, premature labor	
II	Propranolol	C			Yes
II	Atenolol	D	Still commonly used in pregnancy	Higher prevalence of pre-term delivery and small-for-gestational age babies	Caution – cyanosis, bradycardia
II	Metoprolol	C			Yes
III	Ibutilide	C		Teratogenic in supraclinical dosages in animal models	Unknown
III	Sotalol	B	May cause adverse effects similar to beta-blockers, in addition to class III effects	Potential teratogen, fetal death	Yes
III	Amiodarone	D	Used for maternal and fetal tachycardias	Thyroid dysfunction, prolongation of the QT interval, bradycardia, neurodevelopmental delay, and both intrauterine and post-natal growth defects	Of concern – possible hypothyroidism
IV	Verapamil	C	Maternal and fetal supraventricular tachycardia	Fetal bradycardia, heart block, hypotension, death	Yes
IV	Diltiazem	C	Maternal and fetal supraventricular tachycardia. Teratogenic in animal models	Limited data, likely similar to verapamil	Yes
Misc	Adenosine	C		Transient fetal bradycardia	Unknown
Misc	Digoxin	C	Used for maternal and fetal tachyarrhythmia. Long history of use in pregnancy		Yes

AAP: American Academy of Pediatrics (149)

MISCELLANEOUS ANTIARRHYTHMIC AGENTS: DIGOXIN AND ADENOSINE

Adenosine has been shown to be safe and well tolerated in pregnancy for termination of supraventricular arrhythmias dependent on atrioventricular nodal conduction *(19, 20)*. Persistent adverse effects on either mother or fetus have not been described, although transient fetal bradycardia has been reported. It is considered the treatment of choice for acute termination of persistent supraventricular tachycardia refractory to vagal maneuvers *(15, 21, 22)*.

Digoxin has perhaps the longest history of use in pregnancy, and is considered safe, despite FDA category C classification *(23)*. Digoxin crosses the placenta, but is generally found in lower levels in cord blood than in maternal blood, and has not been reported to be teratogenic *(24)*. Digoxin clearance is increased during pregnancy, due to increased renal clearance; and levels may be confusing to interpret, due to the increase in circulating digoxin-like substances late in the third trimester *(25, 26)*. Digoxin also is secreted in breast milk, but is detected in only minute amounts in the infant bloodstream *(26, 27)*.

CLASS I AGENTS (SODIUM CHANNEL BLOCKADE)

Quinidine has a long record of safe use during pregnancy both for arrhythmia and for the treatment of malaria *(28, 29)*. Reported adverse events include mild uterine contractions, premature labor, thrombocytopenia, and fetal cranial nerve VIII toxicity *(15, 30)*. Quinidine is 80% protein-bound; changes in protein concentrations during pregnancy increase complexity when monitoring dosage *(26)*.

Procainamide has the advantage of intravenous dosing, and appears to be safe and effective in arrhythmia management during pregnancy *(31)*. Because of its effectiveness in treatment for both supraventricular and ventricular tachycardias, it is a particularly appropriate choice for the management of undiagnosed wide-complex tachycardias. Procainamide crosses the placenta, but has not been reported to cause adverse effects in the fetus; however, the association with a lupus-like syndrome lessens its usefulness. Although both procainamide and its less active metabolite, *N*-acetyl-procainamide, are secreted in breast milk, the amount that would be ingested by an infant is low, and the drug is considered safe for use during lactation *(32)*.

Disopyramide crosses the placenta, and is found in concentrations of about 40% of maternal levels in the fetus *(33)*. Several reports have linked its use during pregnancy to uterine contractions *(34)*, pre-term labor *(35)*, and in one case report, placental abruption *(36)*. It is therefore considered relatively unappealing for use during pregnancy *(35)*. Disopyramide is secreted in breast milk *(26)*, but is considered compatible for use during breastfeeding.

Lidocaine, used not just for therapy of life-threatening ventricular arrhythmias but for epidural and local anesthesia during labor and delivery, appears to be safe for use in pregnancy *(22)*. It rapidly crosses the placenta, and is found in concentrations of up to 60% of maternal levels *(37)*. Case reports of adverse events have included neonatal toxicity *(38, 39)*; transiently low APGAR scores have been associated with high levels *(40)*. Of particular concern is lidocaine use in cases of fetal stress and hypoxia, since acidosis will increase fetal lidocaine levels *(41)*.

There are few reports concerning the use of mexiletine in pregnancy and postpartum, but it is clear the drug liberally crosses the placenta and is secreted in breast milk *(42–44)*. No teratogenic effects have been reported, although fetal bradycardia, small size for gestational age, and low Apgar scores have been documented *(42–44)*.

Flecainide has been used successfully in pregnancy for the treatment of both supraventricular and ventricular tachycardia *(45–48)*. It actively crosses the placenta, and has been effectively used to treat fetal arrhythmias *(49, 50)*. Due to good fetal outcomes, flecainide is considered quite safe for use in pregnancy, although data are limited. The drug is excreted in breast milk, without deleterious effects having been described *(51)*.

Very few case reports have been published regarding the use of propafenone in pregnancy *(21)*. It has been used successfully in later pregnancy for the control of ventricular arrhythmia, and is transferred across the placenta, as well as into maternal milk at low concentrations *(52, 53)*.

CLASS II (BETA-ADRENERGIC BLOCKING AGENTS)

There are extensive data regarding the use of both selective and nonselective beta-blockers during pregnancy, due to their use in the treatment of hypertension, arrhythmia, hyperthyroidism, hypertrophic cardiomyopathy, and the long QT syndrome *(21, 54)*. In general, beta-blockers are considered safe, yet reports of intrauterine growth retardation, fetal bradycardia, apnea, hypoglycemia, hyperbilirubinemia, and early labor have been linked to their use *(15)*. Through effects on beta-2 adrenergic receptors, beta-blockers reduce umbilical blood flow, increase uterine contractility, and cause peripheral vasodilation, which has led to the suggestion that beta-1 selective drugs may be preferred agents in this class *(54)*. Adverse events in the fetus may occur most commonly in the stressed fetus due to impairment of the fetal response to stress by beta-blockade *(54)*.

Propranolol is the most widely used beta-blocker in pregnancy, and is FDA category C, as are the majority of beta-blockers. Acetabulol and pindolol are FDA category B; atenolol is FDA category D due to a study that demonstrated an increased prevalence of pre-term delivery and infants that were small-for-gestational age *(55)*. Although several studies have not shown a connection between beta-blockers and fetal growth retardation, there is evidence that the use of beta-blockers in the first trimester may increase the risk of this adverse effect *(55, 56)*. Due to pharmacodynamic changes during pregnancy, the dosage of beta-blocker often needs to be significantly increased *(18)*. Most beta-blockers, which are weak bases, do accumulate in breast milk, which is slightly acidic; however, the amount of drug ingested by an infant is usually clinically insignificant *(57, 58)*.

CLASS III AGENTS (PROLONGATION OF REPOLARIZATION)

Sotalol is a class III agent with nonselective beta-blocking properties, and is FDA category B. Small studies in women with hypertension have shown that like other beta-blockers, sotalol crosses the placenta and concentrates in breast milk. Of 12 deliveries where sotalol was used from the mid-second trimester of pregnancy, 8 were uncomplicated, 2 died from congenital anomalies not attributed to sotalol: 1 died of asphyxia, and 1 had transient hypoglycemia *(59–61)*.

Clinical use of dofetilide (FDA category C) during pregnancy has not been reported. Studies in rat models suggest teratogenic potential in early pregnancy, although this does not differ from other class III agents, which after long-term dosing have been shown to produce malformations due to bradycardia/arrhythmia-induced hypoxia *(62, 63)*.

Ibutilide, also FDA category C, prolongs repolarization. It has been described in case reports to have successfully terminated both atrial flutter and atrial fibrillation during pregnancy *(64, 65)*. Chemical conversion allowed avoidance of the sedation necessary for direct current cardioversion in a hypotensive patient *(64)*. No adverse maternal or fetal effects were noted, and the half-life of the drug is short (2–12 h). There are concerns regarding potential toxicity of ibutilide, however, due to animal studies in other class III agents *(62, 66)*.

Amiodarone, FDA category D, has mixed class I, II, III, and IV effects and has been used during all stages of pregnancy for both supraventricular and ventricular tachycardia *(67–72)*. Due to the high iodine content of the drug, the most common adverse effect described in the fetus is thyroid dysfunction; most commonly, this is transient hypothyroidism (9–17%), although goiter and hyperthyroidism have been described *(71, 73–75)*. Both amiodarone and its metabolite, desethyamiodarone, cross the placenta, with concentrations of 10 and 25% that of maternal plasma, respectively *(76)*, although the levels in placental tissue are higher than in maternal plasma *(71)*.

Other reported adverse effects include prolongation of the QT interval *(69)*, bradycardia *(69, 73)*, neurodevelopmental delay *(73, 74)*, and both intrauterine and post natal growth defects *(73)*. In aggregate, it is clear that the use of amiodarone during pregnancy poses potential risk to the fetus. Therefore, its use should be restricted to tachyarrhythmias that are resistant to other drugs or life-threatening.

A relatively high concentration of amiodarone is found in breast milk. There are no reports of adverse consequences from breastfeeding, but it is reasonable to use as low of a dose as possible and to continue to monitor maternal and neonatal thyroid function *(70, 71)*.

CLASS IV (CALCIUM CHANNEL BLOCKING AGENTS)

Verapamil has been used to acutely convert maternal supraventricular tachycardia, and for chronic treatment for supraventricular and ventricular arrhythmia, fetal arrhythmia, premature labor, and preeclampsia *(77–82)*. A limited number of case reports document its safety and efficacy; however, maternal hypotension has been described, and verapamil crosses the placenta *(78, 82)*. Verapamil is effective for treatment of fetal arrhythmia, yet its use has been associated with fetal bradycardia, heart block, hypotension, and even death *(80, 83–85)*. Verapamil is excreted in breast milk in varying concentrations *(77)*.

Little has been published regarding the use of diltiazem during pregnancy *(86)*. In a small series of women with chronic renal disease, diltiazem had beneficial effects in pregnancy, which included decreased maternal proteinuria, fetal growth restriction, and need for labor induction *(87)*.

NONPHARMACOLOGIC THERAPY OF ARRHYTHMIAS DURING PREGNANCY

Cardioversion has been reported to be safe at all trimesters of pregnancy; with standard pad placement the uterus is not within the current pathway, and the fetal fibrillation threshold is high *(88–93)*. Transient fetal bradycardia and distress due to provocation of uterine contraction in the third trimester has been described, and it is recommended that the procedure be performed with fetal rhythm monitoring *(94)*.

Cardiopulmonary resuscitation for the treatment of cardiac arrest during pregnancy is complicated in later trimesters by compression of the inferior vena cava and aorta by the gravid uterus *(15, 95–98)*. The 20-week or later gravid woman is best placed in a left lateral decubitus position, often accomplished by a wedge, or by resting the patient on the knees of a rescuer *(99)*. Airway management and resuscitation pad position can also be complicated by pregnancy. Pregnant patients develop hypoxemia rapidly because of decreased functional residual capacity and increased oxygen demand. Energy and medication dosage recommendations are not changed by the gravid state *(98, 100)*. The success of resuscitation for both the mother and the fetus may depend on emergent caesarean section *(95–98)*.

Successful pregnancies in the setting of a previously implanted pacemaker have been well described *(101–106)*, even when the generator is implanted in the abdominal wall *(107)*. One reported case of recurrent pulmonary emboli during pregnancy was due to pacer wire thrombus *(108)*. Management of a first presentation of complete heart block occurring during pregnancy has varied from close observation without need for pacemaker support, to insertion of a permanent pacemaker system in early pregnancy, to the prolonged use of a temporary wire for pacing through the third trimester and labor *(101–103, 109)*. Implantations of permanent pacemaker systems for symptomatic bradycardia during pregnancy by echocardiographic guidance without the use of fluoroscopy have been reported *(110–112)*.

The presence of an implantable defibrillator, and even ICD shocks, have been reported without complications during pregnancy (113–116). Insertion of defibrillators using minimal fluoroscopy (0.9s) or echocardiographic guidance has also been reported (117, 118). The largest retrospective series of defibrillator patients during pregnancy reported an 18% rate of device-related complications, including pocket tenderness, generator migration, and pericarditis (119). The majority of systems were abdominal, 23% of patients received a shock during pregnancy, and 89% of the babies were born healthy. One infant was stillborn, two were small for gestational age, one had transient hypoglycemia, and one therapeutic abortion occurred, unrelated to the defibrillator (119).

Radiofrequency ablation has been performed during pregnancy in cases of supraventricular arrhythmias refractory to drug management (120–124). A case series of three patients reported a calculated X-ray exposure of the fetus ranging from 118.3 to 515.0 mrad, not taking into account the leaded abdominal protection (123). Two of the three infants were normal at 2 years, and the child with the least amount of radiation exposure (procedure performed at 29 weeks gestation) showed cranial growth retardation at 4 months, despite sonographic normal growth during the pregnancy (123). In another report, successful ablation using intracardiac echocardiographic guidance at 10 weeks gestation resulted in a normal pregnancy (120). Future development of mapping systems limiting radiation exposure will enhance the safety of this therapeutic strategy.

Management of Specific Arrhythmias During Pregnancy

Atrial and ventricular premature beats occurring in the setting of a structurally normal heart are benign, and anxiety related to their existence often responds well to reassurance. Counseling to avoid triggering conditions and exacerbating factors, such as dehydration, caffeine, and sleep deprivation, can also be helpful. If ectopy does not respond to these measures, and is quite bothersome, beta-blockers may be useful.

Atrioventricular node-dependent tachycardias and atrial tachycardia will often respond to nonpharmacologic vagal maneuvers, and drug therapy is only indicated in patients with symptoms refractory to this and avoidance of precipitating factors. Intravenous adenosine or cardioversion can be used for acute management. Digoxin and beta-blockers are the first-line agents for prevention of recurrence; flecainide and propafenone may be useful if these agents fail. Procainamide may be particularly useful acutely for arrhythmias associated with the Wolff-Parkinson-White syndrome.

Atrial flutter and atrial fibrillation can be managed with a rate or rhythm control strategy, similar to in the nonpregnant state, although rate control agents are more appealing for use in pregnancy due to the safety record of digoxin and beta-blockers. As noted above, class IC agents are second-line options.

Ventricular arrhythmia management depends on the underlying heart condition. In patients with a structurally normal heart and idiopathic ventricular tachycardia (VT), beta-blockers are first-line therapy, with class IC agents or sotalol reserved as second-line agents.

In patients with acquired or congenital heart disease, the prognosis can be serious. Patients with long QT or hypertrophic cardiomyopathy may also present during pregnancy with ventricular arrhythmias. Sustained VT may be the initial presentation of peripartum cardiomyopathy or vasospastic coronary artery disease, and requires evaluation after clinical stability is attained. Hemodynamically unstable VT should be treated with emergent cardioversion. If the VT is well tolerated, lidocaine is the first immediate option. Sustained or recurrent VT may require procainamide, flecainide, propafenone, sotalol, or even amiodarone. As noted above, ICD placement and therapy is tolerated in pregnancy.

Asymptomatic bradycardia is best managed conservatively. As noted previously, temporary or permanent pacemakers may be safely inserted during pregnancy, either with minimal radiation and lead abdominal shielding, or echocardiographic guidance.

Management of Specific Conditions During Pregnancy

Wolff-Parkinson-White Syndrome: The incidence of symptomatic arrhythmias associated with manifest pre-excitation appears to increase during pregnancy *(125, 126)*. It is therefore reasonable to offer prophylactic electrophysiology study and ablation to even asymptomatic patients who intend to become pregnant in the future.

Long QT Syndrome: Patients with familial long QT syndrome type 1 (LQT1) have an increased risk of arrhythmic events triggered by adrenergic stimuli; in LQT2, events are often triggered by startle, arousal, or emotional stimuli; and in LQT3 by sleep *(127)*. A retrospective review of the 422 women enrolled in the Long QT Syndrome Registry who had one or more pregnancies revealed no association with cardiac events during pregnancy for probands or first-degree relatives, but an independent association with cardiac events for probands during the postpartum interval (OR, 40.8; 95% CI, 3.1 to 540; $p=0.01$) *(128)*. Treatment with beta-adrenergic blockers was independently associated with a decrease in the risk for cardiac events among probands *(128)*. A later analysis of 391 patients showed that pregnancy itself was associated with a reduced risk of cardiac events, whereas the 9-month postpartum time had an increased risk of cardiac events *(129)*. After the 9-month postpartum period, the risk was similar to the period before the first conception. Genotype analysis of a subset showed that women with the LQT2 genotype were more likely to experience a cardiac event than women with the LQT1 or LQT3 genotype, and confirmed that the cardiac event risk during the high-risk postpartum period was reduced among women using beta-blocker therapy *(129)*.

Hypertrophic Cardiomyopathy: The majority of patients with hypertrophic cardiomyopathy have uneventful pregnancies *(130)*, although sudden death has been reported *(131)*. In a series of 199 live births, the total mortality rate in women with hypertrophic cardiomyopathy was 10 per 1000 live births. The two deaths were in particularly high-risk patients that had been advised to forgo pregnancy. Neither patient had a defibrillator; one died of witnessed sudden death, and one died of arrhythmia during labor *(132)*. Arrhythmias and symptoms other than heart failure were not common during pregnancy: sustained ventricular arrhythmias did not occur in any other of the patients; paroxysmal atrial fibrillation occurred in one; and syncope occurred in one. Patients in these last two categories had also experienced similar and recurrent events before pregnancy *(132)*. In another analysis of 271 pregnancies in 127 patients with hypertrophic cardiomyopathy, no arrhythmias or maternal deaths occurred *(130)*. During pregnancy, 7.1% experienced palpitations and 1.6% reported syncope. These symptoms had occurred prior to pregnancy in all of these patients *(130)*.

Structural Heart Disease: Due to technological developments and improved care over the past several decades, the number of adult women with congenital and acquired heart disease is increasing *(133)*. Surveys of outcomes of pregnancies in affected women reveal a low overall risk of maternal or neonatal mortality, yet significant cardiac and neonatal morbidity *(134)*. A prior history of arrhythmia has been found to be predictive of maternal cardiac complications *(134, 135)*. In women with a history of arrhythmias, the recurrence rate is high *(136)*. In one analysis, 44% (36 of 81 pregnancies) of women developed recurrences of tachyarrhythmias during pregnancy or in the early postpartum period. The recurrence rates in women with a history of supraventricular tachycardia, paroxysmal atrial fibrillation or flutter, and ventricular tachycardia were 50%, 52%, and 27%, respectively. Adverse fetal events occurred more commonly in women who developed antepartum arrhythmias, independent of other maternal and fetal risk factors *(136)*.

The incidence of arrhythmia during pregnancy in patients with repaired congenital heart disease is even higher *(137)*. Of 29 pregnancies in 27 women after cardiac repair, supraventricular tachycardia was identified in 15, ventricular tachycardia in 9, high-grade atrioventricular block in 4, and sick sinus syndrome in 3 *(137)*. Analysis of autonomic function during pregnancy in repaired congenital heart disease patients has revealed a significantly higher incidence of tachyarrhythmia compared with controls and postpartum, coupled with suppression of heart rate variability indices *(138)*. Arrhythmia is a particularly common and important complication during pregnancy in patients after atrial repair for transposition of the great arteries and tetralogy of Fallot *(139–141)*.

Syncope: Syncope is not uncommon during pregnancy. In a survey of normal pregnancies, 4.6% reported experiencing syncope and 10.3% reported recurrent presyncopal episodes sufficient to cause a change in activity or lifestyle *(142)*. Events were not associated with age, race, marital status, hemoglobin levels, blood pressure, occurrence of pregnancy complications, or presence of other underlying medical conditions *(142)*. However, symptoms such as palpitations, dizziness, and syncope are most commonly unrelated to arrhythmia, and the cause for symptoms in most episodes is unclear *(13)*. A comparison of symptomatic pregnant patients to an asymptomatic control group found a higher incidence of frequent ventricular ectopic activity in the symptomatic group, although correlation of symptoms and arrhythmia was seen in only 10% of episodes *(13)*.

Marfan Syndrome: The risk of aortic dissection associated with Marfan syndrome, an inherited connective tissue disorder, has been shown to increase during pregnancy as well as in labor and delivery in high-risk patients *(143, 144)*. In long-term follow-up, sudden arrhythmic death despite beta-blocker therapy has been described in patients with mitral valve prolapse, left ventricular dilatation, and ventricular couplets or tachycardia on Holter monitoring *(145)*. Because of the increased incidence of arrhythmias during pregnancy *(13)*, some have recommended consideration of defibrillator placement in high-risk Marfan syndrome patients prior to conception *(143)*.

LABOR AND DELIVERY

Labor and delivery are associated with significant hemodynamic changes, pain, and anxiety, all of which may increase the risk of arrhythmias. One Holter study of normal, healthy subjects showed that, excluding sinus rhythm variations, only a slight majority of the study subjects had arrhythmia at all; while only 2% had more complex arrhythmias, none of which had any clinical consequences for the mother or the newborn *(146)*. Another similar study revealed a high incidence of isolated atrial premature beats (90%) and ventricular premature beats (50%), which was similar to a comparable group of nonpregnant women in another study, but no sustained arrhythmias *(147)*.

POSTPARTUM AND LACTATION

The actual dose of a particular drug an infant receives when breastfeeding is dependent on several factors: the amount excreted into the breast milk, the daily volume of milk ingested, and the average plasma concentration in the mother *(148)*. Often, the only property known about a particular drug is protein binding. An analysis of infant drug concentration resulting from breastfeeding exposure revealed that for drugs that were at least 85% protein bound, measurable concentrations of drug in the infant did not occur if there was no placental exposure immediately prior to or during delivery. This suggests that knowledge of the protein binding properties of a drug can provide a convenient tool to estimate exposure of an infant to medication from breastfeeding *(148)*.

CONCLUSION

The treatment of arrhythmias in pregnancy is complicated by dynamic changes in maternal physiology and concern for fetal well-being. All antiarrhythmic drugs should be considered potentially toxic to the fetus, and whenever possible, nonpharmacologic measures should be counseled. Drug therapy is indicated only for intolerable symptoms, or if maternal or fetal well-being is compromised.

REFERENCES

1. Gordon MC (2007) Chapter 3 – maternal physiology. In: Obstetrics: normal and problem pregnancies, 5th edn. Churchill Livingstone, an imprint of Elsevier, Philadelphia
2. Theunissen IM, Parer JT (1994) Fluid and electrolytes in pregnancy. Clin Obstet Gynecol 37(1):3–15
3. Lindheimer MD, Davison JM (1995) Osmoregulation, the secretion of arginine vasopressin and its metabolism during pregnancy. Eur J Endocrinol 132(2):133–143
4. Miyamoto S, Shimokawa H, Sumioki H, Touno A, Nakano H (1988) Circadian rhythm of plasma atrial natriuretic peptide, aldosterone, and blood pressure during the third trimester in normal and preeclamptic pregnancies. Am J Obstet Gynecol 158(2):393–399
5. Duvekot JJ, Peeters LL (1994) Maternal cardiovascular hemodynamic adaptation to pregnancy. Obstet Gynecol Surv 49(12 Suppl):S1–S14
6. van Oppen AC, Stigter RH, Bruinse HW (1996) Cardiac output in normal pregnancy: a critical review. Obstet Gynecol 87(2):310–318
7. Hunter S, Robson SC (1992) Adaptation of the maternal heart in pregnancy. Br Heart J 68(6):540–543
8. Clark SL, Cotton DB, Pivarnik JM et al (1991) Position change and central hemodynamic profile during normal third-trimester pregnancy and post partum. Am J Obstet Gynecol 164(3):883–887
9. Clapp JF 3rd, Seaward BL, Sleamaker RH, Hiser J (1988) Maternal physiologic adaptations to early human pregnancy. Am J Obstet Gynecol 159(6):1456–1460
10. Granger JP (2002) Maternal and fetal adaptations during pregnancy: lessons in regulatory and integrative physiology. Am J Physiol Regul Integr Comp Physiol 283(6):R1289–R1292
11. Kametas NA, McAuliffe F, Hancock J, Chambers J, Nicolaides KH (2001) Maternal left ventricular mass and diastolic function during pregnancy. Ultrasound Obstet Gynecol 18(5):460–466
12. Zentner D, du Plessis M, Brennecke S, Wong J, Grigg L, Harrap SB (2009) Deterioration in cardiac systolic and diastolic function late in normal human pregnancy. Clin Sci (Lond) 116(7):599–606
13. Shotan A, Ostrzega E, Mehra A, Johnson JV, Elkayam U (1997) Incidence of arrhythmias in normal pregnancy and relation to palpitations, dizziness, and syncope. Am J Cardiol 79(8):1061–1064
14. Li JM, Nguyen C, Joglar JA, Hamdan MH, Page RL (2008) Frequency and outcome of arrhythmias complicating admission during pregnancy: experience from a high-volume and ethnically-diverse obstetric service. Clin Cardiol 31(11):538–541
15. Joglar JA, Page RL (1999) Treatment of cardiac arrhythmias during pregnancy: safety considerations. Drug Saf 20(1):85–94
16. Walbrandt-Pigarelli DL, Kraus CK, Potter BE (2008) Chapter 81. Pregnancy and lactation: therapeutic considerations. In: Pharmacotherapy: a pathophysiologic approach, 7th edn. McGraw-Hill
17. Hebert MF, Easterling TR, Kirby B et al (2008) Effects of pregnancy on CYP3A and P-glycoprotein activities as measured by disposition of midazolam and digoxin: a University of Washington specialized center of research study. Clin Pharmacol Ther 84(2):248–253
18. Hebert MF, Carr DB, Anderson GD et al (2005) Pharmacokinetics and pharmacodynamics of atenolol during pregnancy and postpartum. J Clin Pharmacol 45(1):25–33
19. Elkayam U, Goodwin TM (1995) Adenosine therapy for supraventricular tachycardia during pregnancy. Am J Cardiol 75(7):521–523
20. Hagley MT, Cole PL (1994) Adenosine use in pregnant women with supraventricular tachycardia. Ann Pharmacother 28(11):1241–1242
21. Joglar JA, Page RL (2001) Antiarrhythmic drugs in pregnancy. Curr Opin Cardiol 16(1):40–45
22. Page RL (1995) Treatment of arrhythmias during pregnancy. Am Heart J 130(4):871–876
23. Warnes CA (2007) Chapter 77 – pregnancy and heart disease. In: Braunwald's heart disease: a textbook of cardiovascular medicine, 8th edn. Philadelphia
24. Rogers MC, Willerson JT, Goldblatt A, Smith TW (1972) Serum digoxin concentrations in the human fetus, neonate and infant. N Engl J Med 287(20):1010–1013
25. Anderson GD (2005) Pregnancy-induced changes in pharmacokinetics: a mechanistic-based approach. Clin Pharmacokinet 44(10):989–1008
26. Lees KR, Rubin PC (1987) Treatment of cardiovascular diseases. Br Med J (Clin Res Ed) 294(6568):358–360
27. Chan V, Tse TF, Wong V (1978) Transfer of digoxin across the placenta and into breast milk. Br J Obstet Gynaecol 85(8):605–609
28. Wong RD, Murthy AR, Mathisen GE, Glover N, Thornton PJ (1992) Treatment of severe falciparum malaria during pregnancy with quinidine and exchange transfusion. Am J Med 92(5):561–562
29. Hill LM, Malkasian GD Jr (1979) The use of quinidine sulfate throughout pregnancy. Obstet Gynecol 54(3):366–368

30. Meyer J, Lackner J, Schochet S (1930) Paroxysmal tachycardia in pregnancy. JAMA 94:1901–1904
31. Allen NM, Page RL (1993) Procainamide administration during pregnancy. Clin Pharm 12(1):58–60
32. Wilson JT, Brown RD, Cherek DR et al (1980) Drug excretion in human breast milk: principles, pharmacokinetics and projected consequences. Clin Pharmacokinet. 5(1):1–66
33. Shaxted EJ, Milton PJ (1979) Disopyramide in pregnancy: a case report. Curr Med Res Opin 6(1):70–72
34. Leonard RF, Braun TE, Levy AM (1978) Initiation of uterine contractions by disopyramide during pregnancy. N Engl J Med 299(2):84–85
35. Tadmor OP, Keren A, Rosenak D et al (1990) The effect of disopyramide on uterine contractions during pregnancy. Am J Obstet Gynecol 162(2):482–486
36. Abbi M, Kriplani A, Singh B (1999) Preterm labor and accidental hemorrhage after disopyramide therapy in pregnancy. A case report. J Reprod Med 44(7):653–655
37. Brown WU, Bell GC, Lurie AO, Weiss B, Scanlon JW, Alper MH (1975) Newborn blood levels of lidocaine and mepivacaine in the first postnatal day following maternal epidural anesthesia. Anesthesiology 42(6):698–707
38. De Praeter C, Vanhaesebrouck P, De Praeter N, Govaert P, Bogaert M, Leroy J (1991) Episiotomy and neonatal lidocaine intoxication. Eur J Pediatr 150(9):685–686
39. Kim WY, Pomerance JJ, Miller AA (1979) Lidocaine intoxication in a newborn following local anesthesia for episiotomy. Pediatrics 64(5):643–645
40. Shnider SM, Way EL (1968) Plasma levels of lidocaine (Xylocaine) in mother and newborn following obstetrical conduction anesthesia: clinical applications. Anesthesiology 29(5):951–958
41. Brown WU Jr, Bell GC, Alper MH (1976) Acidosis, local anesthetics, and the newborn. Obstet Gynecol 48(1):27–30
42. Gregg AR, Tomich PG (1988) Mexilitene use in pregnancy. J Perinatol 8(1):33–35
43. Lownes HE, Ives TJ (1987) Mexiletine use in pregnancy and lactation. Am J Obstet Gynecol 157(2):446–447
44. Timmis AD, Jackson G, Holt DW (1980) Mexiletine for control of ventricular dysrhythmias in pregnancy. Lancet 2(8195 Pt 1):647–648
45. Villanova C, Muriago M, Nava F (1998) Arrhythmogenic right ventricular dysplasia: pregnancy under flecainide treatment. G Ital Cardiol 28(6):691–693
46. Ahmed K, Issawi I, Peddireddy R (1996) Use of flecainide for refractory atrial tachycardia of pregnancy. Am J Crit Care 5(4):306–308
47. Connaughton M, Jenkins BS (1994) Successful use of flecainide to treat new onset maternal ventricular tachycardia in pregnancy. Br Heart J 72(3):297
48. Doig JC, McComb JM, Reid DS (1992) Incessant atrial tachycardia accelerated by pregnancy. Br Heart J 67(3):266–268
49. Gerli S, Clerici G, Mattei A, Di Renzo GC (2006) Flecainide treatment of fetal tachycardia and hydrops fetalis in a twin pregnancy. Ultrasound Obstet Gynecol 28(1):117
50. Allan LD, Chita SK, Sharland GK, Maxwell D, Priestley K (1991) Flecainide in the treatment of fetal tachycardias. Br Heart J 65(1):46–48
51. Wagner X, Jouglard J, Moulin M, Miller AM, Petitjean J, Pisapia A (1990) Coadministration of flecainide acetate and sotalol during pregnancy: lack of teratogenic effects, passage across the placenta, and excretion in human breast milk. Am Heart J 119(3 Pt 1):700–702
52. Braverman AC, Bromley BS, Rutherford JD (1991) New onset ventricular tachycardia during pregnancy. Int J Cardiol 33(3):409–412
53. Libardoni M, Piovan D, Busato E, Padrini R (1991) Transfer of propafenone and 5-OH-propafenone to foetal plasma and maternal milk. Br J Clin Pharmacol 32(4):527–528
54. Frishman WH, Chesner M (1988) Beta-adrenergic blockers in pregnancy. Am Heart J 115(1 Pt 1):147–152
55. Lydakis C, Lip GY, Beevers M, Beevers DG (1999) Atenolol and fetal growth in pregnancies complicated by hypertension. Am J Hypertens 12(6):541–547
56. Lip GY, Beevers M, Churchill D, Shaffer LM, Beevers DG (1997) Effect of atenolol on birth weight. Am J Cardiol 79(10):1436–1438
57. Beardmore KS, Morris JM, Gallery ED (2002) Excretion of antihypertensive medication into human breast milk: a systematic review. Hypertens Pregnancy 21(1):85–95
58. Lindeberg S, Sandstrom B, Lundborg P, Regardh CG (1984) Disposition of the adrenergic blocker metoprolol in the late-pregnant woman, the amniotic fluid, the cord blood and the neonate. Acta Obstet Gynecol Scand Suppl 118:61–64
59. O'Hare MF, Leahey W, Murnaghan GA, McDevitt DG (1983) Pharmacokinetics of sotalol during pregnancy. Eur J Clin Pharmacol 24(4):521–524
60. O'Hare MF, Murnaghan GA, Russell CJ, Leahey WJ, Varma MP, McDevitt DG (1980) Sotalol as a hypotensive agent in pregnancy. Br J Obstet Gynaecol 87(9):814–820
61. O'Hare MF, Russell CJ, Leahey WJ, Varma MP, Murnaghan GA, McDevitt DG (1979) Sotalol in the management of hypertension complicating pregnancy [proceedings]. Br J Clin Pharmacol 8(4):390P–391P

62. Danielsson BR, Skold AC, Azarbayjani F (2001) Class III antiarrhythmics and phenytoin: teratogenicity due to embryonic cardiac dysrhythmia and reoxygenation damage. Curr Pharm Des 7(9):787–802

63. Webster WS, Brown-Woodman PD, Snow MD, Danielsson BR (1996) Teratogenic potential of almokalant, dofetilide, and d-sotalol: drugs with potassium channel blocking activity. Teratology 53(3):168–175

64. Burkart TA, Kron J, Miles WM, Conti JB, Gonzalez MD (2007) Successful termination of atrial flutter by ibutilide during pregnancy. Pacing Clin Electrophysiol 30(2):283–286

65. Kockova R, Kocka V, Kiernan T, Fahy GJ (2007) Ibutilide-induced cardioversion of atrial fibrillation during pregnancy. J Cardiovasc Electrophysiol 18(5):545–547

66. Marks TA, Terry RD (1996) Developmental toxicity of ibutilide fumarate in rats after oral administration. Teratology 54(3):157–164

67. McKenna WJ, Harris L, Rowland E, Whitelaw A, Storey G, Holt D (1983) Amiodarone therapy during pregnancy. Am J Cardiol 51(7):1231–1233

68. Robson DJ, Jeeva Raj MV, Storey GC, Holt DW (1985) Use of amiodarone during pregnancy. Postgrad Med J 61: 75–77

69. Foster CJ, Love HG (1988) Amiodarone in pregnancy. Case report and review of the literature. Int J Cardiol 20(3): 307–316

70. Strunge P, Frandsen J, Andreasen F (1988) Amiodarone during pregnancy. Eur Heart J 9(1):106–109

71. Plomp TA, Vulsma T, de Vijlder JJ (1992) Use of amiodarone during pregnancy. Eur J Obstet Gynecol Reprod Biol 43(3):201–207

72. Valensise H, Civitella C, Garzetti GG, Romanini C (1992) Amiodarone treatment in pregnancy for dilatative cardiomyopathy with ventricular malignant extrasystole and normal maternal and neonatal outcome. Prenat Diagn 12(9): 705–708

73. Magee LA, Downar E, Sermer M, Boulton BC, Allen LC, Koren G (1995) Pregnancy outcome after gestational exposure to amiodarone in Canada. Am J Obstet Gynecol 172(4 Pt 1):1307–1311

74. Bartalena L, Bogazzi F, Braverman LE, Martino E (2001) Effects of amiodarone administration during pregnancy on neonatal thyroid function and subsequent neurodevelopment. J Endocrinol Invest 24(2):116–130

75. Widerhorn J, Bhandari AK, Bughi S, Rahimtoola SH, Elkayam U (1991) Fetal and neonatal adverse effects profile of amiodarone treatment during pregnancy. Am Heart J 122(4 Pt 1):1162–1166

76. Pitcher D, Leather HM, Storey GC, Holt DW (1983) Amiodarone in pregnancy. Lancet 1(8324):597–598

77. Tan HL, Lie KI (2001) Treatment of tachyarrhythmias during pregnancy and lactation. Eur Heart J 22(6):458–464

78. Byerly WG, Hartmann A, Foster DE, Tannenbaum AK (1991) Verapamil in the treatment of maternal paroxysmal supraventricular tachycardia. Ann Emerg Med 20(5):552–554

79. Cleary-Goldman J, Salva CR, Infeld JI, Robinson JN (2003) Verapamil-sensitive idiopathic left ventricular tachycardia in pregnancy. J Matern Fetal Neonatal Med 14(2):132–135

80. Rey E, Duperron L, Gauthier R, Lemay M, Grignon A, LeLorier J (1985) Transplacental treatment of tachycardia-induced fetal heart failure with verapamil and amiodarone: a case report. Am J Obstet Gynecol 153(3): 311–312

81. Rimar JM (1985) Verapamil for fetal supraventricular tachycardia. MCN Am J Matern Child Nurs 10(5):345

82. Klein V, Repke JT (1984) Supraventricular tachycardia in pregnancy: cardioversion with verapamil. Obstet Gynecol 63(3 Suppl):16S–18S

83. Owen J, Colvin EV, Davis RO (1988) Fetal death after successful conversion of fetal supraventricular tachycardia with digoxin and verapamil. Am J Obstet Gynecol 158(5):1169–1170

84. Truccone N, Mariona F (1985) Intrauterine conversion of fetal supraventricular tachycardia with combination of digoxin and verapamil. Pediatr Pharmacol (New York) 5(2):149–153

85. Lilja H, Karlsson K, Lindecrantz K, Sabel KG (1984) Treatment of intrauterine supraventricular tachycardia with digoxin and verapamil. J Perinat Med 12(3):151–154

86. Lubbe WF (1987) Use of diltiazem during pregnancy. N Z Med J 100(818):121

87. Khandelwal M, Kumanova M, Gaughan JP, Reece EA (2002) Role of diltiazem in pregnant women with chronic renal disease. J Matern Fetal Neonatal Med 12(6):408–412

88. Cullhed I (1983) Cardioversion during pregnancy. A case report. Acta Med Scand 214(2):169–172

89. Finlay AY, Edmunds V (1979) D.C. cardioversion in pregnancy. Br J Clin Pract 33(3):88–94

90. Klepper I (1981) Cardioversion in late pregnancy. The anaesthetic management of a case of Wolff-Parkinson-White syndrome. Anaesthesia 36(6):611–616

91. Ogburn PL Jr, Schmidt G, Linman J, Cefalo RC (1982) Paroxysmal tachycardia and cardioversion during pregnancy. J Reprod Med 27(6):359–362

92. Schroeder JS, Harrison DC (1971) Repeated cardioversion during pregnancy. Treatment of refractory paroxysmal atrial tachycardia during 3 successive pregnancies. Am J Cardiol 27(4):445–446

93. Rosemond RL (1993) Cardioversion during pregnancy. JAMA 269(24):3167

94. Barnes EJ, Eben F, Patterson D (2002) Direct current cardioversion during pregnancy should be performed with facilities available for fetal monitoring and emergency caesarean section. BJOG 109(12):1406–1407

95. Atta E, Gardner M (2007) Cardiopulmonary resuscitation in pregnancy. Obstet Gynecol Clin North Am 34(3): 585–597

96. Morris S, Stacey M (2003) Resuscitation in pregnancy. BMJ 327(7426):1277–1279

97. Mallampalli A, Guy E (2005) Cardiac arrest in pregnancy and somatic support after brain death. Crit Care Med 33(10 Suppl):S325–331

98. Part 10.8: Cardiac Arrest Associated With Pregnancy. Circulation. December 13, 2005; 112 (24_suppl):IV-150–IV-153

99. Goodwin AP, Pearce AJ (1992)The human wedge. A manoeuvre to relieve aortocaval compression during resuscitation in late pregnancy. Anaesthesia 47(5):433–434

100. Nanson J, Elcock D, Williams M, Deakin CD (2001) Do physiological changes in pregnancy change defibrillation energy requirements? Br J Anaesth 87(2):237–239

101. Suri V, Keepanasseril A, Aggarwal N, Vijayvergiya R, Chopra S, Rohilla M (2009) Maternal complete heart block in pregnancy: analysis of four cases and review of management. J Obstet Gynaecol Res 35(3):434–437

102. Minassian VA, Jazayeri A (2002) Favorable outcome in a pregnancy with complete fetal heart block and severe bradycardia. Obstet Gynecol 100(5 Pt 2):1087–1089

103. Dalvi BV, Chaudhuri A, Kulkarni HL, Kale PA (1992) Therapeutic guidelines for congenital complete heart block presenting in pregnancy. Obstet Gynecol 79(5 Pt 2):802–804

104. Bemiller CR, Forker AD, Morgan JR (1970) Complete heart block, prosthetic aortic valve, and successful pregnancy. JAMA 214(5):915

105. Ginns HM, Hollinrake K (1970) Complete heart block in pregnancy treated with an internal cardiac pacemaker. J Obstet Gynaecol Br Commonw 77(8):710–712

106. Schonbrun M, Rowland W, Quiroz AC (1966) Complete heart block in pregnancy. Successful use of an intravenous pacemaker in 2 patients during labor. Obstet Gynecol 27(2):243–246

107. Middleton EB, Lee YC (1971) Pregnancy associated with cardiac pacemaker generator implanted in abdominal wall. A case report. Obstet Gynecol 38(2):272–275

108. Bilge M, Guler N, Eryonucu B (1999) Recurrent pulmonary emboli and thrombus attached to a permanently implanted pacemaker wire in pregnancy. Acta Cardiol 54(2):97–99

109. Sharma JB, Malhotra M, Pundir P (2000) Successful pregnancy outcome with cardiac pacemaker after complete heart block. Int J Gynaecol Obstet 68(2):145–146

110. Pedrinazzi C, Gazzaniga P, Durin O, Tovena D, Inama G (2008) Implantation of a permanent pacemaker in a pregnant woman under the guidance of electrophysiologic signals and transthoracic echocardiography. J Cardiovasc Med (Hagerstown) 9(11):1169–1172

111. Antonelli D, Bloch L, Rosenfeld T (1999) Implantation of permanent dual chamber pacemaker in a pregnant woman by transesophageal echocardiographic guidance. Pacing Clin Electrophysiol 22(3):534–535

112. Gudal M, Kervancioglu C, Oral D, Gurel T, Erol C, Sonel A (1987) Permanent pacemaker implantation in a pregnant woman with the guidance of ECG and two-dimensional echocardiography. Pacing Clin Electrophysiol 10(3 Pt 1): 543–545

113. Piper JM, Berkus M, Ridgway LE 3rd (1992) Pregnancy complicated by chronic cardiomyopathy and an automatic implantable cardioverter defibrillator. Am J Obstet Gynecol 167(2):506–507

114. Isaacs JD, Mulholland DH, Hess LW, Allbert JR, Martin RW (1993) Pregnancy in a woman with an automatic implantable cardioverter-defibrillator. A case report. J Reprod Med 38(6):487–488

115. Bonini W, Botto GL, Broffoni T, Dondina C (2000) Pregnancy with an ICD and a documented ICD discharge. Europace 2(1):87–90

116. Olufolabi AJ, Charlton GA, Allen SA, Mettam IM, Roberts PR (2002) Use of implantable cardioverter defibrillator and anti-arrhythmic agents in a parturient. Br J Anaesth 89(4):652–655

117. Abello M, Peinado R, Merino JL et al (2003) Cardioverter defibrillator implantation in a pregnant woman guided with transesophageal echocardiography. Pacing Clin Electrophysiol 26(9):1913–1914

118. Doyle NM, Monga M, Montgomery B, Dougherty AH (2005) Arrhythmogenic right ventricular cardiomyopathy with implantable cardioverter defibrillator placement in pregnancy. J Matern Fetal Neonatal Med 18(2):141–144

119. Natale A, Davidson T, Geiger MJ, Newby K (1997) Implantable cardioverter-defibrillators and pregnancy: a safe combination? Circulation 96(9):2808–2812

120. Bongiorni MG, Di Cori A, Soldati E et al (2008) Radiofrequency catheter ablation of atrioventricular nodal reciprocating tachycardia using intracardiac echocardiography in pregnancy. Europace 10(8):1018–1021

121. Kanjwal Y, Kosinski D, Kanj M, Thomas W, Grubb B (2005) Successful radiofrequency catheter ablation of left lateral accessory pathway using transseptal approach during pregnancy. J Interv Card Electrophysiol 13(3): 239–242

122. Pagad SV, Barmade AB, Toal SC, Vora AM, Lokhandwala YY (2004) 'Rescue' radiofrequency ablation for atrial tachycardia presenting as cardiomyopathy in pregnancy. Indian Heart J 56(3):245–247

123. Bombelli F, Lagona F, Salvati A, Catalfamo L, Ferrari AG, Pappone C (2003) Radiofrequency catheter ablation in drug refractory maternal supraventricular tachycardias in advanced pregnancy. Obstet Gynecol 102(5 Pt 2):1171–1173

124. Dominguez A, Iturralde P, Hermosillo AG, Colin L, Kershenovich S, Garrido LM (1999) Successful radiofrequency ablation of an accessory pathway during pregnancy. Pacing Clin Electrophysiol 22(1 Pt 1):131–134

125. Gleicher N, Meller J, Sandler RZ, Sullum S (1981) Wolff-Parkinson-White syndrome in pregnancy. Obstet Gynecol 58(6):748–752

126. Kounis NG, Zavras GM, Papadaki PJ, Soufras GD, Kitrou MP, Poulos EA (1995) Pregnancy-induced increase of supraventricular arrhythmias in Wolff-Parkinson-White syndrome. Clin Cardiol 18(3):137–140

127. Schwartz PJ, Priori SG, Spazzolini C et al (2001) Genotype-phenotype correlation in the long-QT syndrome: gene-specific triggers for life-threatening arrhythmias. Circulation 103(1):89–95

128. Rashba EJ, Zareba W, Moss AJ et al (1998) Influence of pregnancy on the risk for cardiac events in patients with hereditary long QT syndrome. LQTS investigators. Circulation 97(5):451–456

129. Seth R, Moss AJ, McNitt S et al (2007) Long QT syndrome and pregnancy. J Am Coll Cardiol 49(10):1092–1098

130. Thaman R, Varnava A, Hamid MS et al (2003) Pregnancy related complications in women with hypertrophic cardiomyopathy. Heart 89(7):752–756

131. Pelliccia F, Cianfrocca C, Gaudio C, Reale A (1992) Sudden death during pregnancy in hypertrophic cardiomyopathy. Eur Heart J 13(3):421–423

132. Autore C, Conte MR, Piccininno M et al (2002) Risk associated with pregnancy in hypertrophic cardiomyopathy. J Am Coll Cardiol 40(10):1864–1869

133. Proceedings of the 32ND Bethesda Conference (2001) Care of the adult with congenital heart disease. J Am College Cardiol 37:1161–1198

134. Siu SC, Sermer M, Harrison DA et al (1997) Risk and predictors for pregnancy-related complications in women with heart disease. Circulation 96(9):2789–2794

135. Siu SC, Sermer M, Colman JM et al (2001) Prospective multicenter study of pregnancy outcomes in women with heart disease. Circulation 104(5):515–521

136. Silversides CK, Harris L, Haberer K, Sermer M, Colman JM, Siu SC (2006) Recurrence rates of arrhythmias during pregnancy in women with previous tachyarrhythmia and impact on fetal and neonatal outcomes. Am J Cardiol 97(8):1206–1212

137. Tateno S, Niwa K, Nakazawa M, Akagi T, Shinohara T, Yasuda T (2003) Arrhythmia and conduction disturbances in patients with congenital heart disease during pregnancy: multicenter study. Circ J 67(12):992–997

138. Niwa K, Tateno S, Akagi T et al (2007) Arrhythmia and reduced heart rate variability during pregnancy in women with congenital heart disease and previous reparative surgery. Int J Cardiol 122(2):143–148

139. Drenthen W, Pieper PG, Ploeg M et al (2005) Risk of complications during pregnancy after Senning or Mustard (atrial) repair of complete transposition of the great arteries. Eur Heart J 26(23):2588–2595

140. Megerian G, Bell JG, Huhta JC, Bottalico JN, Weiner S (1994) Pregnancy outcome following Mustard procedure for transposition of the great arteries: a report of five cases and review of the literature. Obstet Gynecol 83(4):512–516

141. Meijer JM, Pieper PG, Drenthen W et al (2005) Pregnancy, fertility, and recurrence risk in corrected tetralogy of Fallot. Heart 91(6):801–805

142. Gibson PS, Powrie R, Pipert J (2001) Prevalence of syncope and recurrent presyncope during pregnancy. Obstet Gynecol Surv 97:S41–S42

143. Goland S, Elkayam U (2009) Cardiovascular problems in pregnant women with marfan syndrome. Circulation 119(4):619–623

144. Meijboom LJ, Vos FE, Timmermans J, Boers GH, Zwinderman AH, Mulder BJ (2005) Pregnancy and aortic root growth in the Marfan syndrome: a prospective study. Eur Heart J 26(9):914–920

145. Yetman AT, Bornemeier RA, McCrindle BW (2003) Long-term outcome in patients with Marfan syndrome: is aortic dissection the only cause of sudden death? J Am Coll Cardiol 41(2):329–332

146. Berlinerblau R, Yessian A, Lichstein E, Haberman S, Oruci E, Jewelewicz R (2001) Maternal arrhythmias of normal labor and delivery. Gynecol Obstet Invest 52(2):128–131

147. Romem A, Romem Y, Katz M, Battler A (2004) Incidence and characteristics of maternal cardiac arrhythmias during labor. Am J Cardiol 93(7):931–933

148. Anderson GD (2006) Using pharmacokinetics to predict the effects of pregnancy and maternal-infant transfer of drugs during lactation. Expert Opin Drug Metab Toxicol 2(6):947–960

149. American Academy of Pediatrics Committee on Drugs (2001) The Transfer of Drugs and Other Chemicals into Human Milk. Pediatrics 108(3):776–789

17 Arrhythmias in Children

Bhavya Trivedi and Ronald Kanter

CONTENTS

Abstract

Most cardiac arrhythmias may occur in the fetus, infant, child, and adolescent as a result of congenital arrhythmia substrates or in response to hemodynamic perturbations related to structural defects or subsequent surgical treatments. Unrelated to surgery, arrhythmias are especially prevalent in persons having Ebstein anomaly of the tricuspid valve, congenitally corrected transposition, or heterotaxy. Atrial arrhythmias are important following the older atrial redirection operations for d-transposition of the great arteries and following the Fontan operation for single ventricle physiology. Catheter ablation of these substrates is now possible using electroanatomic mapping systems and high output radiofrequency generators. Ventricular tachycardia and sudden death are of concern in some patients following surgical repair of tetralogy of Fallot and left ventricular outflow tract obstruction. Among children having structurally normal hearts, atrioventricular reciprocating tachycardia and atrioventricular nodal reentrant tachycardia comprise the majority of tachyarrhythmias in infants and teenagers, respectively. Catheter ablation has largely supplanted pharmacological therapy for supraventricular tachycardias in children older than about 5 years, with results comparable to those in adults. Risk of collateral damage to structures in the growing heart makes catheter ablation less attractive as primary therapy in smaller children. Indications for device implantation are being established for the young and may be applied down to newborns (pacemakers) and older infants (implantable cardioverter-defibrillators). Planning such implantations in children and in patients having congenital heart disease requires careful consideration of somatic growth, cardiac anatomy, and venous caliber.

Key Words: L-transposition of the great arteries; Tricuspid atresia; Ebstein anomaly of the tricuspid valve; Wolff-Parkinson-White syndrome; Atrioventricular septal defect; Heterotaxy; Asplenia; Polysplenia; Atrial septal defect; Ventricular septal defect; Pulmonic stenosis; Aortic stenosis; Sinoatrial node dysfunction; D-transpoistion of the great arteries; Mustard operation; Senning operation; Fontan

From: *Contemporary Cardiology: Management of Cardiac Arrhythmias*
Edited by: Gan-Xin Yan, Peter R. Kowey, DOI 10.1007/978-1-60761-161-5_17
© Springer Science+Business Media, LLC 2011

operation; Intraatrial reentry tachycardia; Ventricular tachycardia; Right bundle branch block; Cox III operation; Tetralogy of Fallot; Congenital atrioventricular block; Acquired atrioventricular block; Nkx2.5 transcription factor; Tbx5 transciption factor; Holt–Oram syndrome; Sudden cardiac death; Atrioventricular reciprocating tachycardia; Atrioventricular nodal reentrant tachycardia; Chaotic atrial tachycardia; Congenital junctional ectopic tachycardia; Post-operative junctional ectopic tachycardia; Radiofrequency catheter ablation; Cryoablation; Electroanatomic mapping; Prospective Assessment after Pediatric Catheter Ablation (PAPCA); Pacemaker; Implantabale cardioverter-defibrillator.

INTRODUCTION

Arrhythmias can occur in children with or without associated congenital heart disease (CHD). Based upon emergency room visits, among children with structurally normal hearts, 0.05% will experience an arrhythmia before the age of 18 *(1)*. Congenital heart defects occur in 0.8% of live births, and certain structural abnormalities are associated with arrhythmias. After surgical repair of many types CHD, fibrosis, chronic hypoxia, hypertrophy, chamber dilation, patches, and suture lines can create a substrate for arrhythmias.

Over the past 20 years, improved awareness of normal children with arrhythmias as well as the increasing prevalence of tachyarrhythmias in children with CHD (due to improved survival/surgical techniques) has resulted in improved medical treatment and the emergence of ablative techniques. Pacemaker and ICD devices are also widely utilized in the management of children and adult congenital patients with arrhythmias. The approach to arrhythmias in children must be framed in the context of somatic growth, cardiac developmental changes, maturation of ion channel expression, and autonomic nervous system influences.

This chapter reviews the most common arrhythmias in children, electrophysiological abnormalities associated with specific congenital heart malformations, post-surgical arrhythmias in patients of all ages having CHD, and pharmacologic and non-pharmacologic therapies for pediatric arrhythmias.

SECTION I: CONGENITAL ABNORMALITIES OF THE SPECIALIZED CONDUCTION SYSTEM

In the primitive heart tube, all cardiomyocytes have automaticity and are capable of initiating the heart beat. During development, most cardiomyocytes mature to become contractile working myocardium, while the cells in the four intersegmental zones retain some of their "primitive" characteristics and later differentiate into the specialized conduction system including the sinoatrial node (SAN), atrioventricular node (AVN), and His–Purkinje network (see Fig. 1) *(2)*. While this "four ring theory" remains controversial, immunohistochemical and molecular markers are beginning to unravel the roles that multiple families of transcription factors play in conduction system development in those anatomic zones, especially the T-box (Tbx2 and Tbx3) and homeodomain (Nkx2.5) families. There is additional contribution of neural crest and epicardium-derived cells, especially to the His bundle and Purkinje fibers *(2)*. The anatomic location and often the function of these structures depend upon the pattern of development of adjacent structures including atrial situs, ventricular looping, and septation. As the right side of the primitive atrium joins the bulbus cordis, a portion of this ring of conduction tissue translates rightward and superiorly effectively positioning the compact AVN adjacent to the central fibrous body above the AV valves (arrow in Fig. 1). The position of the AVN will influence the length and course of the penetrating bundle.

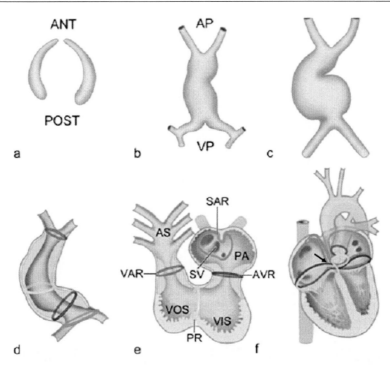

Fig. 1. Contemporary theory of development of the specialized conduction system. (**a**) Paired cardiogenic plates derived from splanchnic mesoderm; (**b**) initially straight heart tube formed from fusion of the cardiogenic plates; (**c**) normal rightward ("dextro") looping of the heart tube; (**d**) following initiation of looping, rings at transitional zones appear; (**e**) during later development and early septation, these rings appear at the putative junctions between chambers: SAR=sinoatrial ring (*teal*), AVR=atrioventricular ring (*blue*), PR=primary ring at the bulboventricular foramen (*yellow*), and ventriculoarterial ring=VAR (*green*); (**f**) position of rings in the developed heart. ANT: anterior; AP: arterial pole; AS: aortic sac; PA: primitive atrium; POST: posterior; SV: sinus venosus; VIS: ventricular inlet segment; VOS: ventricular outlet segment. Adapted with permission from Ref. (*2*).

Levotransposition of the Great Arteries

Levotransposition of the great arteries (L-TGA) is also known as congenitally corrected transposition, since there are both atrioventricular and ventriculoarterial discordance. This results in systemic venous return ultimately being directed to the pulmonary arteries and pulmonary venous return to the aorta. The AV valves form in association with their usual morphological ventricle, resulting in a systemic venous mitral valve and pulmonary venous tricuspid valve. The most common associated structural heart defects include ventricular septal defect (VSD) and pulmonic stenosis. Due to l-looping of the ventricles, the AVN becomes situated anteriorly in the right atrium just lateral to the area of mitral–pulmonary valve continuity. This creates a longer than normal His bundle that courses anterior to the pulmonary valve annulus and then bifurcates into the bundle branches at the crest of the muscular septum. In the presence of a VSD, the His bundle is located at the anterior–superior margin of the defect (see Fig. 2). Dual AVNs may be present with a second, often diminutive node anterior to the coronary sinus (CS) ostium. In rare circumstances, this secondary AVN also connects to the ventricular myocardium via its own penetrating bundle or can have a sling of conduction tissue connecting to the primary anterior AVN (*Mönckeberg sling*).

The anatomic orientation of the conduction tissue in L-TGA creates an ECG pattern with a QS or qR in V_1 and a rS or RS in V_6 (see Fig. 3). There is a greater than expected incidence of mirror-image

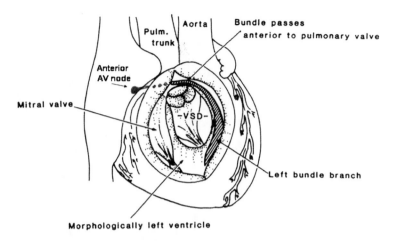

Fig. 2. Congenitally corrected transposition of the great arteries (l-TGA) showing the relationship of the specialized atrioventricular (AV) conduction system to a large ventricular septal defect (VSD).

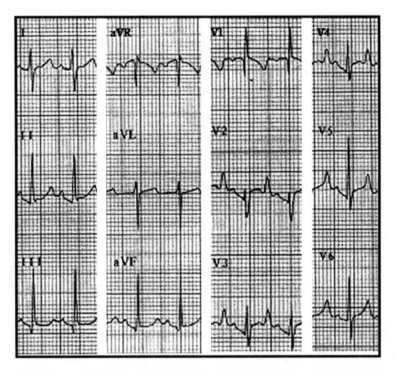

Fig. 3. 12-lead ECG from a 3-year-old having congenitally corrected transposition (l-TGA) and mild pulmonic stenosis, illustrating a septal q wave in V1, absent q wave in V6, and hypertrophy of the right-sided ventricle.

situs inversus with congenitally corrected transposition. In that case, the AVN is located normally at the apex of the triangle of Koch, since the ventricles are d-looped.

The AVN and penetrating bundle are not only malpositioned in l-TGA, but histopathologic studies have demonstrated fibrous infiltration of the elongated His bundle. This may result in complete electrical disruption and AV block. Accordingly, 3.7–18.2% of newborns with l-TGA have congenital complete heart block (CHB) and the remainder carry a 2% per year risk of development of CHB *(3)*. Prophylactic pacemaker placement is not necessary, unless there is significant associated structural abnormalities, or – in a child – if the baseline heart rate is less than 50 beats/min. The postoperative risk of CHB in children undergoing VSD repair is significantly higher in those with l-TGA than in those with ventricular d-looping.

Paroxysmal supraventricular tachycardia (PSVT), usually atrioventricular tachycardia (AVRT), is also more frequent in children with l-TGA compared to normal children. The substrate for AVRT is usually single or multiple accessory AV pathways associated with the left-sided tricuspid valve. This valve may also be malformed, so-called Ebsteinoid malformation. This may lead to significant tricuspid valve regurgitation, atrial enlargement, and an increased risk of atrial tachyarrhythmias in older patients. Adult congenital patients with l-TGA are also at increased risk for symptomatic ventricular tachycardia (VT) *(4, 5)*.

Tricuspid Atresia

In tricuspid atresia, the tricuspid valve does not form, leaving a muscular floor between the right atrium and the right ventricle. In this single ventricle physiology situation, a large atrial septal communication is required for survival. Although these patients cannot be staged to a two-ventricle repair, there may be a right ventricle and outflow tract, depending upon the size of the commonly associated VSD. The AVN is located posteroinferiorly, related to both the muscular plate at the floor of the right atrium and the coronary sinus ostium.

The surface ECG is influenced primarily by the anatomy and hemodynamics, but there typically is right atrial enlargement and minimal right- and prominent left-sided forces. Left axis deviation is present in two-thirds of patients, owing to the course of the specialized conduction system and its relationship to the VSD (see Fig. 4). In 0.29–0.51% there is the appearance of preexcitation, but only 10% of these patients have a true accessory pathway. The term *pseudopreexcitation* is applied to those without an accessory pathway. The true accessory pathways are usually right sided and can be septal. With an older type of Fontan operation involving right atrial appendage to right ventricular outflow connection (Bjork modification), an acquired electrical communication may occur across the suture line, resulting in preexcitation and even AVRT *(6)*. This can be treated with catheter ablation techniques.

Ebstein Anomaly of the Tricuspid Valve

In Ebstein anomaly, there is incomplete delamination of the septal and posterior leaflets of the tricuspid valve from underlying right ventricular myocardium. The combination of leaflet malformation and apical displacement of leaflet coaptation results in tricuspid regurgitation. The functional right atrium may be massively dilated, because it includes the thin-walled, poorly contractile "atrialized" portion of the right ventricle (the region between the leaflet coaptation plane and the normally located plane of the valve annulus) plus the anatomical right atrium. Twenty percent of patients have an accessory AV pathway, which may be manifest. The WPW pattern may be subtle due to relatively slow conduction in atrial myocardium and the inlet portion of the right ventricle. In the absence of WPW pattern, the surface ECG reflects hemodynamic abnormalities and probable hypoplasia of the right bundle branch, with right bundle branch block (RBBB, often with a complex RSR'S' pattern) being a common finding even in those who have had no surgical intervention (see Fig. 5).

Patients with Ebstein anomaly have a high incidence of arrhythmias related to both hemodynamic abnormalities and their accessory connections. Common presentations in children include shortness of breath, cyanosis, and exercise intolerance. In contrast, the most common presenting symptom (42%) in teenagers and adults is arrhythmia. Wolff–Parkinson–White pattern does not seem to contribute

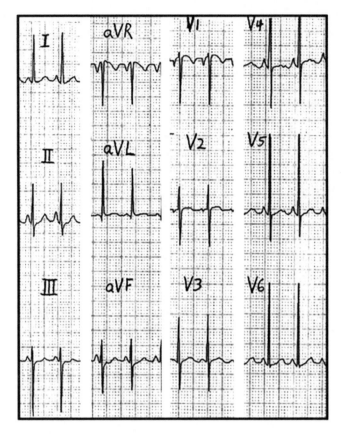

Fig. 4. 12-lead ECG from a 6-month old having tricuspid atresia. Note the relative absence of right-sided forces (rS in V1), short PR interval, right atrial enlargement, and left axis deviation.

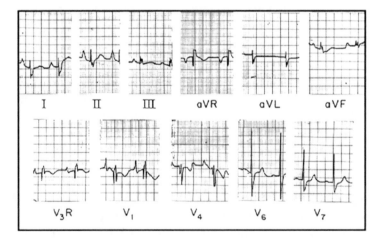

Fig. 5. ECG from a 19-year old having Ebstein anomaly of the tricuspid valve. Note the right atrial enlargement and the complex right bundle branch block pattern (rSR'S' in V1).

to an increased risk of sudden death. Accessory connections are almost always right sided and 50% of affected patients have multiple bypass tracts *(7)*, including the atriofascicular variety of Mahaim fibers. Most pathways are associated with the inferior half of the tricuspid valve annulus (ranging from right posteroseptal to right posterolateral by traditional nomenclature). Catheter ablation is the standard of care in treatment of these accessory pathways with acute success rates of 85% *(7)* but with a higher than usual recurrence rate. The major difficulty with ablative therapy is identification of the true tricuspid valve annulus due to loss of typical anatomic landmarks and presence of fractionated electrograms within the peri-annular right ventricle. Such pacing maneuvers as placement of premature atrial beats into AVRT may be employed to discriminate electrograms. Right coronary angiography can help locate the AV groove and identify the true tricuspid valve annulus. Operators have also reported placement of 2.5 Fr electrode catheters into the right coronary artery to aid in mapping *(8)*.

Atrioventricular Septal Defect

In all variations of atrioventricular septal defect (AVSD), there is no true central fibrous body. Hence, the specialized conduction tissue is always posteroinferiorly displaced from its normal location at the junction of the atrial and ventricular septa, and the AVN is found close to the CS ostium. The elongated penetrating bundle courses inferior to the VSD rim, and there is relative underdevelopment of the left bundle branch, creating the left axis deviation and counterclockwise frontal QRS vector on the surface ECG (see Fig. 6). WPW rarely coexists with AVSD with most accessory pathways being posteroseptal.

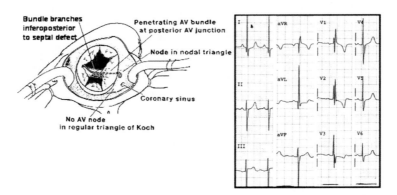

Fig. 6. Composite figure illustrating features of atrioventricular septal defect (AVSD). *Left:* Surgeon's view of the single AV valve from within the open right atrium, demonstrating the location of the specialized AV conduction system. The inferiorly positioned AV node near the coronary sinus ostium gives rise to the penetrating bundle along the margin of the inlet ventricular septal defect. *Right:* 12-lead ECG showing superior QRS axis and right ventricular hypertrophy.

Heterotaxy

Heterotaxy is a broad term encompassing abnormalities of visceral and vascular situs. Although multiple variations in thoracic and abdominal lateralization can exist, two general patterns of malformations are most commonly described; the cardiac-oriented euphemisms, right atrial isomerism ("asplenia"), and left atrial isomerism ("polysplenia") are applied to these. Important cardiac defects coexist with both major categories of heterotaxy (see Fig. 7). Since differentiation of the SAN relies

Right Isomerism   **Left Isomerism**

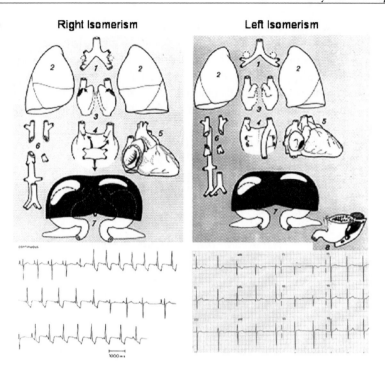

Fig. 7. Composite figure illustrating morphologic and electrocardiologic features of the heterotaxy. *Right isomerism, top:* 1-bilateral eparterial bronchi; 2-bilaterial trilobed lungs; 3-bilateral right atrial appendages with twin sinoatrial nodes (*arrowheads*); 4-total anomalous pulmonary venous connection; 5-AV septal defect with pulmonary atresia; 6-intact inferior vena cava with bilateral superior vena cavae; 7-transverse liver, absent spleen, and abnormal visceral situs. *Right isomerism, bottom:* Continuous rhythm strip showing varying sinus pacemaker, followed by varying PR interval and QRS morphology, representing duplication of the specialized AV conduction system. *Left isomerism, top:* 1-bilateral hyparterial bronchi; 2-bilateral bilobed lungs; 3-bilateral left atrial appendages with absence of sinoatrial node tissue; 4 and 6-ipsilateral pulmonary venous return, interrupted inferior vena cava with azygos continuation to superior vena cava, bilateral superior vena cavae; 5-AV septal defect; 7-transverse liver, abnormal visceral situs; 8-multiple spleens. *Left isomerism, bottom:* 12-lead ECG showing junctional rhythm. (Adapted with permission from: McGraw-Hill, New York, NY. In: Kanter RJ, Knilans T (eds) Pediatric arrhythmias. Hurst's the heart. 2008. pp 1121–1142).

upon formation of the superior caval-to-*right* atrial junction, patients with polysplenia often have low atrial rhythm, junctional rhythm, and other evidence for sinus node dysfunction. In addition, patients having polysplenia may have congenital or develop acquired heart block, independent of other cardiac anomalies such as AVSD or VSD. This is more common in the presence of ventricular l-looping. Conversely, patients having asplenia may have duplication of sinus node tissue with alternating P wave morphologies, each having an inferior axis. In both categories of heterotaxy, the unusually prevalent combination of double outlet right ventricle and AVSD may be associated with duplication of the AV conduction system, even to the extent of double AV nodes, His bundles, and bundle branch systems. This may manifest as gradual shifts in rhythm, involving different P waves, PR intervals, and QRS morphologies. These patients may also have a paroxysmal reentrant tachycardia, utilizing one AV node in the antegrade direction and the other in the retrograde direction, so-called nodo-nodal reentrant tachycardia. This can be treated by catheter ablation of the retrogradedly conducting AV node.

SECTION II: ARRHYTHMIAS ASSOCIATED WITH COMMON CONGENITAL HEART DEFECTS

Atrial Septal Defect

Isolated ostium secundum atrial septal defect (ASD) is the second most common congenital heart defect, excluding bicuspid aortic valve. If left unrepaired into adulthood, chronic left to right shunting with consequent right atrial and right ventricular dilatation leads to an increased incidence of atrial arrhythmias. Sinus node dysfunction has been reported in 22–65% in adults with unrepaired ASDs *(9, 10)*, and almost all patients have ECG evidence of right ventricular conduction delay. For atrial tachyarrhythmias, the primary risk factors are older age at presentation, older age at surgery, higher ratio of pulmonary to systemic blood flow, elevated mean pulmonary artery pressure, pre- or immediate postoperative atrial arrhythmia, and occurrence of immediate postoperative junctional rhythm *(11)*. Atrial flutter and/or atrial fibrillation is seen in 50% of patients who present over age 50 and 80% of patients who present over age 80 *(12)*. Surgical repair or device closure beyond early adulthood does not appear to decrease the risk for atrial flutter or atrial fibrillation. In contrast, only 4% of children will experience an atrial tahcyarrhythmia if they undergo ASD repair under age 11. Catheter ablation of atrial flutter and other macroreentrant atrial tachycardias is effective in nearly all cases with low recurrence rates. The cavotricuspid isthmus, right atriotomy site, and, less commonly, the tissue surrounding the ASD patch are regions of interest to the ablationist.

Since the late 1990s, an ever increasing number of ASDs have been closed with transcatheter devices. In these procedures, transient AV block has been reported in 6% with permanent AV block requiring pacemaker placement in only 0.1% *(13, 14)*. These numbers vary greatly depending on the device (Amplatzer, Helex, Cardioseal). Device closure does not alter the risk of atrial tachyarrhythmias, although the device-related risk of arrhythmia is very low *(15)*.

Ventricular Septal Defect (VSD)

Isolated VSD is the most common congenital heart defect, again, excluding bicuspid aortic valve. The pathophysiology involves volume overload of the right ventricle, pulmonary arteries, left atrium, and left ventricle, proportionate to the amount of left to right shunting. In the case of large defects, if left unrepaired, irreversible pulmonary hypertension is the result; this is so-called Eisenmenger physiology. Among patients having a VSD and enrolled in the Second Natural History Study, there was a 15.3% incidence of SVT (versus 5% of controls) and an even higher incidence of premature ventricular beats *(16)*. More serious ventricular arrhythmias including ventricular couplets, multiform PVCs, and ventricular tachycardia also were observed. Table 1 summarizes the incidence and associated risk factors *(17)* in this patient group. Arrhythmia risk in adults with VSDs has been shown to be independent of VSD size. The causal relationship between VSD and sudden unexplained death (4% incidence) is unclear but is higher than age-matched controls (Table 1), thus warranting close surveillance of patients who have significant hemodynamic alterations. Experience with catheter-delivered device closure of VSDs in older patients is limited but does not appear to be associated with long-term arrhythmias or conduction defects *(18, 19)*. In infants, such devices for perimembranous defects may be associated with AV conduction system damage *(20)*.

Pulmonic Stenosis

The long-term risk of arrhythmia in patients with pulmonic stenosis was also investigated in the Second Natural History Study. Right ventricular outflow obstruction creates RV hypertension and hypertrophy. After surgical or balloon valvotomy, right ventricular volume overload and dilatation from pulmonary insufficiency may occur. The specific effects of these hemodyanamic alterations on arrhythmogenesis in patients having isolated pulmonic stenosis are largely unexplored, in contrast to

Table 1
Serious Ventricular Arrhythmias in Patients Having Ventricular Septal Defect, Pulmonic Stenosis,
or Aortic Stenosis

| Congenital heart defect | Serious ventricular arrhythmias[1] | | | Sudden unexplained death |
	Incidence (%)	Independent risk factors	Odds ratio	Incidence (%)
Ventricular septal defect	31.4	Main pulmonary artery pressure[2]	1.49	4.0
		Age[3]	1.51	
		NYHA class[3]	8.53	
		Cardiomegaly[3]	2.79	
Pulmonic stenosis	29.7	Age[2]	1.05	0.5
		Age[3]	1.04	
		NYHA Class[3]	7.93	
		Cardiomegaly[3]	3.21	
Aortic stenosis	44.8	Left ventricular end-diastolic pressure[2]	2.02	5.4
		Aortic regurgitation[3]	11.70	
		Gender[3]	4.10	
		Prior aortic valve replacement[3]	4.80	

[1] Defined as ventricular couplets, multiform ventricular premature beats, or ventricular tachycardia.
[2] Upon entry into First Natural History Study.
[3] Upon entry into Second Natural History Study *(17)*.
NYHA New York Heart Association.
With permission from Fuster et al. *(119)*, Table 47-1, p 1125.

the extensive data accrued from the pathophysiology resulting from tetralogy of Fallot "repair." We do know that SVT occurred in 18.9% versus 5% of controls in the Second Natural History Study, and this was not related to prior valvotomy *(21)*. More frequent PVCs were associated with prior valvotomy. Serious ventricular arrhythmias, other than ventricular tachycardia, also occurred with high incidence (see Table 1) and were associated with certain preexisting hemodynamic alterations (higher NYHA class, cardiomegaly) but not to degree of stenosis. The incidence of ventricular tachycardia was the same as in controls (2%).

Aortic Stenosis

Aortic stenosis results in left ventricular hypertrophy, reduced left ventricular compliance, and left atrial hypertension. If there is significant associated aortic insufficiency (before or after palliative valvotomy), subendocardial ischemia results from increased wall tension and reduced coronary perfusion gradient. The Second Natural History Study reported a 24.8% incidence of SVT versus 5% of controls independent of prior valvotomy and 13% incidence of PVCs in patients who had undergone valvotomy. There was a very high incidence of serious ventricular arrhythmias (see Table 1) with a 13% incidence of ventricular tachycardia. Unlike pulmonic stenosis, in aortic stenosis the risk of ventricular arrhythmias was associated with severity of obstruction. Concomitant aortic regurgitation appeared to greatly increase the risk of ventricular arrhythmia. These patients have an important incidence of sudden unexplained death (see Table 1). In fact, in Silka's analysis of sudden death risk among adults having all forms of congenital heart disease, aortic stenosis conferred the highest such risk, 5.4/1000 pt-yrs *(22)*.

SECTION III: ARRHYTHMIAS FOLLOWING CONGENITAL HEART SURGERY

Sinoatrial Node Dysfunction (SAND)

Although SAND may occur after any surgery involving an atriotomy, it is most common after Mustard or Senning repair for d-transposition of the great arteries (d-TGA) and after Fontan palliation for patients having a single ventricle. Because the Mustard and Senning procedures were supplanted by the arterial switch operation starting in the mid-1980s, most information regarding SAND is from older studies on adults having undergone these repairs. Most of these patients are now in their third, fourth, and even fifth decades. The Mustard and Senning operations involve creation of atrial baffles using prosthetic material or pericardium (Mustard) or the atrial wall itself (Senning) to redirect the systemic venous return to the sub-pulmonic left ventricle and the pulmonary venous return to the sub-aortic right ventricle. The extensive atrial suture lines may damage the sinus node, perinodal tissues, or the blood supply to these structures (see Fig. 8). The Fontan-style operations have undergone multiple iterations, but all are designed to direct systemic venous return to the pulmonary arteries without an interposed ventricle. Most currently adult-aged "Fontan patients" had undergone an atriopulmonary connection, in which the entire right atrium is included in the systemic venous-to-pulmonary artery circuit (see Fig. 9). These atria become massively dilated, hypertrophic, and fibrotic in response to elevated systemic venous pressure. In most centers, the present surgical strategy in children with single ventricle is to circumvent the atrial mass entirely with an "extracardiac conduit" from the inferior

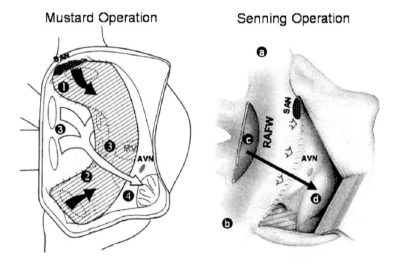

Fig. 8. General anatomic features and anatomic locations of sinoatrial (SAN, *black stippled areas*) and AV nodes (AVN within anterior atrial septal remnant) following Mustard and Senning operations for d-transposition of the great arteries. *Mustard operation:* 1-superior vena cava return; 2-inferior vena cava return; 3-pulmonary venous return (*white arrow* implies direction of flow to tricuspid valve); 4-tricupid valve. ///////, systemic venous baffled region; *gray* MV, mitral valve. *Senning operation:* a-superior vena cava; b-inferior vena cava; c-incision rightward of right pulmonary veins (*black arrow* implies direction of flow to tricuspid valve); d-tricuspid valve. RAFW, right atrial free wall, representing roof over intercaval tube. *Open arrows* represent anterior suture line of right atrial free wall flap to anterior atrial septal remnant. (*Right-sided figure* adapted with permission from: Elsevier, New York, NY. In: Ref. *(33)*).

vena cava to the pulmonary arteries and with a bidirectional Glenn procedure (superior vena cava to pulmonary artery).

Electrophysiologic testing for sinus node function has fallen out of favor. Among Mustard and Fontan patients, older studies showed prolonged sinus node recovery times in >50% and prolonged sinoatrial conduction times in 33–50% of these patients *(23)*.

Patients with SAND may present with fatigue, exercise intolerance, presyncope, or syncope. Asymptomatic patients with signs of sinus node dysfunction on ECG should undergo further non-invasive evaluation with 24-h ambulatory ECGs and all patients who have had extensive atrial surgery should be monitored with 24-h Holters every 2–5 years. Exercise testing is indicated in those with exertional fatigue, syncope, or other symptoms. Sudden, postexercise sinus bradycardia has been well described in Fontan patients. Invasive EP testing is usually not indicated in patients with isolated signs or symptoms of SAND, but those with syncope, presyncope, palpitations, or other paroxysmal events that could also be due to a tachyarrhythmia should undergo formal EP studies to evaluate for VT, SVT, or atrial tachyarrhythmias (see below).

Management of clinically important SAND is with pacemaker implantation. The AHA/ACC/HRS Joint Committee on Pacing *(24)* recommends pacemaker placement in patients with congenital heart disease if they have (1) SAND with correlation of symptoms during age-inappropriate brady-cardia (Class I indication); (2) resting heart rate less than 40 bpm or pauses in ventricular rate longer than 3 sec (class IIa indication; class IIb if after two-ventricle repair of congenital heart disease); or (3) impaired hemodynamics due to sinus bradycardia or loss of AV synchrony (class IIa indication). These recommendations are only guidelines, and many children with less well-defined symptoms such as daytime somnolence and morning headaches may also benefit from atrial pacing.

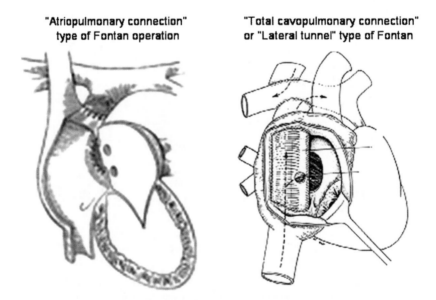

Fig. 9. Diagrams of older (*left*) and newer (*right*) styles of Fontan operations, designed to direct systemic venous return to the pulmonary arteries without an interposed ventricle.

Atrial Tachycardias

Patients who have undergone extensive atrial surgery such as the Mustard, Senning, or Fontan are also at risk for atrial tachycardias, most commonly intraatrial reentry tachycardia (IART). With over 10 years of follow-up, the incidence of IART or typical atrial flutter is as high as 48% in Mustard patients and 57% in Fontan patients. Late sudden death may also occur in Mustard or Senning patients and may be related to 1:1 conduction during atrial flutter. The presence of atrial flutter is associated with an increased risk of sudden death by 4.7-fold ($p<0.01$) (25). With regard to Fontan operations, studies on arrhythmia prevalence must be interpreted in the context of each particular style of Fontan procedure. The incidence of atrial arrhythmias following the lateral tunnel and extracardiac conduit style of Fontan operations does appear to be lower (0–26%) compared to the classic atriopulmonary-type Fontan (12–57%) (26–30). The degree of right atrial enlargement is clearly a risk factor, as are duration of follow-up, history of AV valve surgery, and history of immediate postoperative arrhythmias. The current surgical epoch of the extracardiac conduit Fontan operation partially evolved in order to avoid atrial dilatation and potentially traumatic atrial suture lines. This appears to result in lower incidence of atrial tachycardias and improved hemodynamics.

Because IART may be associated with an increased risk of sudden death in Mustard and Senning patients, therapy should be directed at complete atrial suppression. During an active episode of IART, initial management may involve a transesophageal echocardiogram to evaluate for atrial thrombi, although the incidence of atrial thrombus is low in this patient population. Cardioversion may be effected by either transesophageal or transvenous overdrive pacing termination or by DC cardioversion. Due to the higher risk of thrombus formation in classic and lateral tunnel Fontan patients (31), they should always undergo TEE evaluation prior to rhythm conversion. Also, IART in these patients is less likely to respond to esophageal overdrive pacing.

Catheter ablation of IART is a potentially curative procedure with long-term success rates of up to 80% (32, 33). Antiarrhythmic agents, including sotalol, amiodarone, and dofetilide, are of variable value. Class Ia agents in combination with an AV node blocking drug have fallen out of favor due to cardiac and non-cardiac side effects. Class Ic agents are mostly avoided due to their proarrhythmic risk in this patient group. Antibradycardia pacing may become necessary due to sinus node suppression from any of these drugs. Antitachycardia pacing with a pacemaker or ICD may be efficacious, especially in the Mustard/Senning patients, but inadvertant IART acceleration is a particular hazard in all of these patients.

A surgical approach to IART management in Fontan patients has been championed by several groups. The surgical atrial maze procedure is combined with surgical conversion of the atriopulmonary-style Fontan to an extracardiac conduit and right atrial reduction. Specific lines of conduction block using cryo-energy are created, customized to the various intrinsic anatomies encountered and must include a left atrial maze (Cox III), if the patient has a history of atrial fibrillation (Fig. 10). The anatomic "conversion" component of this operation results in improved hydrodynamics and, eventually, measureable functional status. Antibradycardia pacing is nearly always required in these patients. In several surgical series, at 17–43 months follow-up, IART recurrence is still in the 8–30% range. The operative mortality rate is reported at <10% (34–38). There remains debate among members of the electrophysiology community between transvenous catheter ablation and surgical maze in many of these patients. In general, patients having very large right atria and NYHA class worse than I are best served by the surgical approach.

The catheter ablation technique in Mustard and Senning patients with IART has been described (33, 39). As in anatomically normal hearts, the cavotricuspid isthmus (CTI) is the most common substrate. However, in these patients, this structure is bisected by the inferior portion of the surgically placed baffle. Catheter access to the pulmonary venous side of the CTI may be required for successful ablation and may be achieved by a retroaortic, retro-tricuspid valve approach or by baffle perforation (see Fig. 11).

The ablation procedure is more challenging in Fontan patients due to the presence of multiple tachycardia circuits, difficulty maintaining good catheter contact in massively dilated chambers, and often

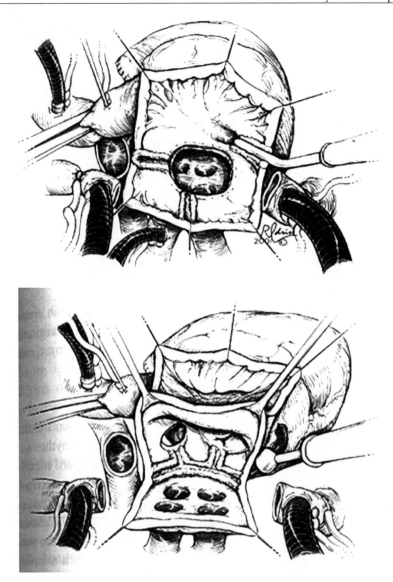

Fig. 10. Typical cryolesions used for the intraoperative maze procedure to treat atrial intraatrial reentry tachycardia arising in the right atrium (*top*) and atrial fibrillation in the left atrium (*bottom*) in patients who had undergone an older Fontan-style operation, at the time of surgical conversion to an extracardiac conduit from inferior vena cava to pulmonary arteries (reproduced with permission from Mavroudis et al. *(120)*, Elsevier, New York, NY).

very thick atrial walls *(40)*. A history of atrial fibrillation and failure to eliminate all tachycardia substrates are associated with reduced rates of success at follow-up *(39)*. Acutely successful ablation of all substrates, the use of irrigated-tipped catheters, and use of electroanatomic mapping systems are associated with clinical success at follow-up *(39)*. Compared with IART in other forms of CHD, identification of ideal ablation targets is more difficult *(41)*. Location of diastolic potentials and concealed entrainment mapping may not be helpful due to lack of specificity, further complicating the ablation procedure. With the atriopulmonary-type Fontan, IART circuits are most often related to the atriopulmonary connection at the right atrial appendage, the cavotricuspid isthmus, or the atriotomy scar *(42)*.

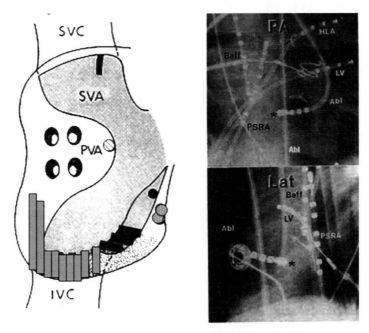

Fig. 11. *Left:* Successful radiofrequency catheter ablation locations for supraventricular tachycardia substrates following Mustard operation for d-transposition of the great arteries. *Gray region,* systemic venous baffle; *stippled region,* cavotricuspid isthmus; *black rectangles,* successful zones in systemic venous atrium for intraatrial reentry tachycardia (IART); *gray rectangles,* successful zones in pulmonary venous atrium for IART; *black circle,* successful location in systemic venous atrium for focal atrial tachycardia (FAT); *gray-hatched circle,* successful location in pulmonary venous atrium for FAT; *gray-stippled circles,* successful location in pulmonary venous atrium for AV nodal reentry tachycardia (AVNRT). *Right:* Posteroanterior (PA) and lateral (Lat) radiographs showing electrode catheter locations during successful radiofrequency ablation of slow inputs to AV node for AVNRT in a Mustard patient. *Asterisk,* tip of ablation catheter; Abl, ablation catheter; Baff, multipole catheter in systemic venous baffle; HLA, high left atrial catheter; LV, left ventricular catheter; PSRA, posteroseptal right atrial catheter (both figures adapted with permission from Elsevier, New York, NY. In: Ref. *(33)*).

Despite the challenges, acute success rates of up to 85% have been reported *(39)* but there is a high likelihood of late recurrence *(43)*. Patients with newer types of Fontans such as the lateral tunnel or extracardiac conduit present a new challenge since venous access to the atria is limited. Transthoracic puncture has been employed as an ablation approach in these patients *(44)*. Irrespective of the method of IART ablation, adjunctive bradycardia pacing and antiarrhythmic drug therapy are still required in a large proportion of these challenging patients.

Ventricular Tachyarrhythmias

Patients who have undergone any type of ventricular surgery are at risk for ventricular arrhythmias. Sudden death has been correlated with ventricular tachycardia in patients following surgery for tetralogy of Fallot and left ventricular outflow tract obstruction, with an overall risk for long-term sudden cardiac death 25–100 times greater than age-matched controls *(22)*. Ventricular tachycardia has been demonstrated in up to 8% of patients having undergone Mustard operation for d-TGA, especially among those having undergone concomitant VSD closure; this probably accounts for at least a portion of the increased sudden death risk in this patient group, as well.

Most data on ventricular arrhythmias following congenital heart surgery are from patients with repaired tetralogy of Fallot, although the results from this patient group can almost certainly be applied to patients having undergone classic Rastelli operation for d-TGA, PS, and VSD; repair of truncus arteriosus; and repair of pulmonary atresia and VSD. Older studies identified older age at repair, prior performance of certain palliative procedures (especially the Potts anastamosis: descending aorta-to-left pulmonary artery anasatamosis), duration since repair, residual outflow tract obstruction, and spontaneous high-grade ventricular ectopy (especially during exercise) as risk factors for clinically important sustained ventricular arrhythmias and sudden death. By the mid-1990s, the advent of catheter ablation and transvenous ICD implantation heralded intensified interest in scientific approaches to risk assessment, so that primary prevention of sudden death could be offered. Perhaps excepting only spontaneous ventricular ectopy, the above risk factors are still relevant, but right and left ventricular systolic dysfunction is now recognized as major risk factors. In many individuals, this results from severe pulmonary valve insufficiency. In those patients, right ventricular dilation combined with right bundle branch block (RBBB) appears to create a vulnerable substrate for ventricular tachycardia and fibrillation. They manifest "electromechanical interaction," with an increased cardiothoracic ratio paralleling certain electrocardiographic changes. Hence, such electrocardiographic features as QRS duration ≥180 msec (45, 46), and rapid rate of QRS duration increase have good predictive value for sudden death risk. Irrespective of ECG findings, significantly reduced right *or* left ventricular ejection fraction is considered worrisome, as well.

If ventricular function and "electromechanical interactions" are acceptable, asymptomatic patients who have high-grade ventricular ectopy during ambulatory monitoring may simply be followed closely or referred for surgical correction of any hemodynamic abnormality (such as compensated pulmonary valve insufficiency). Patients with minor symptoms may be evaluated with event recorders, 24-h ECG, and exercise tests, but invasive electrophysiologic testing is warranted in patients with poor hemodynamics, markedly prolonged QRS duration, concerning paroxysmal palpitations, or syncope. In a multicenter study, inducible ventricular tachycardia during invasive testing has been validated as an important prognostic indicator in repaired tetralogy of Fallot patients (46). Polymorphic ventricular tachycardia had an even worse prognosis than monomorphic. More recently, the same authors showed a similar rate of appropriate ICD discharge in groups implanted for either primary or secondary prevention (47). Hence, as a medical community, we are getting closer to accurate risk assessment in these patients. In patients with inducible or documented sustained monomorphic ventricular tachycardia, radiofrequency catheter ablation and/or ICD placement is indicated. With electroanatomic mapping and standard entrainment techniques, macroreentrant circuits can be identified and successfully ablated. Follow-up electrophysiologic testing at intervals is mandatory, if an ICD is not implanted. We have found a higher than expected recurrence rate in patients having more complex anatomy with even moderately elevated right ventricular systolic pressure, especially when the anatomy involves a right ventricle-to-pulmonary artery conduit. Antiarrhythmic drugs that have historically demonstrated efficacy such as propranolol, phenytoin, mexiletine, sotalol, and amiodarone are now considered adjunctive therapy, in order to limit ICD discharges. ICD implantation is required for patients who have survived resuscitated sudden death, in those who have inducible polymorphic ventricular tachycardia, and, probably, in those having monomorphic ventricular tachycardia and reduced ventricular function.

Postoperative AV Block

Irrespective of initial anatomic abnormality, approximately 90% of patients who undergo right ventricular outflow tract patch or conduit plus VSD repair have residual right bundle branch block (RBBB). Most data regarding RBBB and future conduction abnormalities as well as long-term functional consequences from dyssynchronous ventricular activation are from the cohort of patients with tetralogy of Fallot repair. This repair involves patch closure of a membranous VSD and right ventricular muscle bundle resection to enlarge the infundibulum. Although modern surgical techniques utilize limited ventriculotomies and even transatrial approaches, adults having undergone this repair in child-hood had generally received a very generous ventriculotomy. In this population, 80% have RBBB; 11% have RBBB with left axis deviation; and 3% have RBBB, left axis deviation, and first-degree AV block. Permanent AV block occurs in less than 1% *(48)*, but some patients may have transient complete AV block which is also associated with a risk of late sudden death *(49)*. Occasionally patients with RBBB will develop LBBB later in life and result in complete AV block. Functionally, there is growing concern that dyssynchronous ventricular activation from RBBB may lead to global LV dysfunction *(50)*, a higher risk of ventricular arrhythmias, and reduced exercise capacity *(51)*. Investigations to assess the benefits of right ventricular resynchronization are underway.

Patients with lower conduction system disease may experience symptoms such as presyncope or syncope from transient AV block. Evaluation usually involves ambulatory event recorders but invasive electrophysiologic testing is also helpful for prognosis and decision making. If there is significant HV prolongation or any evidence of block below the His at atrial paced rates less than 120/min then a pacemaker is indicated. In the absence of symptoms, bifascicular or trifascicular block may also require permanent pacing if there is type II second-degree AV block during sinus rhythm, complete AV block, or marked HV prolongation (>100 msec). Alternatively, patients may be followed closely with 24-h ambulatory ECG and exercise testing. With transient postoperative AV block, permanent pacing is indicated in any child with type II second-degree AV block or complete AV block lasting more than 7 days following surgery (class I indication) *(24)*.

SECTION IV: SPECIFIC ARRHYTHMIAS IN CHILDREN AND TEENAGERS

Congenital Atrioventricular Block (CAVB)

Congenital atrioventricular block occurs in 1 in 18,000–22,000 lives births. Approximately two-thirds occur secondary to transplacental passage of anti-ribonucleoprotein antibodies (anti-SSA, Ro; or anti-SSB, La) from women who are ANA positive, though only a minority of these women have active systemic lupus erythematosis, mixed connective tissue disease, or Sjögren syndrome. These antibodies result in an immune-mediated fibroelastic destructive process starting at about 18 weeks of gestation and resulting in third-degree AV block (>90%) and/or sinoatrial node dysfunction (10%). New data identify L-type calcium channels as being targets for these antibodies *(52)*. About 2% of pregnancies in women having these antibodies result in CAVB, but after a first affected infant, that incidence increases to about 15% for subsequent pregnancies. Affected newborns may also have transient rashes or cytopenias. Rarely, AV block does not occur until weeks to a few months post-partum.

Congenital atrioventricular block occurs with a higher than expected incidence in fetuses having certain structural congenital heart defects, especially congenitally corrected transposition and some forms of heterotaxy (particularly, left atrial isomerism or "polysplenia"). Uncommon genetic etiologies, which may or may not have associated structural defects, include mutations in the Nkx2.5 transcription factor gene *(53)* or the Tbx5 transcription factor gene. When the latter is associated with Holt–Oram syndrome, sinoatrial node dysfunction may coexist or predominate *(54)*.

Congenital atrioventricular block is a morbid diagnosis. Considering all fetuses with this diagnosis, the mortality rate is 19–31%, and in the presence of hydrops, 73–100%. The diagnosis of congenital heart block is usually made during fetal ultrasound, and once identified, patients should be observed closely in utero for signs of heart failure and hydrops fetalis. Early delivery and immediate post-birth pacing may be indicated and weighed against the risks of prematurity. Several small studies have suggested failure of progression or even reversal of first- or second-degree AV block with maternally administered steroids such as dexamethasone *(55–57)*, but results are mixed *(58–60)*. Randomized studies of steroid administration with longer term follow-up to determine if progression of AV block is also prevented are currently ongoing. These agents are not helpful once AV block becomes complete.

For fetuses with CAVB who have signs of hydrops or an excessively slow rate (<55 bpm) and in whom early delivery is felt to be highly undesirable, maternal administration of the beta-adrenergic agent, ritodrine, has been reported to be helpful *(61)*.

Once an infant with heart failure is born, aggressive therapy is required for all other aggravating factors, including pleural and pericardial effusions, lung disease of prematurity, and coexisting structural heart defects. Duration of temporary transcutaneous pacing is limited by skin fragility, so placement of temporary transvenous or epicardial wires in the intensive care nursery may be necessary.

Specific indications for permanent pacing in newborns and in children with congenital complete heart block are included in the 2008 guidelines for device-based therapy of cardiac rhythm abnormalities and appear in Table 2 *(62)* . Even asymptomatic adults with congenital complete heart block have a 5% incidence of sudden death at long-term follow-up *(63)*. It has therefore become standard practice to permanently pace all such patients by their late teenage years.

Among patients with congenital complete heart block who require pacing, perhaps up to 10% will develop significant ventricular dysfunction *(64)*. Whether this is due to intrinsic muscle disease related to the initial immune-mediated process, or whether this is purely due to dyssynchronous ventricular depolarization is unknown. Ventricular function benefits from ventricular resynchronization pacing in this patient group *(65)*.

Supraventricular Tachycardia (SVT) and Preexcitation

The ontogeny of SVT subtypes in the pediatric age range indicates that atrioventricular reciprocating tachycardia (AVRT) accounts for 80% of cases in neonates and infants. By the teenage years, AVNRT is as frequent as AVRT. Focal atrial tachycardia and atrial ectopic tachycardia seem to have a constant and low combined incidence of 5–10% of SVT across the entire age spectrum. These data are based upon esophageal EP studies, primarily using the V–A interval during SVT as the major diagnostic criterion.

Antegrade dual AV nodal physiology (based on criteria established in adults) is seen in 50% or fewer pediatric patients with AVNRT *(66)* and may be almost as frequently seen in control patients *(67)*. During diagnostic intracardiac studies, the observation that the AH interval exceeds the pacing cycle length during incremental atrial pacing appears to have better functional correlation with the existence of the typical variety of AVNRT *(68)*.

After the newborn period, the peak age for first occurrence of childhood SVT is about 8 years. With regard to SVT due to AVRT, age at presentation is an important natural history factor. In neonates with WPW, 25–35% will have spontaneous disappearance of their delta wave by 1 year of age, though this does not always predict loss of retrograde accessory pathway function. Indeed, neonates whose SVT has seemingly spontaneously resolved by 1 year of age may have SVT recurrences later in 1/3 of cases. We routinely offer esophageal electrophysiological testing to all 1- to 2-year-old infants whose ECGs have lost preexcitation and who have had no SVT recurrences. We believe that this helps guide continuation of antiarrhythmic drug therapy and prognosis. In contrast, older children with SVT are very unlikely to have spontaneous resolution of their arrhythmia substrate.

Management of children having asymptomatic preexcitation remains controversial. One recent prospective study in children found that 51 of 184 patients (28%) had an arrhythmic event after 20 months of follow-up, with 19 of these cases being potentially "life threatening," including 3 cardiac arrests *(69)*. In this series, independent predictors of life-threatening arrhythmias were antegrade refractory period of accessory pathways (APERP) ≤240 msec and presence of multiple accessory pathways. The shortest preexcited R–R interval during induced atrial fibrillation <220 msec is the most robust predictor of catastrophic events *(70)*. We now routinely recommend esophageal electrophysiological testing in asymptomatic 6- to 10-year-olds having preexcitation, before consenting to allow competitive sports participation. Just as in adults, digoxin therapy may increase the risk of

Table 2
Indications for Pacemaker Implantation in Children, Adolescents, and in Patients Having Congenital Heart Disease

Class I
1. Permanent pacemaker implantation is indicated for advanced second- or third-degree AV block associated with symptomatic bradycardia, ventricular dysfunction, or low cardiac output *(Level of Evidence: C)*.
2. Permanent pacemaker implantation is indicated for SND with correlation of symptoms during age-inappropriate bradycardia. The definition of bradycardia varies with the patient's age and expected heart rate *(Level of Evidence: B)*.
3. Permanent pacemaker implantation is indicated for postoperative advanced second- or third-degree AV block that is not expected to resolve or that persists at least 7 days after cardiac surgery *(Level of Evidence: B)*.
4. Permanent pacemaker implantation is indicated for congenital third-degree AV block with a wide QRS escape rhythm, complex ventricular ectopy, or ventricular dysfunction *(Level of Evidence: B)*.
5. Permanent pacemaker implantation is indicated for congenital third-degree AV block in the infant with a ventricular rate less than 55 bpm or with congenital heart disease and a ventricular rate less than 70 bpm *(Level of Evidence: C)*.

Class IIa
1. Permanent pacemaker implantation is reasonable for patients with congenital heart disease and sinus bradycardia for the prevention of recurrent episodes of intraatrial reentrant tachycardia; SND may be intrinsic or secondary to antiarrhythmic treatment *(Level of Evidence: C)*.
2. Permanent pacemaker implantation is reasonable for congenital third-degree AV block beyond the first year of life with an average heart rate less than 50 bpm, abrupt pauses in ventricular rate that are two or three times the basic cycle length, or associated with symptoms due to chronotropic incompetence *(Level of Evidence: B)*.
3. Permanent pacemaker implantation is reasonable for sinus bradycardia with complex congenital heart disease with a resting heart rate less than 40 bpm or pauses in ventricular rate longer than 3 sec *(Level of Evidence: C)*.
4. Permanent pacemaker implantation is reasonable for patients with congenital heart disease and impaired hemodynamics due to sinus bradycardia or loss of AV synchrony *(Level of Evidence: C)*.
5. Permanent pacemaker implantation is reasonable for unexplained syncope in the patient with prior congenital heart surgery complicated by transient complete heart block with residual fascicular block after a careful evaluation to exclude other causes of syncope *(Level of Evidence: B)*.

Class IIb
1. Permanent pacemaker implantation may be considered for transient postoperative third-degree AV block that reverts to sinus rhythm with residual bifascicular block *(Level of Evidence: C)*.
2. Permanent pacemaker implantation may be considered for congenital third-degree AV block in asymptomatic children or adolescents with an acceptable rate, a narrow QRS complex, and normal ventricular function *(Level of Evidence: B)*.
3. Permanent pacemaker implantation may be considered for asymptomatic sinus bradycardia after biventricular repair of congenital heart disease with a resting heart rate less than 40 bpm or pauses in ventricular rate longer than 3 sec *(Level of Evidence: C)*.

Class III
1. Permanent pacemaker implantation is not indicated for transient postoperative AV block with return of normal AV conduction in the otherwise asymptomatic patient *(Level of Evidence: B)*.
2. Permanent pacemaker implantation is not indicated for asymptomatic bifascicular block with or without first-degree AV block after surgery for congenital heart disease in the absence of prior transient complete AV block *(Level of Evidence: C)*.
3. Permanent pacemaker implantation is not indicated for asymptomatic type I second-degree AV block *(Level of Evidence: C)*.
4. Permanent pacemaker implantation is not indicated for asymptomatic sinus bradycardia with the longest relative risk interval less than 3 sec and a minimum heart rate more than 40 bpm *(Level of Evidence: C)*.

From ACC/AHA/HRS 2008 Guidelines for Device-Based Therapy of Cardiac Rhythm Abnormalities *(62)*.

severe events in patients who develop atrial fibrillation and who also have ventricular preexcitation and is therefore contraindicated in children with SVT and WPW.

Chaotic Atrial Tachycardia

This uncommon arrhythmia is usually referred to as multifocal atrial tachycardia in adults, and among children it occurs mostly in infants less than 1 year of age. One-third of patients tend to present with coexisting respiratory infections and one-third have structural heart disease *(71)*. Diagnosis is based on ECG criteria requiring: (1) more than three ectopic P wave morphologies; (2) irregular P–P intervals; (3) isoelectric baseline between P waves; and (4) rapid atrial and ventricular rate. Some criteria also include absence of a dominant atrial pacemaker. Atrial rates vary from 250 to 600 beats/min while ventricular rates are from 110 to 250 beats/min. Congestive heart failure is not a common presentation, but one-fourth of patients present with tachycardia-induced cardiomyopathy as evidenced by echocardiographic criteria *(71)*. Chaotic atrial tachycardia is not responsive to adenosine, direct current cardioversion, and overdrive pacing suggesting that the mechanism is not reentry. It is thought to be a triggered mechanism but calcium channel blockers have not been shown to be efficacious. Perhaps the best explanation is rapid automaticity with various exit points and multiple reentry wavelets similar to focal atrial fibrillation in adults.

Prognosis for infants with chaotic atrial tachycardia is generally good with most having complete resolution by 1 year of age. Pharmacologic therapy is aimed at control of the ventricular rate with digoxin or an oral calcium channel blocker. Beta blocker therapy may be useful in some patients in whom the ventricular rate cannot be otherwise controlled. Conversion to sinus rhythm may be attempted with agents such as amiodarone, flecainide, or, as is our preference, propafenone. Once in sinus rhythm, therapy may be discontinued after 1 year of age with close follow-up of ambulatory ECGs.

Congenital Junctional Ectopic Tachycardia

Junctional ectopic tachycardia (JET) that begins in the first year of life is considered "congenital." Most cases of congenital JET are sporadic, though a familial predisposition has been demonstrated in some patients *(72)*. Congenital JET may also result from anti-Ro or anti-La antibodies and may even evolve to CAVB *(73)*. Since the ventricular rate varies from 140 to 370 beats/min in this incessant tachycardia, most infants present with heart failure due to tachycardia-induced cardiomyopathy. The ECG diagnostic criteria are (1) narrow QRS tachycardia; (2) AV dissociation; and (3) ventricular rate greater than the atrial rate. JET usually does not terminate with adenosine or cardioversion and thus the mechanism is enhanced automaticity of the AV junction above the bundle branches. Therapy is aimed at control of the ventricular rate, generally to <150 beats/min, which should allow recovery of ventricular function. Pharmacologic therapy with digoxin has been shown to be ineffective and agents such as sotalol, flecainide, propranolol, or propafenone may have some efficacy. However, the most useful medication is amiodarone, which has become the mainstay of therapy for congenital JET. For intractable cases in which pharmacologic therapy fails to control the ventricular rate, catheter ablation of the AV junction with preservation of normal AV conduction has been successfully performed, even in infants *(74, 75)*.

Postoperative Junctional Ectopic Tachycardia

Junctional ectopic tachycardia is the most common postoperative arrhythmia after congenital heart surgery with an incidence of up to 8–10%. It is most commonly associated with repair of tetralogy of Fallot, VSD, or AVCD, though it may be seen after nearly any type of cardiac surgery *(76)*. The mechanisms are thought to be related to transient edema or inflammatory injury to the His bundle from nearby suture lines or to direct traction. When it occurs following Fontan-style operations or repair of total anomalous pulmonary venous return, it almost certainly occurs due to traction from elevated cavitary pressures, as might be related to higher filling pressure or pulmonary hypertension. Longer cardiopulmonary bypass, longer aortic cross clamp times *(77)*, and the level of inotropic support *(78)* are risk factors.

Postoperative JET usually occurs within the first 24 h after surgery and can have serious hemodynamic consequences due to loss of AV synchrony and limited diastolic filling time. Previously reported mortality rates have been as high as 50%, but with early recognition and improvements in management, the mortality rate can be significantly reduced. The aim of therapy is to bring the ventricular rate below 180 in infants and less than 150 in older children. The initial steps in management include correction of electrolyte abnormalities, especially hypokalemia, and reduction in inotropic support as can be tolerated hemodynamically. Moderate hypothermia (32–34°C) has some efficacy, but it requires paralytic drugs and often causes metabolic acidosis. Our institutional policy has been to cool the patient to mild hypothermia (35–36°C) when the initial management fails. The drugs most frequently reported to be efficacious for postoperative JET are procainamide, propafenone, and amiodarone. Although amiodarone is the most widely used agent for the management of JET, practitioners must be aware of the risk of significant hypotension with IV administration. The hypotension can sometimes be managed with administration of IV fluids and calcium. In our opinion, the rate of bolus administration should not be faster than 5 mg/kg over 45 min. Maintenance dosing is then begun. Once the ventricular rate is reduced to less than 180, sequential AV pacing at a slightly faster rate may be initiated for AV synchrony. The older therapy of ventricular "double pacing" is now considered largely antiquated due to the risk of causing ventricular fibrillation. The rhythm will gradually slow to less than the ambient sinus rate over 24–96 h, in most cases. With appropriate management, prognosis is generally good, though patients with JET do have a higher reported postoperative mortality (13.5%) compared to controls (1.7%) *(78)*. Intractable JET may require aggressive support with ECMO or ventricular assist devices and in some extreme cases, ablation of the AV node followed by placement of a permanent dual-chamber pacemaker.

SECTION V: THERAPIES FOR PEDIATRIC ARRHYTHMIAS

Pharmacologic Therapies

Drug therapy has an important role in pediatric arrhythmias despite the primary treatment of catheter ablation for most arrhythmias. Some indications for pharmacologic management include fetal tachyarrhythmias and infant SVT in which catheter ablation carries increased risk, and which may eventually resolve spontaneously. Ventricular arrhythmias in infants and young children with or without congenital heart disease often require antiarrhythmic medications.

Table 3 summarizes the major antiarrhythmic medications and includes information on dosing, pharmacology, and metabolism specific to the pediatric (and in some cases, fetal) population. As with all medications used in children, the bioavailability must be taken into consideration with an understanding of gastrointestinal and hepatic physiology in the young. In general, drugs are less bioavailable in children compared to adults due to relative achlorhydria (until 3 years of age), slower gastric emptying (until 6–8 months of age), and reduced gut motility (until 4 years of age). Most hepatic enzyme systems are immature until at least 6 months of age. This causes reduced biotransformation and first-pass elimination of drugs such as propranolol, lidocaine, amiodarone, and verapamil; thus, their half-lives are longer than in older children and adults. Most antiarrhythmic medications are renally excreted, and this system is also immature until 1 year of age. Pathologic processes in the gut (including mucosal edema), liver, or kidneys due to congestive heart failure, low cardiac output, congenital anomalies, or other causes of organ dysfunction affect drug metabolism similarly in children and adults.

Table 3
Antiarrhythmic Drug Use in Children

Drug	Half-life	Intravenous dosing	Oral dosing	Transplacental passage (%)	Pregnancy category/safety for fetus	Passage in breast milk	Indications
Class Ia							
Disopyramide	4.5–7.8 h	Not available	10–30 mg/kg/d (infants); 10–20 mg/kg/d (children); 6–15 mg/kg/d (adolescents); 400–800 mg/d (adults) q 6 h (regular), q 12 h (sustained release); maximum: 1600 mg/d)	39	C	50–90% maternal blood level; safe for infant	PSVT; AF1; AF; VT in CHD with good ventricular function
Quinidine	30–90 min (sulfate); 3.4–4.0 h (gluconate)	Not recommended	30–60 mg/kg/d (450–900 mg/m²); q 4–6 h; 10 mg/kg/d (adult); 20% higher if gluconate	24–94	C	Reported to occur; safe for infant	Rarely used due to "quinidine syncope"; PSVT; AFI; AF; VT in CHD
Procainamide	1.7 h (children); 2.5–4.7 h (adults) (short acting) 6–7 h (slow release); shorter in children; longer in neonates	10–15 mg/kg over 20 min; maintenance: 30–80 μg/kg/min	50–100 mg/kg/d	25–100	C	Reported to occur; safe for infant	PSVT; AF1; AF; AET; VT in CHD; postoperative JET
Class Ib							
Moricizine	1.5–3.5 h; biologic T 1/2 48 h	Not available	200 mg/m²/d (initial) increase to 600 mg/m²/d; q 8 h	Not known	B	Not known	AET; VT; PSVT

Drug	Half-life	IV	Oral		Pregnancy	Breast milk	Indication
Lidocaine	3.2 h (neonate); 1.5–2 h (children and adults)	1 mg/kg, may repeat twice; maintenance: 20–50 µg/kg/min	Not effective	50	B (fetal bradycardia reported; generally safe for fetus)	40% maternal blood level; safe for infant	VT, especially ischemic
Mexiletine	6.3–11.8 h	Not available	Infants: 8–25 mg/kg/d; children: 4.5–15 mg/kg/d; maximum: 600–1200 mg/d; q 8 h	100 (equivalent to maternal blood level)	C	100% maternal blood level; safe for infant	VT
Phenytoin	75 ± 64 h (premature); 21 ± 12 h (term);; 8 ± 4 h; (1 month); 22 ± 7 h (child–adult)	10–15 mg/kg over 1 h	Load: 15 mg/kg/d q 6 h (day 1), 7.5 mg/kg/d q 6 h (day 2); maintenance: 0–2 weeks: 4–8 mg/kg/d q 12 h; 2 weeks–2 years: 8–12 mg/kg/d q 8 h; 3–12 years: 5–6 mg/kg/d q 12 h; >12 years: 4.5 mg/kg/d q 12 h	Excellent	D (11% have "fetal hydantoin syndrome"; 31% have lesser manifestations)	Safe for infant	VT
Tocainide	15 h (adult)	Not available	Children: 350–700 mg/m^2/d	Not known	C	Not known	VT
Class 1c							
Flecainide	29 h (newborn); 11–12 h (infant); 8 h (children) 12–27 h (adult)	1–2 mg/kg over 5–10 min	1–6 mg/kg/d or 50–150 mg/m^2/d q 8 h (children) & q 12 h (newborn, infant and adult); maximum: 400 mg/d; avoid administration with milk-based formulas in infants	100 (equivalent to maternal blood level)	C	Concentrated (2.3–3.7:1); safe for infant	PSVT; AF1; AF; PJRT; VT; fetal tachycardias; JET

(Continued)

Table 3
(Continued)

Drug	Half-life	Intravenous dosing	Oral dosing	Transplacental passage (%)	Pregnancy category/ safety for fetus	Passage in breast milk	Indications
Propafenone	4.7 ± 1.3 h (extensive metabolizer); 16.8 ± 10.6 h (slow = 10% population); ↑ with time in both groups	0.2 mg/kg q 10 min to effect (max = 2 mg/kg); maintenance: 4–7 µg /kg/min	200–600 mg/m²/d q 6–8 h; maximum: 900 mg/d	Not known	C	Not known	PSVT; AF1; AF; PJRT; VT; infantile CAT; JET
Class II							
Atenolol	16–35 h (newborn); 3.5–7 h (children); 6–9 h (adults)	No pediatric data	0.8–1.5 mg/kg/d q 12–24 h; when used for potentially life-threatening arrhythmia (LQTS), q 12 h recommended	100 maternal blood level	D	Concentrated (1.5–6:8:1); fetal bradycardia	PSVT; rate control in AF1 and AF; VT in normal heart; LQTS
Esmolol	4.5 ± 2.1 min (children); 9 min (adults)	Load: 500 µg/kg over 1 min; maintenance: 50–600 µg /kg/min	Not applicable	Not known	C	Not known	PSVT; rate control in AF1 and AF
Nadolol	20–24 h (adults); shorter in infants and children	Not available	1–2 mg/kg/d q day	Some passage occurs	C (hypoglycemia; symptomatic bradycardia)	Concentrated (3:1); fetal bradycardia	PSVT; rate control in AF1 and AF; VT in normal heart; LQTS

Propranolol	3.9–6.4 h (children); 4–6 h (adults)	0.01–0.15 mg/kg over 5 min	1–5 mg/kg/d q 6–8 h (short acting); q 12–24 h (time release); when used for potentially life-threatening arrhythmia (LQTS), q 12 h recommended	100 maternal blood level	C (IUGR; hypoglycemia; respiratory depression)	64% maternal plasma level; safe for infant	PSVT; rate control in AFl and AF; VT in normal heart; LQTS
Class III							
Amiodarone	8–107 d; biphasic elimination (plasma level 50% after 10 d; rebounds days 12–21; falls again)	Load: 2–5 mg/kg over 20–45 min (repeat as needed); then 0.4–1.0 mg/kg/h	Load: 10 mg/kg/d q 8–12 h (up to 60 mg/kg/d x ≤ 3 d, if necessary); then, 5 mg/kg/d × 2 months; then, wean to 2.5 mg/kg/d	10–25 maternal blood level	D (prematurity 12%; IUGR 21%; hypothyroidism 9%)	Exceeds maternal plasma level; safe for infant	PSVT; AFl; AF; VT; JET; AET
Sotalol	9.5 h (children); 7–18 h (adult); beta-blocking effect longer	Not available	2–8 mg/kg/d or 40–250 mg/m²/d q 8–12 h; maximum dose 640 mg/d; usual adult starting dose: 160 mg/d	5–100 maternal blood level	B (asymptomatic bradycardia)	Concentrated (5:4:1); may not be important	PSVT; AFl; AF; VT
Class IV							
Verapamil	2.5–7 h (infancy); 5–12 h with chronic use	0.1 mg/kg over 2 min (maximum 10 mg); infusion: 5 μ/kg/min; not < 1 year of age	3–10 mg/kg/d q 8 h (short acting); q day (time release)	15–50 maternal level	C	23–100% maternal blood level; safe for infant	PSVT; rate control in AFl and AF; fetal PSVT; occasional forms of VT in normal heart

(Continued)

Table 3
(Continued)

Drug	Half-life	Intravenous dosing	Oral dosing	Transplacental passage (%)	Pregnancy category/safety for fetus	Passage in breast milk	Indications
Digoxin							
Digoxin	61–170 h (premature); 35–45 h (term); 18–25 h (infant); 35 h (child); 38–48 h (adult)	Oral load (three doses/ doses/ 16–24 h): 30 μg/kg (premature), 35 (term), 40–50 (<2 years), 30–40 (>2 years); maintenance: ¼ load / q 12 h; Intravenous dose: 75–80% oral		Similar to maternal level	C	Similar to maternal blood level; safe for infant	PSVT; fetal PSVT
Adenosine							
Adenosine	<5 sec	50–300 μg/kg rapidly	Not applicable	Not applicable	Not applicable	Not applicable	PSVT; SANRT; some FAT; some normal heart VT

AET atrial ectopic tachycardia; *AF* atrial fibrillation; *AFl* atrial flutter; *CAT* chaotic atrial tachycardia; *CHD* congenital heart disease; *FAT* focal atrial tachycardia; *JET* junctional ectopic tachycardia; *LQTS* long QT syndrome; *PJRT* permanent form of junctional reciprocating tachycardia; *PSVT* paroxysmal supraventricular tachycardia; *SANRT* sinoatrial node reentry tachycardia; *VT* ventricular tachycardia; United States FDA Pregnancy Categories: *A* Controlled studies in women fail to demonstrate a risk to the fetus in the first trimester, and the possibility of fetal harm appears remote. *B* Animal studies do not indicate a risk to the fetus and there are no controlled human studies, or animal studies do show an adverse effect on the fetus but well-controlled studies in pregnant women have failed to demonstrate a risk to the fetus. *C* Studies have shown that the drug exerts animal teratogenic or embryocidal effects, but there are no controlled studies in women, or no studies are available in either animals or women. *D* Positive evidence of human fetal risk exists, but benefits in certain situations (e.g., life-threatening situations or serious diseases for which safer drugs cannot be used or are ineffective) may make use of the drug acceptable despite its risks, *X* Studies in animals or humans have demonstrated fetal abnormalities or there is evidence of fetal risk based on human experience, or both, and the risk clearly outweighs any possible benefit.

Adapted and with permission from: Fuster et al. (*119*), Table 47-3, pp 1134–1136.

Catheter Ablation

In many communities, catheter ablation has become first-line therapy for most tachyarrhythmia substrates in older children and teenagers. Radiofrequency catheter ablation (RFA) of cardiac dysrrhythmia substrates in humans has been available for over 20 years, and its efficacy and safety was well defined in children by the Prospective Assessment of Pediatric Catheter Ablation (PAPCA) project *(79)*. Cryoablation has been used for over 10 years and has also been shown to be effective and safe in children with increasing popularity as first-line treatment for dysrhythmia substrates located in the atrial paraseptal region *(80)*. The indications for radiofrequency catheter ablation in pediatric patients based on the 2002 Expert Consensus Conference report are summarized in Table 4 *(81)*.

Due to smaller patient size, there are special considerations when considering catheter ablation in children. For example, in the 3-year-old child, the triangle of Koch is 3–5 mm at its base and 3–6 mm in length, which is not much larger than the lesion size generated by even the smallest available (3 mm tip) radiofrequency ablation catheters. Hence, ablation of septal accessory pathways or AVNRT presents a significant risk in these smaller patients and is generally not electively undertaken. Another anatomic consideration is cardiac wall thickness at the annulus fibrosis, representing the theoretical distance between the epicardial coronary arteries and the endocardial ablation catheter tip. Based upon autopsy specimens, among children less than 7 years of age, this distance is ≤4 mm for 76% of measured sites and ≤5 mm for 96% *(82)*. As observed in adults, the shortest distance is just within the coronary sinus ostium. There are few reports of damage to coronary arteries with catheter ablation in children, though it may go unrecognized more frequently than previously thought *(83, 84)*. Cryoablation may be safer than radiofrequency ablation with regard to coronary injury *(85)*.

If necessary, invasive electrophysiologic testing and catheter ablation can be safely performed in very small patients including infants *(86)*. Even with small femoral vein size, 7 Fr sheaths can be placed and multiple 2 Fr quadripolar electrode catheters can be advanced or a single catheter may be used for both His and right ventricular pacing/recording and for lateral right atrial and coronary sinus pacing/recording. Thus, femoral venous capacity is usually not a limiting factor, since each vein can accommodate up to 5 mm circumference (5 Fr) hardware in children >2.0 kg, 6 Fr if > 3.0 kg, 7 Fr if >5.0 kg, 9 Fr if >10 kg, 11 Fr if >25 kg, and 14 Fr for larger patients. Atrial sensing and pacing may also be performed from the esophagus. Arterial access requires different considerations but is generally avoided with the use of transseptal access to the left side of the heart.

With regard to radiofrequency energy delivery, there does not appear to be a correlation between patient size and impedance load. Thus, the applied power is the same as in adults. Longer duration of radiofrequency lesion application has been shown to correlate with higher complication rates in smaller patients and careful judgment must be employed weighing the risks of ablation and severity of the arrhythmia *(87)*. Growing experience with irrigated-tipped catheters suggest they are also safe and perhaps more effective in congenital heart disease patients with arrhythmia substrates in their thickened atrial walls *(88)*.

Catheter ablation in patients with complex congenital heart disease presents further challenges. Prior to the procedure, review of surgical reports is a prerequisite, and the anatomy must be clearly defined with imaging modalities such as transthoracic/transesophageal echocardiography, CT, and/or MRI. At the time of the procedure, angiography of the vascular and heart structures may be required prior to placement of the electrode catheters. Reduced or altered venous access to the heart should be anticipated due to occluded iliofemoral veins, congenitally interrupted IVC with azygos continuation, or surgically created venous bypass pathways (e.g., bidirectional Glenn procedure, Fontan operation). In patients with inferior vena caval interruption, successful catheter ablation may be performed via hepatic vein cannulation or by the azygos vein *(89, 90)*. Anticipatory knowledge of unusual anatomic locations of important conduction system structures in various congenital heart malformations should

Table 4
Indications for Radiofrequency Catheter Ablation in Pediatric Patients [from the 2002 Expert Consensus Conference Report (80)]

Indications for radiofrequency catheter ablation in pediatric patients

Class I: There is consistent agreement and/or supportive data that catheter ablation is likely to be medically beneficial or helpful for the patient.

1. Wolff–Parkinson–White (WPW) syndrome following an episode of aborted sudden cardiac death.
2. The presence of WPW syndrome associated with syncope when there is a short preexcited R–R interval during atrial fibrillation (preexcited R–R interval, 250 ms) or the antegrade effective refractory period of the AP measured during programmed electrical stimulation is <250 ms.
3. Chronic or recurrent supraventricular tachycardia (SVT) associated with ventricular dysfunction.
4. Recurrent VT that is associated with hemodynamic compromise and is amenable to catheter ablation.

Class IIA: There is a divergence of opinion regarding the benefit or medical necessity of catheter ablation; the majority of opinions/data are in favor of the procedure.

1. Recurrent and/or symptomatic SVT refractory to conventional medical therapy and age >4 years.
2. Impending congenital heart surgery when vascular or chamber access may be restricted following surgery.
3. Chronic (occurring for >6 to 12 months following an initial event) or incessant SVT in the presence of normal ventricular function.
4. Chronic or frequent recurrences of intraatrial reentrant tachycardia (IART).
5. Palpitations with inducible sustained SVT during electrophysiological testing.

Class IIB: There is clear divergence of opinion regarding the need for the procedure.
1. Asymptomatic preexcitation (WPW pattern on an electrocardiograph), age >5 years, with no recognized tachycardia, when the risks and benefits of the procedure and arrhythmia have been clearly explained.
2. SVT, age >5 years, as an alternative to chronic antiarrhythmic therapy which has been effective in control of the arrhythmia.
3. SVT, age <5 years (including infants), when antiarrhythmic medications, including sotalol and amiodarone, are not effective or associated with intolerable side effects.
4. IART, one to three episodes per year, requiring medical intervention.
5. AVN ablation and pacemaker insertion as an alternative therapy for recurrent or intractable IART.
6. One episode of VT associated with hemodynamic compromise and which is amenable to catheter ablation.

Class III: There is an agreement that catheter ablation is not medically indicated and/or the risk of the procedure may be greater than the benefit for the patient.

1. Asymptomatic WPW syndrome, age <5 years.
2. SVT controlled with conventional antiarrhythmic medications, age <5 years.
3. Nonsustained, paroxysmal VT, which is not considered incessant (i.e., present on monitoring for hours at a time or on nearly all strips recorded during any 1-h period) and where no concomitant ventricular dysfunction exists.
4. Episodes of nonsustained SVT that do not require other therapy and/or are minimally symptomatic.

be applied to meticulous electroanatomic mapping. Newer technologies such as intracardiac ultrasound, image fusion, and non-contact balloon array mapping are emerging as useful techniques in patients with congenital heart disease *(32)*. Three-dimensional electroanatomic mapping has been demonstrated to improve success rates for ablation of atrial tachyarrhythmia substrates following congenital heart surgery *(39)* and is now considered requisite technology (see Fig. 12). It may also reduce

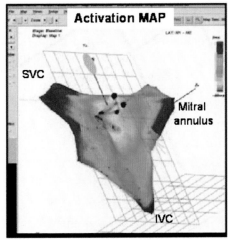
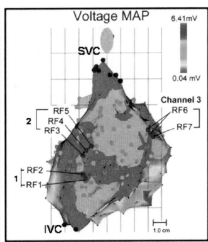

Fig. 12. Electroanatomic maps used to direct catheter ablation of supraventricular tachycardia substrates following complex congenital heart disease. *Left:* Right posterolateral projection of the systemic venous baffle following Senning operation for d-transposition of the great arteries. The earliest focus of focal atrial tachycardia is identified adjacent to baffle suture line from this bipolar isochronal map ("activation map"). *Red* represents earliest activity and violet, latest. *Right:* Right posterolateral projection of a dilated right atrium following atriopulmonary-style Fontan operation. In this bipolar voltage map, electrically inactive regions ("scar") are represented by *gray* and viable tissue by colors ranging from *red* (lowest voltage) to *violet* (highest). Catheter ablation of narrow channels (1–3) of conducting tissue rendered this patient's intraatrial reentry tachycardia non-inducible. IVC, inferior vena cava; RF, radiofrequency lesion; SVC, superior vena cava (*right-sided figure adapted with permission from: Lippincott, Williams, & Wilkins, Philadelphia, PA. In: Ref. (41)).*

or, in some cases, eliminate the need for radiation exposure *(91)* which is always a matter of concern in pediatric patients.

Most catheter ablation procedures in children are performed under general anesthesia. Anesthetic agents such as propofol and isoflurane are commonly used and generally do not suppress arrhythmia inducibility *(92)*. There are minor effects on conduction and refractoriness intervals, which are clinically unimportant *(92)*. Among youngsters having tachycardias using enhanced automaticity as the mechanism (especially AET and some "normal heart VTs"), general anesthesia may render the tachycardia uninducible. Of course, the selection of sedation versus anesthesia needs to be individualized with awareness of coexistent issues such as structural heart disease, other medical issues, and potential airway obstruction. In particular, patients whose heart conditions are especially preload dependent, such as those having cardiomyopathy or "Fontan physiology" may be especially prone to hypotension during general anesthesia. Primary agents such as ketamine may be useful in those instances. Prior to the procedure, age-appropriate reading material, play therapy, and opportunities to network with other children and teenagers who had previously undergone the procedure may be useful.

Overall, the results of catheter ablation in pediatric patients are comparable to results in adult patients. Results from the PAPCA project comprise a large prospective analysis of AV reciprocating tachycardia and AVNRT in patients aged 0–21 years, excluding patients with congenital heart disease *(93)*. The cohort included 481 patients and the acute success rate was 95.7%. For left free wall and right free wall accessory pathways, the success rate was 97.8 and 90.8%, respectively. The procedural complication rate was 4%. Patients were followed for 12 months, and the arrhythmia substrate recurrence rate was 7.0, 9.2, and 10.7% at 2, 6, and 12 months, respectively *(94)*. For individual arrhythmia substrates, the recurrence rates were as follows: 24.6% (right septal pathways), 15.8% (right free wall pathways), 9.3% (left free wall pathways), 4.3% (left septal pathways), and 4.8% (AVNRT). Similar results were reported in other studies of radiofrequency ablation in pediatric patients (95, 96). Cryoablation is becoming more widely applied for pediatric catheter ablation due to relative safety when targeting AVNRT or septal pathways. Reported acute success rate of cryoablation for AVNRT ranges between 83–96% and 60–92% for accessory pathways. Short-term follow-up studies have demonstrated an 8–45% recurrence rate with cryoablation (97–102). Longer applications of cryoenergy may improve success rates (103) and successful ablation of ventricular tachycardia has also been reported with cryoablation (104).

Pacemakers in Children and in Congenital Heart Disease

The indications for permanent pacing in pediatric children have been summarized in Table 2 (62). As with catheter ablation, there are size, developmental, and disease-related considerations with regard to implantable cardiac rhythm devices in pediatric patients. Advances in device and lead design have made it possible to provide rhythm management in the smallest of patients with epicardially placed systems. Several factors have reversed the trend of transvenous lead placement in small children: Steroid-eluting, passive fixation epicardial leads have an excellent long-term track record; newer surgical techniques, including thoracoscopic approaches, have made epicardial lead placement less invasive than in the past; and there is now greater recognition of the long-term adverse impact of failed transvenous leads in patients who still have decades of pacing ahead of them. Indeed, most pediatric electrophysiologists now reserve transvenous lead implantation for children weighing at least 25 kg.

Among patients having repaired or unrepaired congenital heart disease and who require pacing, safe venous access to the heart may be limited by the presence of single ventricle physiology, residual potential right–left shunts, and venous obstruction from prior procedures. As examples, following the Mustard operation, the operator must be certain that there is no superior vena caval baffle obstruction, and that there are no baffle "leaks" (potentiating paradoxical embolization) before placing leads; following the atriopulmonary type of Fontan operation, the operator must be concerned that a new atrial lead may stimulate thrombus formation due to the potential procoagulant state so common in those patients; and following a Rastelli type of operation (right ventricle-to-pulmonary artery conduit and VSD closure as repair of d-TGA, VSD, and pulmonic stenosis; pulmonary atresia and VSD; or truncus arteriosus), even a small residual VSD should make the operator concerned about paradoxical embolization, as the conduit narrows over time, resulting in right ventricular hypertension. "Hybrid procedures" may be performed, in which one lead is transvenous and the other epicardial. Although this was once mostly limited to atriopulmonary-style Fontan patients who had heart block and required an epicardial ventricular lead, this approach is now performed in an effort to provide ventricular resynchronization in young patients having ventricular dysfunction who require a systemic ventricular lead (see Fig. 13).

Ventricular resynchronization pacing is now being applied to certain patients having congenital heart disease and ventricular dysfunction. In the immediate postoperative period (mostly in infants), there is a clear benefit of biventricular pacing using temporary pacing wires for children having poor systemic ventricular function and flagging hemodynamic parameters (105). Evidence-based indications for chronic application of this technology are more difficult to establish than in adults having two anatomically and positionally normal ventricles. Initial multi-institution series of patients having heterogeneous congenital heart defects have shown promising results (106). Those patients having a failing systemic right ventricle and a subpulmonic left ventricle (both d-TGA following Mustard/Senning and l-TGA) appear to benefit with improved indices of conduction synchronization, ventricular function, and NYHA class (107). Use of three-dimensional tissue Doppler techniques are currently being

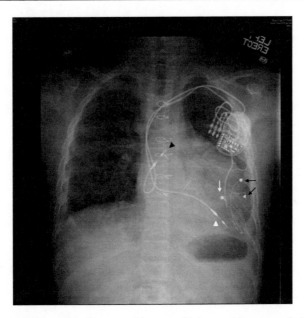

Fig. 13. Posteroanterior chest radiograph from an 11-year-old boy with congenitally corrected transposition (l-TGA) and acquired complete AV block, who is status-post left-sided tricuspid valve replacement and who developed severely diminished systemic ventricular dysfunction 6 years after placement of a transvenous dual chamber pacing system. This figure illustrates a hybrid dual chamber, biventricular pacing system, with an epicardial bipolar lead (*black arrows*) attached to the posterolateral base of the left-sided ventricle and tunneled to the left infraclavicular pacemaker pocket. *White arrow* represents a "spare" unipolar epicardial lead attached to the left-sided ventricle; *black arrowhead* represents the original right atrial lead; and *white arrowhead*, the original right-sided ventricular lead.

applied to patients having a poorly functioning single ventricle in an effort to assess the role of multi-site pacing *(108)*.

In general, children and adolescents adapt well to life with an implanted device and can maintain a healthy self-image given appropriate support from family members and medical professionals. Normalization of lifestyle helps greatly in psychosocial well-being. This includes permission to participate in sports activities as deemed appropriate for the disease. We allow participation in high endurance activities such as basketball, soccer, track, and swimming in patients who are not "pacemaker dependent" while keeping the families informed about potential damage to transvenous leads from excessive shoulder movement. There is general agreement that these patients should be restricted from contact sports.

Implantable Cardioverter/Defibrillators (ICDs)

Implantable cardioverter-defibrillators have been implanted in children and teenagers for prevention of sudden cardiac death over the last 20 years. Silka's original report substantiating the efficacy of ICDs in young patients having cardiomyopathy, primary electrical disease, or congenital heart disease, was primarily concerned with secondary prevention *(109)*. Progress in sudden death risk identification in the patient groups described above has shifted the balance toward implantation for primary prevention. This philosophy has been facilitated by downsizing of hardware and creative and less invasive methods in conductor (sense/pace lead, high-voltage conductors) implantation. However, for children and adults having congenital heart disease, there is no evidence-based reservoir analogous to MADIT or SCD-HeFT from which to "mine" data. Hence, practitioners largely base decisions upon single- or multi-institution retro- or ambispective studies *(46, 110)* or as a "best fit" with adult series of patients having cardiomyopathy or coronary artery disease. Therefore, implantable cardioverter-defibrillator implantation now appears *somewhere* in every treatment algorithm for pediatric patients having hypertrophic cardiomyopathy, restrictive cardiomyopathy, dilated cardiomyopathy, left ventricular noncompaction, arrhythmogenic right ventricular cardiomyopathy, Brugada syndrome, catecholaminergic polymorphic ventricular tachycardia, long QT syndrome; and in all patients having congenital heart disease with ventricular tachyarrhythmias and/or low ejection fraction (<35%?). The efficacy of ICD implantation has also been demonstrated as part of a "bridge" to heart transplantation in some patients with severe cardiac failure and life-threatening arrhythmias *(111)*. The 2008 guidelines for device-based therapy of cardiac rhythm abnormalities include a section on indications for ICD implantation in children and in patients with congenital heart disease (see Table 5) *(62)*.

Table 5
Indications for Implantable Cardioverter-Defibrillators in Children, Adolescents, and in Patients Having Congenital Heart Disease

Class I
1. ICD implantation is indicated in the survivor of cardiac arrest after evaluation to define the cause of the event and to exclude any reversible causes *(Level of Evidence: B)*.
2. ICD implantation is indicated for patients with symptomatic sustained VT in association with congenital heart disease who have undergone hemodynamic and electrophysiological evaluation. Catheter ablation or surgical repair may offer possible alternatives in carefully selected patients *(Level of Evidence: C)*.

Class IIa
ICD implantation is reasonable for patients with congenital heart disease with recurrent syncope of undetermined origin in the presence of either ventricular dysfunction or inducible ventricular arrhythmias at electrophysiological study *(Level of Evidence: B)*.

Class IIb
ICD implantation may be considered for patients with recurrent syncope associated with complex congenital heart disease and advanced systemic ventricular dysfunction when thorough invasive and noninvasive investigations have failed to define a cause *(Level of Evidence: C)*.

Class III
All Class III recommendations that appear in the general document as "indications for implantable cardioverter-defibrillator therapy," apply to pediatric patients and patients with congenital heart disease, and ICD implantation is not indicated in these patient populations *(Level of Evidence: C)*.

From ACC/AHA/HRS 2008 Guidelines for Device-Based Therapy of Cardiac Rhythm Abnormalities *(62)*.

The mitigating factors of small patient size and lack of safe vascular access to the heart mentioned above for pacemakers are amplified for ICDs. Every system requires attachment of a bipolar ventricular lead to the heart for purposes of sensing (mandatory) and pacing (usually desirable) and a conductor capable of delivering high-voltage energy. All of these functions are incorporated into the standard transvenous ventricular lead used with ICDs. When this is not possible, placement of subcutaneous arrays, pericardial patches, and/or coils into a subcutaneous location surrounding the ventricular mass or affixing a transvenous ventricular lead to the pericardium within the pericardial space have proven effective as one (or more) components of the shock vector, with the ICD device as another (see Fig. 14)

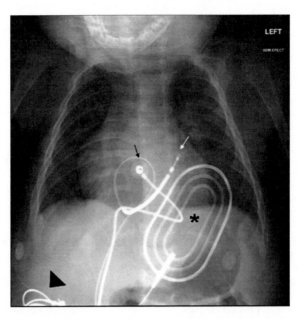

Fig. 14. Posteroanterior chest radiograph from an 8-month-old boy having infant Brugada syndrome and presenting with rapid ventricular tachycardia. The superior aspect of an implantable cardioverter-defibrillator is indicated by the *black arrowhead*. The *black arrow* represents a bipolar, epicardial pace/sense lead attached to the right ventricle. The *white arrow* represents a transvenous-style ventricle lead with coil, which has been attached by its active fixation screw to the posterior pericardium. Due to unacceptably elevated defibrillation threshold at implantation, a pericardial-style patch was placed into the subcutaneous tissue anterior to the heart (*asterisk*). Using the patch as a second conductor, an acceptable defibrillation threshold was achieved.

(112). Using this strategy, we have implanted devices in infants weighing as little as 5 kg. Patients weighing more than 25–30 kg can usually receive transvenous leads and a subclavicular device.

Complications of ICD use in this patient population include lead or high-voltage conductor failure and inappropriate shocks, especially when they are not in standard anatomic locations. Hardware fracture results from repetitive body motion by active youngsters, and somatic growth may shift the ICD device from its original position, potentially altering the shock vector and increasing the defibrillation threshold or even potentiating electrical "shorts." Although retrospective studies have demonstrated a high rate of appropriate ICD discharge *(113)*, the rate of inappropriate shocks in pediatric patients is higher than in adults, ranging from 20 to 50% in published series with mean follow-up of 29–51 months *(114–117)*. Inappropriate discharges result from appropriate sensing of sinus tachycardia or SVT, T wave oversensing, and from conductor damage. Although children having ICDs seem to be generally emotionally resilient *(118)*, at least one study has suggested an increased incidence of anxiety, depression, and reduced activity; and this incidence appears to increase with the number of inappropriate shocks *(113)*. The decision to implant an ICD in a pediatric patient requires open discussion with the family with careful consideration of the risks associated with the cardiac disease versus the risks of inappropriate shocks, device complications, and behavioral factors. With careful patient-specific device programming, pharmacologic therapy, and appropriate atrial and QRS discrimination algorithms the rate of inappropriate discharges from due to ST, atrial arrhythmias, or T wave oversensing can be greatly reduced.

REFERENCES

1. Sacchetti A, Moyer V, Baricella R, Cameron J, Moakes ME (1999) Primary cardiac arrhythmias in children. Pediatr Emerg Care 15:95–98

2. Jongbloed MR, Mahtab EA, Blom NA, Schalij MJ, Gittenberger-de Groot AC (2008) Development of the cardiac conduction system and the possible relation to predilection sites of arrhythmogenesis. Scientific World J 8:239–269

3. Huhta JC, Maloney JD, Ritter DG, Ilstrup DM, Feldt RH (1983) Complete atrioventricular block in patients with atrioventricular discordance. Circulation 67:1374–1377

4. Malhotra S, Patel RN, Mandawat M (2007) A case of congenitally corrected transposition of the great arteries with rare but life-threatening ventricular tachycardia and a coincidental single coronary ostium. J Invasive Cardiol 19: E139–E141

5. Baral VR, Veldtman GR, Yue AM, Duke A, Morgan JM (2004) Successful percutaneous ablation of ventricular tachycardia in congenitally corrected transposition of the great arteries, a case report. J Interv Card Electrophysiol 11:211–215

6. Hager A, Zrenner B, Brodherr-Heberlein S, Steinbauer-Rosenthal I, Schreieck J, Hess J (2005) Congenital and surgically acquired Wolff-Parkinson-White syndrome in patients with tricuspid atresia. J Thorac Cardiovasc Surg 130:48–53

7. Reich JD, Auld D, Hulse E, Sullivan K, Campbell R (1998) The pediatric radiofrequency ablation registry's experience with Ebstein's anomaly. Pediatric electrophysiology society. J Cardiovasc Electrophysiol 9:1370–1377

8. Shah MJ, Jones TK, Cecchin F (2004) Improved localization of right-sided accessory pathways with microcatheter-assisted right coronary artery mapping in children. J Cardiovasc Electrophysiol 15:1238–1243

9. Walker RE, Mayer JE, Alexander ME, Walsh EP, Berul CI (2001) Paucity of sinus node dysfunction following repair of sinus venosus defects in children. Am J Cardiol 87:1223–1226

10. Roos-Hesselink JW, Meijboom FJ, Spitaels SEC et al (2003) Excellent survival and low incidence of arrhythmias, stroke and heart failure long-term after surgical ASD closure at young age – a prospective follow-up study of 21–33 years. Eur Heart J 24:190–197

11. Magnin-Poll I, De Chillou C, Miljoen H, Andronache M, Aliot E (2005) Mechanisms of right atrial tachycardia occurring late after surgical closure of atrial septal defects. J Cardiovasc Electrophysiol 16:681–687

12. Oliver JM, Gallego P, Gonzalez A, Benito F, Mesa JM, Sobrino JA (2002) Predisposing conditions for atrial fibrillation in atrial septal defect with and without operative closure. Am J Cardiol 89:39–43

13. Suda K, Raboisson MJ, Piette E, Dahdah NS, Miro J (2004) Reversible atrioventricular block associated with closure of atrial septal defects using the amplatzer device. J Am College Cardiol 43:1677–1682

14. Chessa M, Carminati M, Butera G et al (2002) Early and late complications associated with transcatheter occlusion of secundum atrial septal defect. J Am College Cardiol 39:1061–1065

15. Silversides CK, Haberer K, Siu SC et al (2008) Predictors of atrial arrhythmias after device closure of secundum type atrial septal defects in adults. Am J Cardiol 101:683–687

16. Kidd L, Driscoll DJ, Gersony WM et al (1993) Second natural history study of congenital heart defects. Results of treatment of patients with ventricular septal defects. Circulation 87:I38–I51

17. Wolfe RR, Driscoll DJ, Gersony WM et al (1993) Arrhythmias in patients with valvar aortic stenosis, valvar pulmonary stenosis, and ventricular septal defect. Results of 24-hour ECG monitoring. Circulation 87:I89–I101

18. Kalra GS, Verma PK, Dhall A, Singh S, Arora R (1999) Transcatheter device closure of ventricular septal defects: immediate results and intermediate-term follow-up. Am Heart J 138:339–344

19. Thanopoulos BD, Rigby ML (2005) Outcome of transcatheter closure of muscular ventricular septal defects with the Amplatzer ventricular septal defect occluder. Heart 91:513–516

20. 2Yip WCL, Zimmerman F, Hijazi ZM (2005) Heart block and empirical therapy after transcatheter closure of perimembranous ventricular septal defect. Catheterization Cardiovasc Interventions 66:436–441

21. Hayes CJ, Gersony WM, Driscoll DJ et al (1993) Second natural history study of congenital heart defects. Results of treatment of patients with pulmonary valvar stenosis. Circulation 87:I28–I37

22. Silka MJ, Hardy BG, Menashe VD, Morris CD (1998) A population-based prospective evaluation of risk of sudden cardiac death after operation for common congenital heart defects. J Am Coll Cardiol 32:245–251

23. Khairy P, Landzberg MJ, Lambert J, O'Donnell CP (2004) Long-term outcomes after the atrial switch for surgical correction of transposition: a meta-analysis comparing the Mustard and Senning procedures. Cardiol Young 14: 284–292

24. Smith SC, Epstein AE, DiMarco JP et al (2008) ACC/AHA/HRS 2008 guidelines for device-based therapy of cardiac rhythm abnormalities: executive summary. Heart Rhythm 5:934–955

25. Gewillig M, Cullen S, Mertens B, Lesaffre E, Deanfield J (1991) Risk factors for arrhythmia and death after Mustard operation for simple transposition of the great arteries. Circulation 84:III187–III192

26. Sugimoto S, Takagi N, Hachiro Y, Abe T (2001) High frequency of arrhythmias after Fontan operation indicates earlier anticoagulant therapy. Int J Cardiol 78:33–39

27. Ghai A, Harris L, Harrison DA, Webb GD, Siu SC (2001) Outcomes of late atrial tachyarrhythmias in adults after the Fontan operation. J Am College Cardiol 37:585–592

28. Stamm C, Friehs I, Mayer JE et al (2001) Long-term results of the lateral tunnel Fontan operation. J Thoracic Cardiovasc Surg 121:28–41

29. Nurnberg JH, Ovroutski S, Alexi-Meskishvili V, Ewert P, Hetzer R, Lange PE (2004) New onset arrhythmias after the extracardiac conduit Fontan operation compared with the intraatrial lateral tunnel procedure: early and midterm results. Ann Thoracic Surg 78:1979–1988

30. Ovroutski S, Dahnert I, Alexi-Meskishvili V, Nurnberg JH, Hetzer R, Lange PE (2001) Preliminary analysis of arrhythmias after the Fontan operation with extracardiac conduit compared with intra-atrial lateral tunnel. Thoracic Cardiovasc Surgeon 49:334–337

31. Varma C, Warr MR, Hendler AL, Paul NS, Webb GD, Therrien J (2003) Prevalence of "silent" pulmonary emboli in adults after the Fontan operation. J Am College Cardiol 41:2252–2258

32. Walsh EP, Cecchin F (2007) Arrhythmias in adult patients with congenital heart disease. Circulation 115:534–545

33. Kanter RJ, Papagiannis J, Carboni MP, Ungerleider RM, Sanders WE, Wharton JM (2000) Radiofrequency catheter ablation of supraventricular tachycardia substrates after mustard and senning operations for d-transposition of the great arteries. J Am Coll Cardiol 35:428–441

34. Agnoletti G, Borghi A, Vignati G, Crupi GC (2003) Fontan conversion to total cavopulmonary connection and arrhythmia ablation: clinical and functional results. Heart 89:193–198

35. Sheikh AM, Tang AT, Roman K et al (2004) The failing Fontan circulation: successful conversion of atriopulmonary connections. J Thorac Cardiovasc Surg 128:60–66

36. Mavroudis C, Deal BJ, Backer CL (2004) Surgery for arrhythmias in children. Int J Cardiol 97(Suppl 1):39–51

37. Weinstein S, Chan D (2005) Extracardiac Fontan conversion, cryoablation, and pacemaker placement for patients with a failed Fontan. Semin Thorac Cardiovasc Surg 17:170–178

38. Morales DL, Dibardino DJ, Braud BE et al (2005) Salvaging the failing Fontan: lateral tunnel versus extracardiac conduit. Ann Thorac Surg 80:1445–1451; discussion 1451–1452

39. Triedman JK, Alexander ME, Love BA et al (2002) Influence of patient factors and ablative technologies on outcomes of radiofrequency ablation of intra-atrial re-entrant tachycardia in patients with congenital heart disease. J Am College Cardiol 39:1827–1835

40. Triedman JK, Alexander ME, Berul CI, Bevilacqua LM, Walsh EP (2001) Electroanatomic mapping of entrained and exit zones in patients with repaired congenital heart disease and intra-atrial reentrant tachycardia. Circulation 103:2060–2065

41. Nakagawa H, Shah N, Matsudaira K et al (2001) Characterization of reentrant circuit in macroreentrant right atrial tachycardia after surgical repair of congenital heart disease – isolated channels between scars allow "focal" ablation. Circulation 103:699–709

42. Collins KK, Love BA, Walsh EP, Saul JP, Epstein MR, Triedman JK (2000) Location of acutely successful radiofrequency catheter ablation of intraatrial reentrant tachycardia in patients with congenital heart disease. Am J Cardiol 86:969–74

43. Kannankeril PJ, Anderson ME, Rottman JN, Wathen MS, Fish FA (2003) Frequency of late recurrence of intra-atrial reentry tachycardia after radiofrequency catheter ablation in patients with congenital heart disease. Am J Cardiol 92:879–881

44. Nehgme RA, Carboni MP, Care J, Murphy JD (2006) Transthoracic percutaneous access for electroanatomic mapping and catheter ablation of atrial tachycardia in patients with a lateral tunnel Fontan. Heart Rhythm 3:37–43

45. Gatzoulis MA, Balaji S, Webber SA et al (2000) Risk factors for arrhythmia and sudden cardiac death late after repair of tetralogy of Fallot: a multicentre study. Lancet 356:975–981

46. Khairy P, Landzberg MJ, Gatzoulis MA et al (2004) Value of programmed ventricular stimulation after tetralogy of Fallot repair – a multicenter study. Circulation 109:1994–2000

47. Khairy P, Harris L, Landzberg MJ et al (2008) Implantable cardioverter-defibrillators in tetralogy of Fallot. Circulation 117:363–370

48. Andersen HO, de Leval MR, Tsang VT, Elliott MJ, Anderson RH, Cook AC (2006) Is complete heart block after surgical closure of ventricular septum defects still an issue? Ann Thoracic Surg 82:948–957

49. Hokanson JS, Moller JH (2001) Significance of early transient complete heart block as a predictor of sudden death late after operative correction of tetralogy of Fallot. Am J Cardiol 87:1271–1277

50. Abd El Rahman MY, Hui W, Yigitbasi M et al (2005) Detection of left ventricular asynchrony in patients with right bundle branch block after repair of tetralogy of Fallot using tissue-Doppler imaging-derived strain. J Am College Cardiol 45:915–921

51. D'Andrea A, Caso P, Sarubbi B et al (2004) Right ventricular myocardial dysfunction in adult patients late after repair of tetralogy of Fallot. Int J Cardiol 94:213–220

52. Qu Y, Xiao GQ, Chen L, Boutjdir M (2001) Autoantibodies from mothers of children with congenital heart block downregulate cardiac L-type Ca channels. J Mol Cell Cardiol 33:1153–1163

53. Jay PY, Harris BS, Buerger A et al (2004) Function follows form: cardiac conduction system defects in Nkx2–5 mutation. Anat Rec A Discov Mol Cell Evol Biol 280:966–972

54. Bossert T, Walther T, Gummert J, Hubald R, Kostelka M, Mohr FW (2002) Cardiac malformations associated with the Holt-Oram syndrome–report on a family and review of the literature. Thorac Cardiovasc Surg 50:312–314

55. Kleinman CS, Nehgme RA (2004) Cardiac arrhythmias in the human fetus. Pediatric Cardiol 25:234–251

56. Raboisson MJ, Fouron JC, Sonesson SE, Nyman M, Proulx F, Gamache S (2005) Fetal Doppler echocardiographic diagnosis and successful steroid therapy of Luciani-Wenckebach phenomenon and endocardial fibroelastosis related to maternal anti-Ro and anti-La antibodies. J Am Soc Echocardiogr 18:375–380

57. Jaeggi ET, Silverman ED, Yoo SJ, Kingdom J (2004) Is immune-mediated complete fetal atrioventricular block reversible by transplacental dexamethasone therapy? Ultrasound Obstetrics Gynecol 23:602–605

58. Fesslova V, Mannarino S, Salice P et al (2003) Neonatal lupus: fetal myocarditis progressing to atrioventricular block in triplets. Lupus 12:775–778

59. Askanase AD, Friedman DM, Copel J et al (2002) Spectrum and progression of conduction abnormalities in infants born to mothers with anti-SSA/Ro-SSB/La antibodies. Lupus 11:145–151

60. Breur J, Visser GHA, Kruize AA, Stoutenbeek P, Meijboom EJ (2004) Treatment of fetal heart block with maternal steroid therapy: case report and review of the literature. Ultrasound Obstetrics Gynecol 24:467–472

61. Matsubara S, Morimatsu Y, Shiraishi H et al (2008) Fetus with heart failure due to congenital atrioventricular block treated by maternally administered ritodrine. Arch Gynecol Obstet 278:85–88

62. Epstein AE, DiMarco JP, Ellenbogen KA et al (2008) ACC/AHA/HRS 2008 guidelines for device-based therapy of cardiac rhythm abnormalities: a report of the American college of cardiology/American heart association task force on practice guidelines (writing committee to revise the acc/aha/naspe 2002 guideline update for implantation of cardiac pacemakers and antiarrhythmia devices) developed in collaboration with the American association for thoracic surgery and society of thoracic surgeons. J Am Coll Cardiol 51:e1–e62

63. Michaelsson M, Jonzon A, Riesenfeld T (1995) Isolated congenital complete atrioventricular block in adult life. A prospective study. Circulation 92:442–449

64. Moak JP, Barron KS, Hougen TJ et al (2001) Congenital heart block: development of late-onset cardiomyopathy, a previously underappreciated sequela. J Am Coll Cardiol 37:238–242

65. Cecchin F, Frangini PA, Brown DW et al (2009) Cardiac resynchronization therapy (and multisite pacing) in pediatrics and congenital heart disease: five years experience in a single institution. J Cardiovasc Electrophysiol 20:58–65

66. Lee PC, Chen SA, Chiang CE, Tai CT, Yu WC, Hwang B (2003) Clinical and electrophysiological characteristics in children with atrioventricular nodal reentrant tachycardia. Pediatr Cardiol 24:6–9

67. Blurton DJ, Dubin AM, Chiesa NA, Van Hare GF, Collins KK (2006) Characterizing dual atrioventricular nodal physiology in pediatric patients with atrioventricular nodal reentrant tachycardia. J Cardiovasc Electrophysiol 17:638–644

68. Kannankeril PJ, Fish FA (2006) Sustained slow pathway conduction: superior to dual atrioventricular node physiology in young patients with atrioventricular nodal reentry tachycardia? Pacing Clin Electrophysiol 29:159–163

69. Santinelli V, Radinovic A, Manguso F et al (2009) The natural history of asymptomatic ventricular pre-excitation a long-term prospective follow-up study of 184 asymptomatic children. J Am Coll Cardiol 53:275–280

70. Bromberg BI, Lindsay BD, Cain ME, Cox JL (1996) Impact of clinical history and electrophysiologic characterization of accessory pathways on management strategies to reduce sudden death among children with Wolff-Parkinson-White syndrome. J Am Coll Cardiol 27:690–695

71. Bradley DJ, Fischbach PS, Law IH, Serwer GA, Dick M (2001) The clinical course of multifocal atrial tachycardia in infants and children. J Am College Cardiol 38:401–408

72. Sarubbi B, Musto B, Ducceschi V et al (2002) Congenital junctional ectopic tachycardia in children and adolescents: a 20 year experience based study. Heart 88:188–190

73. Collins KK, Van Hare GF, Kertesz NJ et al (2009) Pediatric nonpost-operative junctional ectopic tachycardia medical management and interventional therapies. J Am Coll Cardiol 53:690–697

74. Fukuhara H, Nakamura Y, Ohnishi T (2001) Atrial pacing during radiofrequency ablation of junctional ectopic tachycardia – a useful technique for avoiding atrioventricular bloc. Jpn Circ J 65:242–244

75. Bae EJ, Kang SJ, Noh CI, Choi JY, Yun YS (2005) A case of congenital junctional ectopic tachycardia: diagnosis and successful radiofrequency catheter ablation in infancy. Pacing Clin Electrophysiol 28:254–257

76. Batra AS, Chun DS, Johnson TR et al (2006) A prospective analysis of the incidence and risk factors associated with junctional ectopic tachycardia following surgery for congenital heart disease. Pediatr Cardiol 27:51–55

77. Delaney JW, Moltedo JM, Dziura JD, Kopf GS, Snyder CS (2006) Early postoperative arrhythmias after pediatric cardiac surgery. J Thorac Cardiovasc Surg 131:1296–300

78. Andreasen JB, Johnsen SP, Ravn HB (2008) Junctional ectopic tachycardia after surgery for congenital heart disease in children. Intensive Care Med 34:895–902

79. Van Hare GF, Carmelli D, Smith WM et al (2002) Prospective assessment after pediatric cardiac ablation: design and implementation of the multicenter study. Pacing Clin Electrophysiol 25:332–341

80. Perry JC (2006) State-of-the-art pediatric interventional electrophysiology: transvenous cryoablation establishes its niche. Heart Rhythm 3:259–260

81. Friedman RA, Walsh EP, Silka MJ et al (2002) NASPE expert consensus conference: radiofrequency catheter ablation in children with and without congenital heart disease. Report of the writing committee. North American society of pacing and electrophysiology. Pacing Clin Electrophysiol 25:1000–1017

82. Al-Ammouri I, Perry JC (2006) Proximity of coronary arteries to the atrioventricular valve annulus in young patients and implications for ablation procedures. Am J Cardiol 97:1752–175

83. Weiss C, Becker J, Hoffmann M, Willems S (2002) Can radiofrequency current isthmus ablation damage the right coronary artery? Histopathological findings following the use of a long (8 mm) tip electrode. Pacing Clin Electrophysiol 25:860–862

84. Sassone B, Leone O, Martinelli GN, Di Pasquale G (2004) Acute myocardial infarction after radiofrequency catheter ablation of typical atrial flutter: histopathological findings and etiopathogenetic hypothesis. Ital Heart J 5:403–407

85. Lustgarten DL, Bell S, Hardin N, Calame J, Spector PS (2005) Safety and efficacy of epicardial cryoablation in a canine model. Heart Rhythm 2:82–90

86. Kolditz DP, Blom NA, Bokenkamp R, Schalij MJ (2005) Low-energy radiofrequency catheter ablation as therapy for supraventricular tachycardia in a premature neonate. Eur J Pediatr 164:559–562

87. Blaufox AD, Paul T, Saul JP (2004) Radiofrequency catheter ablation in small children: relationship of complications to application dose. Pacing Clin Electrophysiol 27:224–229

88. Blaufox AD, Numan MT, Laohakunakorn P, Knick B, Paul T, Saul JP (2002) Catheter tip cooling during radiofrequency ablation of intra-atrial reentry: effects on power, temperature, and impedance. J Cardiovasc Electrophysiol 13:783–787

89. Emmel M, Sreeram N, Pillekamp F, Boehm W, Brockmeier K (2006) Transhepatic approach for catheter interventions in infants and children with congenital heart disease. Clin Res Cardiol 95:329–333

90. Kilic A, Amasyali B, Kose S, Aytemir K, Kursaklioglu H, Lenk MK (2005) Successful catheter ablation of a right-sided accessory pathway in a child with interruption of the inferior vena cava and azygos continuation. Int Heart J 46:537–541

91. Drago F, Silvetti MS, Di Pino A, Grutter G, Bevilacqua M, Leibovich S (2002) Exclusion of fluoroscopy during ablation treatment of right accessory pathway in children. J Cardiovasc Electrophysiol 13:778–782

92. Erb TO, Kanter RJ, Hall JM, Gan TJ, Kern FH, Schulman SR (2002) Comparison of electrophysiologic effects of propofol and isoflurane-based anesthetics in children undergoing radiofrequency catheter ablation for supraventricular tachycardia. Anesthesiology 96:1386–1394

93. Van Hare GF, Javitz H, Carmelli D et al (2004) Prospective assessment after pediatric cardiac ablation: demographics, medical profiles, and initial outcomes. J Cardiovasc Electrophysiol 15:759–770

94. Van Hare GF, Javitz H, Carmelli D et al (2004) Prospective assessment after pediatric cardiac ablation: recurrence at 1 year after initially successful ablation of supraventricular tachycardia. Heart Rhythm 1:188–196

95. Bae EJ, Ban JE, Lee JA et al (2005) Pediatric radiofrequency catheter ablation: results of initial 100 consecutive cases including congenital heart anomalies. J Korean Med Sci 20:740–746

96. Celiker A, Kafali G, Karagoz T, Ceviz N, Ozer S (2003) The results of electrophysiological study and radio-frequency catheter ablation in pediatric patients with tachyarrhythmia. Turk J Pediatr 45:209–216

97. Papez AL, Al-Ahdab M, Dick M 2nd, Fischbach PS (2006) Transcatheter cryotherapy for the treatment of supraventricular tachyarrhythmias in children: a single center experience. J Interv Card Electrophysiol 15:191–196

98. Miyazaki A, Blaufox AD, Fairbrother DL, Saul JP (2005) Cryo-ablation for septal tachycardia substrates in pediatric patients: mid-term results. J Am Coll Cardiol 45:581–588

99. Kirsh JA, Gross GJ, O'Connor S, Hamilton RM (2005) Transcatheter cryoablation of tachyarrhythmias in children: initial experience from an international registry. J Am Coll Cardiol 45:133–136

100. Kriebel T, Broistedt C, Kroll M, Sigler M, Paul T (2005) Efficacy and safety of cryoenergy in the ablation of atrioventricular reentrant tachycardia substrates in children and adolescents. J Cardiovasc Electrophysiol 16:960–966

101. Drago F, De Santis A, Grutter G, Silvetti MS (2005) Transvenous cryothermal catheter ablation of re-entry circuit located near the atrioventricular junction in pediatric patients: efficacy, safety, and midterm follow-up. J Am Coll Cardiol 45:1096–1103

102. Bar-Cohen Y, Cecchin F, Alexander ME, Berul CI, Triedman JK, Walsh EP (2006) Cryoablation for accessory pathways located near normal conduction tissues or within the coronary venous system in children and young adults. Heart Rhythm 3:253–258

103. Drago F, Silvetti MS, De Santis A, Grutter G, Andrew P (2006) Lengthier cryoablation and a bonus cryoapplication is associated with improved efficacy for cryothermal catheter ablation of supraventricular tachycardias in children. J Interv Card Electrophysiol 16:191–198

104. Moniotte S, Triedman JK, Cecchin F (2008) Successful cryoablation of ventricular tachycardia arising from the proximal right bundle branch in a child. Heart Rhythm 5:142–144

105. Janousek J, Vojtovic P, Hucin B et al (2001) Resynchronization pacing is a useful adjunct to the management of acute heart failure after surgery for congenital heart defects. Am J Cardiol 88:145–152

106. Dubin AM, Janousek J, Rhee E et al (2005) Resynchronization therapy in pediatric and congenital heart disease patients – an international multicenter study. J Am College Cardiol 46:2277–2283

107. Jauvert G, Rousseau-Paziaud J, Villain E et al (2009) Effects of cardiac resynchronization therapy on echocardiographic indices, functional capacity, and clinical outcomes of patients with a systemic right ventricle. Europace 11:184–190

108. Zimmerman FJ, Starr JP, Koenig PR, Smith P, Hijazi ZM, Bacha EA (2003) Acute hemodynamic benefit of multisite ventricular pacing after congenital heart surgery. Ann Thorac Surg 75:1775–1780

109. Silka MJ, Kron J, Dunnigan A, Dick M 2nd (1993) Sudden cardiac death and the use of implantable cardioverter-defibrillators in pediatric patients. The pediatric electrophysiology society. Circulation 87:800–807

110. Spirito P, Bellone P, Harris KM, Bernabo P, Bruzzi P, Maron BJ (2000) Magnitude of left ventricular hypertrophy and risk of sudden death in hypertrophic cardiomyopathy. N Engl J Med 342:1778–1785

111. Dubin AM, Berul CI, Bevilacqua LM et al (2003) The use of implantable cardioverter-defibrillators in pediatric patients awaiting heart transplantation. J Card Fail 9:375–379

112. Stephenson EA, Batra AS, Knilans TK et al (2006) A multicenter experience with novel implantable cardioverter defibrillator configurations in the pediatric and congenital heart disease population. J Cardiovasc Electrophysiol 17:41–46

113. Blom NA (2008) Implantable cardioverter-defibrillators in children. Pacing Clin Electrophysiol 31(Suppl 1):S32–S34

114. Ten Harkel AD, Blom NA, Reimer AG, Tukkie R, Sreeram N, Bink-Boelkens MT (2005) Implantable cardioverter defibrillator implantation in children in The Netherlands. Eur J Pediatr 164:436–441

115. Gradaus R, Wollmann C, Kobe J et al (2004) Potential benefit from implantable cardioverter-defibrillator therapy in children and young adolescents. Heart 90:328–329

116. Stefanelli CB, Bradley DJ, Leroy S, Dick M 2nd, Serwer GA, Fischbach PS (2002) Implantable cardioverter defibrillator therapy for life-threatening arrhythmias in young patients. J Interv Card Electrophysiol 6:235–244

117. Korte T, Koditz H, Niehaus M, Paul T, Tebbenjohanns J (2004) High incidence of appropriate and inappropriate ICD therapies in children and adolescents with implantable cardioverter defibrillator. Pacing Clin Electrophysiol 27:924–932

118. DeMaso DR, Lauretti A, Spieth L et al (2004) Psychosocial factors and quality of life in children and adolescents with implantable cardioverter-defibrillators. Am J Cardiol 93:582–587

119. Fuster V, O'Rourke RA, Walsh RA, Poole-Wilson P (eds) (2008) Hurst's the heart, 12th edn. McGraw-Hill, New York, NY

120. Mavroudis C, Backer CL, Deal BJ, Johnsrude C, Strasburger J (2001) Total cavopulmonary conversion and maze procedure for patients with failure of the Fontan operation. J Thorac Cardiovasc Surg 122:863–871

VI SPECIFIC SYNDROMES

18 Syncope

Ilknur Can and David G. Benditt

CONTENTS

Abstract

Syncope is a syndrome characterized by a relatively sudden, temporary, and self-terminating loss of consciousness. Possible causes of syncope are numerous, but the unifying feature is the underlying pathophysiology; specifically, a temporary inadequacy of cerebral nutrient flow most often due to a fall in systemic arterial pressure. Delineating the underlying etiology of syncope in a given patient is often challenging but is important, since syncope, while even if often relatively benign from a mortality perspective, tends to recur. An inaccurate diagnosis and an incorrect treatment leave the affected individual at risk of physical injury, diminished quality-of-life, and possible restriction from employment or avocation; furthermore, a life-threatening problem may be missed (e.g., cardiac syncope, channelopathies). In the majority of patients presenting with syncope a careful history, physical examination, ECG, and possibly an echocardiogram are sufficient to establish the diagnosis with substantial certainty. The most common example is when the history is indicative of one of the neurally mediated reflex faints (i.e., vasovagal, carotid sinus, or situational syncope). However, although the medical history is the physician's most valuable tool in the initial syncope assessment, its value is undermined if it is inadequate in detail and/or the patient cannot provide a reliable description of events (e.g., children, patients with cognitive impairment). In these latter cases or if the initial evaluation is inconclusive, selective application of further diagnostic tests (e.g., ambulatory ECG monitoring, head-up tilt test) is needed. As a rule assessment should be lead by physicians who take a particular interest in the syncope evaluation. In this regard, more widespread development of syncope management units (SMUs) and rapid access syncope/falls clinics is strongly encouraged; together, they have been shown to reduce both hospital costs and number of undiagnosed cases.

Key Words: Syncope; carotid sinus syndrome; fainting; neural reflex syncope; vasodepressor; arrhythmia; vasodilatation; hypotension; cerebral hypoperfusion; orthostatic; tachycardia; vasovagal

From: *Contemporary Cardiology: Management of Cardiac Arrhythmias*
Edited by: Gan-Xin Yan, Peter R. Kowey, DOI 10.1007/978-1-60761-161-5_18
© Springer Science+Business Media, LLC 2011

syncope; pseudosyncope; bradycardia; ECG monitors; transient loss of consciousness (TLOC); fludrocortisone; loop-recorders; tilt-table; midodrine; beta-blocker.

Syncope is a syndrome characterized by a relatively sudden, temporary, and self-terminating loss of consciousness. Possible causes of syncope are numerous, but the unifying feature is the underlying pathophysiology; specifically, a temporary inadequacy of cerebral nutrient flow most often due to a fall in systemic arterial pressure below the minimum needed to sustain cerebral blood flow.

Despite the fact that syncope is relatively common *(1–3)*, it is only one of many possible explanations for suspected episodic transient loss of consciousness (TLOC) (Fig. 1). Consequently, the diagnostic evaluation of a patient who presents with an apparent self-terminating collapse or "blackout" should start not with assuming that it was "syncope", but should be initiated more broadly with consideration of a range of possible causes for real (e.g., seizures and concussion) or seemingly real (e.g., narcolepsy and certain psychogenic disturbances) TLOC *(1)* (Table 1).

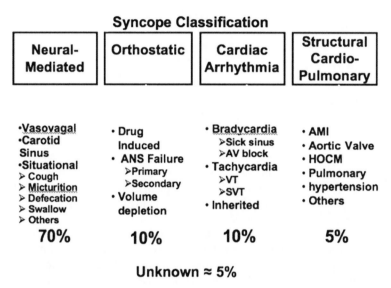

Fig. 1. Classification of syncope and approximate frequency of occurrence in published studies. As a rule the causes on the *left side* of the figure are most frequent and the likelihood of possible cause of syncope decreases as one move towards the *right side* of the figure.

Table 1
Pathophysiological Differences Among Causes of Real or Seemingly Real TLOC

Condition	Basic pathophysiology
Syncope	Transient self-terminating insufficiency of cerebral nutrient perfusion
Concussion	Head trauma
Epilepsy	Primary electrical disturbance of cerebral function
Intoxication	Self-terminating depression of cerebral function by excess of specific agent (e.g., alcohol, psychotropic drugs)
Metabolic	Self-terminating depression of cerebral function by metabolic disturbance (e.g., hypoglycemia)
Psychogenic	Not true TLOC, mechanisms unknown (pseudosyncope, pseudoseizure)

ESSENTIAL FEATURES OF SYNCOPE

Loss of Consciousness

True loss of consciousness is the "sine qua non" of syncope. Its occurrence can only be derived from the history taken from the patient and/or from those who witnessed the episode(s). In this regard, "consciousness" is a complex concept that lies beyond the scope of this chapter. However, physicians usually have a "working" definition that suffices for most clinical purposes. In essence, loss of consciousness implies not only loss of awareness and appropriate responsiveness to external stimuli but also loss of postural tone. Consequently, if standing, the fainter falls down; if seated he or she slumps over. Only rarely does syncope occur with the patient supine or prone; such cases suggest that a hemodynamically serious tachy- or bradyarrhythmia has occurred.

Occasionally, symptoms may suggest that "syncope" is imminent, but the full TLOC picture does not evolve at that time. This circumstance, which physicians may consider as being a "near-syncope", is usually described by patients as "dizziness" or "lightheadedness". However, these latter complaints (especially in the elderly) are nonspecific and may be due to an ill-defined functional cerebral disturbance triggered by a less severe transient hypotension than that needed to cause a complete faint. One should not assume that all complaints of "lightheadedness" are "near-syncope". Distinguishing transient functional disturbances of cerebral function due to modest hypoperfusion from "lightheadeness" of non-specific origin is often difficult.

If the history indicates that there has not been loss of consciousness associated with the "spell", then "true" syncope is excluded. On the other hand, one can be misled. Due to lack of recall, cognitive impairment (especially in elderly "fallers") or embarrassment, the patient may deny having lost consciousness. Reports from witnesses may prove essential to clarify the story. Often, however, despite best efforts, whether true loss of consciousness has occurred remains unclear, and it is not possible to distinguish a faint from other conditions (e.g., an accidental fall).

Onset is Relatively Rapid

The timing of events surrounding an apparent syncope is unreliable, as many fainters either do not experience or have no recall of premonitory symptoms, or are incapable of assessing the passage of time accurately. Nonetheless, true syncope tends to be characterized by a relatively abrupt onset, perhaps within 10–20 sec of warning symptoms.

Recovery is Spontaneous, Complete, and Usually Prompt

A spontaneous, complete, and prompt recovery from the faint excludes a number of nonsyncope conditions that may cause TLOC, but which do not self-terminate promptly or require medical intervention. Examples include coma, intoxicated states, and stroke (which may cause loss of consciousness in some instances). On the other hand, in certain forms of syncope, particularly the vasovagal faint, recovery while rapid, may be accompanied by fatigue, and a general sense of diminished energy for a lengthy period of time (often hours in duration).

Underlying Mechanism is Transient Global Cerebral Hypoperfusion

Cerebral hypoperfusion differentiates "true syncope" from loss of consciousness due to trauma (e.g., concussion), seizures (epilepsy), intoxications, or metabolic disturbances. Both trauma and epilepsy may lead to loss of consciousness with complete and spontaneous recovery, but their origins are not inadequacy of cerebral perfusion. With regard to differentiating syncope from epilepsy, the aspect that causes most confusion is abnormal motor activity. Jerky movements of the arms and legs for a brief period of time (sometimes referred to as "convulsive syncope") is not unusual in syncope; non-expert bystanders may incorrectly interpret these movements as a "seizure" or a "fit". However, jerky movements during a faint differ from those accompanying epilepsy; they are of shorter duration, tend to occur after rather than before collapse, do not have tonic-clonic features, and are briefer in duration.

INITIAL EVALUATION

Among patients in whom TLOC is deemed to be due to "true" syncope, the next step is thorough evaluation of the underlying cause (Fig. 2). The goal should be to determine the cause of syncope with sufficient confidence to provide a reliable assessment of prognosis, recurrence risk, and treatment options.

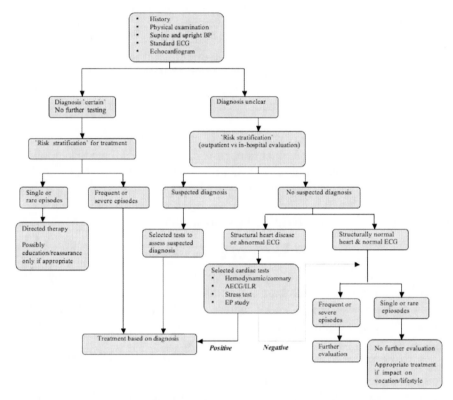

Fig. 2. Initial evaluation and further management strategy of syncope based on European Society of Cardiology Task Force Guidelines (1). ECG, electrocardiogram; BP; blood pressure; AECG, ambulatory electrocardiogram; ILR, implantable loop recorder; EP, electrophysiologic.

The initial evaluation alone will permit an experienced physician to determine, with a high level of confidence, the cause of syncope in a substantial proportion of patients. As a rule, the initial evaluation begins with a comprehensive medical history including detailed description of symptomatic events. We recommend beginning with obtaining details of the most recent episode, and then going backward one-by-one with the expectation that a pattern will emerge. Additionaly, careful note should be made of patient's co-morbidities (for example diabetic neuropathy, autonomic dysfunction), drug therapy (including recent dose changes), and family history. A pre-prepared patient questionnaire may prove helpful to save time and still acquire the needed details. Additional steps at this stage include physical examination, electrocardiogram (ECG), and often an echocardiogram.

Although the medical history is the physician's most valuable tool in the initial syncope assessment, its value is undermined if the patient cannot provide a reliable description of events. Elderly patients and those with cognitive impairment may not remember or accurately relate crucial details. In other cases, patients may not volunteer information because of risk of losing jobs, avocations, or driving privileges. Consequently, family members, friends, and witnesses to symptomatic events should be included in the history-taking process, whenever possible.

Not infrequently the history alone is diagnostic of the cause of syncope and no further testing is needed. The most common example is when the history is indicative of a "classic" vasovagal faint or one of the so-called "situational" neurally mediated reflex faints. In such cases, an experienced physician can feel comfortable that the basis for symptoms has been established, and can proceed with appropriate treatment steps.

Among the most important factors to identify in the patient with suspected syncope is whether he/she has a history of or physical findings suggesting the presence of underlying structural heart disease. In this regard, the inclusion of an echocardiogram as part of the initial evaluation of suspected syncope patients can be valuable. The presence of heart disease is an independent predictor of a "cardiac cause" for syncope (i.e., a primary arrhythmic cause or a cause based on a structural cardiac abnormality leading to a transient hemodynamic disturbance), with a sensitivity of 95% and a specificity of 45%; by contrast, the absence of heart disease excludes a cardiac cause of syncope in 97% of the patients (4).

Syncope in conjunction with exertion raises special concerns. In particular, if the faint occurs in "full flight", one must consider the possibility of structural and/or dynamic heart lesions producing a relatively "fixed" cardiac output in the setting of vascular dilatation (e.g., severe aortic or mitral valvular stenosis, hypertrophic cardiomyopathy). However, syncope during or early following exercise (even moderate exertion such as climbing stairs) can also occur in patients with severe autonomic dysfunction (e.g., pure autonomic failure) in whom vascular control is unable to maintain adequate cerebral perfusion pressure (the presence of neck and shoulder pain in a "clothes hanger distribution" is an uncommon but important suggestion of autonomic failure syndrome). In addition, on rare occasions syncope accompanying exertion may occur as a consequence of a neurally mediated reflex faint (i.e., post-exertional variant of vasovagal faint); however, in these latter cases the faint typically occurs shortly after completion of, not during, the exercise.

DOES MANAGEMENT REQUIRE ADMISSION TO HOSPITAL?

Even after the emergency departmnent (ED) physician or general practitioner has concluded that "syncope" was the most likely cause of TLOC, clinical assessment may remain a challenge for several reasons. First, the affected individual is usually asymptomatic on arrival for medical attention, and as a result the physician has no direct "acute event observations" to work with. Second, the victim (especially if in an older age group) may not be able to provide a detailed history of the circumstances. Third, the event(s) may not have been witnessed; or if witnessed, the observer may not be able to recollect sufficient detail. Finally, as noted earlier syncope has many possible causes ranging from relatively benign to potentially life-threatening arrhythmias. Sorting through the possibilities may be time-consuming, and consequently not feasible given time limitations in an urgent care setting. Therefore, the physician almost always must determine whether the affected individual needs in-hospital evaluation or can be referred to an outpatient syncope evaluation clinic; in general, the issue that determines the answer to this question is most often concern regarding the individual's immediate mortality risk, potential for physical injury (e.g., falls risk), the patient's ability to care for him/herself, and to a lesser extent the issue of whether certain treatments inherently require in-hospital initiation.

The outcome of the "hospitalization versus outpatient management" decision has many implications, including life-style and economic concerns for the patient, health care system management issues (e.g. bed availability, hospital costs, and laboratory utilization), and ultimately impact on the broader healthcare system. In this regard utilization of syncope management units, guideline-based softwares, and personnel training has been shown to reduce hospitalization rates, in-hospital stays, number of tests performed, and mean cost per diagnosis (5, 6).

In instances when the etiology of syncope has been diagnosed after initial clinical evaluation, need for hospitalization depends in part on the immediate risk posed by the underlying problem, and in addition on the treatment proposed. Thus, for example, patients with syncope accompanying complete heart block, ventricular tachycardia, acute aortic dissection, or pulmonary embolism should be admitted to the hospital and preferably to an ECG monitored unit. On the other hand, most vasovagal fainters can be sent home after careful discussion of the nature of the problem and simple preventative maneuvers (e.g., hydration, avoidance of hot crowded environments, etc.); syncope evaluation clinic follow-up suffices in most of these cases.

The following provides an overview of common circumstances for which hospitalization is recommended or conversely is usually not needed.

Patients at High Risk

Several markers identify syncope patients who should be considered for in-hospital evaluation. Syncope associated with symptoms suggestive of acute myocardial ischemia or acute aortic dissection, signs or biochemical evidence (i.e., elevated brain natriuretic peptide, BNP) of congestive heart failure, and/or suspicion of hemodynamically concerning underlying structural heart disease (e.g., valvular aortic stenosis, pulmonary hypertension) have the highest immediate mortality risk. At similar high risk are the syncope patients with certain electrocardiographic (ECG) abnormalities, including high-grade AV block, cardiac pauses >3 sec, preexcitation syndromes (e.g., Wolff-Parkinson-White Syndrome), or suspected ventricular tachycardia including torsade de pointes (i.e., marked QT interval prolongation). Patients with syncope during exercise, and syncope causing motor vehicle or major work accidents or severe injury, should also be evaluated in the hospital.

Patients with Intermediate Risk

Syncope associated at age >50 years, history of structural heart disease but without signs of active consequences of disease, certain ECG abnormalities (e.g., bundle-branch block, Q wave), family history of sudden death, cardiac devices without evidence of dysfunction, symptoms not consistent with vasovagal or reflex-mediated syncope, and physician's judgment that a cardiac syncope is possible constitute the patient group with intermediate risk for adverse outcome.

At present, guidelines for management of intermediate risk cases are ill-defined. However, we recommend that an ED-based observation unit may be useful initially; if there are no particiularly worrisome physical examination, x-ray, ECG or biochemical findings after 4–6 h they could be managed without hospital admission. These patients should be referred to and promptly seen (typically <72 h) in a syncope evaluation clinic.

Patients with Low Risk

Patients in this group typically have no evidence of structural heart disease and have a normal baseline ECG. The syncope is considered of a "relatively benign" nature in terms of mortality risk (although "falls" and injury risk remains a concern). As a rule, syncope in thsese cases is of neurally-mediated reflex or orthostatic cause. However, rarer conditions that are more worrisome may present with a normal ECG; these include long QT syndromes, Brugada syndrome, and other less well-defined channelopathies.

Low-risk patients can generally be stabilized in the ED or clinic. Most can be reassured regarding immediate mortality risk, but early further assessment in a "syncope/falls" clinic is recommended.

SYNCOPE MANAGEMENT UNITS (SMUs)

Syncope management units have been advocated by the ESC Syncope Task Force as a means of enhancing the management process for syncope patients while reducing cost. Such a "unit" might take several forms. In most institutions, the SMU is a "virtual unit" consisting mainly of a working relationship among several key medical specialties (usually cardiac electrophysiology, neurology, general medicine, and geriatrics). In some hospitals the SMU may be a physical space, incorporating an observation unit and possibly an outpatient facility. Currently, however, SMUs remain a relatively infrequent finding.

An as yet incompletely answered question is whether structured guideline-directed SMU care can help solve the problem of too many low- and intermediate-risk syncope patients being admitted to hospital where they often are submitted to unneeded expensive diagnostic tests. However, recent prospective observational studies suggest that a positive benefit is likely. For instance, the SEEDS study *(5)* was a single-center, unblinded randomized study in which 103 patients were randomized to "standard care" or SMU after initial assessment. The study found that a presumptive diagnosis of the cause of syncope was significantly increased from 10% in the "standard care" patients to 67% among those who underwent SMU evaluation; hospital admission was reduced from 98% among the "standard care" patients to 43% among the SMU patients. Furthermore, the total length of patient-hospital days was reduced by >50% for patients in the SMU group. In the Evaluation of Guidelines in Syncope Study-2 (EGSYS-2), the application of guidelines to clinical circumstances was facilitated by the use of purpose-designed software in addition to personnel training at test sites *(6)*. A definite diagnosis was established in 98% of cases, with the initial evaluation (history, physical examination, and electrocardiogram) establishing a diagnosis in 50% of cases. The investigators further compared the outcomes of 745 patients managed with this "standardized care" system to 929 patients managed with usual care. In the group designated to "standardized-care", hospitalizations were fewer, in-hospital stay was shorter, fewer tests were performed per patient, and cost per patient and mean cost per diagnosis were lower.

CLASSIFICATION OF THE CAUSES OF SYNCOPE

Given the many possible causes for syncope, it is crucial that the practitioner approach the problem in an organized manner (Fig. 2). Unfortunately though, even after careful assessment it may not be possible to assign a single cause for fainting. Patients often have multiple comorbidities, and consequently several equally probable causes of fainting (or several conditions may act together to cause the faint). Thus, while individuals with severe heart disease may nonetheless be susceptible to vasovagal faints, they may also suffer transient tachyarrhythmias, high-grade atrioventricular (AV) block, or even the effects of being excessively medicated. Thus, the physician must not readily accept an observed abnormality as either the certain cause or the sole cause of fainting in a given individual.

Neurally Mediated Reflex Syncope

The neurally mediated reflex syncope (NMS) syndromes have three common variations: vasovagal syncope (the most frequent of all causes of fainting and often termed the "common faint"), carotid sinus syndrome, and the so-called "situational faints". The principal pathophysiological mechanism of these faints is the triggering of a neural reflex resulting in both hypotension due to vaso- and venodilation (including the splanchnic bed) and an inappropriate chronotropic response (occasionally resulting in severe bradycardia or asystole, but at other times causing a "relative" bradycardia in which the heart rate is less than expected for the degree of hypotension) *(7, 8)*. Both vascular dilatation and/or brady-cardia may diminish arterial pressure sufficiently (below cerebrovascular autoregulatory capability) to compromise perfusion to the brain, thereby causing syncope; however, the contribution of each of these two factors to systemic hypotension and cerebral hypoperfusion may vary considerably among patients and probably even within patients at different times.

VASOVAGAL SYNCOPE (COMMON FAINT)

The reflexes that cause vasovagal syncope are thought to be universal, and consequently it is believed that such faints may occur in anybody; about 20–30% of the population report events in their lifetime. However, it seems that certain individuals are particularly susceptible, although susceptibility may vary during their lives. In any case, vasovagal syncope may be triggered by prolonged periods of upright posture, relative dehydration, excessively warm confining environments, extreme emotions, or acute pain. Common places for these events are religious services, restaurants, and long queues. Warning symptoms may occur, and include feeling: hot or cold, sweaty, tachycardic, short of air, loss of hearing, nausea, and change in breathing pattern. Physical findings often reported by bystanders in these cases (if the physician actively elicits the information) include pallor ("white as a ghost", "death-like"), a cold "clammy" feel to the affected individual's skin, and confusion or marked fatigue on the part of the victim after return of consciousness. If "jerky" motor activity is reported (often mistaken as "seizures"), it occurs after loss of consciousness and is brief and incoordinate in character.

After the faint, if the patient is permitted to remain recumbent, recovery typically is prompt. How-ever, as noted earlier, a period of post-event fatigue is quite common. Further, since warning symptoms may not always be present, or at least not recollected after the fact, and, if the medical history does not otherwise provide sufficient basis to make the diagnosis, selected testing may be needed. Most often, head-up tilt-table testing (HUT) has been used to help support a diagnosis of vasovagal syncope *(9–11)*. Such testing, in the absence of pharmacological provocation, has a specificity of approximately 90% (sensitivity cannot be stated absent a "gold standard") *(12)*. However, if the history is "typical" for vasovagal syncope, HUT is not needed unless used to teach the patient about warning symptoms so they become aware of future events.

CAROTID SINUS SYNDROME

Carotid sinus syndrome (CSS) and carotid sinus hypersensitivity (CSH) are two distinctly differ-ent entities. The first is a clinical syndrome resulting in syncope or near-syncope due to bradycardia and/or vasodilatation secondary to hypersensitivity of the carotid sinus baroreceptor. CSH, on the other hand, is the physiologic observation that may or may not have any clinical sequelae; only if CSH is responsible for syncope is the patient diagnosed with CSS.

Syncope in CSS is thought to be triggered by accidental manipulation of the neck that results in external pressure on the carotid sinus baroreceptors. The susceptible individual can often be demon-strated to exhibit carotid sinus hypersensitivity (CSH, a pause >3–5 sec in conjunction with a separate vasodepressor response as noted earlier) during deliberate diagnostic carotid sinus massage applied by a suitably experienced physician *(13, 14)*.

Physiologically, pressure on the region of carotid artery bifurcation produces a reflex causing decrease in blood pressure and heart rate. In most individuals the effect is minor. However, in those with CSH (usually older male patients >65 years of age, possibly with some age-related imbalance of carotid sinus afferent signals to the brain), the impact is more dramatic resulting in a prolonged bradycardic event and a concomitant period of vasodilatation (Fig. 3). The outcome can be sufficient diminution of cerebral blood flow to cause syncope, although in the laboratory syncope is only repro-duced if the carotid region is massaged while the patient is in an upright posture such as on a head-up tilt table.

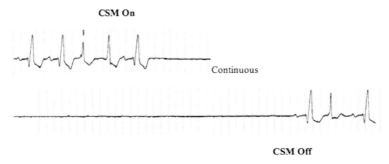

Fig. 3. ECG recording illustrating prolonged cardiac pause induced by carotid sinus massage (CSM) in a patient with suspected carotid sinus syndrome. The pause duration is approximately 9.2 sec.

SITUATIONAL SYNCOPE

The "situational" faints are essentially identical to conventional vasovagal faint except that the trigger is peripheral and identifiable. Thus, these faints include micturition syncope, defecation syncope, deglutition, or swallowing syncope, etc. Cough may also trigger reflex hypotension although other nonreflex mechanisms for cough syncope have been proposed as well *(15)*. In any case, situational faints are diagnosed by their distinctive history; it is both difficult and usually unnecessary to evaluate these fainters in the clinical laboratory.

Orthostatic Syncope (Postural or Orthostatic Intolerance Syncope Syndromes)

Orthostatic hypotension (OH) leading to syncope (orthostatic syncope) is one aspect of orthostatic intolerance syndrome. The other frequently encountered condition in this group is postural orthostatic tachycardia syndrome (POTS).

As its name implies, orthostatic syncope occurs as a result of transient excessive cerebral hypotension that may occur when susceptible individuals arise from a lying or sitting to a standing position *(16, 17)*. Two basic forms are recognized. The first is so-called "immediate hypotension". This occurs almost immediately upon "active" standing, and can be observed in young healthy individuals as well as in older patients. In fact, many healthy individuals experience a minor form of "immediate hypotension" as evidenced by the need to support himself or herself momentarily as they stand up. Essentially, in these instances, "immediate hypotension" causes a transient self-limited "gray-out". However, immediate hypotension may not always be benign; instability and falls are a risk in more frail individuals, and frank syncope can also occur. The second form of orthostatic hypotension is the delayed form. Symptoms usually occur several moments after standing up. The patient has already walked some distance, then collapses. The cause in both cases is deemed to be failure of autonomic nervous system to respond to a sudden upright posture, but the delayed form tends not to reverse until gravity intervenes (i.e., the patient has fallen). Lack of autonomic system response can be due to either extrinsic factors or primary autonomic failure. Extrinsic factors include dehydration from prolonged exposure to hot environments, inadequate fluid intake, or excessive use of diuretics, antihypertensives, or vasodilators. Additional extrinsic factors include chronic diseases such as diabetes, alcohol abuse, or other agents that induce a peripheral neuropathy and thereby predispose patients to orthostatic syncope. Less commonly, orthostatic hypotension is the result of a primary autonomic failure with inadequate reflex adaptations to upright posture *(18)*. These latter conditions include multisystem atrophy and Parkinson's disease *(19)*.

Cardiac Arrhythmias as Primary Cause of Syncope

Primary cardiac arrhythmias (i.e., those that are not secondary to neural-reflex events discussed earlier) are less commonly the cause of syncope than is either neurally mediated reflex faints or orthostatic hypotension. However, given the propensity for arrhythmias to accompany other health conditions, and especially structural heart disease, the prognosis associated with arrhythmic syncope is of concern. On the other hand, the principal driver of prognosis in most of these cases is not the syncope per se, but the nature and severity of the underlying disease.

Cardiac arrhythmias may be the primary cause of syncope if the heart rate becomes too fast (tachyarrhythmias), or conversely too slow (bradyarrhythmias), to maintain stable cerebral nutrient flow. Either or both may occur as a result of "intrinsic" disease of the cardiac conduction system, or as a consequence of structural cardiac or cardiopulmonary disease.

Determining which, if any, of the cardiac arrhythmias are responsible for syncope in a given individual can be difficult, especially if symptomatic events are infrequent. Electrophysiological (EP) testing may be helpful in some cases, but often the findings are non-specific. Consequently, prolonged ambulatory electrocardiographic (ECG) monitoring may be more effective in order to better define symptom-arrhythmia concordance. In this regard, external event recorders, mobile cardiac outpatient telemetry, and implantable loop recorders have become very valuable diagnostic aids.

Sinus Node Dysfunction and Atrioventricular (AV) Conduction Disorders

Syncope in patients with "sinus node dysfunction" may be due to either brady- or tachyarrhythmias. Thus, while sinus/junctional bradycardia, sinus arrest or a sinus pause are common, paroxysmal atrial tachyarrhythmias fall into this category as well. In either case, the heart rate (HR) may be inadequate to support adequate cerebral blood flow. In some instances, both brady- and tachycardia may be contributory; for example, an abrupt spontaneous termination of an atrial tachycardia may be followed by long asystolic pause prior to recovery of the sinus mechanism.

Paroxysmal or persistent atrioventricular (AV) block can cause severe bradycardia and thereby lead to syncope *(20)*. In practical terms, if a patient is found to have Mobitz type II second-degree AV block, third-degree AV block, or alternating left and right bundle branch block, a basis for syncope can be made with reasonable certainty and generally warrant pacemaker implantation *(21)*. However, the diagnosis remains inferential absent direct symptom-ECG documentation.

Absent a direct symptom-arrhythmia correlation, a tentative causative diagnosis can be made if ventricular pauses >3 sec are recorded when the patient is awake, or if Mobitz type II second-degree or third-degree (i.e., complete or "high grade") AV block is discovered. In the setting of nothing more than bifascicular block or nonspecific intra-ventricular conduction delay, a cause cannot be assigned; invasive EP study may be helpful *(22)*. In all of these cases, substantial underlying structural heart disease is often present. Consequently, it is important to consider concomitant susceptibility to tachyarrhythmias as a cause of symptoms.

Supraventricular and Ventricular Tachyarrhythmias

In one report, supraventricular tachycardia (SVT) accounted for 15% of syncope patients and ventricular tachycardia (VT) was responsible for 20% of syncope patients referred for EP testing *(23)*. Due to referral bias, these percentages are likely overestimates of the true prevalence of these causes in the community. In our laboratory, SVT accounts for fewer than 5% of syncope referrals and VT for at most 10%.

When syncope does occur in the setting of SVT, symptoms tend to occur at the onset of the tachycardia, before peripheral vessels have a chance to constrict. Factors that increase risk of syncope during SVT include high heart rate, reduced circulating volume status (i.e., relative dehydration), upright posture, presence of structural heart disease (especially with diminished ejection fraction, or significant valvular or other outflow obstruction), and delayed or inadequate peripheral vascular responsiveness *(24)*. In regard to the last point, reflex responses may be undermined by commonly prescribed drugs, such as beta-adrenergic blockers, vasodilators, and diuretics.

Ventricular tachyarrhythmias (VT) tend to be more closely associated with syncope than are SVTs primarily due to the fact that most VTs occur in the setting of more severe heart disease (i.e., one less capable of maintaining blood pressure when stressed). Thus, VT occurring in the setting of ischemic heart disease, valvular heart disease, dilated or obstructive cardiomyopathies, or arrhythmogenic right ventricular dysplasia (ARVD) may cause syncope. However, polymorphous VT causing syncope also occurs in some individuals with structurally relatively normal hearts, particularly in the setting of so-called "channelopathies" (e.g., long-QT syndrome, Brugada syndrome, short-QT syndrome, and idiopathic ventricular fibrillation [including those with recently described infero-lateral ST segment "early repolarization"]). Risk stratification recommendations for patients suspected of having these conditions remains in evolution. For example, the value of electrophysiological study to assess risk in Brugada syndrome remains a controversial topic, and no definitive statement can be offered at this time.

Cardiovascular and Cardiopulmonary Disease as Cause of Syncope

Syncope may occur as a direct result of severe underlying cardiac or cardiopulmonary disease, although a concomitant neural reflex contribution also likely plays a role. Perhaps, the best examples are severe aortic stenosis or hypertrophic obstructive cardiomyopathy (HOCM). However, as causes of syncope, these are relatively rare circumstances.

The more common scenarios in which structural disease is seemingly associated with triggering syncope in adult patients without congenital heart disease are acute coronary syndromes (ACS), acute myocardial infarction, acute aortic dissection, and severe pulmonary hypertension *(25, 26)*. In each of these cases, despite the potential for important hemodynamic consequences of the conditions, it is also believed that the syncope is primarily a product of neurally mediated reflexes secondary to pain, or excessive central mechano-receptor activation, rather than a direct hemodynamic effect of the lesion. Thus, in the case of valvar aortic stenosis or dynamic left ventricular outflow obstruction (e.g., HOCM), an inappropriate peripheral vascular response to increased left ventricular wall stress may occur during exertion. While this may have merit in normal physiology, it can have calamitous consequences in the setting of a relatively "fixed" aortic valve outflow limitation *(27, 28)*.

Despite obvious hemodynamic limitations imposed by structural heart and cardiopulmonary disease, it must always be borne in mind that syncope due to arrhythmia is far more common than syncope due to the structural components. Further, arrhythmias are often worrisome markers of sudden death risk in these patients.

Cerebrovascular Disease and Related Conditions as Cause of Syncope

Cerebrovascular disease and related conditions are very rare causes of syncope. Evaluation of these conditions should be reserved to those few instances in which there is strong medical history evidence favoring the possibility. Otherwise, much energy will be wasted and unnecesssary expense incurred with low probability of success.

In order for syncope to occur as a result of cerebrovascular disease, large areas of both cerebral cortices or at a minimum critical zones within the reticular activating system (RAS) must be rendered hypoperfused. Thus, it is possible that vascular spasm associated with migraines may cause syncope. However, in most migraineurs, the extracranial vessels are principally involved; and if syncope occurs, it is is vasovagal or orthostatic in nature as discussed later. Similarly, carotid distribution transient ischemic attacks (TIAs) do not cause syncope unless all other cerebral blood vessels are obstructed. Thus, carotid TIAs may present with focal neurological deficit, but not global cerebral hypoperfusion with syncope. The effort and expense wasted on pursuing TIAs as a cause of syncope cannot be underestimated, and every effort should be made to minimize this error.

Vertebrobasilar TIAs are extremely rare, but more likely to present as apparent syncopal episodes than are carotid distribtion TIAs. Furthermore, vertebrobasilar TIAs usually are marked by other symptoms (e.g., vertigo) indicative of posterior circulation compromise.

Subclavian steal is both a rare condition and a very rare cause of syncope. Symptoms tend to occur when patients are exercising using the affected arm. Because of its rarity, it should only be considered when other causes have been eliminated *(29)*.

Migraines are probably the most important condition in this category *(30, 31)*. However, as a rule (absent vertebrobasilar involvement), migraines do not cause syncope directly. Evidence suggests that migraine-related syncope is in fact neurally mediated reflex syncope in the vast majority of cases. Additionally, in individuals who suffer from migraine, syncope of an orthostatic nature occurs statistically more often than in nonmigraineurs *(32)*. These attacks do not occur at the same time as the migraine attacks, however, and so they can usually be readily distinguished.

Syncope Mimics and Pseudosyncope

There are two important groups of conditions that may present with real or apparent TLOC but that should not be considered as "syncope". First of this group are conditions which cause true TLOC, but their mechanism differs from true syncope. We categorize these as "non-syncope TLOC", with epilepsy being the most important example, but trauma leading to concussion (such as might occur after an accidental fall in an older patient) being important as well. Second are conditions in which consciousness is never really lost. These we term "pseudosyncope", and the most important cause is psychiatric conversion disorders. Malingering might also present as pseudosyncope, but this seems to be rare.

Pseudosyncope is a relatively common problem that deserves additional attention. As a rule, it is unassociated with any changes in heart rate or blood pressure. Most often the cause of pseudosyncope is psychiatric in nature, with the key suggestive finding on history-taking being a very high frequency of "symptomatic attacks". The frequency may be as high as many episodes per day or per week, and is much greater than that of a true syncope, although these patients may in fact have occasional "true" faints as well. Further, pseudosyncope rarely results in serious injury.

As the name implies, pseudosyncope does not manifest true TLOC, but the history from the patient and witnesses might suggest that it had. In this setting the history-taker must be both experienced and alert in order to make the necessary distinction. In many cases the diagnosis is one of exclusion after other causes of presumed TLOC have been eliminated.

Three psychiatric disorders are typically associated with pseudosyncope: conversion disorders, factitious disorders, and malingering. "Drop attacks" also belong in the "pseudosyncope" group as true loss of consciousness does not occur. The "drop attack" is an uncommon condition in which postural tone is lost abruptly and patients (most often females) fall to the ground. Consciousness is never lost and the history-taker can determine this by careful questioning of the patient's recollection during the attack. Nevertheless, these episodes can be mistaken for syncope. The basis for "drop attacks" is unclear.

SPECIFIC DIAGNOSTIC TESTING PROCEDURES

The following provides an overview of certain potentially useful diagnostic tests for assessing the cause of syncope, recognizing that often none or at most only a few are needed in the majority of syncope evaluations. The goal is to obtain a tentative diagnosis during the initial clinic evaluation, and use selected tests only as necessary to confirm a suspected diagnosis.

Carotid Sinus Massage (CSM)

CSM is used as a means of confirming a suspected diagnosis of carotid sinus syndrome (CSS). Continuous ECG and blood pressure monitoring must be used. After baseline measurements, the carotid artery one side is firmly massaged for 5–10 sec at the anterior margin of the sternocleidomastoid muscle. After 1 or 2 min a second massage is performed on the opposite side if the initial massage fails to yield a "positive" result. CSM with the patient in an upright posture on a tilt-table may help unmask CSS. Similarly, atropine (1 mg) administartion can be used to assess the contribution of vasodepressor component if an "asystolic" response is produced.

The response to carotid sinus massage is classified as cardioinhibitory (i.e., asystole), vasodepressive (fall in systolic blood pressure), or mixed. The mixed response is defined as asystole lasting ≥ 3 sec and a decline in systolic blood pressure of ≥ 50 mmHg (1). As a general rule, CSS is supported if the history is favorable and CSM results are positive.

Two methods for diagnostic application of CSM have been described. In the first method, CSM is applied only in the supine position for no more than 5 sec, and the test is considered positive if there is a ventricular pause ≥ 3 sec and/or a fall of systolic blood pressure ≥ 50 mmHg. The drawback of this method is that the diagnosis may be missed in about one-third of cases if only supine massage is performed (33). In the second method, CSM is performed with the patient being initially supine and then in an upright position (usually on a tilt-table). The objective of the second method is to reproduce symptoms.

CSM is generally believed to be a safe test, complications are rare; and when they do occur, the consequences are transient in most instances. The main complications are neurological and range from 0.17% to 0.45% in different studies (34, 35). The contraindications to CSM include patients with TIAs or strokes within the past three months, or the presence of carotid bruits unless carotid Doppler studies convincingly exclude significant carotid artery narrowing (35). European Society of Cardiology guidelines recommend CSM be performed in patients over 40 years of age with syncope of unknown etiology after the initial evaluation and the test is considered positive if syncope is reproduced during or immediately after massage in the presence of asystole longer than 3 sec and/or a fall in systolic blood pressure of 50 mmHg or more (1).

Electrocardiographic (ECG) Documentation

Since, cardiac arrhythmias are a frequent cause of syncope, a 12-lead ECG is essential to the initial evaluation. The ECG can give a hint of underlying structural conduction system disease (e.g., bundle branch block) or alert the physician to certain specific arrhythmogenic states (e.g., prior myocardial infarction, long QT syndrome, Brugada syndrome, preexcitation syndromes, AV block). On the other hand, the sampling period of the 12-lead ECG is too short to permit a true symptom–rhythm correlation. Similarly, the exercise ECG test has limited diagnostic utility in evaluation of syncope, unless symptoms are clearly related to exercise. On the other hand, exercise testing may prove helpful in selected cases if findings reveal rate-dependent AV block, exercise-induced tachyarrhythmias, or marked chronotropic incompetence (36, 37). In addition, if autonomic failure is suspected, exercise testing may unmask exercise-induced hypotension due to inability of the vascular system to react appropriately in the presence of exertion-triggered vasodilatation

As discussed earlier, if an arrhythmia is suspected to be the cause of syncope, extended-duration cardiac monitoring is needed in order to have a chance of obtaining a diagnostic symptom-arrhythmia correlation (the "gold standard"). Conventional ECG "event" recorders, Mobile Cardiac Outpatient Telemetry (MCOT, Cardionet Inc., San Diego, CA), and insertable loop recorders (ILR) (Reveal®, Medtronic Inc., Minneapolis, MN; Sleuth®, Transoma Medical, St Paul, MN; SJM Confirm®, St Jude Medical, St Paul, MN) are possible options in this category. MCOT has the particular advantage of both detecting and automatically transmitting symptomatic and potentially important asymptomatic (e.g., non-sustained VT, arrhythmias during sleep). However, like conventional "event" recorders, MCOT systems are not likely to be tolerated for more than 2–3 weeks. ILRs have the potential for providing recordings for up to 3 years, and recent evolution of this technology permits wireless transmission of ECG events without the need for patient interaction.

Recent opinion favors earlier use of long-term monitoring in the syncope evaluation strategy than was initially the case. Unfortunately, in the United States, many insurors insist that a standard "Holter-type" recording be done first, despite the usual futility and lack of cost-effectiveness of such a step.

Echocardiography

While echocardiography rarely provides a definitive basis for syncope, it is of value in helping to determine whether there is evidence of potentially contributing underlying structural heart disease. This is important as the presence of structural heart disease has an important impact on subsequent diagnostic strategy and ultimately on prognosis. Consequently, obtaining an echocardiogram is justifiable early in the evaluation – perhaps as part of the "initial" evaluation – if structural heart disease cannot be excluded by physical examination alone.

Head Up Tilt Table (HUT) Testing

HUT testing is useful in patients to help confirm a diagnosis of vasovagal syncope when the medical history is not "classical" (1). Conversely, if the medical history is clear, such testing adds no new diagnostic information. On the other hand, if HUT reproduces the faint, the experience may prove helpful to the patient to be more alert to warning symptoms. Such testing may also provide the patient some confidence that the physician has indeed arrived at the correct diagnosis.

HUT methodology is described in detail elsewhere (1, 11). In brief, the patient is gently secured on a tilt-table with feet resting on a foot plate. Continuous ECG and blood pressure (usually noninvasive, but preferably not using a sphygmomanometer) recordings are initiated. The table is then tilted at an angle of 60–70° for durations of 20–45 min (depending on the center preference) unless syncope occurs earlier. If syncope has not been triggered by drug-free tilt, pharmacological provocation (e.g., isoproterenol, edrophonium, nitroglycerin) can be used. By way of example, the popular so-called "Italian Protocol" entails an initial drug-free tilt duration of 20 min at 70°, followed if necessary by one dose of 0.4 mg sublingual nitroglycerin spray.

HUT testing can be used to confirm a suspected diagnosis of vasovagal syncope. However, HUT has limited reproducibility, and does not always cause the same hemodynamic abnormality observed during spontaneous faints in the same patient. Consequently, HUT should not be used to ascertain effectiveness of treatment interventions.

Invasive Electrophysiological Testing

EP study is appropriate when the initial evaluation points towards a primary cardiac rhythm abnormality or a conduction disturbance, and the diagnosis needs to be confirmed. The most common scenarios are: (1) assessment of suspected infra-nodal conduction system disease, (2) evaluation of suspected susceptibility to paroxysmal SVT, and (3) induction of VT in susceptible individuals.

Neurological Studies

Studies such as head CT and MRI are low yield in syncope patients and their use is strongly discouraged. These studies are best reserved for cases in which there is concern that syncope may have resulted in head injury. Alternatively, they may be helpful in non-syncope TLOC patients who demonstrate persistent focal neurological deficits, carotid bruits etc.

TREATMENT

Treatment of the syncope patient may be divided into two parts. The first is management of an acute syncopal event. Although physicians are only infrequently involved in this aspect of care, treatment of the acute episode requires protection of the patient from injury, assuring that the victim is placed safely in a gravitationally neutral position and documenting adequacy of respiration and circulation. Thereafter, recovery is spontaneous. The second part is prevention of syncope recurrences. Inasmuch as physicians are most often responsible for this element of patient care, it is on this aspect that we have focused the treatment section of this review, and the reader is referred to a recent review of this subject *(38)*.

Vasovagal Syncope

As noted earlier, the vasovagal faint is the most frequent condition in this group. Situational faints are also very common, and from a practical perspective these two types of neurally mediated reflex faints can be treated in a similar fashion.

In most cases, vasovagal syncope or situational faints are a solitary or at most very infrequent event. Therefore, most patients need little more than reassurance and education about the "benign" nature of this condition from a mortaliy perspective. Modification or discontinuation of potentially contributory drug treatment for concomitant conditions is reasonable, as is identifying (in order to hopefully avoid in the future) apparent triggers. In addition, it is important to identify and treat psychological and/or psychiatric factors that may contribute to exacerbating symptom susceptibility. In this regard, a high prevalence of minor psychiatric disorders has been reported in patients with vasovagal syncope (VVS) *(39)*.

In certain individuals vasovagal or "situational" faints become quite frequent and thereby adversely alter quality of life, as well as exposing the individual to risk of trauma. In these cases additional treatment steps may be necessary, including:

1. Avoiding those environments that seem to provoke episodes.
2. Being alert to warning symptoms such as feeling of being hot or cold, sweaty, clammy, short of breath, or nauseated. The goal is to educate susceptible individuals to recognize impending events and take action in order to prevent the episodes (e.g., sitting or lying down with feet elevated). Similarly, if a patient knows that sight of blood could bring about a vasovagal faint, he/she may either avoid the situation or possibly be preconditioned to perform maneuvers to prevent the faint (e.g., aggressive hydration, arm-tensing, leg crossing).
3. Incorporate fluids rich in salts and electrolytes into the daily diet. Examples would include sport drinks (although avoiding high calorie versions) and salt tablets.If these initial steps prove inadequate, then the treatment strategy can be expanded to include as needed : (1) physical techniques to improve orthostatic tolerance, (2) pharmacologic interventions to prevent depletion of intra-vascular volume and/or enhance arterial and venous tone and block the sympathetic neural excitation that often is the initial feature of the evolving faint, and (3) cardiac pacing to avert bradycardia (albeit infrequently).

Physical Techniques to Improve Orthostatic Tolerance

TILT TRAINING (STANDING TRAINING)

Tilt-training (better termed "standing-training") is a form of physical therapy intended to "desensitize" and/or "re-train" abnormal responses to normal conditions that trigger syncope, most notably orthostatic stress. It has been advocated as a useful nonpharmacologic treatment for vasovagal syncope as well as other orthostatic intolerance syndromes *(40)*. Originally, the "tilt-training" concept used repeated exposure to postural stress by means of daily in-hospital tilt-table tests until syncope was no longer inducible. Currently, the method we advocate entails home "standing training" consisting of the patient standing with the upper back positioned lightly against a wall or a corner (preferably using a carpeted floor and no sharp-edged objects near-by) without moving arms or legs for progressively longer periods of stationary upright posture. Initially, the recommended standing duration is 3–5 min twice daily; the duration is then gradually lengthened every 3–4 days to as much as 30–40 min twice daily.

Tilt-training has anecdotally proven helpful if undertaken twice daily for periods of 8–12 weeks, with subsequent maintenance 3–4 times weekly thereafter. Nonrandomized studies suggest that tilt-training reduces NMS susceptibility if undertaken consistently *(38, 41–43)*. However, controlled studies are less supportive of benefit and the treatment is hampered by low compliance *(38)*.

PHYSICAL COUNTER PRESSURE MANEUVERS

Physical counter pressure maneuvers (CPMs) are used primarily to interrupt evolving syncope attacks. Several PCM options are available: leg-crossing alone (Fig. 4), leg-crossing with lower body muscle tensing, arm-tugging maneuver (by pulling apart gripped hands) (Fig. 5), or squeezing of the fists or of a "stress ball". Thus, the patient initiates one or other of these maneuvers when he or she first recognizes onset of presyncope warning symptoms. Considerable evidence supports the observation that CPMs are able to increase blood pressure at least transiently, thereby "buying" the affected individual some time to avoid an abrupt collapse *(38, 44–46)* and seek a safe a safe position (i.e., become seated, pull their vehicle off the road, etc.). CPMs should be considered a first-line recommendation for patients with VVS who are capable of recognizing premonitory symptoms.

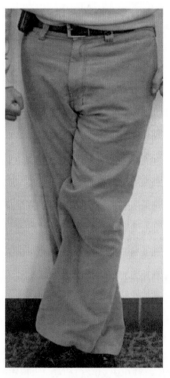

Fig. 4. The leg crossing maneuver consists of crossing the legs in standing position with tensing of leg, abdominal, and buttock muscles. The legs are firmly squeezed together.

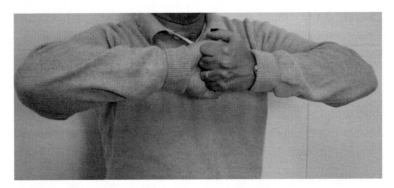

Fig. 5. Arm tensing consists of isometric contraction of the two arms performed by gripping one hand with the other and concurrently abducting the arms.

HEAD-UP SLEEPING

Sleeping with the head of the bed elevated provides nocturnal postural stress that has long been advocated for treatment of orthostatic hypotension, but may be similarly proposed in vasovagal fainters (especially as adjunctive therapy in those who cannot take added salt due to comorbid conditions [e.g., heart failure, hypertension] or who do not respond to other non-pharmacological interventions). The head of the patient's bed is raised to 5–20°. However, there is no data showing sustained benefit in the long-term. Further, compliance may be a problem, since spouses may not care for sleeping in this manner.

Pharmacological Therapy to Improve Orthostatic Intolerance

Volume expansion has long been the foundation of medical therapy for NMS syndromes; conventional approaches entail increased dietary salt and electrolyte-rich sport drinks (although it is wise to avoid many high-caloric "sport" drinks). The primary safety concern is induction of hypertension. Fortunately, this is uncommon in younger patients, but becomes a real concern in older patients.

A number of more conventional pharmacologic agents have been proposed for preventing vasovagal syncope. However, efficacy of most of them have not been supported in randomized, controlled trials. Examples of such medications include fludrocortisone, beta-adrenergic blocking drugs, vasoconstrictor agents (e.g., midodrine), and serotonin re-uptake inhibitors.

Midodrine: Midodrine is a pro-drug, the active metabolite of which is a peripherally active alpha-agonist used to ameliorate the reduction in peripheral sympathetic neural outflow that causes venous pooling and vasodepression, which are central to vasovagal syncope. The drug stimulates both arterial and venous systems with minimal direct central nervous system or cardiac effects *(47)*. Midodrine has been most extensively studied in patients with orthostatic hypotension *(48)*, but has also been shown to be effective in vasovagal syncope *(47)*.

Midodrine therapy can be started with 2.5 mg three times daily with the maximum dose being 10–15 mg three times daily, largely during the daytime hours when the patient needs to be upright, pursuing the activities of daily life (i.e., shortly before or upon arising in the morning, midday, and late afternoon). Doses may be given in 3-hour intervals, if required, to control symptoms, but generally not more frequently.

Midodrine is reasonably well tolerated with dose-related and easily reversible side effects. The most potentially serious adverse reaction associated with midodrine is supine hypertension. The feelings of paresthesia, pruritus, piloerection, tingling of the scalp, and chills are associated with the action of midodrine on the alpha-adrenergic receptors of the hair follicles. Urinary urgency, retention, and frequency are associated with the action of midodrine on the alpha-receptors of the bladder neck.

Fludrocortisone: Fludrocortisone is a mineralocorticoid used to facilitate salt and water retention as an adjunct to the increase of dietary salt. As a rule the drug is well tolerated at 1–2 mg/day. However, potassium depletion is a concern, and potassium concentration in the blood should be periodically assessed.

Beta-adrenergic blockers: Beta-blockers were initially advocated based on the theoetical view that they would moderate the early-phase sympathetic activation associated with the evolving vasovagal faint. However, while evidence tends to suggest that this theoretical benefit may not readily translate into clinical effectiveness in all patients, such an approach may be helpful in those individuals with seemingly high levels of sympathetic excitation.

Serotonin re-uptake inhibitors: The basis for using serotonin re-uptake inhibitors in vasovagal is not well substantiated. Nevertheless, anecdotal reports have benefit have been published. We only recommend their use in patients in whom a depressive overlay may be contributing to symptoms.

Permanent Pacemakers

Cardiac pacing has received considerable study as a potential treatment option in patients experiencing very frequent vasovagal faints. However, despite early favorable reports, placebo-controlled prospective trials in which all enrolled patients received pacemakers did not show a statistically significant benefit from pacing *(49, 50)*. A recent meta-analysis *(51)* concluded that blinded trials do not show a benefit. Thus, pacing is not considered mainstream therapy for preventing vasovagal syncope; it may, however, reduce the morbidity by prolonging the warning phase and allowing the fainter to seek a safe position. In general, pacemaker therapy should not be embarked upon lightly in vasovagal fainters, and should only be considered in patients in whom recurrent events despite standard treatment have been documented to correlate with bradycardia during long-term ECG monitoring.

CAROTID SINUS SYNDROME (CSS)

As discussed earlier, CSS is a special form of neurally mediated reflex syncope that tends to occur in older individuals. In such cases, the value of lifestyle interventions as sole treatment is unknown. Therefore, while it may be prudent to include avoidance of tight collars and neckties, and abrupt neck movements in the treatment strategy, early initiation of cardiac pacing is probably an essential component of therapy *(1)*. CSS is the only form of neurally mediated syncope in which pacing has proved very effective. However, many of these patients exhibit a prominent vasodepressor response as well as cardioinhibition, and may therefore continue to experience symptoms (usually "dizziness" rather than syncope) despite the presence of a cardiac pacemaker. The vasodepressor aspect may need to be addressed as in the vasovagal fainter (see earlier discussion)

SITUATIONAL SYNCOPE

Avoiding or ameliorating the triggering event is the basic treatment for most forms of neurally mediated situational syncope. Sometimes, though the trigger is readily recognized, suppressing it might not be easily accomplished (e.g., cough trigger in a patient with chronic obstructive pulmonary disease). As in the case of defaection or post-micturition syncope, it is impossible to avoid exposure to the triggering situation (i.e., bowel movement, bladder emptying). In the latter situation, certain general treatment strategies may be advocated, including maintenance of central volume, protected posture (sitting rather than standing), slower changes of posture (e.g., waiting after a bowel movement before arising). Certain additional advice may be helpful in specific conditions, such as use of stool softeners in patients with defaecation syncope, avoidance of excessive fluid intake (especially alcohol) just prior to bedtime in post-micturition syncope, and elimination of cold drinks in "swallow" syncope.

ORTHOSTATIC SYNCOPE

Treatment of orthostatic syncope and other orthostatic intolerance syndromes, such as postural orthostatic tachycardia syndrome (POTS), parallels the strategy discussed earlier for vasovagal faints. POTS will not be discussed further here, and treatment of orthostatic syncope will focus on the "delayed" form since it is clinically much more important than is the "immediate" form.

Typical delayed orthostatic syncope differ from vasovagal syncope in several respects: (1) the duration of treatment is likely to be longer, (2) affected individuals are typically older and more frail making physical maneuvers more difficult to employ, and (3) patients are more prone to supine hypertension, thereby complicating the overall treatment strategy. In any event, treatment for the prevention of orthostatic syncope should focus initially on maintenance of hydration and physical maneuvers as discussed in the section on neurally mediated reflex syncope.

In many cases, syncope associated with postural change may be caused by low circulating plasma volume, or inadequate vascular constriction upon moving to the upright posture (often drug-induced), or both. Consequently, one of the basic tenets of treatment is expanding central circulating volume (i.e., encouraging increased salt and volume intake to the extent that this does not induce supine hypertension). Additionally, affected individuals should be instructed to try and avoid certain predisposing conditions (e.g., prolonged exposure to hot environments) or medications that decrease volume status (e.g., diuretics) or that impair vasoconstriction (e.g., vasodilators, beta-adrenergic blockers). In some severe cases, use of vasoconstrictors (like midodrine) or volume expanders (e.g., fludrocortisone) may be necessary to maintain adequate cerebral perfusion. Finally, patients who exhibit poor autonomic function may benefit from progressive standing-training (discussed earlier), counter-pressure clothing such as fitted stockings and abdominal compression devices.

A special case is the patient with severe pure autonomic failure. In these situations, bolus water intake, especially before arising from bed in the morning, may result in a substantial and sustained increase in blood pressure *(52)*. On the other hand, these same individuals tend to be very susceptible to supine hypertension. In such cases it may be necessary to tailor the treatment prescription to include salt, volume, and midodrine early in the day and antihypertensive at night. Bear in mind, however, the patient may be at risk if they get up in the middle of the night. A "walker" at the bedside or use of a bedside commode may be needed.

PRIMARY CARDIAC ARRHYTHMIAS

The treatment of cardiac arrhythmias causing syncope is determined by the specific arrhythmia that is deemed to be at fault. Given the numerous possibilities and the many factors that go into selecting appropriate therapies for these arrhythmias, only a brief overview is provided here. Greater detail will be found in the most recent ESC syncope task force guideline documents *(1)*.

Sinus Node Dysfunction (SND)

SND may cause syncope either due to bradycardia or tachycardia mechanisms as discussed earlier. When a temporal correlation between syncope and bradycardia has been established, pacemaker implantation is the treatment of choice. In the case of tachyarrhythmia-induced syncope, both antiarrhythmic drugs and ablation are reasonable treatment considerations. The final choice depends on specific clinical circumstances and patient preferences.

Atrioventricular (AV) Conduction Disorders

Treatment of AV conduction system disease in syncope patients does not differ measurably from their treatment in other patients. However, once again it is crucial to obtain concordance between syncopal episodes and bradycardia. If such a correlation is found and the cause of AV block is irreversible, pacemaker implantation is a class I indication.

Supraventricular Tachycardia

When SVT is known to provoke hypotension and therefore syncope, transcatheter ablation is the treatment of choice in most cases. Drug therapy remains an option, however, given the high success rate with ablation and its ready availability, the ablation track seems more desirable. Finally, in the case of refractory symptomatic atrial tachyarrhythmias (particularly atrial fibrillation) with rapid ventricular rates, treatment by AV junction (His bundle) ablation and placement of a permanent pacemaker has proved to be safe and highly effective *(53)*.

Ventricular Tachyarrhythmias

Syncope patients with ischemic heart disease or dilated cardiomyopathies and severely diminished left ventricular function (i.e., LV ejection fractions <35%), and often some element of heart failure, have a high mortality rate and are indicated for ICD therapy. As alluded to earlier, however, syncope may not be prevented by ICD treatment since the devices must take time before intervening with pacing or shock treatment *(54)*. Consequently, in these syncope patients concomitant antiarrhythmic drug therapy and/or ablation may be needed. In arrhythmogenic right ventricular dysplasia (ARVD), treatment strategies are controversial. Medical treatment has not been found to be very effective. Furthermore, since there are potentially many regions of the heart that are affected, long-term efficacy of transcatheter ablation is limited. Therefore, syncope patients with ARVD, in whom ventricular tachyarrhythmias have been documented, may be best served by placement of an ICD. Once again, however, syncope may not necessarily be completely averted and concomitant medications may be needed.

Syncope may also be associated with paroxysmal ventricular tachyarrhythmias other than in the setting of cardiomyopathies. Perhaps, the most important of these is torsades-de-pointe occurring in conjunction with the abnormal repolarization states. Long QT syndrome, Brugada syndrome, and other "channelopathies" are increasingly recognized as causes of syncope due to polymorphous VT (so-called "torsades de pointe"). The management of these arrhythmias is not discussed in detail here. However, therapy incorporates both avoidance of drugs that predispose to aggravating the problem, along with use of ICDs (to diminish sudden death risk) and beta-adrenergic blockade depending on the specific circumstance.

Tachyarrhythmias arising from the right ventricular outflow tract (RVOT) or left ventricular outflow tract (LVOT), or from the intraventricular fascicular system or bundle-branch system (i.e., bundle-branch reentry), are infrequent causes of syncope. However, when they are responsible for symptoms, transcatheter ablation is probably the treatment of choice.

Structural Cardiovascular or Cardiopulmonary Disease

In these conditions, syncope may be only one subset of symptomology being experienced by the patient. Correction or amelioration of the structural lesion is usually the treatment of choice. As an example, patients with valvular aortic stenosis, atrial myxoma, and congenital cardiac anomalies benefit from a direct corrective approach. In other cases, such as primary pulmonary hypertension or restrictive cardiomyopathy, the structural lesions are not correctable but medical therapy may ameliorate the problem sufficiently to prevent syncope recurrences.

In the case of hypertrophic obstructive cardiomyopathy (HOCM), modification of the outflow gradients surgically may be accompanied by substantial risk and morbidity, but becomes a necessity when medical therapy is not effective. If it is clear that syncope is due to the obstruction (as opposed to arrhythmias discussed earlier), cardiac pacing to diminish dynamic outflow gradients and transcatheter alcohol septal ablation may prove helpful, but the utility of this approach remains controversial.

CONCLUSION

Syncope is a form of transient loss of consciousness (TLOC) that is brief in duration, self-limited, and due to a transient and spontaneously reversible cerebral hypoperfusion. Syncope has many possible causes; delineating the underlying etiology in a given patient is often challenging but is important since syncope, while often relatively benign from a mortality perspective in the vast majority of cases, tends to recur. Inadequate treatment leaves the affected individual subject to risk of physical injury, resulting from falls or accidents, diminished quality-of-life, and possible restriction from employment or avocation.

In the majority of patients presenting with syncope, a careful history and physical examination is sufficient to establish the diagnosis with substantial certainty. The most common example is when the history is indicative of one of the neurally mediated reflex faints; vasovagal (common faint), carotid sinus, or situational syncope. In other instances, when the initial evaluation is inconclusive, further assessment is needed. More widespread development of syncope management units (SMUs) and rapid access syncope/falls clinics is strongly encouraged; together, they have been shown to reduce both hospital costs and number of undiagnosed cases.

POTENTIAL CONFLICTS OF INTEREST

Dr Can: No conflicts to disclose.

Dr Benditt: Discloses consulting relationship with and equity position in Boston Scientific Inc., Cardionet Inc., Medtronic Inc., St Jude Medical Inc., and Transoma Inc.

REFERENCES

1. Brignole M, Alboni P, Benditt D et al (2004) Task force on syncope, European society of cardiology. guidelines on management (diagnosis and treatment) of syncope – update 2004. Executive summary. Europace 6:467–537
2. Quinn JV, Stiell IG, McDermott DA et al (2004) Derivation of the San Francisco syncope rule to predict patients with short-term serious outcomes. Ann Emerg Med 43:224–232
3. Blanc JJ, L'Her C, Touiza A et al (2002) Prospective evaluation and outcome of patients admitted for syncope over a 1 year period. Eur Heart J 23:815–820
4. Alboni P, Brignole M, Menozzi C et al (2001) The diagnostic value of history in patients with syncope with or without heart disease. J Am Coll Cardiol 37:1921–1928
5. Shen WK, Decker WW, Smars PA et al (2004) Syncope evaluation in the emergency department study (SEEDS): a multidisciplinary approach to syncope management. Circulation 110:3636–3645
6. Brignole M, Menozzi C, Bartoletti A et al (2006) A new management of syncope: prospective systematic guideline-based evaluation of patients referred urgently to general hospitals. Eur Heart J 27:76–82
7. Serletis A, Rose S, Sheldon AG et al (2006) Vasovagal syncope in medical students and their first degree relatives. Eur Heart J 27:1965–1970
8. Lewis T (1932) Lecture on vasovagal syncope and carotid sinus mechanism. BMJ 1:873–876
9. Abi-Samra F, Maloney JD, Fouad-Tarazi FM et al (1988) The usefulness of head-up tilt testing and hemodynamic investigations in the workup of syncope of unknown origin. Pacing Clin Electrophysiol 11:1202–1214
10. Almquist A, Goldenberg IF, Milstein S et al (1989) Provocation of bradycardia and hypotension by isoproterenol and upright posture in patients with unexplained syncope. N Engl J Med 320:346–351
11. Benditt DG, Ferguson DW, Grubb BP et al (1996) Tilt table testing for assessing syncope. J Am Coll Cardiol 28:263–275
12. Sutton R, Petersen ME (1995) The clinical spectrum of neurocardiogenic syncope. J Cardiovasc Electrophysiol 6:569–576

13. Brignole M, Menozzi C, Gianfranchi L et al (1991) Neurally mediated syncope detected by carotid sinus massage and head-up tilt test in sick sinus syndrome. Am J Cardiol 68:1032–1036
14. Morley CA, Sutton R (1984) Carotid sinus syncope. Int J Cardiol 6:287–293
15. Benditt DG, Samniah N, Pham S et al (2005) Effect of cough on heart rate and blood pressure in patients with "cough syncope". Heart Rhythm 2:807–813
16. Bannister R (1979) Chronic autonomic failure with postural hypotension. Lancet 2:404–406
17. Low PA, Opfer-Gehrking TL, McPhee BR et al (1995) Prospective evaluation of clinical characteristics of orthostatic hypotension. Mayo Clin Proc 70:617–622
18. Mathias CJ, Bannister R (1999) Clinical features and evaluation of the primary chronic autonomic failure syndromes. In: Bannister R, Mathias CJ (eds) Autonomic failure : a textbook of clinical disorders of the autonomic nervous system, 4th edn. University Press, Oxford, New York, p 562
19. Koike Y, Takahashi A (1997) Autonomic dysfunction in Parkinson's disease. Eur Neurol 38(Suppl 2):8–12
20. Moya A (2006) Cardiac arrhythmias and conduction system disease as a primary cause of syncope. In: Benditt DG, Brignole M, Raviele A, Wieling W (eds) The evaluation and treatment of syncope : a handbook for clinical practice, 2nd edn. Blackwell, Malden, MA, pp 301–305
21. Epstein AE, DiMarco JP, Ellenbogen KA et al (2008) ACC/AHA/HRS 2008 guidelines for device-based therapy of cardiac rhythm abnormalities: a report of the American college of Cardiology/American heart association task force on practice guidelines (writing committee to revise the ACC/AHA/NASPE 2002 guideline update for implantation of cardiac pacemakers and antiarrhythmia devices): developed in collaboration with the american association for thoracic surgery and society of thoracic surgeons. Circulation 117:e350–e408
22. Morady F, Higgins J, Peters RW et al (1984) Electrophysiologic testing in bundle branch block and unexplained syncope. Am J Cardiol 54:587–591
23. Camm AJ, Lau CP (1988) Syncope of undetermined origin: diagnosis and management. Prog Cardiol 139–156
24. Leitch JW, Klein GJ, Yee R et al (1992) Syncope associated with supraventricular tachycardia. an expression of tachy-cardia rate or vasomotor response? Circulation 85:1064–1071
25. Dixon MS, Thomas P, Sheridan DJ (1988)Syncope as the presentation of unstable angina. Int J Cardiol 19:125–129
26. Pathy MS (1967) Clinical presentation of myocardial infarction in the elderly. Br Heart J 29:190–199
27. Mark AL (1983) The Bezold-Jarisch reflex revisited: clinical implications of inhibitory reflexes originating in the heart. J Am Coll Cardiol 1:90–102
28. Prasad K, Williams L, Campbell R et al (2008) Episodic syncope in hypertrophic cardiomyopathy: evidence for inap-propriate vasodilation. Heart 94:1312–1317
29. Hadjipetrou P, Cox S, Piemonte T et al (1999) Percutaneous revascularization of atherosclerotic obstruction of aortic arch vessels. J Am Coll Cardiol 33:1238–1245
30. Shechter A, Stewart WF, Silberstein SD et al (2002) Migraine and autonomic nervous system function: a population-based, case-control study. Neurology 58:422–427
31. Silberstein SD (2000) Practice parameter: evidence-based guidelines for migraine headache (an evidence-based review): report of the quality standards subcommittee of the American academy of neurology. Neurology 55:754–762
32. Thijs RD, Kruit MC, van Buchem MA et al (2006) Syncope in migraine: the population-based CAMERA study. Neu-rology 66:1034–1037
33. Parry SW, Richardson DA, O'Shea D et al (2000) Diagnosis of carotid sinus hypersensitivity in older adults: carotid sinus massage in the upright position is essential. Heart 83:22–23
34. Puggioni E, Guiducci V, Brignole M et al (2002) Results and complications of the carotid sinus massage performed according to the 'methods of symptoms'. Am J Cardiol 89:599–601
35. Munro N, McIntosh S, Lawson J et al (1994) The incidence of complications after carotid sinus massage in older patients with syncope. J Am Geriatr Soc 42:1248–1251
36. Sakaguchi S, Shultz JJ, Remole SC et al (1995) Syncope associated with exercise, a manifestation of neurally mediated syncope. Am J Cardiol 75:476–481
37. Calkins H, Shyr Y, Frumin H et al (1995) The value of the clinical history in the differentiation of syncope due to ventricular tachycardia, atrioventricular block, and neurocardiogenic syncope. Am J Med 98:365–373
38. Benditt DG, Nguyen JT (2009) Syncope: therapeutic approaches. J Am Coll Cardiol 53:1741–51
39. Leftheriotis D, Michopoulos I, Flevari P et al (2008) Minor psychiatric disorders and syncope: the role of psychopathol-ogy in the expression of vasovagal reflex. Psychother Psychosom 77:372–376
40. Ector H, Reybrouck T, Heidbuchel H et al (1998) Tilt training: a new treatment for recurrent neurocardiogenic syncope and severe orthostatic intolerance. Pacing Clin Electrophysiol 21(1 Pt 2):193–196
41. Di Girolamo E, Di Iorio C, Leonzio L et al (1999) Usefulness of a tilt training program for the prevention of refractory neurocardiogenic syncope in adolescents. A controlled study. Circulation 100:1798–1801
42. Reybrouck T, Heidbüchel H, Van De Werf F et al (2002) Long-term follow-up results of tilt training therapy in patients with recurrent neurocardiogenic syncope. Pacing Clin Electrophysiol 25:1441–1446

43. Abe H, Kondo S, Kohshi K et al (2002) Usefulness of orthostatic self-training for the prevention of neurocardiogenic syncope. Pacing Clin Electrophysiol 25:1454–1458

44. Krediet CT, van Dijk N, Linzer M, et al. (2002) Management of vasovagal syncope: controlling or aborting faints by leg crossing and muscle tensing. Circulation 106:1684–9

45. Brignole M, Croci F, Menozzi C et al (2002) Isometric arm counter-pressure maneuvers to abort impending vasovagal syncope. J Am Coll Cardiol 40:2053–2059

46. van Dijk N, Quartieri F, Blanc J-J et al (2006) PC-Trial Investigators. Effectiveness of physical counterpressure maneuvers in preventing vasovagal syncope: the physical counterpressure manoeuvres trial (PC-Trial). J Am Coll Cardiol 48:1652–1657

47. Kaufmann H, Saadia D, Voustianiouk A (2002) Midodrine in neurally mediated syncope: a double-blind, randomized, crossover study. Ann Neurol 52:342–345

48. Jankovic J, Gilden JL, Hiner BC et al (1993) Neurogenic orthostatic hypotension: a double-blind, placebo-controlled study with midodrine. Am J Med 95:38–48

49. Connolly SJ, Sheldon R, Thorpe KE et al (2003) VPS II Investigators. Pacemaker therapy for prevention of syncope in patients with recurrent severe vasovagal syncope: second vasovagal pacemaker study (VPS II): a randomized trial. JAMA 289:2224–2229

50. Raviele A, Giada F, Menozzi C et al (2004) Vasovagal syncope and pacing trial investigators. a randomized, double-blind, placebo-controlled study of permanent cardiac pacing for the treatment of recurrent tilt-induced vasovagal syncope. The vasovagal syncope and pacing trial (SYNPACE). Eur Heart J 25:1741–1748

51. Sud S, Massel D, Klein GJ et al (2007) The expectation effect and cardiac pacing for refractory vasovagal syncope. Am J Med 120:54–62

52. Young TM, Mathias CJ (2004) The effects of water ingestion on orthostatic hypotension in two groups of chronic autonomic failure: multiple system atrophy and pure autonomic failure. J Neurol Neurosurg Psychiatry 75:1737–1741

53. Ozcan C, Jahangir A, Friedman PA et al (2001) Long-term survival after ablation of the atrioventricular node and implantation of a permanent pacemaker in patients with atrial fibrillation. N Engl J Med 344:1043–1051

54. Olshansky B, Poole JE, Johnson G et al (2008) Syncope predicts the outcome of cardiomyopathy patients: analysis of the SCD-HeFT study. J Am Coll Cardiol 51:1277–1282

19 Long QT Syndrome

Jonathan N. Johnson and Michael J. Ackerman

CONTENTS

Abstract

Over the past half century, LQTS has matriculated through several critical milestones including its sentinel clinical description, clinical diagnostic scorecard, pathogenetic discovery, decade of research-based genetic testing and genotype–phenotype correlations, and clinical availability of genetic testing. In this chapter, we will discuss the history, epidemiology, and clinical presentations of congenital long QT syndrome (LQTS). We will clarify current diagnostic approaches to LQTS, including clinical history and specific diagnostic testing. Treatment strategies including pharmacologic and surgical techniques will be examined, as well as the role of individualized treatment for the LQTS patient. Finally, preventative strategies will be discussed, including athletic participation.

Key Words: Beta-blockers; denervation therapy; electrocardiogram; epinephrine QT stress test; genetic testing; internal cardioverter defibrillator; ion channels; long QT syndrome; potassium channel; QT interval; sodium channel; sudden death; syncope; T wave alternans.

INTRODUCTION

In 1957, Drs. Anton Jervell and Fred Lange-Nielsen described a Norwegian family of six children, of whom four had congenital sensorineural hearing loss, recurrent syncope during exercise or emotion, and a prolonged QT interval on a 12-lead electrocardiogram (ECG). Three of the four affected children died suddenly at the ages of 4, 5, and 9 years *(1)*. The family history was consistent with an autosomal recessive pattern of inheritance. Drs. Romano *(2)* and Ward *(3)* each separately described a clinical syndrome of sudden death during exercise and emotion in 1963 and 1964, respectively, in an autosomal dominant pattern of inheritance. These patients had normal hearing, and presented with QT interval prolongation, syncope, and sudden death. These two forms of congenital long QT Syndrome (LQTS)

From: *Contemporary Cardiology: Management of Cardiac Arrhythmias*
Edited by: Gan-Xin Yan, Peter R. Kowey, DOI 10.1007/978-1-60761-161-5_19
© Springer Science+Business Media, LLC 2011

were coined as the autosomal recessive Jervell and Lange-Nielsen syndrome (JLNS) and the autosomal dominant Romano-Ward syndrome (RWS).

Our scientific understanding of the heritable arrhythmia syndromes, particularly LQTS, was significantly advanced in 1995 with the discovery of mutations in genes encoding cardiac ion channels as the pathogenic basis of LQTS *(4–6)*. Now less than 15 years after that momentous discovery, LQTS genetic testing has completed its maturation from discovery to translation to clinical availability (2004) and recognition as a clinical test with diagnostic, prognostic, and therapeutic implications *(7)*. Presently, LQTS is recognized as a collection of genetically distinct, arrhythmogenic "channelopathies", resulting from hundreds of mutations in 13 distinct LQTS-susceptibility genes *(8)* (Table 1). These mutations generally involve either loss-of-function potassium channel mutations or gain-of-function sodium channel mutations *(4–6)*.

Table 1
Molecular Basis of Long QT Syndrome

Long QT subtype	Gene	Chromosome	Protein	Relative patient frequency
LQT1	KCNQ1	11p15.5	Kv7.1	30–35%
LQT2	KCNH2	7q35–36	Kv11.1	25–30%
LQT3	SCN5A	3p21–p24	NaV1.5	5–10%
LQT4	ANKB	4q25–q27	Ankyrin B	Rare
LQT5	KCNE1	21q22.1	MinK	Rare
LQT6	KCNE2	7q35–36	MiRP1	Rare
LQT7 (ATS1)	KCNJ2	17q23	Kir2.1	Rare
LQT8 (TS1)	CACNA1C	12p13.3	CaV1.2	Rare
LQT9	CAV3	3p25	Caveolin-3	Rare
LQT10	SCN4B	11q23.3	NaV1.5 beta 4 subunit	Rare
LQT11	AKAP9	7q21–q22	Yotiao	Rare
LQT12	SNTA1	20q11.2	Syntrophin-alpha 1	Rare
LQT13	KCNJ5	11q23.3–24.3	Kir3.4	Rare

ATS Andersen-Tawil Syndrome, *TS* Timothy Syndrome

Overall, approximately 75% of patients with strong clinical evidence of LQTS have identifiable disease causing mutations in one of the three canonical LQTS-susceptibility genes that encode critical cardiac channel alpha subunits *(9–12)*: the *KCNQ1*-encoded I_{Ks} (Kv7.1) potassium channel causing type 1 LQTS (LQT1), accounting for 30–35% of LQTS *(6)*, *KCNH2*-encoded I_{Kr} (Kv11.1) potassium channel causing LQT2 and accounting for 25–30% of LQTS *(4)*, and the *SCN5A*-encoded I_{Na} (Nav1.5) sodium channel causing LQT3 and accounting for 5–10% of LQTS *(5)*. The nine minor LQTS-susceptibility genes explain only 5% of LQTS and involve perturbations in genes that encode key *c*hannel *i*nteracting *p*roteins or ChiPs, including *KCNE1* (LQT5) *(13)* and *KCNE2* (LQT6) *(14)* which encode potassium channel beta subunits, SCN4B (LQT10) *(11)* which encodes the sodium channel beta-4 subunit, *ANKB* (ankyrin B, LQT4) *(15)*, *CAV3* (caveolin-3, LQT9) *(16)*, and *SNTA1* (syntrophin α1, LQT12) *(12)* all which encode for structural membrane scaffolding proteins, and *AKAP9* (yotiao, LQT11) *(10)* which encodes a key regulator of the I_{Ks} potassium channel (Table 1).

The majority of patients with diagnosed LQTS will have the autosomal dominant form (RWS). As such, this chapter will focus mostly on this form of LQTS and its three most common genotypes: LQT1, LQT2, and LQT3. We will also briefly discuss the complex multisystem variants that include abnormal cardiac repolarization, such as Andersen-Tawil syndrome (ATS1) *(17)* and Timothy syndrome (TS1 or LQT8) *(18)*. Finally, we will examine acquired long QT syndrome, a functional mimicker of congenital LQTS with its own unique and profound implications.

EPIDEMIOLOGY

Congenital LQTS affects as many 1 in 2500 persons *(19)* and may be responsible for approximately 20% of autopsy negative sudden unexplained death in the young *(20)* and 10% of sudden infant death syndrome (SIDS) *(21)*.

Although approximately 5–10% of LQTS-causative mutations are de novo (sporadic), autosomal dominant LQTS is the most common inherited form of LQTS, accounting for over 90% of LQTS cases. Females and males are equally affected, and every child of an affected parent has a ~50% chance of inheriting the particular LQTS-susceptibility mutation. JLNS, the extremely rare autosomal recessive form of inherited LQTS, affects approximately 1 per million persons. JLNS similarly affects females and males equally, carries a more severe cardiac phenotype than RWS, and is associated with sensorineural congenital deafness *(22)*. Unlike RWS which requires a single mutation for pathogenicity, JLNS results from homozygous or compound heterozygous mutations in the I_{Ks} potassium channel alpha (Kv7.1) or beta (minK) subunit. JLNS type 1 (JLN1) arises from double mutations in the *KCNQ1* gene, whereas type 2 (JLN2) involves double mutations in the *KCNE1* gene. Notably, the cardiac phenotype in JLNS is a dominant trait, and both parents of a child with JLNS are thus obligate-affected individuals, at least genetically, for autosomal dominant LQTS. However, curiously, the parents are usually asymptomatic and do not typically have significant QT prolongation. In contrast, the characteristic deafness seen in JLNS is a recessive trait, thus the parents are not affected. The deafness arises from ineffective potassium homeostasis of the endolymph in the inner ear that is precipitated by essentially complete knock-out of Kv7.1 channels localizing in the endolymph.

CLINICAL PRESENTATION

The clinical course of a patient with LQTS is highly variable. Patients can remain asymptomatic for a lifetime or can suffer premature sudden cardiac death (SCD) in utero, during infancy, or anytime throughout childhood and adulthood. Around 50% of LQTS patients who have a known causative LQTS mutation (genotype-positive LQTS) will never have a symptom attributable to LQTS. Further, many patients with genetic LQTS will not show overt QT prolongation, and are referred to as having either "concealed" LQTS or "normal QT interval" LQTS. In fact, 27% of patients with genetically proven LQTS have a resting QTc < 440 msec *(9)*. While patients with "concealed" LQTS are at lower risk of cardiac events compared to patients with a QTc >500 msec *(23–27)*, it is nevertheless possible (albeit extremely rare) to have SCD as a sentinel event despite hosting a "low-risk" QTc.

The most common presenting symptoms for a patient with LQTS are recurrent syncope, "seizures", and SCD *(8)*. For the 50% who will experience at least one LQTS-triggered cardiac event, syncope is the most frequent symptom, occurring most commonly during the first three decades of life. These symptoms arise secondary to LQTS' trademark dysrhythmia known as *torsades de pointes* (TdP) *(8)*. The outcome of TdP depends on whether the heart rhythm spontaneously reverts to normal rhythm or if the patient is defibrillated back to normal rhythm before death occurs *(28, 29)*. Most often, TdP is self-terminating with less than 5% of LQTS patients presenting with sudden death or aborted cardiac arrest as their sentinel event. Among those experiencing LQTS-triggered SCD, approximately half may have had a pre-mortem warning of spontaneously terminating TdP (i.e., "torsadogenic syncope").

About 50% of symptomatic probands experience their first cardiac event by 12 years of age, increasing to 90% by 40 years of age *(30)*. Events are most commonly related to physical activity or emotional stress, with around 50% of patients presenting with activity- or emotion-related syncope, seizures, or palpitations. A faint that is triggered by emotion or activity should be considered potentially "torsadogenic" until convinced otherwise, and LQTS needs to be considered during the evaluation. In fact, among patients with LQTS, an assessment of a history for "torsadogenic syncope" (not vasovagal syncope) is the most significant risk factor from a sudden death primary prevention perspective, exceeding the other traditional risk factors of QTc, gender, and genotype *(26)*. Males are more likely to experience their first cardiac event in childhood, with risk decreasing after puberty, whereas females tend to have a later onset of symptoms usually beginning in adolescence and adulthood. Furthermore, approximately 10% of LQTS females experience their first cardiac event during the postpartum period *(31)*.

The clinical evaluation of LQTS has been advanced considerably by the discovery of specific genotype–phenotype relationships. These relationships can assist the physician in choosing correct assessment strategies, expanding personal risk stratification, and tailoring individualized genotype-directed treatment strategies.

Type 1 LQTS (LQT1)

Patients with LQT1 tend to have events triggered by physical or emotional exertion, including swimming, running, anger, fright, and startle *(32)*. Swimming is a relatively specific LQT1- arrhythmogenic trigger, and a personal history or an extended family history of a near drowning plus documented QT prolongation should be viewed as LQT1 until proven otherwise *(33)*. However, if the resting QTc is normal, strong consideration should be instead given to another channelopathy, catecholaminergic polymorphic ventricular tachycardia (CPVT), before invoking and pursuing "concealed" LQT1. The I_{Ks} channel that is mutated in LQT1 patients is reactive to adrenergic stimulation. Thus, instead of the QT interval shortening in response to increased heart rate as seen in normal patients, the ventricular myocyte's action potential paradoxically lengthens during exercise and during early recovery. This cellular dysregulation is exploited for diagnostic purposes with treadmill stress testing and the epinephrine QT stress test discussed later. Patients with LQT1 tend to have a prolonged T wave duration or a broad-based T wave pattern on 12-lead ECG (Fig. 1) *(34, 35)*.

Genotype-Suggestive ECG Patterns

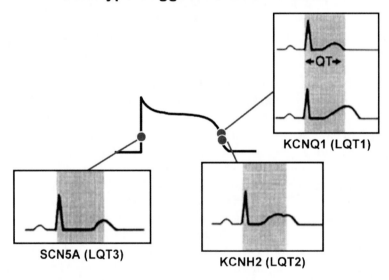

Fig. 1. Genotype-specific/suggestive findings of the 12-lead electrocardiogram evident in LQTS genotypes LQT1, LQT2, and LQT3.

Type 2 LQTS (LQT2)

Patients with LQT2 have more events in association with auditory stimuli, such as the ringing of a telephone or alarm clock *(36)*. Post-partum events in LQTS are significantly more common in LQT2 as compared to other LQTS genotypes *(37)*. Up to 15% of LQT2 patients may have events during rest or sleep, providing some overlap with LQT3. We recently showed that patients with LQT2 also have an increased propensity for a history of seizure activity, which may or may not be related to their cardiac arrhythmogenic phenotype *(38)*. Patients with LQT2 have characteristic bifid T waves in the inferior and lateral leads (Fig. 1) *(34, 35)*. Patients with homozygous mutations of *KCNH2* may exhibit 2:1 AV block, indicating a high-risk phenotype.

Type 3 LQTS (LQT3)

Compared to LQT1 and LQT2 patients, LQT3 patients tend to have more events during rest or sleep. While patients have a lower frequency of LQTS-related cardiac events, they are predisposed to a higher lethality/event rate *(39)*. Like homozygous LQT2 patients, LQT3 patients may exhibit 2:1 AV block, which also indicates a high-risk phenotype. The ECG from patients with LQT3 tends to display long ST isoelectric segments with normal T waves (Fig. 1) *(34, 35)*. However, although pre-genetic test predictions based upon careful inspection of the ECG can start the evaluation, such predictions must be buttressed by the genetic test result. Clinically, the most common mimicker of the LQT3-looking ECG is derived from patients with the most common LQTS genotype (LQT1). As will be discussed later, the treatment strategies for LQT1 and LQT3 are quite different.

DIAGNOSIS

In 1985, Schwartz et al. proposed the first diagnostic criteria for LQTS *(40)* with major criteria including the presence of a QTc > 440 msec (a value exceeded by 2.5% of all infants and by 10–20% of all adolescents and adults), stress-induced syncope, and family members with LQTS, and minor criteria that included the presence of congenital deafness, episodes of T-wave alternans, bradycardia in children, and abnormal ventricular repolarization. These criteria were updated in 1993 with a point system based on various QTc values (Table 2) *(41)*. The calculated "Schwartz score" (more correctly the "Schwartz-Moss-Vincent-Crampton score") designates clinical probability of LQTS with three potential diagnostic outcomes; $\leq$ 1 point implies a low probability of LQTS, 2 or 3 points gives an intermediate probability of LQTS, and $\geq$ 3.5 points designates a high probability of LQTS. The positive predictive value of a modified "Schwartz score" $\geq$ 3.5 is quite good, and this diagnostic scorecard still provides a useful schematic for evaluation of index cases.

The LQTS diagnostic score, however, is not useful for the assessment of relatives/family members who may have genotype-positive/phenotype-negative LQTS (i.e., "concealed LQTS"). The clinical phenotypic penetrance of LQTS may be as low as 25% in some families. Although the risk of SCD is extremely low for patients with concealed LQTS, their correct identification enables the implementation of several preventative strategies that are discussed in the treatment section. Here, confirmatory genetic testing is the only definitive diagnostic test for family members of a patient with a known LQTS-causative mutation, as the cumulative diagnostic score and 12-lead ECG will not accurately expose this subpopulation of low-risk, concealed LQTS.

It is important to understand the currently available clinical tests, in terms of both diagnostic and prognostic utility, that are often used when LQTS is in the differential diagnosis. These tests are summarized below.

The 12-Lead Electrocardiogram (ECG)

Despite the possibility that more interpretive mishaps and errors have occurred with this test than any other *(42, 43)*, the ECG remains the cornerstone of the LQTS evaluation. Central to its assessment is the ability to accurately measure the QTc. Computer-derived measurements are fraught with errors, particularly in patients with complex T-wave and U-wave arrangements *(42, 44)*. As such, the

Table 2
Schwartz Score for LQTS Diagnostic Criteria

LQTS Clinical Probability Score Card (i.e., "Schwartz/Moss/Vincent/Crampton Score")

Finding	Points
History	
Clinical history of syncope[a]	
Without stress	1
With stress	2
Congenital deafness	0.5
Family history of LQTS[b]	1
Unexplained sudden death in a 1st-degree family member <age 30[b]	0.5
ECG	
Corrected QT interval (Bazett's formula)	
450 msec (in males)	1
460–470 msec	2
$\geq$480 msec	3
Torsade de pointes[a]	2
T wave alternans	1
$\geq$3 leads with notched T waves	1
Bradycardia (<2nd percentile for age)	0.5
≤ 1 = low probability; 1 < score < 4 = intermediate probability; ≥ 4 = high probability	

[a]Syncope and torsade de pointes are mutually exclusive

[b]Cannot count the same family member for both criteria

Adapted from Ref. *(41)*

computer's QTc cannot be relied upon when a diagnosis of LQTS is in question, and *must* be verified manually. However, even experienced cardiologists may have difficulty in accurately and independently measuring the QTc *(43)*.

The QT interval is defined as the time duration between the onset of the QRS complex and the end of the T-wave as it returns to baseline (Fig. 2a), ideally measured using either lead II or lead V5 of the 12-lead ECG. There are no standards for interpreting prolonged QT intervals from Holter or 24/48-hour ambulatory monitoring records, and thus QTc assessment by ambulatory monitoring is not typically utilized to make a diagnosis of LQTS *(16)*. Whilst numerous methodologies for correcting QT intervals for heart rate have been proposed *(45–47)*, the most universally utilized method is that described by Bazett *(48)*, who calculated the QTc as the QT interval divided by the square root of the preceding RR interval (Fig. 2a). At normal heart rates this formula is useful; however, it underestimates and overestimates the QTc at extreme low and high heart rates respectively. In the presence of sinus arrhythmia, the interpreting physician should calculate an average QTc from analysis of the entire 12-lead ECG rhythm strip *(49)*. Although prior authors have recommended applying Bazett's formula to the QT interval following the shortest available RR interval *(50)*, this will result in a marked overestimation of cardiac repolarization, leading to overdiagnosis. On the other hand, using only the longest RR interval may underestimate the duration of cardiac repolarization.

The U-wave is a common ECG finding that vexes QTc interpretations. A U-wave distinctly separate from and much smaller than the preceding T-wave should be excluded from the QT interval measurement *(51)*. If such U waves are included, the QTc will be inflated by as much as 80–200 msec, and unnecessarily cause an incorrect LQTS diagnosis *(16)*. To avoid U wave inflations, many specialists recommend a method where the end of the T-wave is considered to be the intersection of the tangent to the steepest slope of the last limb of the T-wave and the baseline (Fig. 2b) *(44, 52)*. This "teach-the-tangent" method, which we also refer to as "avoid-the-tail", when taught to a cohort

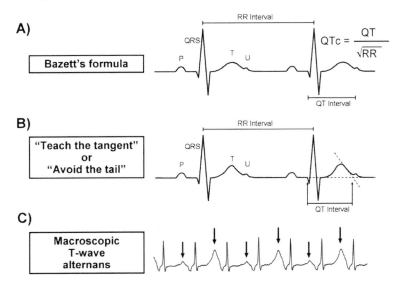

Fig. 2. (a) Diagrammatic representation of two cardiac cycles, with the calculation of the QTc identified using the Bazett formula. (b) Diagrammatic representation of two cardiac cycles, with identification of the "teach-the-tangent" method of QTc measurement as described by Postema et al. *(44)*. (c) Macroscopic T-wave alternans as noted on electrocardiography.

of medical students, resulted in significantly improved accuracy of LQTS diagnosis, even compared to experienced clinicians *(44)*.

"Normal" QTc values on the 12-lead ECG range between 350 and 440 msec *(51, 53)*, but as will be discussed, the use of QTc > 440 msec as indicative of QT prolongation will result in a mini-epidemic of LQTS overdiagnosis. The wide overlap between LQTS and normalcy remains a significant diagnostic challenge. While the diagnosis is readily suggested in a patient with a QTc persistently greater than 500 msec (especially if accompanied by typical LQTS-related cardiac events), physicians are frequently confronted with patients diagnosed with "borderline" LQTS. These patients may not give an LQTS-specific history or complaint, and instead may have received an ECG for variety of reasons. A pronouncement of "borderline" QT prolongation is commonly given when a patient has a QTc value between 440 and 480 msec *(53)*. Within this range however, there is a significant "overlap zone," an area in which it is unclear purely based on the ECG whether or not a patient actually has LQTS (Fig. 3). Fully 15% of the general population may have a QTc residing in the "borderline range" *(42)*. However, over 25% of patients harboring an LQTS-causing mutation have a QTc < 440 msec *(9)*. Due to this overlap, it is easy to appreciate why LQTS can be both over- and underdiagnosed. Care has to be taken to avoid overdiagnosing post-pubertal females who tend to have a slightly longer QTc compared to males *(54)*.

Figure 3 depicts the distribution of QTc values among healthy post-pubertal adult men and women as well as the QTc distribution seen for all genotype-positive patients evaluated in Mayo Clinic's LQTS clinic. The presence of a QTc < 400 msec is > 99% sensitive in indicating a normal patient. Likewise, a QTc ≥ 480 msec typically indicates abnormal repolarization, which could be due to either acquired or congenital LQTS. The overlap zone between 400 and 480 msec is the source of many referrals and confusion amongst physicians. It is important to understand the differences between the normal QTc distribution in healthy subjects and the distribution of the 1 in 2500 LQTS-affected persons (Fig. 3). For example, an asymptomatic patient without an LQTS-specific family history and a QTc of 450 msec is 500 times more likely to be normal than have concealed LQTS. It is true that patients with concealed LQTS (again, defined as a genotype-positive patient with a normal ECG) can experience

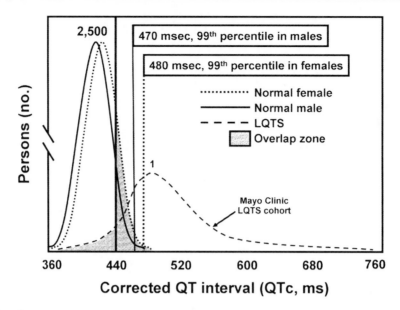

Fig. 3. QTc distribution in health and LQTS. Adapted from Taggart et al. *(42).*

cardiac events, including sudden death. Therefore, although the risk of sudden death in a patient with concealed LQTS is rare, it is not indicative of the absence of risk.

Although the latest 2009 ECG position statement from the ACC coins a QTc $\geq$ 450 msec (males) and $\geq$ 460 msec (females) as prolonged *(55)*, these are dangerous QTc cutoff values from the perspective of screening for a 1:2500 person condition known as LQTS where those particular QTc values will have a < 1% positive predictive value on their own. This provides a chance to admonish cardiologists in training and physicians in general to resist the rapid reflex of going from an ECG rendition of "borderline QT prolongation" to a clinical diagnosis of "possible LQTS". From a LQTS screening standpoint only, a QTc cutoff value > 480 msec may maximize the utility of the ECG as a screening test where the objective would be to catch patients with higher risk LQTS (QTc > 500 msec) while trying to minimize the onslaught of false-positives.

In addition to the QTc, specific T-wave and ST segment findings can help the shrewd clinician in an LQTS evaluation, even in the presence of a normal or borderline QTc *(34)*. Examples of possible LQTS-associated morphologies include T waves that are wide-based and slowly generated, biphasic or bifid, notched, sinusoidal oscillation, low-amplitude bumps on the down-slope T-wave limb, indistinct termination, or simply delayed. We typically look for T-wave abnormalities in the lateral precordial leads where the presence of notched T waves might tip-off the presence of LQTS. The type of T-wave notching may also be helpful. Previous reports have classified notching into grade 1 (G1) notches, which occur at or below the apex no matter the amplitude, and grade 2 (G2) notches, which occur above the apex *(56)*. G2 notches are more specific but are infrequent, and when present often suggest LQT2. G2 notching identified during low-dose epinephrine infusion can also unmask patients with concealed LQT2 *(57)*. However, the cardiologist must be cautious not to over-interpret T-wave changes observed in the precordial leads V2 and V3 as potentially pathogenic in nature, as T-waves in these leads are highly variable in the non-LQTS general population, especially among adolescents in general and adolescent women in particular.

The presence of macrovoltage and microvoltage T wave alternans (TWA, Fig. 2c) may confer prognostic implications as an at-risk finding, but its clinical utility is minimal overall secondary to its infrequent sighting. TWA is the beat-to-beat alternation of the morphology and amplitude of the T wave. It can be a marker of electrical instability and regional repolarization heterogeneity, and is associated with an increased risk of cardiac events *(58, 59)*. Several investigators have reported the use of QT dispersion (QTd), defined as the difference between the maximal and minimal QT intervals in the 12 standard leads. It is thought to potentially represent spatial repolarization *(60)*. QTd is reportedly increased in LQTS patients compared to normal patients, and there is a difference in QTd between mutation carriers and unaffected family members *(61–63)*. However, the potential diagnostic utility of QTd to make a distinction between LQTS and normal is unknown, and it is rarely used clinically.

Exercise Testing

Normally, repolarization becomes more efficient during exercise, hence the expected shortening of the QT and QTc with exercise stress testing. In contrast, patients with LQTS have been observed to have "attenuated QTc shortening" with exercise, particularly patients with LQT1 *(64)*. Additionally, the QT has been shown to lengthen abnormally during the recovery phase of exercise in patients with LQTS *(65)*. While failure of appropriate shortening is relatively diagnostic in patients with LQT1, the presence of normal shortening of the QT interval during exercise does not rule out other LQTS genotypes *(66)*. While most research of exercise testing in LQTS patients has been performed on patients with an obviously prolonged QTc at rest, provocative testing is most often utilized in the diagnosis of patients with concealed LQTS, where it can distinguish concealed LQTS from normalcy.

Other findings on exercise testing are uncommon in patients with LQTS. Exercise-induced ventricular ectopy is exceedingly rare. The presence of ventricular ectopy including premature ventricular contractions, in bigeminy or as couplets, or bidirectional ventricular tachycardia, is much more suggestive of catecholaminergic polymorphic ventricular tachycardia than LQTS. The presence of macro- or microvoltage TWA at rest or during provocative testing can indicate increased risk in LQTS *(67)*. Macrovoltage TWA is extremely rare, having been witnessed only twice in the over 1000 treadmill/epinephrine QT stress tests that we have performed. Microvoltage TWA studies have not been clinically helpful in our experience and are no longer performed at our LQTS clinic.

Epinephrine QT Stress Test

Like exercise testing, the epinephrine QT stress test has been shown to be particularly helpful in unmasking patients with concealed LQT1. Patients with LQT1 typically show a paradoxical lengthening of repolarization, measured by the QTc (Shimizu bolus protocol) or the absolute QT interval (Ackerman/Mayo continuous infusion protocol) during intravenous epinephrine infusion *(67, 68)*. The presence of paradoxical lengthening (> 30 msec) of the QT interval is suggestive (75% positive predictive value) of concealed LQT1 with the Mayo protocol *(69)*. The absence of paradoxical QT lengthening is not effective in diagnosing other LQTS genotypes. It is critical to note that, as one might expect, the presence of concurrent beta-blockade will affect the outcome and interpretation of the epinephrine QT stress test.

We also use epinephrine QT stress testing in patients with novel LQT1-associated mutations. This allows us to physiologically challenge the patient's potassium channel function, and provide an independent confirmation of the novel mutation's pathogenicity, using the 96% negative predictive value of the test. In other words, both treadmill and epinephrine stress testing represent in vivo functional challenges to assess the integrity of the I_{Ks} (Kv7.1) channel pathway where loss-of-function mutations compromise the ability of this key channel to respond to sympathetic stimulation and accentuate its phase 3 repolarizing force.

Molecular Genetic Testing

After the sentinel discovery of LQTS as a cardiac channelopathy in 1995, LQTS genetic testing was performed in several research laboratories for research and "pseudo-clinical" purposes for the next decade. Then, in 2004, a commercially available genetic test called FAMILION™ was introduced (Clinical Data, Inc, New Haven, CT). This clinical genetic test includes the comprehensive open reading frame analysis of the translated exons for the 3 canonical LQTS-susceptibility genes and several of the minor genes. A second commercial genetic test has also been introduced recently (GeneDx, Inc, Gaithersburg, MD). A list of indications for LQTS genetic testing is summarized in Table 3.

Table 3
Considerations for LQTS Genetic Testing

1. Unequivocal and unexplained QT prolongation (QTc > 500 msec)
2. Clinically suspected LQTS regardless of (a) baseline QTc or (b) history of prior genetic testing, either research-based or commercial/clinical.
3. All first-degree relatives of a genotype-positive index case of LQTS regardless of their screening ECG, with subsequent distantly-related family testing depending on results.
4. Postmortem genetic testing for autopsy-negative sudden unexplained death (debatable)
5. Patients with a history of drug-induced torsades (debatable)
6. Postmortem genetic testing in victims of sudden infant death syndrome (debatable)

QTc Corrected QT Interval, *LQTS* Congenital Long QT Syndrome

The current generation LQTS clinical genetic tests will be positive about 75% of the time in patients with clinically definite LQTS *(70–72)*. This is clinically helpful, both in determination of appropriate treatment as well as in guiding diagnosis for potentially affected family members. About 5–10% of LQTS probands have spontaneous germline mutations. Conversely, approximately 5% of genotype-positive LQTS patients will have more than one mutation *(70)*, and these patients typically have a more severe arrhythmogenic phenotype *(73)*. Therefore, it is critical that comprehensive genetic testing is performed, even after finding a single potentially causative mutation, as other mutations may be present and drive therapy in a different direction.

Considering that 25% of patients with "no doubt about it" LQTS will have a negative LQTS genetic test, genetic testing, as a stand alone test, can not exclude LQTS. Secondary to the fear of "missing" this potentially fatal disease, many patients are given a clinical diagnosis of LQTS despite a low or intermediate diagnostic assessment. In our experience, 44% of patients who had LQTS genetic testing despite an intermediate probability "Schwartz score" had a positive genetic test, changing their diagnosis from clinical indeterminate to genetically possible/probable *(72)*.

On the other hand, indiscriminate use of LQTS genetic testing (i.e., screening) rather than its proper story-driven indications would result in a tremendous number of false positives. Unlike nearly all of the 1500+ genetic tests that are clinically available, the background frequency of rare genetic variation that could be viewed as "possible deleterious mutations" or "variants of uncertain significance" is known for only a handful of disease genes including the breast cancer-associated genes and the major LQTS-susceptibility genes *(74, 75)*. This has been extended with an analysis of over 1300 reportedly healthy volunteers whereby approximately 4% of whites and 6–8% of non-whites hosted a rare genetic variant that would have to be classified currently as a possible (maybe) disease-contributing mutation *(76)*. Juxtaposed to the expected frequency of 75% for cases of robust LQTS, this implies that even among the purest of case mutation results, there is a 5–10% chance that the mutation elicited for the patient with highest pre-test probability is nevertheless a "false positive". Importantly, mutation type and mutation location strongly inform the probability of pathogenicity for the current generation genetic test *(76)*. Like the probabilistic nature of virtually every clinical test that we utilize, genetic testing is slowly being grasped by the clinician community as a probabilistic, rather than deterministic, test that must be carefully scrutinized and interpreted.

MANAGEMENT

The key in understanding potential management strategies in LQTS rests with proper interpretation of clinical and genetic testing, and in appropriate risk stratification. For the entire population of LQTS, the annual mortality is < 1%/year, but may increase to 5–8%/year in the highest risk subsets of patients.

Risk Stratification

Due to the inherent heterogeneity of LQTS, the phenotypic expression of LQTS may vary from a purely asymptomatic life to premature sudden cardiac death (SCD) despite intervention. Any patient who has a personal history of recurrent cardiac arrest carries an increased risk of subsequent SCD (77). Except for the subset that presents with aborted cardiac arrest as the sentinel event where there is near universal agreement that an implantable cardioverter defibrillator (ICD) is indicated for such a patient, primary prevention risk stratification attempts to determine which patients will experience life-threatening events in the future.

Factors associated with increased risk in LQTS-triggered SCD include a QTc >500 msec, a history of LQTS-related symptoms (especially syncope and aborted cardiac arrest), the LQT2 or LQT3 genotype, concurrent 2:1 AV block, and post-pubertal females (78). In particular, an LQTS-triggered cardiac event such as syncope occurring in the first 5 years of life suggests a severe LQTS cardiac phenotype, and syncope in the first year of life portends a poor prognosis (79). The risk of cardiac events is higher in males until they reach pubertal age, and is higher in females once they reach adult age (80). As such, asymptomatic males over the age of 20 years of life are at a particularly low risk of having cardiac events, especially among males with C-terminal localizing, haploinsufficient LQT1-associated mutations (80–82). Unlike males, asymptomatic females carry a continued risk for cardiac events into adulthood, especially in the post-partum period (31). Patients with the autosomal recessive JLNS are also a high risk subset.

Patients with LQT1 have the greatest number of LQTS-triggered events, with 60% of patients having a history of syncope, aborted cardiac arrest, and sudden death (39). Around 40% of patients with LQT2 have a history of these LQTS-related events, with LQT3 patients having the fewest cardiac events of the genotypes (18%) (32, 39, 83). Despite the different event frequencies, the mortality rate is similar among the 3 genotypes. Hence, the so-called "lethality per event" rate is highest in patients with LQT3.

The correct distinction between vasovagal syncope and "torsadogenic syncope" is critical. Syncope with a prodrome, occurring in common situations including overheating/dehydration, venipuncture, prolonged standing, or during micturition, is much more indicative of vasovagal syncope, although there may be overlap. A history of syncope deemed to be "torsadogenic syncope" should be viewed as a strong sudden death warning sign prompting aggressive therapy though certainly not a self-sufficient indication for a prophylactic ICD (26). A family history of SCD, while important in the screening of potential LQTS patients, does not appear to confer risk among the surviving genotype positive or clinically apparent LQTS family members (84). Similarly, a negative family history for SCD should not invoke a conclusion towards a favorable outcome.

As discussed above, a QTc > 500 msec, particularly in the presence of LQTS-related symptoms, is associated with a relative risk ranging from 2 to 4 for a LQTS-triggered cardiac event of syncope or worse (23–27, 81). There is a distinct direct relationship between clinical risk and degree of QT prolongation; the higher the QTc, the higher the clinical risk. Despite this however, there is essentially no QTc value at which there is absolutely zero risk.

T-wave notching is more common in symptomatic patients, and may be useful in prognosis (85). Macroscopic TWA (Fig. 2c) on the 12-lead ECG is a marker of severe electrical lability in patients with LQTS, and may be of prognostic significance (58, 59). However, macroscopic TWA is rare, and the relationship between degree of TWA and risk of SCD is unknown (79). There currently is no role for invasive electrophysiology studies for the purposes of LQTS risk stratification, as the majority of LQTS patients will not exhibit arrhythmias during programmed electrical stimulation *(86)*.

Treatment

First and foremost, all patients with LQTS, either in a congenital or acquired form, should be counseled to avoid all medications known to aggravate the QT interval as a drug-mediated side effect. A list of the most common offenders is shown in Table 4. The University of Arizona maintains an updated list of all known QT-prolonging medications at www.qtdrugs.org. If there is a clear medical necessity for a listed medication, there should be a careful assessment of risks and benefits of administering the medication, as well as appropriate monitoring while on such medication(s).

Table 4
Common Medications that Prolong the QT Interval

Class	*Medication*
Anti-arrhythmics	
	Amiodarone
	Dofetilide
	Procainamide
	Quinidine
	Sotalol
Antibiotics	
	Azithromycin
	Erythromycin
	Gatifloxacin
	Levofloxacin
	Moxifloxacin
Motility agents	
	Cisapride (withdrawn)
	Domperidone (withdrawn)
Narcotics	
	Methadone
Psychotropics	
	Haloperidol
	Phenothiazine
	Thioridazine
	Tricyclic antidepressants

The ultimate goal for the treatment of LQTS is to prevent SCD secondary to TdP with failure to spontaneously convert back to normal sinus rhythm. Given the risk of mortality in LQTS, all previously symptomatic patients should be treated. However, the vast majority of even symptomatic LQTS can be treated pharmacologically. The full spectrum of therapeutic options includes pharmacologic, denervation, device, and preventative treatment measures. Indeed, recent years have shown a trend towards increased use of the most aggressive but more definitive treatment option, the ICD. Given the potential risk/benefit ratios of invasive treatments, particularly in children, it is the physician's imperative to offer individualized treatment plans. In any case, it is a near universal recommendation that any patient who survives LQTS-triggered aborted cardiac arrest should receive an ICD as secondary prevention.

The treatment of asymptomatic LQTS patients is a matter of continued debate. It is true that in older studies, up to 9% of patients had a cardiac arrest as their first symptom/manifestation of LQTS *(87)*, and that 4% of patients asymptomatic at the time of diagnosis later died suddenly. With these findings, it became common for all patients with LQTS to be treated regardless of symptomatology, particularly young patients *(88)*. Once a patient has been diagnosed with LQTS, due to the >90% inherited nature of the disease, all first-degree relatives should be screened, with treatment offered on an individual basis *(89)*. Further, all patients should be seen by a physician well-versed in the intricacies of LQTS.

Medical therapy, particularly pharmacologic, should be considered for ALL asymptomatic patients with manifest QT prolongation (QTc > 480 msec). Asymptomatic males over the age of 40 years with LQT1, especially those with lower risk LQT1-associated mutations, may not need any active intervention, only QT-drug avoidance and other simple preventative measures *(23)*. This profile indicates the "near-zero" risk subpopulation of LQTS.

Medications

In LQT1 and LQT2, as well as most cases of genotype-negative LQTS, beta-blocker therapy has been and should be the first-line therapy *(77)*. Beta-blockers have been shown to reduce the frequency of sudden death and ventricular arrhythmias, as well as reduce symptoms in patients with LQTS *(87, 90)*. In one study, mortality was significantly reduced to less than 2% in LQTS patients treated with beta-blockers *(77)*. At Mayo Clinic's LQTS Clinic, infants with LQTS are generally started on liquid propranolol, which is typically dosed three times a day (every 6 h has been advised by others but this has not been shown to be necessary). Liquid nadolol can be used twice daily but has a relatively short (2–4 week) shelf-life. Generally, nadolol has been our drug of choice because of its long half-life and the ability to dose once daily (especially after age 10 or so), thereby contributing favorably to compliance. However, a lateral move to propranolol or its long-acting version (Inderal) can be made without hesitation if there are unacceptable side effects to see if a different beta-blocker is better tolerated.

Although atenolol continues to be one of the most frequent beta-blockers prescribed on the outside, it is not used in our program. Among the centers with the largest LQTS experience, nadolol and propranolol/Inderal are the preferred beta-blockers (Table 5) and atenolol is viewed as potentially inferior *(91)*. At this point in time, it is unclear whether atenolol is intrinsically a suboptimal beta-blocker or whether it has been pharmacokinetically misused. Patients still tend to arrive on atenolol dosed once daily when its pharmacokinetic properties require twice daily dosing to provide 24-hour protection. Regardless, each patient should have an individualized recommendation regarding which beta-blocker medication to use if indicated, taking into account the method of administration, dosing schedule, potential benefits, and side effects.

Table 5
Preferred Medications and Suggested Dosages for the Management of LQTS

Class	Medication	Dosage	Dose frequency
Beta-blockers	Nadolol	1–2.0 mg/kg/day	Once daily (Twice daily until around 10 years)
	Propranolol	3–4 mg/kg/day	Three times daily or twice daily with long acting form (Inderal, LA)
Sodium-channel blockers			
	Mexiletine	~10–15 mg/kg/day	Three times daily
	Flecainide	1–6 mg/kg/day	Three times daily
	Ranolazine	Up to 1000 mg/dose (adults)	Twice daily

Overall, beta-blockers are the only pharmacotherapeutic agents that can be used alone for the two most common subtypes of LQTS (LQT1 and LQT2) and for those patients with genotype-negative

LQTS. Other medications are not typically used as "stand alone" therapies. Calcium channel blockers like verapamil or potassium channel openers like nicorandil may be used in patients with recurrent ICD discharges despite beta-blocker therapy and surgical denervation. As will be discussed later, pharmacological targeting with late sodium current blockers may be a stand alone pharmacologic option for patients with LQT3.

Pacing

Many spontaneous arrhythmias in LQTS are pause-dependent, where the sentinel arrhythmia of TdP is preceded by the sudden increase in cycle length *(92)*. LQTS patients may have slower resting heart rates, and beta-blocker therapy can worsen bradycardia and potentiate the chance of a long-short-long type of pause. Cardiac pacing can prevent pause-dependent TdP, especially in LQT2 patients *(93)*. It does not, however, reduce the risk of sudden death in high-risk patients *(93)*. When considered, pacing should seldom be stand alone therapy as it is usually used in conjunction with beta-blocker therapy *(94)*. Potential indications for pacing in LQTS patients include those with preexisting AV block and those with a history/Holter evidence of pause-dependent arrhythmias. Specific recommendations for device programming and pacing strategies are well summarized by Viskin et al. *(94)*. In our clinical practice, if a pacemaker is considered due to a perceived high patient risk, we typically will place an implantable defibrillator/pacemaker instead of an isolated pacemaker. Over the past 10 years, no LQTS patient has received an isolated pacemaker in Mayo's LQTS Clinic.

Implantable Cardioverter-Defibrillator (ICD)

The ICD represents one of the most significant medical advances of our time, enabling a subset of the population to survive potentially lethal arrhythmias while maintaining routine activities of daily life. The current indications for ICD placement in LQTS patients are summarized in Fig. 4. Contrary to popular belief and the seeming trend in the United States towards universal ICD therapy in LQTS, < 15% of the > 500 LQTS patients followed in our LQTS Clinic have an ICD. Indeed, the vast majority of LQTS patients can and should be managed without an ICD. As mentioned previously, ICD therapy is almost universally recommended as secondary prevention following an aborted cardiac arrest *(95–97)*.

The use of ICD therapy as primary prevention is debatable and open to personal interpretation and patient preference. ICD therapy as primary prevention is often recommended in cases where beta-blockade may significantly reduce, but not eradicate, the risk of sudden death *(26, 98)*. Family history

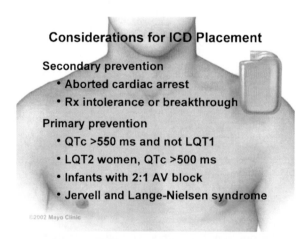

Fig. 4. Current considerations for ICD therapy in LQTS. Adapted from Ackerman et al. *(121)*.

of sudden death, despite current listing as a class IIb indication for ICD therapy, is not supported by evidence as an independent indication for ICD placement *(84)*. As shown in Fig. 4, risk factors that warrant consideration of a prophylactic ICD include a LQTS-triggered cardiac event despite adequate beta blocker therapy both in terms of drug and dose *(26)*, intolerance of primary pharmacotherapy, severe QT prolongation (QTc > 550 msec) without the LQT1 genotype *(97, 99)*, and infants with 2:1 AV block *(87)*. In addition, patients with JLNS, especially those with type 1 JLNS *(100)*, probably warrant a prophylactic ICD due to their severe cardiac phenotype.

Many patients with the LQT3 genotype have received ICDs , including nearly 50% of the LQT3 patients at Mayo, due to LQT3's comparatively higher lethality/event rate *(39, 98, 101)*. This has been called into question recently, and remains a controversial issue *(102)*. If an ICD is needed, we typically place a single lead ICD system. If pacing is going to be used as an adjuvant therapy, then a dual chamber pacemaker/ICD should be implanted. No matter the scenario, it is key that all risk-benefit ratios be weighed without bias, with patients and families being as fully informed as possible.

Left Cardiac Sympathetic Denervation (LCSD)

Left cardiac sympathetic denervation (LCSD) involves resection of the lower half of the left stellate ganglion and the left-sided sympathetic chain at the level of T2, T3, and T4 *(103, 104)*. Resection of the lower half of the stellate ganglion is critical; removal of T2-T4 only will not provide the same antifibrillatory effect and should be considered an incomplete denervation *(105)*. LCSD can be performed using open thoracotomy or via video-assisted thoracic surgery (VATS), depending on surgeon preference. The rationale behind denervation therapy is based on evidence that the left-sided cardiac sympathetic nerves have a very high arrhythmogenic potential *(106, 107)*, and may carry increased activity in patients with LQTS *(107)*. There are now several well-published studies showing a significant decrease in events in LQTS patients after LCSD *(104, 106, 108)*. Further, LCSD's antifibrillatory effect appears to be relatively substrate independent with demonstrated efficacy seen in patients with both genotype positive and genotype negative LQTS as well as the three major LQTS genotypes. Here, the predicted efficacy is LQT1 > LQT3 > LQT2, but this ranking awaits confirmation. Schwartz has recommended that LCSD be considered in all LQTS patients who have syncope despite adequate β-blocker therapy, as well as in patients with arrhythmia storms and recurrent ICD shocks *(109)*.

Mortality associated with LCSD is near zero at most experienced centers and the complication of Horner's syndrome is seldom seen (< 5%). A list of current indications for videoscopic denervation

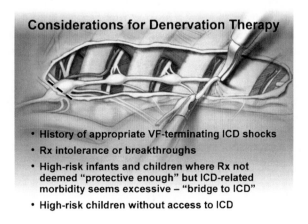

Considerations for Denervation Therapy

- History of appropriate VF-terminating ICD shocks
- Rx intolerance or breakthroughs
- High-risk infants and children where Rx not deemed "protective enough" but ICD-related morbidity seems excessive – "bridge to ICD"
- High-risk children without access to ICD

Fig. 5. Current considerations for LCSD in LQTS.

therapy/LCSD in our institution is shown in Fig. 5 *(104)*. While initially reserved for patients with multiple VF-terminating ICD therapies (secondary prevention denervation therapy), LCSD is now offered as an alternative to ICD for patients with beta-blocker intolerance and as a "bridge to ICD" in patients such as infants and small children where ICD placement is associated with higher complication rates. In addition, LCSD may be used as a treatment strategy for patients where ICDs are either unavailable or unattainable.

Gene-Specific Therapy

LQT1: Patients with LQT1 are significantly protected by the use of beta-blocker therapy, particularly since many of their cardiac events are typically induced by adrenergic stimulation *(99)*. LCSD can be used if events including syncope occur despite beta-blocker therapy *(108)*. A prophylactic ICD should be least frequent among patients with LQT1.

LQT2: Patients with LQT2 are also protected well by beta-blockade, but tend to have more breakthrough events compared to LQT1 patients *(77)*. Medical augmentation of potassium channel function using medications including nicorandil is of unclear significance, and these are not typically used. LCSD can be used in patients with breakthrough events. In high-risk patients (females, QTc > 500 msec), prophylactic ICD may be considered, typically with single lead ICD therapy. Potassium supplementation and/or pharmacological attempts to increase serum potassium (i.e., spironolactone) may enhance cardiac repolarization and have been utilized *(110)*. To date, however, spironolactone pharmacotherapy has not been needed at our institution.

LQT3: Fortunately LQT3 is the least common (5–10%) among the three canonical LQTS genotypes, as management of LQT3 continues to vex LQTS specialists. The combination of its highest lethality per event label and concerns regarding insufficient protection afforded by beta-blocker therapy has compelled a high use of prophylactic ICD. However, propranolol therapy with or without mexiletine/flecainide/ranolazine may provide a cogent, gene-tailored treatment option for the low/moderate risk LQT3 patient. Propranolol is specifically advocated because in addition to its beta blocking properties, it is a weak blocker of late sodium current *(111)*. This component of its mechanism of action may explain why clinically, pro-arrhythmias from beta blocker therapy have not been observed among LQT3 patients when the cellular in vitro data suggests this possibility of beta blocker-mediated LQT3-related cardiac events *(101)*. Historically, the largest LQTS programs treating the largest number of this subpopulation of LQT3 patients have utilized propranolol as the preferred beta blocker.

Regarding direct targeting of the late sodium current, this must be carefully monitored and individualized as not all LQT3-susceptibility mutations are created equal. For example, those LQT3 mutations that result in isolated accentuation of late sodium current could conceivably be "medically cured" by blocking the pathological current, thereby restoring repolarization to more normal like conditions which has been demonstrated for both dogs and humans *(112, 113)*. As indicated previously, however, although it makes sense as an effective anti-arrhythmic treatment strategy, there are no studies to date demonstrating a survival benefit with this approach. In addition, given that some LQT3 mutations exhibit a hybrid, loss- and gain-of-function phenotype, it is conceivable that late sodium channel blocker therapy could unmask and accentuate the loss-of-function side of the equation and precipitate a Brugada-like phase 2 re-entrant mechanism. This possibility serves as a clear reminder that management of all LQTS patients and LQT3 patients specifically must be carefully scrutinized and individualized. This disease truly personifies the call for personalized/individualized medicine.

PREVENTION

As discussed above, it is critical for patients to consult their doctor before taking any medications. Medications known to prolong the QT interval must be avoided. If a medication is required that has known QT-aggravating potential, the physician and patient/family need to perform a careful risk/benefit analysis. If an alternative medication exists with similar efficacy but without the QT side effect, then that medication should be used. Common situations where this may arise includes the use of Albuterol in treating asthma and the use of Ritalin or other stimulant therapies in treating attention deficit disorder. Again, the physician and patient/family need to weight the risks/benefits carefully, recognizing the life-changing potential and risks of these medications. Over the past 10 years, we have not seen a single albuterol-triggered or stimulant-triggered cardiac event among the subpopulation of our patients with LQTS where jointly we concluded that continued use of such medications had a favorable benefit to risk ratio.

Physicians should inform patients and family members of several key preventative health measures for patients with LQTS, unrelated to the above pharmacotherapeutic and surgical therapies. Healthy sleep and dietary habits, as in other disease processes, are important and should not be overlooked. Hypokalemia can precipitate an LQTS-related cardiac event, and thus a potassium-enriched diet may be helpful. During gastrointestinal illnesses, hydration and electrolyte replacement is important to avoid hypokalemia and other electrolyte disturbances. Patients should be cautioned against drinking excessive amounts of grapefruit juice, especially purple grapefruit juice, as it contains a chemical that inhibits the I_{Kr} potassium channel and can prolong the QT interval in a mechanism similar to that of drug-induced QT prolongation (114). Over-the-counter supplements including cesium chloride or amphetamine-like agents should be avoided (115).

Patients with LQTS, especially those with LQT2, should avoid or at least minimize sources of loud auditory triggers in their home and workplace (i.e., telephones or alarm clocks), particularly during sleep (109, 116, 117). This is often forgotten for patients in the hospital setting, when the recurrent alarms in patients' rooms can trigger events. An identification card, necklace, or bracelet should be carried or worn at all times, to let emergency response personnel know of their diagnosis and allow for quicker activation of appropriate therapy. All families should consider having an automatic external defibrillator (AED) at home, and this should accompany the family whenever possible on vacations, car trips, athletic outings, etc. Appropriate maintenance and checkups should be performed on the AED to ensure that it will be ready whenever needed. Most schools now have AEDs in place as standard equipment, but this should be assessed by the family during the process of school enrollment. Family members should be trained in CPR, and all should be taught how to administer a precordial thump prior to chest compressions. In LQTS, this "artificial" commotio cordis might restore sinus rhythm in some patients and prevent significant morbidity (118). Although we continue to recommend a personal AED as part of our overarching sudden death safety net strategy, there has not been an AED use among any patient managed in our comprehensive LQTS Clinic at now > 5000 patient-years.

The issue of competitive athletic participation for the athlete with LQTS remains complex and controversial. The 36th Bethesda Conference guidelines were published in 2005 (119). Competitive sports disqualification was advised for any patient, regardless of underlying genotype or QTc, with a history of out of hospital cardiac arrest or LQTS-related syncopal episode. Asymptomatic patients with a QTc over 470 in males or over 480 msec in females were recommended limitation to the class IA sports (billiards, bowling, cricket, curling, golf, riflery). Loosening of the restrictions was supported (from a guideline perspective) for asymptomatic LQT3 patients, as well as for asymptomatic genotype-positive LQTS patients with QTc values in the overlapping/borderline range, except for competitive swimming in athletes with concealed LQT1 (119). The European Society of Cardiology (ESC) in 2006 published a similar set of athletic activity guidelines (120). Disqualification was advised for LQTS athletes who were symptomatic, had a prolonged QT interval (over 440–470 msec in men, over 460–480 msec in women), or were carriers of a known genetic mutation. Patients considered at "low-risk" for cardiac events were allowed participation in light to moderate leisure activity. All sports involving sudden bursts of activity or genotype-specific triggers were absolutely contraindicated. In contrast to the Bethesda Conference guidelines, the ESC recommended disqualification even for patients with concealed LQTS (i.e., positive gene test only) *(120)*.

All guidelines withstanding, it is important to avoid the temptation to advise avoidance of activity altogether. The risk of obesity and early-onset diabetes are higher in sedentary individuals, and we certainly do not want to create a collection of new diseases by limiting exercise. We support continuation of most recreational activity for our LQTS patients, avoiding of course genotype-specific triggers such as swimming in patients with LQT1. Each patient and family should have a clear understanding of what is currently known about the risks and benefits of athletic activity in LQTS. In Mayo's LQTS Clinic, we prefer the role of "informer/educator" rather than a mere "if in doubt, kick them out" approach to this very complex issue. Rather than mandating disqualification, we respect patient/family autonomy whereby each patient and family should be fully involved in the decision-making process and be allowed to make an informed decision even if such a decision runs contrary to the published guidelines. This approach has guided our LQTS Clinic for the past decade and notably about half of families have chosen disqualification and half have chosen continued participation. To date, there have been no competitive sports precipitated cardiac events in the latter.

CONCLUSIONS

Over the past half century, LQTS has matriculated through several critical milestones including its sentinel clinical description, clinical diagnostic scorecard, pathogenetic discovery, decade of research-based genetic testing and genotype–phenotype correlations, and clinical availability of genetic testing. With all the diagnostic tools now available, the physician must be not only a wiser user but also a wiser interpreter of these tests in order to accurately recognize the presence/absence of LQTS, and if present, to tailor an informed and individualized treatment strategy.

CONFLICTS OF INTEREST

Dr. Ackerman is a consultant for PGxHealth with respect to the FAMILION™ genetic tests for cardiac ion channel mutations and hypertrophic cardiomyopathy. Intellectual property derived from MJA's research program resulted in license agreements in 2004 between Mayo Clinic Health Solutions (formerly Mayo Medical Ventures) and PGxHealth (formerly Genaissance Pharmaceuticals).

REFERENCES

1. Jervell A, Lange-Nielsen F (1957) Congenital deaf-mutism, functional heart disease with prolongation of the QT interval, and sudden death. Am Heart J 54
2. Romano C, Gemme G, Pongiglione R (1963) Aritmie cardiache rare dell'eta'pediatrica. II. Accessi sincopali per fibrillazione ventricolare parossistica. Clin Peditr (Bologna) 45:656–683
3. Ward OC (1964) A new famillial cardiac syndrome in children. J Irish Med Assoc 54:103–106
4. Curran, ME, Splawski I, Timothy KW et al (1995) A molecular basis for cardiac arrhythmia: HERG mutations cause long QT syndrome. Cell 80:795–803
5. Wang Q, Shen J, Splawski I et al (1995) SCN5A mutations associated with an inherited cardiac arrhythmia, long QT syndrome. Cell 80:805–811
6. Wang Q, Curran ME, Splawski I et al (1996) Positional cloning of a novel potassium channel gene: KVLQT1 mutations cause cardiac arrhythmias. Nat Genet 12:17–23
7. Zipes DP, Camm AJ, Borggrefe M et al (2006) ACC/AHA/ESC 2006 guidelines for management of patients with ventricular arrhythmias and the prevention of sudden cardiac death: a report of the American college of cardiology/American heart association task force and the European society of cardiology committee for practice guidelines (writing committee to develop guidelines for management of patients with ventricular arrhythmias and the prevention of sudden cardiac death). J Am Coll Cardiol 48:1064–1108
8. Ackerman MJ (2004) Cardiac channelopathies: it's in the genes. Nat Med 10:463–464

9. Tester DJ, Will ML, Haglund CM et al (2006) Effect of clinical phenotype on yield of long QT syndrome genetic testing. J Am Coll Cardiol 47:764–768

10. Chen L, Marquardt ML, Tester DJ et al (2007) Mutation of an A-kinase-anchoring protein causes long-QT syndrome. Proc Natl Acad Sci USA 104:20990–20995

11. Medeiros-Domingo, A, Kaku, T, Tester, DJ et al (2007) SCN4B-encoded sodium channel beta4 subunit in congenital long-QT syndrome. Circulation 116:134–142

12. Ueda K, Valdivia C, Medeiros-Domingo A et al (2008) Syntrophin mutation associated with long QT syndrome through activation of the nNOS-SCN5A macromolecular complex. Proc Natl Acad Sci USA 105:9355–9360

13. Splawski I, Tristani-Firouzi M, Lehmann MH et al (1997) Mutations in the hminK gene cause long QT syndrome and suppress IKs function. Nat Genet 17:338–340

14. Abbott GW, Sesti F, Splawski I et al (1999) MiRP1 forms IKr potassium channels with HERG and is associated with cardiac arrhythmia. Cell 97:175–187

15. Mohler PJ, Schott JJ, Gramolini AO et al (2003) Ankyrin-B mutation causes type 4 long-QT cardiac arrhythmia and sudden cardiac death. Nature 421:634–639

16. Vatta M, Ackerman MJ, Ye B et al (2006) Mutant caveolin-3 induces persistent late sodium current and is associated with long-QT syndrome. Circulation 114:2104–2112

17. Zhang L, Benson DW, Tristani-Firouzi M et al (2005) Electrocardiographic features in Andersen-Tawil syndrome patients with KCNJ2 mutations: characteristic T-U-wave patterns predict the KCNJ2 genotype. Circulation 111: 2720–2726

18. Splawski I, Timothy KW, Sharpe LM et al (2004) Ca(V)1.2 calcium channel dysfunction causes a multisystem disorder including arrhythmia and autism. Cell 119:19–31

19. Schwartz PJ, Stramba-Badiale M, Crotti L et al (2009) Prevalence of the congenital long-QT syndrome. Circulation 120:1761–1767

20. Tester DJ, Ackerman MJ (2007) Postmortem long QT syndrome genetic testing for sudden unexplained death in the young. J Am Coll Cardiol 49:240–246

21. Arnestad M, Crotti L, Rognum TO et al (2007) Prevalence of long-QT syndrome gene variants in sudden infant death syndrome. Circulation 115:361–367

22. Goldenberg I, Moss AJ, Zareba W et al (2006) Clinical course and risk stratification of patients affected with the Jervell and Lange-Nielsen syndrome. J Cardiovasc Electrophysiol 17:1161–1168

23. Goldenberg I, Moss AJ, Bradley J et al (2008) Long-QT syndrome after age 40. Circulation 117:2192–2201

24. Goldenberg I, Moss AJ, Peterson DR et al (2008) Risk factors for aborted cardiac arrest and sudden cardiac death in children with the congenital long-QT syndrome. Circulation 117:2184–2191

25. Spazzolini C, Mullally J, Moss AJ et al (2009) Clinical implications for patients with long QT syndrome who experience a cardiac event during infancy. J Am Coll Cardiol 54:832–837

26. Hobbs JB, Peterson DR, Moss AJ et al (2006) Risk of aborted cardiac arrest or sudden cardiac death during adolescence in the long-QT syndrome. JAMA 296:1249–1254

27. Sauer AJ, Moss AJ, McNitt S et al (2007) Long QT syndrome in adults. J Am Coll Cardiol 49:329–337

28. Moss AJ, Robinson JL (1992) Clinical aspects of the idiopathic long QT syndrome. Ann NY Acad Sci 644:103–111

29. Vincent GM, Timothy K, Fox J et al (1999) The inherited long QT syndrome: from ion channel to bedside. Cardiol Rev 7:44–55

30. Moss AJ, Schwartz PJ, Crampton RS et al (1991) The long QT syndrome. Prospective longitudinal study of 328 families. Circulation 84:1136–1144

31. Rashba EJ, Zareba W, Moss AJ et al (1998) Influence of pregnancy on the risk for cardiac events in patients with hereditary long QT syndrome. LQTS investigators. Circulation 97:451–456

32. Schwartz PJ, Priori SG, Spazzolini C et al (2001) Genotype-phenotype correlation in the long-QT syndrome: gene-specific triggers for life-threatening arrhythmias. Circulation 103:89–95

33. Ackerman MJ, Tester DJ, Porter CJ (1999) Swimming, a gene-specific arrhythmogenic trigger for inherited long QT syndrome. Mayo Clin Proc 74:1088–1094

34. Moss AJ, Zareba W, Benhorin J et al (1995) ECG T-wave patterns in genetically distinct forms of the hereditary long QT syndrome. Circulation 92:2929–2934

35. Zhang L, Timothy KW, Vincent GM et al (2000) Spectrum of ST-T-wave patterns and repolarization parameters in congenital long-QT syndrome: ECG findings identify genotypes. Circulation 102:2849–2855

36. Wilde AA, Jongbloed RJ, Doevendans PA et al (1999) Auditory stimuli as a trigger for arrhythmic events differentiate HERG-related (LQTS2) patients from KVLQT1-related patients (LQTS1). J Am Coll Cardiol 33:327–332

37. Khositseth A, Tester DJ, Will ML et al (2004) Identification of a common genetic substrate underlying postpartum cardiac events in congenital long QT syndrome. Heart Rhythm 1:60–64

38. Johnson JN, Hofman N, Haglund CM et al (2009) Identification of a possible pathogenic link between congenital long QT syndrome and epilepsy. Neurology 72:224–231

39. Zareba W, Moss AJ, Schwartz PJ et al (1998) Influence of genotype on the clinical course of the long-QT syndrome. International long-QT syndrome registry research group. N Engl J Med 339:960–965

40. Schwartz PJ (1985) Idiopathic long QT syndrome: progress and questions. Am Heart J 109:399–411

41. Schwartz PJ, Moss AJ, Vincent GM et al (1993) Diagnostic criteria for the long QT syndrome. An update. Circulation 88:782–784

42. Taggart NW, Haglund CM, Tester DJ et al (2007) Diagnostic miscues in congenital long-QT syndrome. Circulation 115:2613–2620

43. Viskin S, Rosovski U, Sands AJ et al (2005) Inaccurate electrocardiographic interpretation of long QT: the majority of physicians cannot recognize a long QT when they see one. Heart Rhythm 2:569–574

44. Postema PG, De Jong JS, Van der Bilt IA et al (2008) Accurate electrocardiographic assessment of the QT interval: teach the tangent. Heart Rhythm 5:1015–1018

45. Davey P (1999) A new physiological method for heart rate correction of the QT interval. Heart 82:183–186

46. Sagie A, Larson MG, Goldberg RJ et al (1992) An improved method for adjusting the QT interval for heart rate (the Framingham heart study). Am J Cardiol 70:797–801

47. Fridericia L (1920) The duration of systole in the electrocardiogram of normal subjects and of patients with heart disease. Acta Medica Scandinavica 469–486

48. Bazett H (1920) An analysis of the time-relations of electrocardiograms. Heart 353–370

49. Vincent GM, Richard J (2001) Calculation of the QTc interval during sinus arrhythmia in patients suspected to have long QT syndrome. Circulation 104:II-690–II-691

50. Martin AB, Perry JC, Robinson JL et al (1995) Calculation of QTc duration and variability in the presence of sinus arrhythmia. Am J Cardiol 75:950–952

51. Goldenberg I, Moss AJ, Zareba W (2006) QT interval: how to measure it and what is "normal". J Cardiovasc Electrophysiol 17:333–336

52. Basavarajaiah S, Wilson M, Whyte G et al (2007) Prevalence and significance of an isolated long QT interval in elite athletes. Eur Heart J 28:2944–2949

53. Levine E, Rosero SZ, Budzikowski AS et al (2008) Congenital long QT syndrome: considerations for primary care physicians. Cleve Clin J Med 75:591–600

54. Merri M, Benhorin J, Alberti M et al (1989) Electrocardiographic quantitation of ventricular repolarization. Circulation 80:1301–1308

55. Rautaharju PM, Surawicz B, Gettes LS et al (2009) AHA/ACCF/HRS recommendations for the standardization and interpretation of the electrocardiogram: part IV: the ST segment, T and U waves, and the QT interval: a scientific statement from the American heart association electrocardiography and arrhythmias committee, council on clinical cardiology; the American college of cardiology foundation; and the heart rhythm society. Endorsed by the international society for computerized electrocardiology. J Am Coll Cardiol 53:982–991

56. Lupoglazoff JM, Denjoy I, Berthet M et al (2001) Notched T waves on Holter recordings enhance detection of patients with LQt2 (HERG) mutations. Circulation 103:1095–1101

57. Khositseth A, Hejlik J, Shen WK et al (2005) Epinephrine-induced T-wave notching in congenital long QT syndrome. Heart Rhythm 2:141–146

58. Schwartz PJ, Malliani A (1975) Electrical alternation of the T-wave: clinical and experimental evidence of its relationship with the sympathetic nervous system and with the long Q-T syndrome. Am Heart J 89:45–50

59. Zareba W, Moss AJ, le Cessie S et al (1994) T wave alternans in idiopathic long QT syndrome. J Am Coll Cardiol 23:1541–1546

60. Napolitano C, Priori SG, Schwartz PJ (2000) Significance of QT dispersion in the long QT syndrome. Prog Cardiovasc Dis 42:345–350

61. Day CP, McComb JM, Campbell RW (1990) QT dispersion: an indication of arrhythmia risk in patients with long QT intervals. Br Heart J 63:342–344

62. Priori SG, Napolitano C, Diehl L et al (1994) Dispersion of the QT interval. A marker of therapeutic efficacy in the idiopathic long QT syndrome. Circulation 89:1681–1689

63. Moennig G, Schulze-Bahr E, Wedekind H et al (2001) Clinical value of electrocardiographic parameters in genotyped individuals with familial long QT syndrome. Pacing Clin Electrophysiol 24:406–415

64. Vincent GM, Jaiswal D, Timothy KW (1991) Effects of exercise on heart rate, QT, QTc and QT/QS2 in the Romano-Ward inherited long QT syndrome. Am J Cardiol 68:498–503

65. Swan H, Toivonen L, Viitasalo M (1998) Rate adaptation of QT intervals during and after exercise in children with congenital long QT syndrome. Eur Heart J 19:508–513

66. Schwartz PJ, Priori SG, Locati EH et al (1995) Long QT syndrome patients with mutations of the SCN5A and HERG genes have differential responses to Na$^+$ channel blockade and to increases in heart rate. Implications for gene-specific therapy. Circulation 92:3381–3386

67. Ackerman MJ, Khositseth A, Tester DJ, Hejlik J, Shen WK, Porter CJ (2002) Epinephrine-induced QT interval prolongation: a gene-specific paradoxical response in congenital long QT syndrome. Mayo Clin Proc 77:413–421

68. ShimizuW, Noda T, Takaki H et al (2003) Epinephrine unmasks latent mutation carriers with LQT1 form of congenital long-QT syndrome. J Am College Cardiol 41:633–642

69. Vyas H, Hejlik J, Ackerman MJ (2006) Epinephrine QT stress testing in the evaluation of congenital long-QT syndrome: diagnostic accuracy of the paradoxical QT response. Circulation 113:1385–1392

70. TesterDJ, Will ML, Haglund CM et al (2005) Compendium of cardiac channel mutations in 541 consecutive unrelated patients referred for long QT syndrome genetic testing. Heart Rhythm 2:507–517

71. Napolitano C, Priori SG, Schwartz PJ et al (2005) Genetic testing in the long QT syndrome: development and validation of an efficient approach to genotyping in clinical practice [see comment]. JAMA 294:2975–2980

72. Tester DJ, Will ML, Haglund CM et al (2006) Effect of clinical phenotype on yield of long QT syndrome genetic testing. J Am College Cardiol 47:764–768

73. Westenskow P, Splawski I, Timothy KW et al (2004) Compound mutations: a common cause of severe long-QT syndrome. Circulation 109:1834–1841

74. Ackerman MJ, Splawski I, Makielski JC et al (2004) Spectrum and prevalence of cardiac sodium channel variants among black, white, Asian, and Hispanic individuals: implications for arrhythmogenic susceptibility and Brugada/long QT syndrome genetic testing. Heart Rhythm 1:600–607

75. Ackerman MJ, Tester DJ, Jones GS et al (2003) Ethnic differences in cardiac potassium channel variants: implications for genetic susceptibility to sudden cardiac death and genetic testing for congenital long QT syndrome. Mayo Clin Proc 78:1479–1487

76. Kapa S, Tester DJ, Salisbury BA et al (2009) Genetic testing for long QT syndrome: distinuishing pathogenic mutations from benign variants. Circulation 120:1752–1760

77. Moss AJ, Zareba W, Hall WJ et al (2000) Effectiveness and limitations of beta-blocker therapy in congenital long-QT syndrome. Circulation 101:616–623

78. Priori SG, Schwartz PJ, Napolitano C et al (2003) Risk stratification in the long-QT syndrome. N Engl J Med 348: 1866–1874

79. Priori SG, Aliot E, Blomstrom-Lundqvist C et al (2001) Task force on sudden cardiac death of the European society of cardiology. Eur Heart J 22:1374–1450

80. Locati EH, Zareba W, Moss AJ et al (1998) Age- and sex-related differences in clinical manifestations in patients with congenital long-QT syndrome: findings from the international LQTS registry. Circulation 97:2237–2244

81. Priori SG, Schwartz PJ, Napolitano C et al (2003) Risk stratification in the long-QT syndrome. N Engl J Med 348: 1866–1874

82. Moss AJ, Shimizu W, Wilde AA et al (2007) Clinical aspects of type-1 long-QT syndrome by location, coding type, and biophysical function of mutations involving the KCNQ1 gene. Circulation 115:2481–2489

83. Zareba W, Moss AJ, Schwartz PJ et al (1998) Influence of genotype on the clinical course of the long-QT syndrome. International long-QT syndrome registry research group. N Engl J Med 339:960–965

84. Kaufman ES, McNitt S, Moss AJ et al (2008) Risk of death in the long QT syndrome when a sibling has died. Heart Rhythm 5:831–836

85. Malfatto G, Beria G, Sala S et al (1994) Quantitative analysis of T wave abnormalities and their prognostic implications in the idiopathic long QT syndrome. J Am Coll Cardiol 23:296–301

86. Bhandari AK, Shapiro WA, Morady F et al (1985) Electrophysiologic testing in patients with the long QT syndrome. Circulation 71:63–71

87. Garson A Jr, Dick M 2nd, Fournier A et al (1993) The long QT syndrome in children. An international study of 287 patients. Circulation 87:1866–1872

88. Priori SG, Maugeri FS, Schwartz PJ (1998) The risk of sudden death as first cardiac event in asymptomatic patients with the long QT syndrome (abstract). Circulation 98(Suppl I):777

89. Ackerman MJ (1998) The long QT syndrome: ion channel diseases of the heart. Mayo Clin Proc 73:250–269

90. Schwartz PJ (1997) The long QT syndrome. Curr Probl Cardiol 22:297–351

91. Chatrath R, Bell CM, Ackerman MJ (2004) Beta-blocker therapy failures in symptomatic probands with genotyped long-QT syndrome. Pediatr Cardiol 25:459–465

92. Viskin S, Fish R, Zeltser D et al (2000) Arrhythmias in the congenital long QT syndrome: how often is torsade de pointes pause dependent? Heart 83:661–666

93. Dorostkar PC, Eldar M, Belhassen B et al (1999) Long-term follow-up of patients with long-QT syndrome treated with beta-blockers and continuous pacing. Circulation 100:2431–2436

94. Viskin S (2000) Cardiac pacing in the long QT syndrome: review of available data and practical recommendations. J Cardiovasc Electrophysiol 11:593–600

95. Chatrath R, Porter CJ, Ackerman MJ (2002) Role of transvenous implantable cardioverter-defibrillators in preventing sudden cardiac death in children, adolescents, and young adults. Mayo Clin Proc 77:226–231

96. Zareba W, Moss AJ, Daubert JP et al (2003) Implantable cardioverter defibrillator in high-risk long QT syndrome patients. J Cardiovasc Electrophysiol 14:337–341

97. Monnig G, Kobe J, Loher A et al (2005) Implantable cardioverter-defibrillator therapy in patients with congenital long-QT syndrome: a long-term follow-up. Heart Rhythm 2:497–504

98. Moss AJ, Zareba W, Hall WJ et al (2000) Effectiveness and limitations of beta-blocker therapy in congenital long-QT syndrome. Circulation 101:616–623

99. Villain E, Denjoy I, Lupoglazoff JM et al (2004) Low incidence of cardiac events with B-blocking therapy in children with long QT syndrome. Eur Heart J 25:1405–1411

100. Schwartz PJ, Spazzolini C, Crotti L et al (2006) The Jervell and Lange-Nielsen syndrome: natural history, molecular basis, and clinical outcome. Circulation 113:783–790

101. Shimizu W, Antzelevitch C (2000) Differential effects of beta-adrenergic agonists and antagonists in LQT1, LQT2 and LQT3 models of the long QT syndrome. J Am Coll Cardiol 35:778–786

102. Schwartz PJ, Spazzolini C, Crotti L (2009) All LQT3 patients need an ICD: true or false? Heart Rhythm 6:113–120

103. Moss AJ, McDonald J (1971) Unilateral cervicothoracic sympathetic ganglionectomy for the treatment of long QT interval syndrome. N Engl J Med 285:903–904

104. Collura CA, Johnson JN, Moir C et al (2009) Left cardiac sympathetic denervation for the treatment of long QT syndrome and catecholaminergic polymorphic ventricular tachycardia using video-assisted thoracic surgery. Heart Rhythm 6:752–759

105. Schwartz PJ, Priori SG, Cerrone M et al (2004) Left cardiac sympathetic denervation in the management of high-risk patients affected by the long-QT syndrome. Circulation 109:1826–1833

106. Moss AJ, McDonald J (1971) Unilateral cervicothoracic sympathetic ganglionectomy for the treatment of long QT interval syndrome. N Engl J Med 285:903–904

107. Schwartz PJ, Locati E (1985) The idiopathic long QT syndrome: pathogenetic mechanisms and therapy. Eur Heart J 6(Suppl D):103–114

108. Schwartz PJ, Priori SG, Cerrone M et al (2004) Left cardiac sympathetic denervation in the management of high-risk patients affected by the long-QT syndrome. Circulation 109:1826–1833

109. Schwartz PJ (2006) The congenital long QT syndromes from genotype to phenotype: clinical implications. J Inter Med 259:39–47

110. Etheridge SP, Compton SJ, Tristani-Firouzi M et al (2003) A new oral therapy for long QT syndrome: long-term oral potassium improves repolarization in patients with HERG mutations. J Am Coll Cardiol 42:1777–1782

111. Bankston JR, Kass RS (2009) Molecular determinants of local anesthetic action of beta-blocking drugs: implications for therapeutic management of long QT syndrome variant 3. J Mol Cell Cardiol 48:246–253

112. Schwartz PJ, Priori SG, Locati EH et al (1995) Long QT syndrome patients with mutations of the SCN5A and HERG genes have differential responses to Na$^+$ channel blockade and to increases in heart rate. Implications for gene-specific therapy. Circulation 92:3381–3386

113. Shimizu W, Antzelevitch C (1997) Sodium channel block with mexiletine is effective in reducing dispersion of repolarization and preventing torsade des pointes in LQT2 and LQT3 models of the long-QT syndrome. Circulation 96:2038–2047

114. Fitzgerald PT, Ackerman MJ (2005) Drug-induced torsades de pointes: the evolving role of pharmacogenetics. Heart Rhythm 2:S30–S37

115. Vyas H, Johnson K, Houlihan R et al (2006) Acquired long QT syndrome secondary to cesium chloride supplement. Altern Complement Med 12:1011–1014

116. Moss AJ, Robinson JL, Gessman L et al (1999) Comparison of clinical and genetic variables of cardiac events associated with loud noise versus swimming among subjects with the long QT syndrome. Am J Cardiol 84:876–879

117. Schwartz PJ, Priori SG, Spazzolini C et al (2001) Genotype-phenotype correlation in the long-QT syndrome: gene-specific triggers for life-threatening arrhythmias. Circulation 103:89–95

118. Caldwell G, Millar G, Quinn E et al (1985) Simple mechanical methods for cardioversion: defence of the precordial thump and cough version. Br Med J (Clin Res Ed) 291:627–630

119. Zipes DP, Ackerman MJ, Estes NA 3rd et al (2005) Task Force 7: arrhythmias. J Am Coll Cardiol 45:1354–1363

120. Heidbuchel H, Corrado D, Biffi A et al (2006) Recommendations for participation in leisure-time physical activity and competitive sports of patients with arrhythmias and potentially arrhythmogenic conditions. Part II: ventricular arrhythmias, channelopathies and implantable defibrillators. Eur J Cardiovasc Prev Rehabil 13:676–686

121. Ackerman et al (2008) Congenital long QT syndrome. In Electrical diseases of the heart; genetics, mechanisms, treatment, prevention. Springer, New York, NY, pp 462–482

20 Short QT Syndrome: Clinical Presentation, Molecular, Genetic, Cellular, and Ionic Basis

Chinmay Patel, Gan-Xin Yan, and Charles Antzelevitch

Contents

Abstract

Short QT Syndrome is a recently recognized inherited channelopathy responsible for sudden cardiac death (SCD) in individuals with a structurally normal heart. It is characterized by abnormally short QTc interval (<360 msec) on the electrocardiogram seen in conjunction with a family history of atrial and/or ventricular fibrillation. It is a genetically heterogeneous disease with mutations in five different genes encoding cardiac ion channels linked to familial or sporadic cases. Based on the chronology of discovery, gain-of-function mutations in *KCNH2*, *KCNQ1*, and *KCNJ2* have been labeled SQT1, SQT2 and SQT3, respectively. In addition, loss-of-function mutations in two calcium channel genes *CACNA1C* and *CACNB2B* have been linked to a new clinical entity characterized by a SQTS and Brugada syndrome phenotype. These have been designated as SQT4 and SQT5, respectively. SCD is a common presenting symptom and has been reported as early as the first year of life, suggesting that SQTS may be responsible for some cases of sudden infant death. Amplified transmural dispersion of repolarization along with abbreviation of the refractory period is thought to underlie the cellular basis for arrhythmogenesis in SQTS. Implantation of an implantable cardioverter defibrillator is recommended for both primary and secondary prevention of SCD. Data regarding a pharmacologic approach to therapy are limited, but quinidine has been identified as being of benefit. This chapter provides an overview of the available literature.

Key Words: Short QT syndrome; sudden cardiac death; sudden infant death syndrome; atrial fibrillation; idiopathic ventricular tachycardia; syncope; channelopathy; transmural dispersion of repolarization;

From: *Contemporary Cardiology: Management of Cardiac Arrhythmias*
Edited by: Gan-Xin Yan, Peter R. Kowey, DOI 10.1007/978-1-60761-161-5_20
© Springer Science+Business Media, LLC 2011

QT interval; $T_{peak}-T_{end}$/QT ratio; I_{Kr}; I_{Ks}; I_{to}; I_{K1}; I_{Ca}; quinidine; sotalol; HERG; KCNQ1; KCNJ2; CACNA1C; CACNB2b.

Short QT Syndrome (SQTS) is a recently recognized inherited channelopathy responsible for sudden cardiac death (SCD) in individuals with a structurally normal heart. In contrast to long QT syndrome, ion channel defects associated with SQTS lead to abnormal abbreviation of repolarization, predisposing affected individuals to a risk of atrial and ventricular arrhythmias. Since its first report in 2000, significant progress has been achieved in defining the molecular, genetic, and cellular basis of SQTS and therapeutic approaches. SQTS is genetically heterogeneous disease. So far, mutation in five different genes encoding various cardiac ion channels has been causally linked to SQTS. Data regarding genotype–phenotype correlation and genotype-specific treatment are promising but limited, primarily due to the paucity of clinical cases. The clinical presentation, diagnostic approach, and treatment modalities for SQTS are discussed in this chapter based on available data.

HISTORICAL BACKGROUND

Algra et al. in 1993 first proposed that shorter than normal QT intervals (<400 msec) are associated with 2.4-fold increased risk for SCD (1). Abnormally short QT interval observed before and after runs of VT/VF has been reported anecdotally (2, 3). Interestingly, certain species of kangaroo known to have high incidence of SCD display abnormally short QT interval as a normal ECG feature (4, 5). SQTS was first described as a new clinical entity by Gussak et al. (6), who reported four patients with extremely short QT interval in association with paroxysmal atrial fibrillation and SCD. In 2003, Gaita and his colleagues (7) provided further description of six patients of SQTS in two unrelated European families with a strong family history of sudden death in association with short QT interval on ECG. Since then nearly 100 cases of SQTS have been reported and existence of this novel channelopathy has been validated.

HOW SHORT IS TOO SHORT?

The upper limit of normal QT interval is now fairly well defined, but the lower limit of the normal QT interval and the value below which it could be considered arrhythmogenic remains unclear. The ECGs of the first few SQTS patients described by Gussak and colleagues showed extremely short QT and QTc intervals of less than 300 msec. In coming years, patients with SQTS with QT interval longer than 300 msec have been reported; however, in most cases the QT and QTc interval have been less than 360 msec.

To define the lower limit of the QT interval, many experts refer to a landmark study by Rautaharju et al. (8), who investigated distribution of normal QT interval in 14,379 healthy individuals. He established the formula by which the QT interval can be predicted as QT predicted (QTp) = 656/(1+ heart rate/100). In his study, prevalence of QT interval shorter than 88% of QTp (QT/QTp <88%, which is equivalent to two standard deviations below the mean) was 0.03%. Based on his observation, we recommend that QT interval less than 88% of QTp (two standard deviations below mean predicted value) at a particular heart rate may be considered as a short QT interval. For example, at heart rate of 60 beats/min (bpm), per Rautaharju's formula, QTp will be 410 msec; 88% of QTp (410 msec) would be 360 msec. Thus a QTc of 360 msec or shorter may be considered a short QT interval. QT interval values less than 80% of QTp may be considered extremely short (which is equivalent 320 msec at heart rate 60).

DEFINITION, DIAGNOSIS, AND DIFFERENTIAL DIAGNOSIS

SQTS can be best defined as congenital, inherited, primary electrical disorder of the heart characterized by abnormally short QT interval on surface ECG (<360 msec) and increased proclivity to develop atrial and/or ventricular tachyarrhythmia due to abbreviated refractoriness *(9–12)*.

Before arriving at a diagnosis of SQTS, secondary causes of short QT interval like hyperkalemia, acidosis, hypercalcemia, hyperthermia, effect of drugs like digitalis, effect of acetylecholine or catecholamine, and abbreviation of QT interval related to activation of K_{ATP} current need to be ruled out (Table 1). A rare but interesting paradoxical ECG phenomenon called deceleration-dependent shortening of QT interval (DDSQTI) should also be considered in the differential diagnosis of SQTS *(13)*. A strong parasympathetic stimulation to the heart can lead to bradycardia and concurrent activation of myocardial K_{ACh} channels. In such cases, the QT interval abbreviates paradoxically with a decrease in heart rate instead of lengthening (Fig. 1). Such shortening of QT interval may be transient and should resolve as parasympathetic tone decreases.

Table 1
Secondary Causes of SQT Interval on ECG

Hyperkalemia
Hypercalcemia
Hyperthermia
Acidosis
Effect of catecholamine
Activation of K_{Ach}
Activation of K_{ATP}
Effects of drugs like digitalis

A comprehensive battery of tests as recommended in guidelines from the Joint Steering Committees of UCARE and IVF-US *(14)*, including and not limited to resting ECG, exercise stress testing, echocardiogram, 24-h Holter monitoring; cardiac MRI should be performed to rule out presence of any organic heart disease. Paroxysmal atrial fibrillation is very common in patients with SQTS, hence diagnosis of SQTS should be considered in young individuals with lone atrial fibrillation with shorter than normal QT intervals. A history of arrhythmic symptoms or family history of lone atrial fibrillation, primary or resuscitated VF or SCD may provide additional clues. The isolated presence of short QT interval without associated arrhythmogenic complication warrants further interrogation to rule out SQTS.

A typical ECG associated with SQTS is shown in Fig. 2a, and includes the following features *(6, 7, 15)*:

1. Abnormally short QT interval, usually <360 msec with a range of 220–360 msec.
2. Absence of ST segment.
3. Tall and peaked T waves in the precordial leads which can be positive or negative, symmetrical or asymmetrical.
4. Poor rate adaptation of QT interval (diminished rate dependence) *(16)*.
5. Prolonged T_{peak}–T_{end} interval and T_{peak}–T_{end}/QT ratio *(17, 18)*.

In cases of SQT4 and SQT5, short QT intervals may appear together with a Brugada-type ST segment elevation in the right precordial leads V1–V3 at baseline or after administration of a potent sodium channel blocker (Fig. 2) *(19)*.

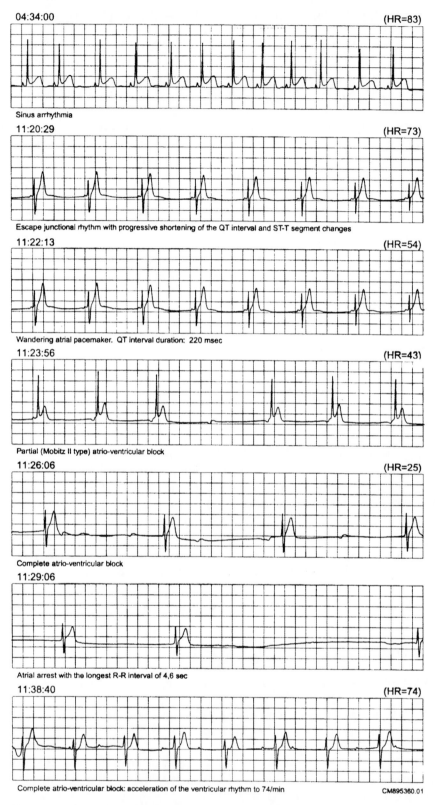

Fig. 1. Deceleration-dependent shortening of QT interval. As the rhythm changes from sinus arrhythmia to atrial arrest, heart rate progressively decreases. This is accompanied by paradoxical progressive shortening of the QT interval. Reproduced from Ref. *(6)*, with permission.

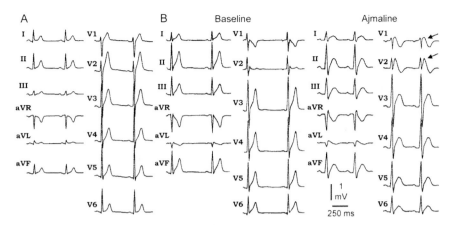

Fig. 2. (a) A 12-lead ECG showing characteristic ECG features of SQTS. **(b)** A 12-lead ECG showing characteristic ECG features of new clinical entity with combined ECG phenotype of Brugada syndrome in addition to SQTS. Note that ECG shows Brugada-type ST elevation in V1 and V2 after administration of ajmaline in addition to abbreviated QT intervals. (Modified from Refs. *(15)* and *(19)*, with permission).

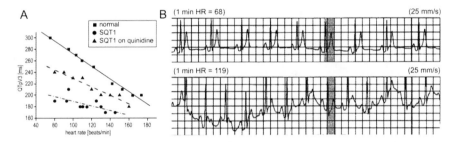

Fig. 3. (a) Reduced rate adaptation of QT interval. The QT–RR relationship is less linear and its slope is less steep in SQTS patient as compared to controls. Quinidine restores the relationship toward control values. QTpV3 denotes the interval from the beginning of QRS complex to peak of T wave, measured in lead V3 (Reproduced from Ref. *(16)*, with permission). **(b)** Holter monitoring showing impaired adjustment of QT interval with change in heart rate.

When the diagnosis of SQTS is suspected, a resting 12-lead ECG should be performed at a heart rate within normal limits, preferably less than 80 beats/min. In patients with SQTS, QT–RR relationship is less steep and less linear (Fig. 3) *(16)*. In other words, the QT interval fails to lengthen appropriately with a decrease in the heart rate. As a consequence, QT correction using Bazzett's or comparable formulas will overcorrect at initially fast rates, leading to a false negative diagnosis. Overnight Holter monitoring or long-term ECG monitoring may prove helpful in such cases. Although T waves are generally positive and symmetric (SQT1 and 2), asymmetric T waves with less steep ascending limb followed by a rapid descending limb has been reported in SQT3 *(20)*. In most cases, a distinct ST segment is short or absent with the T wave originating from the S wave.

MOLECULAR GENETICS

SQTS is a genetically heterogeneous disease. Mutations in five different genes (three gain of function and two loss of function) encoding different cardiac ion channels have been identified and termed SQT1 to SQT5 based on the chronology of their discovery (Table 2). SQT1 and SQT3–5 have been

Table 2
Genetic Basis of SQTS

Subtype	Inheritance	Locus	Ion channel	Gene	Electrophysiologic characteristic of mutant current/channel	Net effect of mutation
SQT1	AD	7q35	I_{Kr}	KCNH2, HERG	Shift of voltage dependence of inactivation of IKr by +90 mV out of the range of the action potential	Gain of function of I_{Kr}
SQT2	AD	11p15	I_{Ks}	KCNQ1, KvLQT1	Shift of voltage dependence of activation of I_{Ks} by −20 mV and acceleration of activation kinetics	Gain of function of I_{Ks}
SQT3	AD	17q23.1–24.2	I_{K1}	KCNJ2, Kir2.1	Increase in outward I_{K1} current at potentials between −75 and −45 mV	Gain of function of I_{K1}
SQT4	AD	12p13.3	I_{Ca}	CACNA1C, $Ca_v 1.2$	Decrease in amplitude of the inward	Loss of function of
SQT5	AD	10p12.33	I_{Ca}	CACNB2b, $Ca_v \beta_{2b}$	calcium current	I_{Ca}

reported in familial setting and SQT2 is reported only in a single patient in a sporadic setting. Mode of transmission of SQTS traits is autosomal dominant. The genes involved in SQTS are the same as those responsible for LQTS; however, the net effect of the mutations in SQTS is to increase repolarizing forces, an effect opposite to that encountered in LQTS.

CLINICAL PRESENTATION

The clinical presentation of SQTS is variable and many patients are asymptomatic. The initial presentation and further clinical course vary between different families and even within different members of the same family. In the largest available case series of SQTS, Giustetto et al. *(15)* described the clinical presentation of 29 patients with SQTS. Approximately 25% had a mutation in *KCNH2* (SQT1) and no mutation was found in the rest of the patients. Mutations in *KCNQ1* and *KCNJ2* were not detected and *CACNA1c* and *CACNB2b* were not screened. In this case series, the first manifestation of the disease was reported at an age as young as 1 month or as old as 80 years. About 62% of the patients were symptomatic. Cardiac arrest was the most frequently (34%) reported symptom and was the presenting symptom in about 28% patients. Cardiac arrest had occurred in the first month of life in two patients, suggesting that SQTS may be one of the causes of sudden infant death syndrome (SIDS). Palpitations were the second most frequently reported symptom (31%) followed by syncope (24%). AF was the first presenting symptom in about 17% of the patients. Many patients had frequent ventricular extra systoles. About 38% patients were asymptomatic and were diagnosed based on strong family history of arrhythmic symptoms including SCD, a common finding in familial forms of SQTS.

The circumstances of onset of symptoms are highly variable and episodes of SCD have been reported following loud noise, at rest, during exercises, and during daily activities.

The only reported SQT2 patient is a 70-year-old male who was successfully resuscitated after an episode of ventricular fibrillation *(21)*. There are two reported cases of SQT3 – a 5-year-old female child who was asymptomatic and a 35-year-old father, who had frequent episodes of sudden awakening at night with seizure-like activity followed by shortness of breath and palpitations *(20)*.

SQT4 has thus far been reported in two different patients of two unrelated families *(19)*: a 41-year-old male with a family history of SCD, who presented with AF and a QTc of 346 msec and a 44-year male with SQT4 with a family history of syncope and SCD, who was recently also diagnosed with fascioscapulohumeral muscular dystrophy. SQT5 has been described in seven patients belonging to a family of European descent *(19)*. The proband, a 25-year-old male presented with a QTc of 330 msec and had an episode of aborted SCD. His 23-year-old brother had frequent syncope as well. The rest of the family was asymptomatic.

Most patients with SQTS have QTc ≤ 340 msec with a range of 210–320 msec. However, in patients with SQT4 and SQT5, a clinical entity with ECG phenotype of Brugada syndrome and SQTS, QTc intervals are little longer (340–360 msec). No correlation thus far has been identified between the magnitude of QT interval abbreviation and risk of arrhythmic events *(15)*.

ELECTROPHYSIOLOGICAL STUDY

Upon invasive electrophysiological testing (EP), SQTS patients characteristically show extremely short atrial and ventricular effective refractory periods (ERP) regardless of genotype *(7, 15, 19–21)*. The ventricular ERP measured at the right ventricular apex varies between 140 and 180 msec at cycle length of 500–600 msec and 130 and 180 msec at pacing cycle length of 400–430 msec. Atrial ERP measured in the high lateral right atrium varies between 120 and 180 msec at cycle length of 600 msec. The programmed electrical stimulation with two to three premature stimuli up to the refractoriness induced AF and VF in many patients. The inducibility of VF at EP study in SQTS patients is about 60%. Moreover, in the case series presented by Giustetto et al. *(15)*, VF was inducible at EP study in only 3/6 patient with clinically documented VF, suggesting that sensitivity of EP study for inducibility of VF may be as low as 50%.

CELLULAR BASIS OF ARRHYTHMOGENESIS IN SQTS

The QT interval is determined by the ventricular action potential duration, which in turn is dependent on delicate balance of currents active during the repolarization phases of the action potential. An increase in net outward current, due to either a reduction in inward depolarizing currents like I_{Na} and I_{Ca} or augmentation of outward repolarizing currents such as I_{to}, I_{K1}, I_{K-ATP}, I_{ACh}, I_{Kr}, and I_{Ks} or combination of thereof, can shift the balance favoring early repolarization, thus leading to abbreviation of action potential duration, refractoriness, and QT interval. Available data suggest that abbreviation of the action potential in SQTS is heterogeneous with preferential abbreviation of either epicardial *(22)* or endocardial *(23)* cells as compared to sub-endocardial M cells, thereby causing an increase in transmural dispersion of repolarization (TDR). Dispersion of repolarization serves as substrate, and abbreviation of wavelength (product of refractory period and conduction velocity) promotes the maintenance of reentry under conditions of SQTS. The trigger responsible for generating the premature beat that precipitaties the rapid polymorphic VT in SQTS is not known but is believed to involve a phase 2 reentry or late phase 3 early afterdepolarization mechanisms. These mechanisms give rise to short-coupled R-on-T extrasystoles *(24)*.

Recent reports have shown that while electrical repolarization in SQTS patient is abbreviated, mechanical contraction is not, leading to electromechanical dissociation *(25)*. A ventricular extrasystole in such milieu has been shown to induce incomplete tetanus in kangaroos *(26, 27)*.

A gain-of-function mutation augments outward potassium current in SQT1–3 *(20, 21, 28)* and a loss-of-function mutation reduces I_{Ca-L} in SQT4–5 *(19)*. T_{peak}–T_{end}/QT ratio, an electrocardiographic index of spatial dispersion of repoarlization, is significantly augmented in most cases of SQTS, suggesting an increase in TDR at the cellular level *(17, 18)*. Interestingly, this ratio is more amplified in patients who are symptomatic *(29)*. The increase in TDR is known to predispose to phase 2 reentry may be responsible for the closely coupled premature ventricular extrasystole that precedes the onset of polymorphic VT in SQTS patients (Fig. 4) *(30, 31)*.

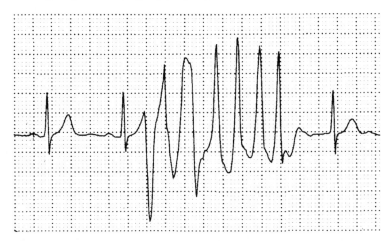

Fig. 4. Holter monitoring showing self-terminating polymorphic VT in a patient with SQTS. The coupling interval of the first beat of pVT is very short. (Modified from Ref. *(30)*, with permission).

TREATMENT IN SQTS

ICD

SQTS patients are at a very high risk for SCD. ICD implantation is strongly recommended for both primary and secondary prevention of SCD, unless absolutely contraindicated or refused by the patient *(12)*. It should be kept in mind that because the sensitivity of inducibility of VF is only 50%, failure to induce VF during EP study does not rule out future risk of SCD *(15, 31)*. Accordingly, a negative EP study should not defer a clinician's decision to implant an ICD. The decision to implant an ICD should be based purely on clinical grounds rather than inducibility of VT/VF. The effectiveness of an ICD in aborting episodes of VF has been reported in a primary prevention setting *(31)*.

Oversensing of the T wave is a frequent clinical problem encountered in patients with SQTS who receive an ICD *(32)*. The tall, peaked, and closely coupled T wave are often mistakenly sensed as R wave, leading to inappropriate ICD shocks. Reprogramming the decay delay, the sensitivity, or both generally prevents such inappropriate discharges. Caution must be exercised to avoid programming modifications that prevent the detection of lethal ventricular tachyarrhythmia.

Pharmacological Therapy

Pharmacological therapy may be used as an adjunct to ICD. It may be used as a primary treatment modality in cases of patient's refusal to receive ICD, absolute contraindication to ICD, or in very young patients in whom ICD implantation is problematic.

Data regarding pharmacological therapy in SQTS is very limited and much of it pertains to patients with SQT1. In six SQT1 patients, Gaita et al. *(33)* tested four different antiarrhythmic drugs: flecainide, sotalol, ibutilide, and hydroquinidine.

Surprisingly, only hydroquinidine normalized the QT, increased ventricular ERP, and rendered VF noninducible while Class IC and III antiarrhythmic drugs failed to do so. In addition, quinidine restored QT–RR relationship toward normal *(16)*. In a 1-year follow-up, patient treated with hydroquinidine remained asymptomatic and no further episodes of ventricular arrhythmia were detected. Similarly disopyramide has proved to be effective in prolonging the QT interval and restoring the ventricular effective refractory period towards normal *(34)*. Amiodarone has been shown to prolong the QT interval in two patients with SQTS of unknown genotype *(30, 35)*.

The failure of Class IC and pure Class III antiarrhythmic drugs in SQT1 is due to the fact that N588K mutation desensitizes the IKr channel to these agents. The inactivated state of the channel normally stabilizes the interaction of Class III agents such as sotalol and flecainide with the channel. The N588K missense mutation by eliminating the inactivated state of the channel reduces the affinity of the drugs for the I_{Kr} channel *(28)*. Consistent with clinical findings, heterologous expression systems have shown that N588K mutation reduces the affinity of the mutant channel for E-4031 and D-sotalol by 11.5- and 20-folds, respectively *(28, 36–38)*. However, the affinity for quinidine is reduced by only by 3.5- to 5.8-fold, affinity for disopyramide was reduced by 1.5-fold *(36)*, and for amiodarone by 4.1-fold *(39)*.

The efficacy of quinidine in SQT1 is due to its interaction with the activated state of the IKr channel as well as the fact that it blocks multiple K currents including I_{to}, I_{K1}, I_{Kr}, and I_{Ks}. Its multi-ion channel inhibition suggests that it should be effective in other forms of SQTS, particularly SQT4 and SQT5 where its I_{to} block may provide a therapeutic edge over other antiarrhythmic drugs by reducing the substrate and trigger for Brugada syndrome. Prolongation of the QT interval by quinidine has been reported in one patient with SQT4 *(19)*. Class III antiarrhythmic drugs would be expected to be effective in patients with SQT2 and SQT3; however, clinical data are not available as yet.

AF is another common clinical problem in SQTS. Some patients with SQTS exhibit only AF *(40)*. Propafenone and quinidine have been shown to be therapeutically effective *(11)*.

CONCLUSIONS

The short QT syndrome is a rare channelopathy associated with SCD in individuals with structurally normal heart. Timely diagnosis and treatment can significantly improve the overall prognosis of the patient and family members. In contrast to its mirror image disorder LQTS, there is scarcity of data regarding clinical presentation, diagnosis, genotype–phenotype correlation, risk stratification and treatment of SQTS. However, considerable progress has been made in terms of defining the molecular genetic and cellular basis of arrhythmogenesis since the first description of SQTS in 2000. ICD is recommended as first-line treatment for both primary and secondary prevention of SCD. There is little information about the long-term effectiveness of pharmacologic therapy and it is best reserved as an adjunct to ICD treatment. Quinidine has thus far proved to be the most effective pharmacotherapeutic agent.

REFERENCES

1. Algra A, Tijssen JGP, Roelandt JRTC, Pool J, Lubsen J (1993) QT interval variables from 24-hour electrocardiography and the 2-year risk of sudden death. Br Heart J 70:43–48
2. Fei L, Camm AJ (1995) Shortening of the QT interval immediately preceding the onset of idiopathic spontaneous ventricular tachycardia. Am Heart J 130(4):915–917
3. Kontny F, Dale J (1990) Self-terminating idiopathic ventricular fibrillation presenting as syncope: a 40-year follow-up report. J Intern Med 227:211–213
4. Campbell TJ (1989) Characteristics of cardiac action potentials in marsupials. J Comp Physiol [B] 158(6):759–762

5. Rezakhani A, Webster JD, Atwell RB (1986) The electrocardiogram of the eastern grey kangaroo (*Macropus giganteus*). Aust Vet J 63(9):310–312

6. Gussak I, Brugada P, Brugada J et al (2000) Idiopathic short QT interval: a new clinical syndrome? Cardiology 94(2): 99–102

7. Gaita F, Giustetto C, Bianchi F et al (2003) Short QT syndrome: a familial cause of sudden death. Circulation 108(8):965–970

8. Rautaharju PM, Zhou SH, Wong S et al (1992) Sex differences in the evolution of the electrocardiographic QT interval with age. Can J Cardiol 8(7):690–695

9. Gussak I, Antzelevitch C, Goodman D, Bjerregaard P (2003) Short QT interval: ECG phenomenon and clinical syndrome. In: Gussak I, Antzelevitch C (eds) Cardiac repolarization. bridging basic and clinical sciences. Humana, Totowa, NJ, pp 497–506

10. Gussak I, Bjerregaard P (2005) Short QT syndrome-5 years of progress. J Electrocardiol 38(4):375–377

11. Bjerregaard P, Gussak I (2005) Short QT Syndrome. Ann Noninvasive Electrocardiol 10(4):436–440

12. Bjerregaard P, Gussak I (2005) Short QT syndrome: mechanisms, diagnosis and treatment. Nat Clin Pract Cardiovasc Med 2(2):84–87

13. Gussak I, Liebl N, Nouri S, Bjerregaard P, Zimmerman F, Chaitman BR (1999) Deceleration-dependent shortening of the QT interval: a new electrocardiographic phenomenon? Clin Cardiol 22(2):124–126

14. Survivors of out-of-hospital cardiac arrest with apparently normal heart (1997) Need for definition and standardized clinical evaluation. Consensus Statement of the joint steering committees of the unexplained cardiac arrest registry of Europe and of the idiopathic ventricular fibrillation registry of the United States. Circulation 95(1):265–272

15. Giustetto C, Di MF, Wolpert C et al (2006) Short QT syndrome: clinical findings and diagnostic-therapeutic implications. Eur Heart J 27(20):2440–2447

16. Wolpert C, Schimpf R, Giustetto C et al (2005) Further insights into the effect of quinidine in short QT syndrome caused by a mutation in HERG. J Cardiovasc Electrophysiol 16(1):54–58

17. Anttonen O, Vaananen H, Junttila J, Huikuri HV, Viitasalo M (2008) Electrocardiographic transmural dispersion of repolarization in patients with inherited short QT syndrome. Ann Noninvasive Electrocardiol 13(3):295–300

18. Gupta P, Patel C, Patel H et al (2008) T(p-e)/QT ratio as an index of arrhythmogenesis. J Electrocardiol 41(6):567–574

19. Antzelevitch C, Pollevick GD, Cordeiro JM et al (2007) Loss-of-function mutations in the cardiac calcium channel underlie a new clinical entity characterized by ST-segment elevation, short QT intervals, and sudden cardiac death. Circulation 115(4):442–449

20. Priori SG, Pandit SV, Rivolta I et al (2005) A novel form of short QT syndrome (SQT3) is caused by a mutation in the KCNJ2 gene. Circ Res 96:800–807

21. Bellocq C, Van Ginneken AC, Bezzina CR et al (2004) Mutation in the KCNQ1 gene leading to the short QT-interval syndrome. Circulation 109(20):2394–2397

22. Patel C, Antzelevitch C (2008) Cellular basis for arrhythmogenesis in an experimental model of the SQT1 form of the short QT syndrome. Heart Rhythm 5(4):585–590

23. Extramiana F, Antzelevitch C (2004) Amplified transmural dispersion of repolarization as the basis for arrhythmogenesis in a canine ventricular-wedge model of short QT syndrome. Circulation 110:3661–3666

24. Burashnikov A, Antzelevitch C (2006) Late-phase 3 EAD. A unique mechanism contributing to initiation of atrial fibrillation. PACE 29(3):290–295

25. Schimpf R, Antzelevitch C, Haghi D et al (2008) Electromechanical coupling in patients with the short QT syndrome: further insights into the mechanoelectrical hypothesis of the U wave. Heart Rhythm 5(2):241–245

26. O'Rourke MF, Avolio AP, Nichols WW (1996) The kangaroo as a model for the study of hypertrophic cardiomyopathy in man. Cardiovasc Res 20(6):398–402

27. Sugishita Y, Iida K, O'Rourke MF et al (1990) Echocardiographic and electrocardiographic study of the normal kangaroo heart. Aust NZ J Med 20(2):160–165

28. Brugada R, Hong K, Dumaine R et al (2004) Sudden death associated with short-QT syndrome linked to mutations in HERG. Circulation 109(1):30–35

29. Anttonen O, Junttila MJ, Maury P et al (2009) Differences in twelve-lead electrocardiogram between symptomatic and asymptomatic subjects with short QT interval. Heart Rhythm 6(2):267–271

30. Lu LX, Zhou W, Zhang X, Cao Q, Yu K, Zhu C (2006) Short QT syndrome: a case report and review of literature. Resuscitation 71(1):115–121

31. Schimpf R, Bauersfeld U, Gaita F, Wolpert C (2005) Short QT syndrome: successful prevention of sudden cardiac death in an adolescent by implantable cardioverter-defibrillator treatment for primary prophylaxis. Heart Rhythm 2(4): 416–417

32. Schimpf R, Wolpert C, Bianchi F et al (2003) Congenital short QT syndrome and implantable cardioverter defibrillator treatment: inherent risk for inappropriate shock delivery. J Cardiovasc Electrophysiol 14(12):1273–1277

33. Gaita F, Giustetto C, Bianchi F et al (2004) Short QT syndrome: pharmacological treatment. J Am Coll Cardiol 43(8):1494–1499

34. Schimpf R, Veltmann C, Giustetto C, Gaita F, Borggrefe M, Wolpert C (2007) In vivo effects of mutant HERG K+ channel inhibition by disopyramide in patients with a short QT-1 syndrome: a pilot study. J Cardiovasc Electrophysiol 18(11):1157–1160

35. Mizobuchi M, Enjoji Y, Yamamoto R et al (2008) Nifekalant and disopyramide in a patient with short QT syndrome: evaluation of pharmacological effects and electrophysiological properties. Pacing Clin Electrophysiol 31(9):1229–1232

36. McPate MJ, Duncan RS, Witchel HJ, Hancox JC (2006) Disopyramide is an effective inhibitor of mutant HERG K+ channels involved in variant 1 short QT syndrome. J Mol Cell Cardiol 41(3):563–566

37. Cordeiro JM, Brugada R, Hong K, Antzelevitch C, Dumaine R (2004) Short QT syndrome mutation in HERG abolishes inactivation. Biophys J 86:134a

38. Cordeiro JM, Brugada R, Wu YS, Hong K, Dumaine R (2005) Modulation of I_{Kr} inactivation by mutation N588K in KCNH2: a link to arrhythmogenesis in short QT syndrome. Cardiovasc Res 67(3):498–509

39. McPate MJ, Duncan RS, Hancox JC, Witchel HJ (2008) Pharmacology of the short QT syndrome N588K-hERG K^+ channel mutation: differential impact on selected class I and class III antiarrhythmic drugs. Br J Pharmacol 155(6): 957–966

40. Hong K, Bjerregaard P, Gussak I, Brugada R (2005) Short QT syndrome and atrial fibrillation caused by mutation in KCNH2. J Cardiovasc Electrophysiol 16(4):394–396

21 J Wave Syndromes

Jianfang Lian, Peter R. Kowey, and Gan-Xin Yan

CONTENTS

Abstract

J wave syndromes are a collection of clinical entities characterized by accentuation of the I_{to}-mediated J wave, early repolarization and ST segment elevation. Although the risks of sudden cardiac death of these syndromes differ with respect to the magnitude and location of abnormal J wave manifestation and ST segment elevation, they share with a common ionic and cellular mechanism and their responses to heart rate and autonomic influences are similar. The congenital forms of J wave syndromes include early repolarization syndrome, which can be categorized into three subtypes according to J wave location and the risk of arrhythmogenesis, and the Brugada syndrome. J wave syndromes can be acquired in certain pathological conditions with augmentation of J-wave like hypothermia and acute ST segment elevation myocardial infarction. In the chapter, we attempt to summarize current state of knowledge about J-wave syndromes, bridging basic and clinical aspects.

Key Words: J wave syndrome; early repolarization; Brugada syndrome; transient outward current; L-type calcium current; hypothermia; ST segment elevation myocardial infarction; polymorphic ventricular tachycardia; idiopathic ventricular fibrillation; ventricular fibrillation; sudden cardiac death; right bundle branch block; epicardium; endocardium; action potential spike and dome; transmural voltage gradient; dispersion of repolarization; 4-aminopyridine; isoproterenol; procainamide; pilsicainide; propafenone; flecainide; sodium channel blockers; quinidine; amiodarone; β-blockers; ST-segment elevation; phase 2 reentry; trigger; ECG; implantable cardioverter defibrillator; R-on-T extrasystoles.

The J wave is a deflection with a dome or hump morphology immediately following the QRS complex of the surface ECG. It is also referred to as the Osborn wave because of Osborn's landmark description in the early 1950s *(1)*. The clinical and arrhythmogenic significance of J wave abnormal-

From: *Contemporary Cardiology: Management of Cardiac Arrhythmias*
Edited by: Gan-Xin Yan, Peter R. Kowey, DOI 10.1007/978-1-60761-161-5_21
© Springer Science+Business Media, LLC 2011

ities was largely ignored until a report by Yan and Antzelevitch in 1996 elucidating the ionic and cellular basis of J wave, pointing out its potential role in life-threatening ventricular arrhythmias *(2)*. An increasing amount of evidence has since been advanced, indicating that the early repolarization (ER) pattern and the Brugada syndrome (BrS) are mechanistically linked to abnormalities in the manifestation of the transient outward current (I_{to})-mediated J wave. In addition, J wave abnormalities may be also involved in arrhythmogenesis associated with hypothermia and the acute phase of ST segment elevation myocardial infarction (STEMI).

Although BrS and ER patterns differ with respect to the magnitude and location of abnormal J wave manifestation, they can be considered to represent a variable spectrum of phenotypic expression that we and others have proposed be termed J wave syndromes *(3–7)*. Here, we attempt to summarize the current state of knowledge about J -wave syndromes, bridging basic and clinical aspects.

HISTORICAL PERSPECTIVE OF J WAVE AND J WAVE SYNDROMES

The J wave was first described by Kraus in animal experiments involving hypercalcemia in 1920 *(8)*. Tomashewski et al. provided a description of the hypothermic J wave as a slowly inscribed deflection between the QRS complex and the ST segment of the ECG in an accidentally frozen man in 1938 *(9)*. In 1953, Osborn further characterized what he called a "current of injury" in dogs that were acidotic and hypothermic, and that went into ventricular fibrillation at rectal temperatures less than 25°C *(1)*. This so-called "current of injury" was later called the Osborn Wave *(10)*.

In 1936, Shipley and Hallaran first described ER pattern related to J wave on the ECG. They described J deflection as slurring or notching of the terminal part of QRS complex and considered it and associated ER as a normal variant after evaluating the four-lead electrocardiogram of 200 healthy young men and women *(11)*. This electrocardiographic phenomenon was ascribed to accelerated ventricular repolarization with a 2% prevalence in healthy adults. In 1961, Wasserburger and coworkers further defined ER as an elevated take-off of the ST segment at the J junction of the QRS complex varying from 1 to 4 mm from the isoelectric line accompanied by downward concavity of the ST segment and symmetrically limbed T wave, often of large amplitude in mid to left precordial leads *(12)*. In subsequent years, several investigators sought to characterize the clinical importance of the electrocardiographic ER pattern and failed to find any immediate and long-term consequences *(13)*.

Possible association of J wave and arrhythmias was first reported in 1984 when Otto and coworkers reported three survivors of sudden cardiac death that occurred during sleep. These were young Southeast Asian male refugees who appeared to have structurally normal hearts. The only ECG manifestation in these patients that was potentially related to sudden cardiac death was a prominent J wave accompanied by ST segment elevation although the authors failed to recognize this ECG marker *(14)*. Ventricular fibrillation was readily induced in these three patients during electrophysiological study. But the authors were perplexed that ventricular fibrillation was inhibited by quinidine and not procanimide, even though both drugs are class Ia antiarrhythmic agents. This puzzle remained unresolved until 1990s when the ionic and cellular basis for J wave was defined *(2, 15)*.

The phenomenon of death in males during sleep is well known in many Asian countries. In the Philippine capital city Manila, a total of 722 apparently healthy young males died during sleep from 1948 to 1982 from a disease then called "Bangungut" (to rise and moan during sleep) *(16)*. The incidence is as high as 26 per 100,000 per year in Manila and some areas of Thailand *(16, 17)*. Locals believe that widow ghosts might seduce and spirit the young and handsome males away during their sleep, and many men therefore wear women's clothes in their sleep to mislead the widow ghosts (Fig. 1).

In the 1980s, the US Center for Disease Control received approximately 120 case reports of sudden cardiac death (SCD) in Southeast Asian refugees living in the United States *(18)*. These victims who

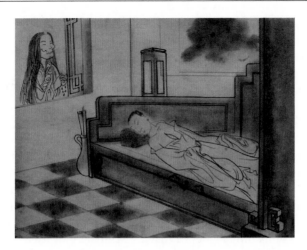

Fig. 1. Sudden death of apparent young healthy males in Southeast Asia remained a mystery over many centuries. Local people believed that widow ghosts might seduce and spirit the males away during their sleep, and men therefore wear women's clothes in their sleep to mislead the widow ghosts.

had died during their sleep were young males without a history of any cardiac disease by autopsy. Several sudden cardiac death cases in which the ECGs exhibited prominent J waves in the inferior leads were reported by Aizawa et al., although the authors considered J waves as intraventricular conduction delay at that time *(19, 20)*.

In 1992, the Brugada brothers published a landmark study describing eight similar sudden cardiac death patients in whom the ECG revealed "right bundle branch block" and ST segment elevation limited in the precordial leads V1 to V3 in the absence of ischemic or other structural disease *(21)*. In 1996, we and others named this entity "Brugada syndrome" (BrS) *(2, 22)*. The Brugada syndrome has attracted great interest because of its high incidence in many parts of the world and its association with high risk of sudden death, especially in males as they enter their third and fourth decades of life. In many cases of BrS the "right bundle branch block" appears without an S wave in the left precordial leads, suggesting that in these cases the RBBB is apparent and that the R' represents accentuation of the J wave.

In 2000, Yan's group reported recurrent ventricular fibrillation in a Vietnamese male whose ECG showed prominent J wave with ST segment elevation in inferior leads without structural heart diseases or myocardial ischemia, postulating that ER is mechanistically linked to BrS *(23)*. Shortly afterwards, Takagi et al. provided further evidence in support of this hypothesis *(24)*. More solid evidence was provided by two reports in the New England Journal of Medicine in 2008. Both Haissaguerre and coworkers *(25)* and Nam and coworkers *(6)* demonstrated a definite association between J waves with ER pattern and ventricular fibrillation. All of these clinical observations have suggested a critical role for the J wave in the pathogenesis of many different forms of idiopathic ventricular fibrillation *(4, 23, 26–29)*.

IONIC AND CELLULAR MECHANISMS FOR THE J WAVE AND ASSOCIATED ARRHYTHMOGENESIS

In the late 1980s, Antzelevitch et al. first proposed a difference in repolarization phases 1 and 2 of the action potential between the ventricular epicardium and the endocardium as the basis for the ECG J wave *(15, 30)*. The ventricular epicardium commonly displays action potentials with a relatively prominent notch or spike and dome mediated by the 4-aminopyridine–sensitive transient outward current (I_{to}). Ventricular endocardium, on the other hand, exhibits a much smaller I_{to}-mediated action potential spike and dome *(2, 15)*. In 1996, Yan and Antzelevitch first provided direct evidence in support of the hypothesis that the difference in I_{to}-mediated action potential spike and dome between ventricular epicardium and endocardium is able to produce a transmural voltage gradient during the initial repolarization phase that contributes to genesis of a J wave on the ECG *(2)*. Therefore, factors that influence I_{to} kinetics or ventricular activation sequence can modify the manifestation of the J wave on the ECG. For example, because of its slow recovery from inactivation, I_{to} is reduced following an acceleration of heart rate, resulting in a decrease in the magnitude of the J wave *(31)*.

The I_{to}-mediated epicardial action potential notch including spike and dome is sensitive to changes in net repolarizing current. An increase in net repolarizing current, due either to a decrease of inward currents or augmentation of outward currents, accentuates the notch leading to augmentation of the J wave. A further increase in net repolarizing current can result in partial or complete loss of the action potential dome, leading to a transmural voltage gradient that manifests as ST segment elevation *(32–34)*. This was the first compelling evidence that ST segment elevation can occur in the absence of myocardial ischemia or other structural heart diseases.

Because accentuation of the action potential notch and loss of the dome are due to an outward shift of currents secondary to either a decrease in inward currents (I_{Na} and I_{Ca}) or an increase in outward potassium currents, sodium channel blockers (e.g., procainamide, pilsicainide, propafenone and fle-

A. Early Repolarization Syndrome in a Healthy Young Male

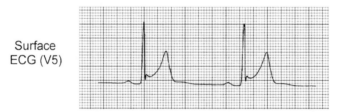

B. Canine Ventricular Action Potentials and ECG

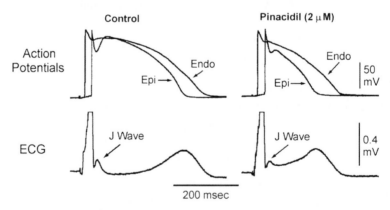

Fig. 2. Cellular basis for the ER. (a) Surface ECG (lead V5) recorded from a 17-year-old healthy African American male. Note the presence of a small J wave and marked ST segment elevation. (b) Simultaneous recording of transmembrane action potentials from epicardial (Epi) and endocardial (Endo) regions and a transmural ECG in an isolated arterially perfused canine left ventricular wedge. A J wave in the transmural ECG is manifest due to the presence of an action potential notch in epicardium but not endocardium. Pinacidil (2 μM), an ATP-sensitive potassium channel opener, causes depression of the action potential dome in epicardium, resulting in ST segment elevation in the ECG resembling the early repolarization syndrome. Reprinted from Yan et al. *(31)*, with permission.

Table 1
J wave Syndromes: Similarities and Differences

	Inherited				Acquired	
	ER in lateral	ER in inferior	Global ER		Ischemia-mediated	Hypothermia-mediated
	Type 1	Type 2	Type 3	Brugada syndrome (Type 4)	VF	VF
Anatomic location responsible for chief EP manifestations	Anterolateral left ventricle	Inferior left ventricle	Left and right ventricles	Right ventricle	Left and right ventricles	Left and right ventricles
Leads displaying J point/ J wave abnormalities	I, V4-V6	II, III, aVF	Global	V1–V3	Any of 12 leads	Any of the 12 leads
Response of J wave amplitude/ST elevation to:						
Bradycardia	Increase	Increase	Increase	Increase	NA	NA
Na+ channel blockers	N/A	Increase	N/A	Increase	NA	NA
Sex dominance	Male	Male	Male	Male	Male	Either gender
VF	Rare	Yes	Yes, VF Storms	Yes	Yes	Yes
Response to quinidine	Normalization of J point elevation and inhibition of VT/VF	Normalization of J point elevation and inhibition of VT/VF	Limited data; Normalization of J point elevation and inhibition of VT/VF	Normalization of J point elevation and inhibition of VT/VF	Limited data	Inhibition of VT/VF
Response to isoproterenol	Normalization of J point elevation and inhibition of VT/VF	Normalization of J point elevation and inhibition of VT/VF	Limited data;	Normalization of J point elevation and inhibition of VT/VF	N/A	N/A
Gene mutations	CACNA1C, CACNB2B	KCNJ8, CACNA1C, CACNB2B	CACNA1C	SCN5A, CACNA1C, CACNB2B, GPD1-L, SCN1B, KCNE3, SCN3B, KCNJ8	SCN5A	N/A

Modified from Antzelevitch et al. with permission (7)

cainide), which can cause loss of the epicardial action potential dome under condition of a prominent I_{to}, can be used to induce or unmask ST segment elevation in patients with concealed J wave syndromes (35, 36). Sodium channel blockers like quinidine that also inhibits I_{to} can restore the epicardial action potential dome and, therefore, normalize ST segment elevation (32). In addition, sympathetic and parasympathetic tone influences ST-segment elevation via effects on inward and outward currents active in action potential phases 1 and 2 (22).

Since ST elevation in the presence of a prominent J wave is the consequence of loss of the I_{to}-mediated epicardial action potential dome (i.e., shortening and depression of the plateau phase) secondary to an outward shift of the currents, early repolarization almost always co-exists. The degree of accentuation of the action potential notch leading to loss of the dome depends on the magnitude of I_{to} (31, 32). When I_{to} is relatively small, as it is in the left ventricular epicardium, an outward shift of current causes partial loss of the dome that is associated with only mild action potential shortening and dispersion of repolarization (Fig. 2b). This is seen in patients with ER in lateral precordial leads that is considered benign (Fig. 2a, Table 1). When I_{to} is prominent, as it is in the right ventricular epicardium, an outward shift of current causes phase 1 of the action potential to progress to more negative potentials at which the L-type calcium current ($I_{Ca,L}$) fails to activate, leading to an *all-or-none* repolarization and loss of the dome. Loss of the action potential dome is usually heterogeneous, resulting in marked abbreviation of the action potential at some sites but not others. The dome can then propagate from regions where it is maintained to regions where it is lost, giving rise to a very

A.   J wave and Associated Ventricular Tachycardia in a Patient

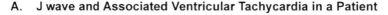

B.   Phase 2 Reentry and Ventricular Tachycardia in a Canine Ventricular Preparation

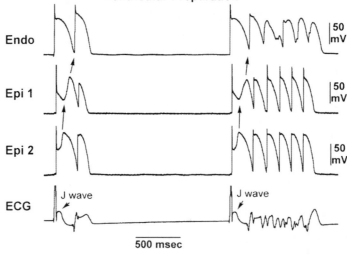

Fig. 3. J wave-mediated arrhythmogenesis. (a) Development of VF in a patient with prominent J waves in lead II (reprinted from Aizawa et al. (20), with permission). (b) VF initiated by phase 2 reentry in a canine right ventricular wedge in the presence of 2.5 μmol/L of pinacidil. Action potentials (AP) were simultaneously recorded from two epicardial sites (Epi₁ and Epi₂) and one Endo site. Loss of the AP dome in Epi₁ but not in Epi₂ led to phase 2 reentry capable of initiating VF (modified from Yan et al. (31) with permission).

closely coupled extrasystole via a mechanism that is termed phase 2 reentry (Fig. 3) *(31, 32)*. The extrasystole produced via phase 2 reentry occurs *always* on the preceding T wave resulting in an R-on-T phenomenon. This in turn can initiate polymorphic ventricular tachycardia (VT) or ventricular fibrillation (VF).

CLINICAL AND ECG FEATURES OF J WAVE SYNDROMES

J wave syndromes can be inherited, like BrS and ER syndrome, or acquired. The clinical and ECG features of the J wave syndromes, including BrS, three subtypes of the ER, and acquired forms, are summarized in Table 1.

It is important to point out that the clinical and ECG features of inherited J wave syndromes may co-exist in an individual patient or among members of the same family. For example, in a family reported by Takagi et al., one patient with recurrent syncope and inducible VF displayed ER in the inferior leads whereas his brother had a typical Brugada-like ECG pattern with ST segment elevation in the right precordial leads *(37)*. SCN5A mutations have been associated with ST segment elevation in the right precordial leads as well as the inferior leads *(38, 39)*. Not surprisingly, acceleration of heart rate during exercise is reported to result in a parallel reduction of J wave amplitude and ST segment elevation in the inferior as well as left precordial leads *(23)*. The common link among these clinical entities is the I_{to}-mediated J wave and associated ST-segment elevation *(3, 4, 31, 40, 41)*.

The fact that J wave syndromes represent a variable spectrum of phenotypic expression including the Brugada syndrome and ER is better demonstrated in a case reported by Qi et al. (Fig. 4) *(29)*. The 12 lead ECG was of a 34-year-old Chinese man admitted following a cardiac arrest and recurrent VF. Myocardial infarction was ruled out and cardiac examination and laboratory tests, including echocardiogram and cardiac catheterization were normal. Prominent J waves and ST segment elevation were observed in almost all ECG leads, displaying the ECG features of all of inherited J wave syndromes: BrS and variants of ER. An ER pattern was apparent in leads I, II, aVL, aVF, and V4 to V6. A saddleback ST segment elevation suggestive of BrS in the right precordial leads V_2 to V_3 (thick arrows) was associated with R-on-T extrasystoles, likely due to phase 2 reentry *(open arrows)*. The beat following the compensatory pause after the extrasystolic beat displayed a coved ST segment elevation characteristic of BrS *(thin arrows)*.

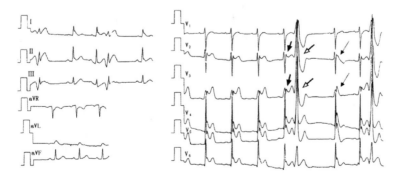

Fig. 4. Body surface ECG obtained from a 34-year-old Chinese man who survived cardiac arrest displayed global J waves and ST segment elevation and ER. Prominent J waves and ST segment elevation are seen in almost all leads. Reprinted from Qi et al. *(29)*, with permission.

THE BRUGADA SYNDROME

The BrS, a clinical entity described by Josep and Pedro Brugada in 1992, is associated with a high risk of sudden cardiac arrest *(21)*. The ECG features of the Brugada patient includes an accentuated J wave imitating right branch bundle block (RBBB) and ST segment elevation in the right precordial leads (V_1–V_3) *(21, 22)*.

As one of the J wave syndromes, the ECG characteristics and clinical outcomes of the BrS are dictated by the ionic and cellular mechanism responsible for the manifestation of the epicardial action potential notch. This governs the appearance of the J wave. ST segment elevation in BrS patients is significantly influenced by heart rate and autonomic tone *(22)* and its coved morphology, which represents a highly accentuated epicardial action potential notch that can readily result in loss of the epicardial action potential dome. The syndrome is associated with a high incidence of sudden cardiac death.

Genetic Basis for BrS

Mutations in *SCN5A* ($Na_v1.5$, BrS1) have been reported in approximately 15% of BrS probands. *CACNA1C*($Ca_v1.2$, BrS3) and *CACNB2b*($Ca_v\beta2b$, BrS4) mutations have been found in 6.7% and 4.8%, respectively. Mutations in glycerol-3-phosphate dehydrogenase 1-like enzyme gene (*GPD1L*, BrS2), *SCN1B* (β_1-subunit of sodium channel, BrS5), *KCNE3* (MiRP2; BrS6), and *SCN3B* (β3-subunit of sodium channel, BrS7) are rare *(42–47)*. These genetic defects lead to the development of BrS either due to loss of function of inward currents (sodium (I_{Na}) or L-type calcium (I_{ca}) current), or gain of function of outward currents like transient outward current (I_{to}). However, approximately 60–70% of BrS probands are genotype-negative *(48)*.

Clinical Characteristics and Epidemiology

The Brugada syndrome manifests clinically during adulthood. The average age at the time of initial diagnosis or sudden death is 40 ± 15 year old *(49)*. This syndrome appears to 8–10 times more frequently in males than in females, and is estimated to be responsible for about 20% of sudden deaths in patients with structurally normal hearts. Because the Brugada ECG pattern is often concealed, it is difficult to estimate its true prevalence in the general population. In a Japanese study, Brugada type 1 ECG was observed in 12/10,000 inhabitants. Nondiagnostic type 2 and 3 Brugada waves (see Fig. 5) were more prevalent (58/10,000 population) *(50)*. VT/VF in the Brugada patients is bradycardia-dependent, and therefore sudden cardiac death often occurs during sleep.

Atrial fibrillation is reported in 10–20% of Brugada cases *(51)*. Atrioventricular (AV) nodal reentrant tachycardia and Wolff-Parkinson-White syndrome have also been described *(52)*. Slow atrial conduction as well as atrial standstill have been reported in association with the syndrome *(39, 53)*. Prolonged HV intervals may be seen during electrophysiology study.

Diagnostic Criteria and Recommendations

Three types of repolarization patterns in the right precordial leads V1 to V3 are considered as ECG markers of the Brugada syndrome (Table 2 and Fig. 5) *(54)*. Type 1 ST-segment elevation is diagnostic of the Brugada syndrome and is characterized by a coved ST-segment elevation ≥ 2 mm (0.2 mV) followed by a negative T wave. Type 2 ECG has a saddleback morphology with a high take-off ST-segment elevation of ≥ 2 mm. Type 3 pattern has either a saddleback or coved appearance with an ST-segment elevation of <1 mm. Dynamic changes from one to other types may be observed sequentially in the same patient or following the introduction of specific drugs. Type 2 and 3 ST-segment elevation should not be considered diagnostic of the Brugada syndrome.

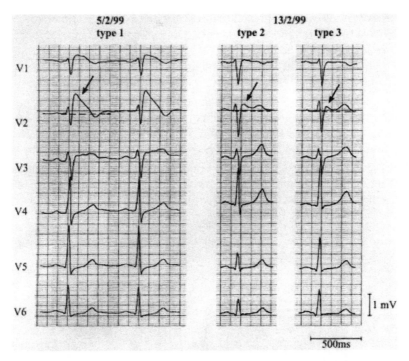

Fig. 5. Three Types of ST-segment elevation generally observed in patients with the Brugada syndrome. Shown are precordial leads recorded from a patient diagnosed with the Brugada syndrome. Note the dynamic ECG changes occurring over a period of 2 days. The *left panel* shows a clear type 1 ECG that is characterized by coved ST elevation and negative T waves. A saddleback ST segment elevation (type 2) is observed on February 7, 1999. The ST segment is partially normalized on February 13, 1999, showing a type 3 ECG. Reprinted from Wilde et al. with permission *(54)*.

Table 2
Diagnostic Criteria for Brugada Syndrome ST-Segment Abnormality in Leads V1–V3

	Type 1	*Type 2*	*Type 3*
J-points	≥2 mm	≥2 mm	≥2 mm
T-wave	Negative	Positive or biphasic	Positive
ST–T configuration	Coved type	Saddleback	Saddleback
ST segment (terminal portion)	Gradually descending	Elevated ≥1 mm	Elevated ≤1 mm

From Wilde et al. *(54)* with permission

The Brugada syndrome is definitively diagnosed when a spontaneous or drug-induced type 1 pattern is observed in more than one right precordial lead (V1 to V3) in conjunction with one of the followings: documented VF, polymorphic ventricular tachycardia, a family history of sudden cardiac death at <45 years old, coved-type ECGs in family members, inducibility of VT with programmed electrical stimulation (PES), syncope, or nocturnal agonal respiration *(41, 55)*. Diagnosis of the Brugada syndrome is also established when a type 2 or 3 ST-segment elevation in more than one right precordial leads under baseline conditions is converted to the diagnostic type 1 pattern upon exposure to a sodium channel blocker (ST-segment elevation should be ≥2 mm). One or more of the clinical criteria described above should also be present. However, drug-induced conversion of a type 3 to type 2 pattern is inconclusive for the diagnosis of the Brugada syndrome *(55)*.

Drug challenge for diagnosis of the Brugada syndrome should be accompanied by continuous ECG recording and should be terminated when the diagnostic type 1 Brugada ECG becomes obvious, when R-on-T premature ventricular beats or other arrhythmias occur, or when the QRS widens to 130% of baseline *(56)*. Intravenous infusion of sodium channel blockers may cause hypotension and arrhythmias. Therefore, the drug challenge test should be performed in a hospital setting equipped for resuscitation. The commonly used sodium channel blockers for the drug challenge test include procanimide (10 mg/kg over 10 min IV), pilsicainide (1 mg/kg over 10 min IV), or ajmalin (1 mg/kg over 5 min IV) *(55)*. Placement of the right precordial leads up to the 2nd intercostal spaces increases the sensitivity of detecting the Brugada ECG waves in some patients, both in the presence or in the absence of a drug challenge (Fig. 6) *(57, 58)*. However, an increase in the sensitivity may increase the chances of a

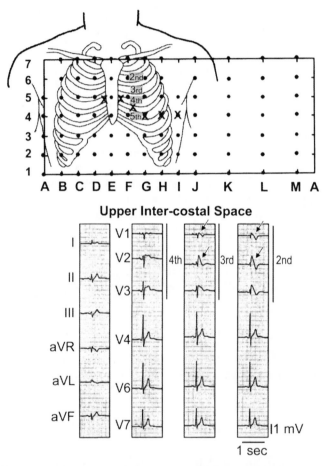

Fig. 6. Shift of right precordial leads to 2nd and 3rd intercostal space unmasks a Brugada type 1 ECG. *(Top)* Plot of 87 unipolar electrode sites *(dots)* and of six percordial electrocardiograms (ECG) *(crosses)*. Eighty seven-lead points are arranged in a lattice-like pattern (13×7 matrix), except for four lead points on both mid-axillary lines and covered the entire thoracic surface. V1 and V2 leads of the ECG are located between D5 and E5, and between E5 and F5, respectively, whereas V4, V5, and V6 are coincident with G4, H4, and I4, repectively. *(Bottom)* Twelve-leads electrocardiograms (ECG) in a patient with Brugada syndrome. Type 2 saddleback ST segment elevation was obesrved in V1 and V2 of the standard 12-lead ECG (4th intercostal space), whereas typical Type 1 coved-type ST segment evelation was apparent in V1 and V2 recorded from the 2nd and 3rd intercostal space *(arrows)*. Modified from Antzelevitch et al. *(55)* with permission.

false-positive result. ST elevation particularly when it is relatively minor may be nonspecific, and so the diagnosis of the Brugada syndrome should be made with care. Some forms of ST segment elevation in the right precordial leads may be simply the consequence of intraventricular conduction delay *(31)*. Upslope instead of downslope from the J point to the onset of T wave suggests that ST elevation is unlikely unrelated to J wave and, therefore, represents the Brugada syndrome.

Risk Stratification and Current Recommendations

Brugada syndrome survivors of cardiac arrest are at a high risk for recurrence and should be protected by an implantable cardioverter defibrillator (ICD). Patients with a history of syncope and spontaneous type 1 ECG, i.e., coved ST segment elevation and negative T waves in more than one of right precordial leads, are at a higher risk as well. However, risk stratification of asymptomatic Brugada syndrome patients is debatable *(59–63)*. Several invasive and noninvasive parameters have been proposed for identification of patients at risk of sudden death, including induciblility of VT/VF with ventricular programmed stimulation, observation for the spontaneous type 1 pattern, and testing for late potentials *(64–66)*.

Therapeutic Recommendations for Brugada Syndrome

ICD implantation is the only proven effective treatment for the Brugada syndrome. Current recommendations for ICD implantation *(55)* are summarized in Table 3.

Table 3
Indications for ICD Implantation in Patients with Brugada Syndrome

	Cardiac events	*Type 1 Brugada wave*	*Family history of SCD*	*EPS*
Class I	Aborted SCD	Occurs spontaneously	±	Not Indicated
	Aborted SCD	Induced during drug challenge test	±	Not Indicated
	Syncope/seizure/NAR*	Occurs spontaneously	±	Not Indicated
Class IIa	–	Occurs spontaneously	Suspected due to BrS	+
	Syncope/seizure/NAR*	Induced during drug challenge test	±	Not indicated

*Clear extracardiac causes must be ruled out; ± with or without; – negative; + positive; *SCD* sudden cardiac death; *NAR* nocturnal agonal respiration; *EPS* electrophysiology study

Although ICD implantation is the mainstay of therapy for the Brugada syndrome, pharmacotherapy may be required for specific cases such as patients who are not suitable for ICD implantation and those with frequent ICD firings. Antiarrhythmic agents such as amiodarone and β-blockers have been shown to be ineffective. Quinidine may exert a therapeutic action via its I_{to}-blocking property *(32)*. Clinical efficacy of quinidine in normalizing ST-segment elevation in patients with the Brugada syndrome has been reported *(67–69)*. Quinidine has also been shown to be effective in suppressing arrhythmias in an infant who was too young to receive an ICD *(70)*. Relatively high doses of quinidine at 1200–1500 mg daily are recommended *(71)*.

EARLY REPOLARIZATION

The ER pattern is characterized by a distinct J wave or J point elevation, concave upward ST segment elevation most commonly found in the inferior and left precordial leads V_4–V_6. The ER pattern has long been considered to be a "benign" ECG manifestation that is more commonly seen in young healthy men and athletes *(12, 34, 72)*. However, there is accumulating evidence that the ER pattern may be associated with a risk of VF, depending on the ER location, magnitude of J wave, and ST elevation (6, 23–25).

The ST segment elevation responsible for the ER pattern is thought to be generated by depression of the left ventricular epicardial action potential dome, identical to that in the Brugada syndrome (31) but by itself not sufficient to give rise to repolarization heterogeneities necessary for the development of reentrant tachycardia. The outward shift in the balance of current responsible for the ER pattern may nevertheless facilitate the development of phase 2 reentry and VF in the presence of other provocative forces. A weaker I_{to} permits a partial loss of the epicardial action potential dome in the left ventricular epicardial lateral free wall that manifests as the ER in lateral precordial leads (31). Because only mild to moderate action potential shortening occurs under these conditions, phase 2 reentry is unlikely to occur. However, in the presence of a more intense I_{to} as found in the right ventricle, or perhaps in the left ventricular infero-posterior region, or with a greater outward shift of current in the left ventricle, all-or-none repolarization can occur, giving rise to phase 2 reentry and VT/VF (Figs. 2 and 3).

Genetic Basis for ER

The genetic basis for ER is not well defined. Consistent with the findings that I_{K-ATP} activation can generate an ER pattern in canine ventricular wedge preparations, a rare variant in KCNJ8, responsible for the pore forming subunit of the I_{K-ATP} channel has recently been reported in a patient with ER (73). However, the functional study of the gene mutation is not available as yet. Preliminary reports by Antzelevitch's group have also identified loss-of-function mutations in the subunits of the cardiac L-type calcium channel in patients with ER (74).

Epidemiology

Data in a most recent study showed that an ER pattern occurs in 5.8% of middle-aged subjects (44±8 years), 3.5% in the inferiors leads, and 2.4% in the lateral leads (75). ER is more common in young men, perhaps especially those who are athletic. The incidence is lower in white and higher in young black males and Asians (76, 77). There is a decreasing incidence with advancing age. Although the condition was considered benign, a number of cases previously labeled as idiopathic ventricular fibrillation, particularly in Asian males, have recently been associated with J wave and ER in the inferior leads (14, 19, 20, 23, 78).

There is accumulating evidence that the ER pattern may be associated with a risk of VF, depending on the ER location, magnitude of J wave, and ST elevation (75). A recent multicenter study has shown that ER in the inferolateral leads was more frequent in case subjects with idiopathic ventricular fibrillation than in control subjects (31% vs. 5%, p<0.001) (25, 78). During a mean (±SD) follow-up of 61±50 months, defibrillator monitoring showed a higher incidence of recurrent ventricular fibrillation in case subjects with a repolarization abnormality than in those without such an abnormality (hazard ratio, 2.1; 95% confidence interval, 1.2–3.5; p = 0.008) (25). The incidence of ER as a potential cause of sudden cardiac death may be underestimated because of spontaneous fluctuation in the J wave inscription, and the rare opportunity to document arrhythmia initiation when repolarization changes are maximal.

Clinical Characteristics

The ER pattern can be divided into three subtypes (Table 1): type 1 is associated with an ER pattern predominantly in the lateral precordial leads that is relatively benign; type 2 is more malignant with an ER pattern predominantly seen in inferior leads (23–25, 75); type 3 is a global ER pattern with accentuation of J waves (6, 29). In fact, the Brugada syndrome can be considered as type 4.

The arrhythmic potential of a global ER pattern and ER in inferior leads was suggested in several clinical reports (23, 29, 79), and highlighted in recent studies by Haissaguerre et al. (25), Nam et al.

(6, 80) and Tikkanen et al. *(75)*. Haissaguerre and co-workers reviewed data from 206 case subjects with IVF from 22 centers and compared them to 412 healthy control subjects *(25)*. They reported a more prevalent ER pattern in subjects with idiopathic ventricular fibrillation as compared to control subjects. They found that patients with IVF who had an ER pattern on ECG were more likely to have a history of syncope and sudden cardiac arrest during sleep than those without the ER pattern. An ER and sudden cardiac death was therefore presented in this report by Haissaguerre and co-workers *(25)* as well as in an adjoining report by Nam and coworkers *(6)*, and subsequent reports from Rosso et al. *(78)* and Tikkanen et al. *(75)*.

These observations suggest that the substrate responsible for the development of malignant arrhythmias associated with ER is identical to those responsible for BrS. However, the ECG features, while reminiscent of BrS, do not fully satisfy all of the diagnostic criteria for BrS *(6)*. Salient diagnostic features of BrS such as provocation by sodium channel blockers were rarely observed in these patients *(6, 80)*. This may be due to the fact that a relatively smaller I_{to} in the left ventricle compared with the right ventricle renders the left ventricular epicardium action potential more resistant to complete loss of the action potential dome *(31)*. Although the ECG findings do not fulfill the classic patterns of BrS, they closely match important ECG features of BrS in many aspects: (1) exercise, quinidine and isoproterenol tend to normalize the ST segment elevation in ER; (2) accentuated J waves is pause-and bradycardia-dependent; and (3) a short coupled extrasystoles is able to initiate polymorphic VT/VF.

Therapy

At present, the most reliable treatment is ICD implantation for patients with documented ventricular fibrillation or cardiac arrest. Unlike the Brugada syndrome, invasive and noninvasive parameters regarding the prognosis of the ER are not available in the asymptomatic patients. Although not a sensitive marker for SCD because of its high prevalence in the general population, ER, when observed in patients with syncope or a family history of sudden cardiac death, may be indicative of risk, suggesting that these patients should be followed closely. The available data suggest that transient J wave augmentation followed by R-on-T extrasystoles, or a change in T wave, particularly a negative T wave in the inferior leads or globally, portends a high risk for VF in patients with ER *(19, 20, 29)*.

Although an ICD is the only effective treatment, drug therapy may be necessary for preventing frequent episodes of VF and reducing ICD shock burden in electrical storm. Isoproterenol is thought to be helpful by increasing I_{Ca-L} current to restore epicardial action potential dome, thus decreasing the electrical gradient on the epicardial surface and suppressing phase 2 reentry *(2, 31)*. Quinidine, a class Ia antiarrhythmic drug with an I_{to}-blocking property, may be a better drug therapy for suppressing VF in ER patients with electrical storm by direct inhibition of I_{to} *(32)*, although it has not been properly studied for this purpose.

HYPOTHERMIA

The appearance of a prominent J wave in the ECG is considered pathognomonic of hypothermia. They may manifest diffusely in all leads or be confined to selected leads. Rarely, hypothermia can induce ECG changes that mimic the BrS *(81)*.

Profound hypothermia can lead to the development of VF. In dogs with profound hypothermia (reduction of body temperature by 5–10°C), intravenous infusion of quinidine, which inhibits I_{to}, is effective in preventing VF *(82)*. However, it seems that there is no significant gender dominance in the appearance of hypothermia-induced VF (Table 1).

VF IN THE ACUTE OF ST SEGMENT ELEVATION MYOCARDIAL INFARCTION (STEMI)

Sudden cardiac death (SCD) accounts for more than 60% of all cardiac deaths, with annual deaths in excess of 400,000 in the United States *(83)*. Most SCDs occur in the setting of coronary artery disease. Interestingly, there are a number of similarities between the ECG and clinical features of acute myocardial ischemia and those of ER and BrS *(14, 23, 29, 32, 84–86)*. Prominent J waves on the ECG has been reported to occur in association with acute myocardial ischemia *(87, 88)*.

Clinical observations suggest an association between I_{to} density and the risk of primary VF during the acute phase of ST elevation myocardial infarction. For example, women with coronary heart disease have only a quarter of the risk for sudden cardiac death as compared to men *(89)*. This may be due, in part, to a more prominent I_{to} in males versus females, which is thought to be responsible for the predominance of J wave syndromes in men (Table 1) *(90)*. Similarly, the incidence of primary VF is higher in patients with acute myocardial infarction who have right ventricular involvement (8.4%) than those without (2.7%), or with an anterior myocardial infarction (5.0%) *(91)*. This may be due to the fact that I_{to} is much more prominent in the right ventricle or in adjacent myocardial tissue like the left ventricular inferoposterior region or left ventricular free wall epicardium *(92, 93)*.

Taken together, these observations suggest that the fundamental mechanisms responsible for ST segment elevation and the initiation of VF are similar in the early phases of acute myocardial ischemia and the inherited J wave syndromes in which phase 2 reentry functions as a trigger and enhanced dispersion of repolarization as substrate for the development of VF *(3)*.

J WAVE SYNDROMES

Because of the similarity in ECG characteristics, clinical outcomes, and risk factors, and the fact that these entities share a common arrhythmic platform related to amplification of I_{to}-mediated J waves, which appear to be governed by similar ionic and cellular mechanisms, we and others consider it appropriate to group these congenital and acquired syndromes and entities under the heading of J wave syndromes (Table 1) *(3–7)*.

Our hypothesis is that an outward shift in net repolarizing current due to a decrease in sodium or calcium channel currents, or an increase in I_{to}, $I_{K–ATP}$, $I_{K–ACh}$, or other outward currents, can give rise to J wave syndromes, which includes BrS, ER, hypothermia- and STEMI-induced VF (Table 1). The particular phenotype depends on what part of the heart is principally affected, the amplitude of the I_{to}-mediated J wave, and what specific ion channels are involved.

We view the J wave syndromes as a spectrum of disorders that involve accentuation of the I_{to}-mediated epicardial action potential notch in different regions of heart, leading to the development of prominent J waves, ER, and ST segment elevation on the ECG *(7)*. Phase 2 reentry as the trigger and enhanced dispersion of repolarization as the substrate, are the common mechanisms for the development of polymorphic VT/VF in J wave syndromes.

REFERENCES

1. Osborn JJ (1953) Experimental hypothermia: respiratory and blood pH changes in relation to cardiac function. Am J Physiol 175:389–398
2. Yan GX, Antzelevitch C (1996) Cellular basis for the electrocardiographic J wave. Circulation 93(2):372–379
3. Yan GX, Joshi A, Guo D, Hlaing T, Martin J, Xu X et al (2004) Phase 2 reentry as a trigger to initiate ventricular fibrillation during early acute myocardial ischemia. Circulation 110(9):1036–1041
4. Shu J, Zhu T, Yang L, Cui C, Yan GX (2005) ST-segment elevation in the early repolarization syndrome, idiopathic ventricular fibrillation, and the Brugada syndrome: cellular and clinical linkage. J Electrocardiol 38(4 Suppl):26–32

5. Hlaing T, DiMino T, Kowey PR, Yan GX (2005) ECG repolarization waves: their genesis and clinical implications. Ann Noninvasive Electrocardiol 10(2):211–223

6. Nam GB, Kim YH, Antzelevitch C (2008) Augmentation of J waves and electrical storms in patients with early repolarization. N Engl J Med 358(19):2078–2079

7. Antzelevitch C, Yan GX (2010) J wave syndromes. Heart Rhythm 7(4): 549–558

8. Kraus F (1920) Ueber die wirkung des kalziums auf den kreislauf. Dtsch Med Wochenschr 46:201–203

9. Tomaszewski W (1938) Changement electrocardiographiques observes chez un homme mort de froid. Arch Mal Coeur Vaiss 31:525–528

10. Abbott JA, Cheitlin MD (1976) The nonspecific camel-hump sign. JAMA 235(4):413–414

11. Shipley RA, Hallaran WR (1936) The four lead electrocardiogram in 200 normal men and women. Am Heart J 11: 325–345

12. Wasserburger RH, Alt WJ (1961) The normal RS-T segment elevation variant. Am J Cardiol 8:184–192

13. Kambara H, Phillips J (1976) Long-term evaluation of early repolarization syndrome (normal variant RS-T segment elevation). Am J Cardiol 38(2):157–156

14. Otto CM, Tauxe RV, Cobb LA, Greene HL, Gross BW, Werner JA et al (1984) Ventricular fibrillation causes sudden death in Southeast Asian immigrants. Ann Intern Med 101(1):45–47

15. Antzelevitch C, Sicouri S, Litovsky SH, Lukas A, Krishnan SC, Di Diego JM et al (1991) Heterogeneity within the ventricular wall. Electrophysiology and pharmacology of epicardial, endocardial, and M cells. Circ Res 69(6): 1427–1449

16. Munger RG, Booton EA (1998) Bangungut in Manila: sudden and unexplained death in sleep of adult Filipinos. Int J Epidemiol 27(4):677–684

17. Nademanee K, Veerakul G, Nimmannit S, Chaowakul V, Bhuripanyo K, Likittanasombat K et al (1997) Arrhythmogenic marker for the sudden unexplained death syndrome in Thai men. Circulation 96(8):2595–2600

18. Centers for Disease Control (CDC) (1981) Sudden, unexpected, nocturnal deaths among Southeast Asian refugees. MMWR Morb Mortal Wkly Rep 30:581–584

19. Aizawa Y, Tamura M, Chinushi M, Niwano S, Kusano Y, Naitoh N et al (1992) An attempt at electrical catheter ablation of the arrhythmogenic area in idiopathic ventricular fibrillation. Am Heart J 123(1):257–260

20. Aizawa Y, Tamura M, Chinushi M, Naitoh N, Uchiyama H, Kusano Y et al (1993) Idiopathic ventricular fibrillation and bradycardia-dependent intraventricular block. Am Heart J 126(6):1473–1474

21. Brugada P, Brugada J (1992) Right bundle branch block, persistent ST segment elevation and sudden cardiac death: a distinct clinical and electrocardiographic syndrome. A multicenter report. J Am Coll Cardiol 20(6):1391–1396

22. Miyazaki T, Mitamura H, Miyoshi S, Soejima K, Aizawa Y, Ogawa S (1996) Autonomic and antiarrhythmic drug modulation of ST segment elevation in patients with Brugada syndrome. J Am Coll Cardiol 27(5):1061–1070

23. Kalla H, Yan GX, Marinchak R (2000) Ventricular fibrillation in a patient with prominent J (Osborn) waves and ST segment elevation in the inferior electrocardiographic leads: a Brugada syndrome variant? J Cardiovasc Electrophysiol 11(1):95–98

24. Takagi M, Aihara N, Takaki H, Taguchi A, Shimizu W, Kurita T et al (2000) Clinical characteristics of patients with spontaneous or inducible ventricular fibrillation without apparent heart disease presenting with J wave and ST segment elevation in inferior leads. J Cardiovasc Electrophysiol 11(8):844–848

25. Haissaguerre M, Derval N, Sacher F, Jesel L, Deisenhofer I, de Roy L et al (2008) Sudden cardiac arrest associated with early repolarization. N Engl J Med 358(19):2016–2023

26. Geller JC, Reek S, Goette A, Klein HU (2001) Spontaneous episode of polymorphic ventricular tachycardia in a patient with intermittent Brugada syndrome. J Cardiovasc Electrophysiol 12(9):1094

27. Komiya N, Imanishi R, Kawano H, Shibata R, Moriya M, Fukae S et al (2006) Ventricular fibrillation in a patient with prominent j wave in the inferior and lateral electrocardiographic leads after gastrostomy. Pacing Clin Electrophysiol 29(9):1022–1024

28. Riera AR, Ferreira C, Schapachnik E, Sanches PC, Moffa PJ (2004) Brugada syndrome with atypical ECG: downsloping ST-segment elevation in inferior leads. J Electrocardiol 37(2):101–104

29. Qi X, Sun F, An X (2004) A case of Brugada syndrome with ST segment elevation through entire precordial leads. Chin J Cardiol 32:272–273

30. Litovsky SH, Antzelevitch C (1988) Transient outward current prominent in canine ventricular epicardium but not endocardium. Circ Res 62(1):116–126

31. Yan GX, Lankipalli RS, Burke JF, Musco S, Kowey PR (2003) Ventricular repolarization components on the electrocardiogram: cellular basis and clinical significance. J Am Coll Cardiol 42(3):401–409

32. Yan GX, Antzelevitch C (1999) Cellular basis for the Brugada syndrome and other mechanisms of arrhythmogenesis associated with ST-segment elevation. Circulation 100(15):1660–1666

33. Antzelevitch C, Yan GX (2000) Cellular and ionic mechanisms responsible for the Brugada syndrome. J Electrocardiol 33(Suppl):33–39

34. Yan GX, Martin J (2003) Electrocardiographic T wave: a symbol of transmural dispersion of repolarization in the ventricles. J Cardiovasc Electrophysiol 14(6):639–640

35. Brugada J, Brugada R, Brugada P (2000) Pharmacological and device approach to therapy of inherited cardiac diseases associated with cardiac arrhythmias and sudden death. Electrocardiol Suppl:41–47

36. Morita H, Morita ST, Nagase S, Banba K, Nishii N, Tani Y et al (2003) Ventricular arrhythmia induced by sodium channel blocker in patients with Brugada syndrome. J Am Coll Cardiol 42(9):1624–1631

37. Matsuo K, Shimizu W, Kurita T, Inagaki M, Aihara N, Kamakura S (1998) Dynamic changes of 12-lead electrocardio-grams in a patient with Brugada syndrome. J Cardiovasc Electrophysiol 9(5):508–512

38. Potet F, Mabo P, Le Coq G, Probst V, Schott JJ, Airaud F et al (2003) Novel brugada SCN5A mutation leading to ST segment elevation in the inferior or the right precordial leads. J Cardiovasc Electrophysiol 14(2):200–203

39. Takehara N, Makita N, Kawabe J (2004) A cardiac sodium channel mutation identified in Brugada syndrome associated with atrial standstill. J Intern Med 255:137–142

40. Viskin S, Antzelevitch C (2005) The cardiologists' worst nightmare sudden death from "benign" ventricular arrhythmias. J Am Coll Cardiol 46(7):1295–1297

41. Antzelevitch C (2006) Brugada syndrome. Pacing Clin Electrophysiol 29(10):1130–1159

42. Chen Q, Kirsch GE, Zhang D, Brugada R, Brugada J, Brugada P et al (1998) Genetic basis and molecular mechanism for idiopathic ventricular fibrillation. Nature 392(6673):293–296

43. Schulze-Bahr E, Eckardt L, Breithardt G, Seidl K, Wichter T, Wolpert C et al (2003) Sodium channel gene (SCN5A) mutations in 44 index patients with Brugada syndrome: different incidences in familial and sporadic disease. Hum Mutat 21(6):651–652

44. London B, Michalec M, Mehdi H, Zhu X, Kerchner L, Sanyal S et al (2007) Mutation in glycerol-3-phosphate dehydrogenase 1 like gene (GPD1-L) decreases cardiac Na$^+$ current and causes inherited arrhythmias. Circulation 116(20):2260–2268

45. Antzelevitch C, Pollevick GD, Cordeiro JM, Casis O, Sanguinetti MC, Aizawa Y et al (2007) Loss-of-function mutations in the cardiac calcium channel underlie a new clinical entity characterized by ST-segment elevation, short QT intervals, and sudden cardiac death. Circulation 115(4):442–449

46. Watanabe H, Koopmann TT, Le Scouarnec S, Yang T, Ingram CR, Schott JJ et al (2008) Sodium channel beta1 sub-unit mutations associated with Brugada syndrome and cardiac conduction disease in humans. J Clin Invest 118(6): 2260–2268

47. Hu D, Barajas-Martinez H, Burashnikov E, Springer M, Wu Y, Varro A et al (2009) A mutation in the beta 3 subunit of the cardiac sodium channel associated with Brugada ECG phenotype. Circ Cardiovasc Genet 2(3):270–278

48. Boussy T, Paparella G, de Asmundis C, Sarkozy A, Chierchia GB, Brugada J et al (2008) Genetic basis of ventricular arrhythmias. Cardiol Clin 26(3):335–353

49. Antzelevitch C, Brugada P, Brugada J, Brugada R (2005) Brugada syndrome: from cell to bedside. Curr Probl Cardiol 30(1):9–54

50. Miyasaka Y, Tsuji H, Yamada K, Tokunaga S, Saito D, Imuro Y et al (2001) Prevalence and mortality of the Brugada-type electrocardiogram in one city in Japan. J Am Coll Cardiol 38(3):771–774

51. Morita H, Kusano-Fukushima K, Nagase S, Fujimoto Y, Hisamatsu K, Fujio H et al (2002) Atrial fibrillation and atrial vulnerability in patients with Brugada syndrome. J Am Coll Cardiol 40(8):1437–1444

52. Eckardt L, Kirchhof P, Johna R, Haverkamp W, Breithardt G, Borggrefe M (2001) Wolff-Parkinson-White syndrome associated with Brugada syndrome. Pacing Clin Electrophysiol 24(9 Pt 1):1423–1424

53. Morita H, Fukushima-Kusano K, Nagase S, Miyaji K, Hiramatsu S, Banba K et al (2004) Sinus node function in patients with Brugada-type ECG. Circ J 68(5):473–476

54. Wilde AA, Antzelevitch C, Borggrefe M, Brugada J, Brugada R, Brugada P et al (2002) Proposed diagnostic criteria for the Brugada syndrome: consensus report. Circulation 106(19):2514–2519

55. Antzelevitch C, Brugada P, Borggrefe M, Brugada J, Brugada R, Corrado D et al (2005) Brugada syndrome: report of the second consensus conference: endorsed by the Heart rhythm society and the European heart rhythm association. Circulation 111(5):659–670

56. Shimizu W, Antzelevitch C, SK, Kurita T, Taguchi A, Aihara N et al (2000) Effect of sodium channel blockers on ST segment, QRS duration, and corrected QT interval in patients with Brugada syndrome. J Cardiovasc Electrophysiol 11:1320–1329

57. Shimizu W, Matsuo K, Takagi M, Tanabe Y, Aiba T, Taguchi A et al (2000) Body surface distribution and response to drugs of ST segment elevation in Brugada syndrome: clinical implication of eighty-seven-lead body surface potential mapping and its application to twelve-lead electrocardiograms. J Cardiovasc Electrophysiol 11(4):396–404

58. Sangwatanaroj S, Prechawat S, Sunsaneewitayakul B, Sitthisook S, Tosukhowong P, Tungsanga K (2001) New elec-trocardiographic leads and the procainamide test for the detection of the Brugada sign in sudden unexplained death syndrome survivors and their relatives. Eur Heart J 22(24):2290–2296

59. Brugada J, Brugada R, Antzelevitch C, Towbin J, Nademanee K, Brugada P (2002) Long-term follow-up of individuals with the electrocardiographic pattern of right bundle-branch block and ST-segment elevation in precordial leads V1 to V3. Circulation 105(1):73–78

60. Priori SG, Napolitano C, Gasparini M, Pappone C, Della BP, Giordano U et al (2002) Natural history of Brugada syndrome: insights for risk stratification and management. Circulation 105(11):1342–1347

61. Brugada P, Brugada R, Brugada J (2005) Should patients with an asymptomatic Brugada electrocardiogram undergo pharmacological and electrophysiological testing? Circulation 112(2):279–292

62. Priori SG, Napolitano C (2005) Management of patients with Brugada syndrome should not be based on programmed electrical stimulation. Circulation 112:285–291

63. Eckardt L, Probst V, Smits JP, Bahr ES, Wolpert C, Schimpf R et al (2005) Long-term prognosis of individuals with right precordial ST-segment-elevation Brugada syndrome. Circulation 111(3):257–263

64. Atarashi H, Ogawa S (2003) New ECG criteria for high-risk Brugada syndrome. Circ J 67(1):8–10

65. Morita H, Takenaka-Morita S, Fukushima-Kusano K, Kobayashi M, Nagase S, Kakishita M et al (2003) Risk stratification for asymptomatic patients with Brugada syndrome. Circ J 67(4):312–316

66. Huang Z, Patel C, Li W, Xie Q, Wu R, Zhang L et al (2009) Role of signal-averaged electrocardiograms in arrhythmic risk stratification of patients with Brugada syndrome: a prospective study. Heart Rhythm 6(8):1156–1162

67. Belhassen B, Viskin S, Antzelevitch C (2002) The Brugada syndrome: is an implantable cardioverter defibrillator the only therapeutic option? Pacing Clin Electrophysiol 25(11):1634–1640

68. Alings M, Dekker L, Sadee A, Wilde A (2001) Quinidine induced electrocardiographic normalization in two patients with Brugada syndrome. Pacing Clin Electrophysiol 24(9 Pt 1):1420–1422

69. Marquez MF, Rivera J, Hermosillo AG, Iturralde P, Colin L, Moragrega JL et al (2005) Arrhythmic storm responsive to quinidine in a patient with Brugada syndrome and vasovagal syncope. Pacing Clin Electrophysiol 28(8):870–873

70. Probst V, Evain S, Gournay V, Marie A, Schott JJ, Boisseau P et al (2006) Monomorphic ventricular tachycardia due to Brugada syndrome successfully treated by hydroquinidine therapy in a 3-year-old child. J Cardiovasc Electrophysiol 17(1):97–100

71. Hermida JS, Denjoy I, Clerc J, Extramiana F, Jarry G, Milliez P et al (2004) Hydroquinidine therapy in Brugada syndrome. J Am Coll Cardiol 43(10):1853–1860

72. Mehta MC, Jain AC (1995) Early repolarization on scalar electrocardiogram. Am J Med Sci 309(6):305–311

73. Haissaguerre M, Chatel S, Sacher F, Weerasooriya R, Probst V, Loussouarn G et al (2009) Ventricular fibrillation with prominent early repolarization associated with a rare variant of KCNJ8/KATP channel. J Cardiovasc Electrophysiol 20(1):93–98

74. Burashnikov E, Pfeifer R, Borggrefe M, Eldar M, Glikson M, Haissaguerre M et al (2009) Mutations in the cardiac L-type calcium channel associated with inherited sudden cardiac death syndromes. Circulation 120:S573

75. Tikkanen JT, Anttonen O, Junttila MJ, Aro AL, Kerola T, Rissanen HA et al (2009) Long-term outcome associated with early repolarization on electrocardiography. N Engl J Med 361(26):2529–2537

76. Klatsky AL, Oehm R, Cooper RA, Udaltsova N, Armstrong MA (2003) The early repolarization normal variant electrocardiogram: correlates and consequences. Am J Med 115(3):171–177

77. Mehta M, Jain AC, Mehta A (1999) Early repolarization. Clin Cardiol 22(2):59–65

78. Rosso R, Kogan E, Belhassen B, Rozovski U, Scheinman MM, Zeltser D et al (2008) J-point elevation in survivors of primary ventricular fibrillation and matched control subjects: incidence and clinical significance. J Am Coll Cardiol 52(15):1231–1238

79. Letsas KP, Efremidis M, Pappas LK, Gavrielatos G, Markou V, Sideris A et al (2007) Early repolarization syndrome: is it always benign? Int J Cardiol 114(3):390–392

80. Nam GB, Ko KH, Kim J, Park KM, Rhee KS, Choi KJ et al (2009) Mode of onset of ventricular fibrillation in patients with early repolarization pattern vs. Brugada syndrome. Eur Heart J in press

81. Ansari E, Cook JR (2003) Profound hypothermia mimicking a Brugada type ECG. J Electrocardiol 36(3):257–260

82. Johnson P, Lesage A, Floyd WL, Young WG Jr, Sealy WC (1960) Prevention of ventricular fibrillation during profound hypothermia by quinidine. Ann Surg 151:490–495

83. Zheng ZJ, Croft JB, Giles WH, Mensah GA (2001) Sudden cardiac death in the United States, 1989 to 1998. Circulation 104(18):2158–2163

84. Yan GX, Kowey PR (2000) ST segment elevation and sudden cardiac death: from the Brugada syndrome to acute myocardial ischemia. J Cardiovasc Electrophysiol 11:1330–1332

85. Di Diego JM, Fish JM, Antzelevitch C (2005) Brugada syndrome and ischemia-induced ST-segment elevation. Similarities and differences. J Electrocardiol 38(4 Suppl):14–17

86. Haissaguerre M, Sacher F, Nogami A, Komiya N, Bernard A, Probst V et al (2009) Characteristics of recurrent ventricular fibrillation associated with inferolateral early repolarization role of drug therapy. J Am Coll Cardiol 53(7):612–619

87. Shinde R, Shinde S, Makhale C, Grant P, Sathe S, Durairaj M et al (2007) Occurrence of "J waves" in 12-lead ECG as a marker of acute ischemia and their cellular basis. Pacing Clin Electrophysiol 30(6):817–819

88. Jastrzebski M, Kukla P (2009) Ischemic J wave: novel risk marker for ventricular fibrillation? Heart Rhythm 6(6): 829–835

89. Kannel WB, Wilson PW, D'Agostino RB, Cobb J (1998) Sudden coronary death in women. Am Heart J 136(2):205–212

90. Di Diego JM, Cordeiro JM, Goodrow RJ, Fish JM, Zygmunt AC, Perez GJ et al (2002) Ionic and cellular basis for the predominance of the Brugada syndrome phenotype in males. Circulation 106(15):2004–2011

91. Mehta SR, Eikelboom JW, Natarajan MK, Diaz R, Yi C, Gibbons RJ et al (2001) Impact of right ventricular involvement on mortality and morbidity in patients with inferior myocardial infarction. J Am Coll Cardiol 37(1):37–43

92. Peschar M, de Swart H, Michels KJ, Reneman RS, Prinzen FW (2003) Left ventricular septal and apex pacing for optimal pump function in canine hearts. J Am Coll Cardiol 41(7):1218–1226

93. Di Diego JM, Sun ZQ, Antzelevitch C (1996) I(to) and action potential notch are smaller in left vs. right canine ventricular epicardium. Am J Physiol 271(2 Pt 2):H548–H561

Subject Index

From: *Contemporary Cardiology: Management of Cardiac Arrhythmias*
Edited by: Gan-Xin Yan, Peter R. Kowey, DOI 10.1007/978-1-60761-161-5
© Springer Science+Business Media, LLC 2011